Textbook of
Oral Embryology and Histology

Textbook of
Oral Embryology and Histology

Editor

B Sivapathasundharam
MDS (Oral Pathology) FIAOMP FISDR FIAFO
Principal and Professor
Department of Oral Pathology
Priyadarshini Dental College and Hospital
Pandur, Thiruvallur
Tamil Nadu, India

Forewords

WM Tilakaratne
Yeshwant B Rawal

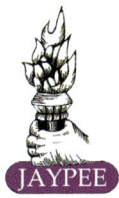

JAYPEE BROTHERS MEDICAL PUBLISHERS
The Health Sciences Publisher
New Delhi | London

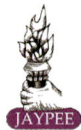 **Jaypee Brothers Medical Publishers (P) Ltd**

Headquarters
Jaypee Brothers Medical Publishers (P) Ltd
EMCA House, 23/23-B
Ansari Road, Daryaganj
New Delhi 110 002, India
Landline: +91-11-23272143, +91-11-23272703
+91-11-23282021, +91-11-23245672
Email: jaypee@jaypeebrothers.com

Corporate Office
Jaypee Brothers Medical Publishers (P) Ltd
4838/24, Ansari Road, Daryaganj
New Delhi 110 002, India
Phone: +91-11-43574357
Fax: +91-11-43574314
Email: jaypee@jaypeebrothers.com

Overseas Office
J.P. Medical Ltd
83 Victoria Street, London
SW1H 0HW (UK)
Phone: +44 20 3170 8910
Fax: +44 (0)20 3008 6180
Email: info@jpmedpub.com

Website: www.jaypeebrothers.com
Website: www.jaypeedigital.com

© 2023, Jaypee Brothers Medical Publishers

The views and opinions expressed in this book are solely those of the original contributor(s)/author(s) and do not necessarily represent those of editor(s) and publisher of the book.

All rights reserved. No part of this publication may be reproduced, stored or transmitted in any form or by any means, electronic, mechanical, photocopying, recording or otherwise, without the prior permission in writing of the publishers.

All brand names and product names used in this book are trade names, service marks, trademarks or registered trademarks of their respective owners. The publisher is not associated with any product or vendor mentioned in this book.

Medical knowledge and practice change constantly. This book is designed to provide accurate, authoritative information about the subject matter in question. However, readers are advised to check the most current information available on procedures included and check information from the manufacturer of each product to be administered, to verify the recommended dose, formula, method and duration of administration, adverse effects and contraindications. It is the responsibility of the practitioner to take all appropriate safety precautions. Neither the publisher nor the author(s)/editor(s) assume any liability for any injury and/or damage to persons or property arising from or related to use of material in this book.

This book is sold on the understanding that the publisher is not engaged in providing professional medical services. If such advice or services are required, the services of a competent medical professional should be sought.

Every effort has been made where necessary to contact holders of copyright to obtain permission to reproduce copyright material. If any have been inadvertently overlooked, the publisher will be pleased to make the necessary arrangements at the first opportunity.

Inquiries for bulk sales may be solicited at: jaypee@jaypeebrothers.com

Textbook of Oral Embryology and Histology

First Edition: 2019

Second Edition: **2023**

ISBN 978-93-5465-932-4

Printed at: Samrat Offset Pvt. Ltd.

Dedicated to

*The optimists of the future of dentistry
and
to my wife Dr S Rohini who supports me continuously in all my academic pursuits.*

Contributors

Anil Sukumaran B MDS PhD FRCPath FDS RCPS (Glas) FDS RCS (Ed) FICD FPFA
Professor and Senior Consultant
Oral Health Institute
Hamad Medical Corporation/Qatar University
Doha, Qatar

Doddabasavaiah Basavapur Nandini
Professor
Department of Oral Pathology
Dental College
RIMS, Imphal, Manipur, India

Einstein T Bertin A MDS
Principal and Professor
Department of Oral Pathology
Thai Moogambigai Dental College
Dr MGR Educational and research Institute
Chennai, Tamil Nadu, India

Govind Rajkumar MDS
Professor and Head
Department of Oral Pathology
Vishnu Dental College
Bhimavaram, Andhra Pradesh, India

Gururaj N MDS
Professor and Head
Department of Oral Pathology
CSI College of Dental Sciences and Research
Madurai, Tamil Nadu, India

Kavitha B MDS
Professor and Head
Department of Oral Pathology and Microbiology
Meenakshi Academy of Higher Education and Research
Faculty of Dentistry
Meenakshi Ammal Dental College
Chennai, Tamil Nadu, India

Logeswari Jayamani MDS
Associate Professor
Department of Oral Pathology and Microbiology
Meenakshi Academy of Higher Education and Research
Faculty of Dentistry
Meenakshi Ammal Dental College
Chennai, Tamil Nadu, India

Mahesh Verma MDS MBA PhD
Vice Chancellor
Guru Gobind Singh Indraprastha University
New Delhi, India

Mandana Darafsh Donoghue MDS
Director
OMFP Center
Belagavi, Karnataka, India

Manimaran K MDS
Oral and Maxillofacial Surgeon
Coimbatore, Tamil Nadu, India

Manoj Prabhakar MDS
Associate Professor
Department of Oral Pathology and Microbiology
Meenakshi Academy of Higher Education and Research
Faculty of Dentistry
Meenakshi Ammal Dental College
Chennai, Tamil Nadu, India

Pratibha Ramani MDS DNB PhD
Professor and Head
Department of Oral Pathology and Microbiology
Saveetha Dental College and Hospitals
Chennai, Tamil Nadu, India

Preethi Murali MDS
Professor
Department of Oral Pathology and Microbiology
Meenakshi Academy of Higher Education and Research
Faculty of Dentistry
Meenakshi Ammal Dental College
Chennai, Tamil Nadu, India

Preethi S MDS
Mandeveli
Chennai, Tamil Nadu, India

Priya Kumar MDS MBA
Associate Professor
Department of Oral Pathology
Maulana Azad Institute of Dental Sciences
New Delhi, India

Protyusha Guha Biswas MDS
Assistant Professor
Department of Oral Pathology and Microbiology
Meenakshi Academy of Higher Education and Research
Faculty of Dentistry
Meenakshi Ammal Dental College
Chennai, Tamil Nadu, India

Punnya V Angadi MDS DNB PhD
Professor and Head
Department of Oral Pathology
KLE VK Institute of Dental Sciences
KLE Academy of Higher Education
Belagavi, Karnataka, India

Sabarinath B MDS
Assistant Professor
Department of Oral Pathology and Microbiology
Meenakshi Academy of Higher Education and Research
Faculty of Dentistry
Meenakshi Ammal Dental College
Chennai, Tamil Nadu, India

Shankaranarayanan S MDS (Deceased)
Director
Mother Cell Regenerative Centre
Trichy, Tamil Nadu, India

Sivapathasundharam B MDS FIAOMP FISDR FIAFO
Principal and Professor
Department of Oral pathology
Priyadarshini Dental College and Hospital
Pandur, Thiruvallur, Tamil Nadu, India

Vijayashree RJ MDS
Assistant Professor
Department of Oral Pathology and Microbiology
Meenakshi Academy of Higher Education and Research
Faculty of Dentistry
Meenakshi Ammal Dental College
Chennai, Tamil Nadu, India

Foreword

It is with great pleasure that I write the foreword for the second edition of the book titled *Textbook of Oral Embryology and Histology* authored by Professor B Sivapathasundharam, Principal and Professor, Department of Oral Pathology, Priyadarshini Dental College and Hospital, Pandur, Thiruvallur, Tamil Nadu, India, Affiliated to The Tamil Nadu Dr MGR Medical University, Chennai, Tamil Nadu, India. I am convinced that he has used his extensive experience as an academic and a researcher to compile this very comprehensive and elaborate text on the subject. There is ample evidence from his illustrious career that he is one of the most appropriate writers to produce a book of this nature. I am sure his wide range of academic capabilities and editorial experience has helped him to compile this comprehensive textbook very successfully. Knowledge of basic structure and the development of the oral tissues is very essential for the understanding of the disease process, their diagnosis and management. This book explains in detail about the microscopic structure of all the dental hard and soft tissues and their development in simple language. It also includes chapters on temporomandibular joint, maxillary sinus, lymphatic system and salivary glands. Separate section is devoted for related topics like evolution of teeth and jaws, stem cells, histochemistry of oral tissues and preparation of tissues for histological examination.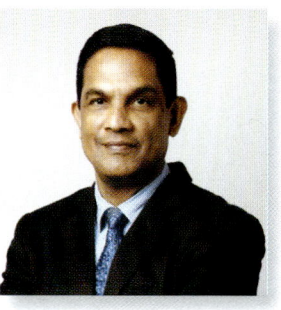

In the new edition, the entire text is updated to include the recent findings in oral embryology and histology in the literature. In addition, each chapter is complemented with a summary, titled as "Points to Remember" along with MCQs. Similar to the previous edition the text is presented in a reader-friendly manner with suitable photomicrographs, electron micrographs, line diagrams and flowcharts. Many clinical photographs, photomicrographs, flowcharts and schematic diagrams are used throughout this book for better understanding. I am sure that this book will cater the needs of the undergraduate students of dentistry and will serve as a reference book for the postgraduate dental students and students of medicine.

I am sure that the *Textbook of Oral Embryology and Histology* will be a highly rated reference text among all categories of students in the years to come.

WM Tilakaratne BDS, MS, FDSRCS, FRCPath, PhD
Professor and Senior Consultant in Oral Pathology
Department of Oral and Maxillofacial Clinical Sciences
Associate Dean/International affairs
Faculty of Dentistry
University of Malaya
Malaysia
Past President: International Association of Oral Pathologists

Foreword

What makes for a good textbook in the field of Oral Histology, Anatomy and Embryology? The organization of material should be visually appealing, the flow of content must be logical, the content should be adequate and contemporary, the material should be supported by appropriate illustrations, tables, flowcharts, figures and diagrams, the index should be comprehensive and key points must be highlighted and the readers understanding of the material must be challenged at the end of each chapter. The second edition of the *Textbook of Oral Embryology and Histology* authored by Professor B Sivapathasundharam fulfills the criteria listed above.

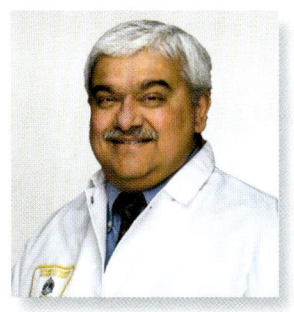

I have known Professor B Sivapathasundharam since 1990. I am acutely aware of his ability to author the second edition of this textbook. In this edition, he has delved into his extensive experience as an academician and oral and maxillofacial pathologist, to infuse the textbook with the quality that students of dentistry and dental hygiene, students in graduate dental programs, and practicing dentists will find unparalleled on the topic.

Allow me to support my enthusiasm for Professor B Sivapathasundharam's textbook. Beginning with an overview of oral hard and soft tissue, and basics of embryology, the content progresses to the development of the face and oral cavity including teeth. It continues to chapters on all dental hard tissue, the periodontal ligament, alveolar bone, the temporomandibular joint, oral soft tissue including the salivary glands, and lymphatics. I was pleasantly surprised to find chapters on age changes, stem cells, and evolution of teeth and jaws. A textbook of histology is incomplete without a chapter on laboratory techniques. Further, this textbook also has an excellent collection of easy-to-understand appendices followed by an extensive glossary of terms, schematic illustrations, and a comprehensive index.

Professor B Sivapathasundharam has given the second edition of this textbook considerable time and thought, and the product is exceptional. This textbook is a must read for all dental students, students in postgraduate residency programs including oral and maxillofacial pathology. A copy of this text will serve as a ready reference for all dental surgeons and specialists including physicians and medical students with an interest in oral histology and embryology. This textbook will be a "must have" addition to medical and dental libraries. I am eager for its release so I can buy myself a copy.

Yeshwant B Rawal BDS MDS MS and Cert in Oral & Maxillofacial Pathology
Fellow, American Academy of Oral & Maxillofacial Pathology
Diplomate and Director, American Board of Oral & Maxillofacial Pathology
Professor, Department of Surgical Sciences
Marquette University School of Dentistry
Milwaukee, Wisconsin, USA

Preface to the Second Edition

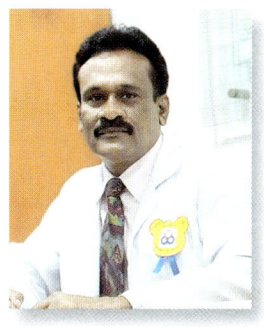

Though the basics of histology continue to be same, the advances in molecular techniques, immunohistochemical methods, and the like make the text on the subject of histology and embryology a dynamic one. However it should be accepted that in spite of the advancements in science and technology many events in the development and growth are unexplored and beyond our perception.

In this edition, the entire text is updated to include the recent findings in oral embryology and histology. Each chapter is complemented with a summary, titled as "Points to Remember" along with MCQs. Similar to the previous edition the text is presented in a reader-friendly manner with suitable photomicrographs, line diagrams and flowcharts. A separate section for the histologic diagrams is added. Comparison tables, glossary and other ready reckoners presented in Appendix 1 is expanded.

I am sure that this book will cater the needs of the undergraduate students of dentistry and will serve as a reference book for the postgraduate dental students and students of medicine. As usual the publisher has given exceptional care in its beautiful user-friendly presentation.

B Sivapathasundharam

Preface to the First Edition

Knowledge about development and structure of orofacial tissues is indispensable for any branch of dentistry. Though few fundamental aspects of developmental biology remain the same, the vast explosion in molecular genetics has changed our perception towards the understanding of many developmental processes. This evolving and intriguing nature of orodental embryology and histology, has been my biggest fascination throughout my teaching career for the past three decades. The molecular interactions and their synchronization in development and function excite me forever. I cannot but stay amazed at the system that governs the biological interplay of developmental processes. I wonder and humbly bow to the Almighty, who has created this universe and regulates everything to the minutest detail.

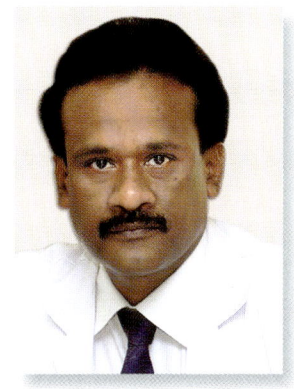

My dream, to write a book of veritable and dependable quality in the subject of 'Oral Embryology and Oral Histology', to cater to the needs of teachers and students of dentistry in India and abroad, has come true today. Many eminent academicians from our country and beyond have contributed to this book, to achieve this goal. With a humble tribute to my teachers Prof Dr Viswanathan and Prof Dr TR Saraswathi, who taught me 'Oral Histology and Oral Pathology', I have made a sincere attempt to execute this project to near perfection.

The text has been presented in a simple, lucid, and reader-friendly manner, supported by photomicrographs, drawings, and flowcharts. The contemporary views and the molecular aspects have been highlighted in colored boxes. The clinical implications have been discussed at the end of each chapter. Comparison tables and glossary have been added at the end of the book for easy reference. A chapter on 'Stem Cells' has been included since stem cell therapy has gained much importance in the recent past. The publisher has given special care to the esthetic presentation. I hope the readers will enjoy growing in knowledge, with this book.

B Sivapathasundharam

Acknowledgments

I am most grateful to the textual and photographic contributors of this book, who are acknowledged in the relevant chapters and legends. I owe a debt of thanks to my former colleagues Dr B Kavitha, Dr M Preethi, Dr B Sabarinath, Dr K Karthik and Dr T Padmapriya, for their advice and suggestions on the content. Special thanks to Dr J Logeswari, for her constructive criticism in building up the text and drafting the chapters. I sincerely acknowledge the help rendered by Dr Manoj Prabhakar for the photographs and photomicrographs and Dr Priyadharshini, Dr D Amal Steffi, Dr E Abigail Viola of Meenakshi Ammal Dental College and Dr Niveditha of Priyadarshini Dental College for converting my ideas into beautiful scientific drawings. I thank Dr S Ramya and Dr U Suganya, for preparing the tables and diagrams. My special thanks to Dr RJ Vijayashree, for her dedicated and tireless help in correcting the language and proofreading.

I like to especially thank my wife, Dr S Rohini, for her continuous help, support and encouragement and sacrificing our personal and family time in bringing out this book.

Also, I like to extend my gratitude to Thiru VG Raajendran, Chairman and Tmt Indira Raajendran, Managing Director, Indira Group of Educational Institutions, Thiruvallur, Tamil Nadu, for encouraging and supporting me to write this book. My thanks are due to my colleagues of Priyadarshini Dental College and Hospital, Pandur, Thiruvallur, Tamil Nadu, for sharing my administrative workload during the preparation of this edition.

Finally, my grateful thanks to Shri Jitendar P Vij (Group Chairman), Mr Ankit Vij (Managing Director), Mr MS Mani (Group President), Dr Madhu Choudhary (Director–Educational Publishing), Ms Pooja Bhandari (Production Head), Ms Sunita Katla (Executive Assistant to Group Chairman and Publishing Manager), Ms Samina Khan (Executive Assistant to Director–Educational Publishing), Dr Aditya Tayal (Team Lead-UG Publishing), Mr Rajesh Sharma (Production Coordinator), Ms Seema Dogra (Cover Visualizer), Mr Kulwant Singh (Typesetter), Mr Nitin Bhardwaj (Graphic Designer), Mr Vakil Khan (Proofreader), for making my dream come true by publishing this book and bringing out the second edition.

Contents

Chapter 1: Overview of Oral Tissues   1
B Sivapathasundharam
- Enamel *3*
- Dentin *3*
- Pulp *3*
- Cementum *3*
- Periodontium *4*
- Maxillary Sinus *4*
- Oral Mucous Membrane *4*
- Salivary Gland *4*
- Temporomandibular Joint *4*
- Microscopic Structures of Oral Tissues *5*
- Eruption and Shedding *5*
- Cell Signaling *6*

Chapter 2: General Embryology   8
B Sivapathasundharam
- Fertilization *9*
- Cleavage *9*
- Formation of Bilaminar Germ Disk *9*
- Prochordal Plate and Trilaminar Germ Disk Formation *9*
- Formation of Neural Crest Cells *11*
- Folding of the Embryo *13*
- Development of Branchial Arches *13*
- Fate of Pharyngeal Clefts *13*

Chapter 3: Development of Face, Palate and Tongue   17
B Sivapathasundharam, Manoj Prabhakar
- Development of Face *17*
- Development of Palate *18*
- Development of Tongue *21*
- Clinical Considerations *21*

Chapter 4: Development of Tooth   25
B Sivapathasundharam, Logeswari Jayamani
- Dental Lamina *26*
- Vestibular Lamina *27*
- Tooth Development *28*
- Apposition and Hard Tissue Formation *36*
- Root Formation *36*
- Clinical Considerations *37*

Chapter 5: Enamel   44
Mandana Darafsh Donoghue, B Sivapathasundharam, RJ Vijayashree
- Physical Properties *44*
- Chemical Composition *45*
- Structure of Enamel *46*
- Hypomineralized Structures of Enamel *49*
- Surface Structures of Enamel *51*
- Amelogenesis *52*
- Age Changes *59*
- Clinical Considerations *59*

Chapter 6: Dentin   66
B Sivapathasundharam
- Physical Properties *66*
- Chemical Composition *67*
- Histology of Dentin *68*
- Structural Patterns of Dentin *72*
- Dentin Sensitivity *76*
- Dentinogenesis *77*
- Clinical Considerations *79*

Chapter 7: Pulp   83
B Sivapathasundharam
- Structure of Pulp *84*
- Cells of the Pulp *88*
- Intercellular Substance *89*
- Functions of Pulp *91*
- Development of Pulp *91*
- Age Changes *92*
- Clinical Considerations *92*

Chapter 8: Cementum   97
Punnya V Angadi, B Sivapathasundharam
- Physical Properties *98*
- Chemical Composition *98*
- Cells of Cementum *99*
- Fibers of the Cementum *101*
- Structure *102*
- Classification of Cementum *103*
- Cementogenesis *103*

- ❖ Cementoid *106*
- ❖ Incremental Lines of Cementum *106*
- ❖ Hyaline Layer of Hopewell–Smith *107*
- ❖ Cementodentinal Junction *107*
- ❖ Cementoenamel Junction *107*
- ❖ Functions of Cementum *108*
- ❖ Age Changes *108*
- ❖ Clinical Considerations *109*

Chapter 9: Periodontal Ligament 113

Anil Sukumaran, B Sivapathasundharam
- ❖ Development of Periodontium *114*
- ❖ Structure of Periodontium *116*
- ❖ Periodontal Fibers *118*
- ❖ Interstitial Tissue *121*
- ❖ Ground Substance *122*
- ❖ Functions of the Periodontal Ligament *122*
- ❖ Age Changes *122*
- ❖ Clinical Considerations *123*

Chapter 10: Alveolar Bone 128

B Sivapathasundharam
- ❖ Physical Properties *129*
- ❖ Chemical Composition *129*
- ❖ Classification of Bones *129*
- ❖ Formation of Bone *133*
- ❖ Cells of the Bone *136*
- ❖ Bone Remodeling *140*
- ❖ Alveolar Bone *141*
- ❖ Development of Maxilla and Mandible *141*
- ❖ Development of Alveolar Process *145*
- ❖ Structure of Alveolar Bone *145*
- ❖ Remodeling of Alveolar Bone *146*
- ❖ Age Changes *147*
- ❖ Clinical Considerations *147*

Chapter 11: Tooth Eruption 153

B Sivapathasundharam, Logeswari Jayamani
- ❖ Eruption *155*
- ❖ Pattern of Tooth Movement *155*
- ❖ Histology of Tooth Movement *157*
- ❖ Theories of Tooth Eruption *159*
- ❖ Clinical Considerations *161*

Chapter 12: Shedding 165

B Sivapathasundharam
- ❖ Order of Shedding *166*
- ❖ Mechanism of Shedding *167*
- ❖ Histology of Shedding *167*
- ❖ Clinical Considerations *170*

Chapter 13: Oral Mucous Membrane 174

B Sivapathasundharam, Preethi S
- ❖ Functions of Oral Mucous Membrane *174*
- ❖ Boundaries of the Oral Cavity *175*
- ❖ Clinical Appearance and Regional Variations *175*
- ❖ Classification of Oral Mucosa *177*
- ❖ Components of the Oral Mucosa *177*
- ❖ Masticatory Mucosa *193*
- ❖ Lining Mucosa *201*
- ❖ Specialized Mucosa *204*
- ❖ Development of the Oral Mucosa *208*
- ❖ Age Changes *208*
- ❖ Clinical Considerations *209*

Chapter 14: Salivary Glands 216

Pratibha Ramani, Einstein T Bertin, B Sivapathasundharam
- ❖ Glands *216*
- ❖ Classification of Glands *216*
- ❖ Salivary Glands *220*
- ❖ Classification of Salivary Glands *220*
- ❖ Development of Salivary Gland *220*
- ❖ Histology of Salivary Glands *224*
- ❖ Myoepithelial Cells (Basket Cells) *226*
- ❖ Other Cells *229*
- ❖ Ductal System *229*
- ❖ Connective Tissue Component of the Gland *231*
- ❖ Formation and Secretion of Saliva *231*
- ❖ Ductal Modification of Saliva *232*
- ❖ Composition of Saliva *232*
- ❖ Properties of Saliva *233*
- ❖ Functions of Saliva *233*
- ❖ Major Salivary Glands *234*
- ❖ Minor Salivary Glands *236*
- ❖ Tubarial Glands—The New Salivary Gland Organs? *237*
- ❖ Clinical Considerations *237*

Chapter 15: Temporomandibular Joint 241

B Sivapathasundharam, Gururaj N
- ❖ Development of Temporomandibular Joint *242*
- ❖ Gross Anatomy and Microscopic Structure of the Temporomandibular Joint *243*
- ❖ Blood Supply *248*
- ❖ Nerve Supply *248*
- ❖ Functions of Temporomandibular Joint *248*
- ❖ Clinical Considerations *249*

Chapter 16: Maxillary Sinus 253

B Sivapathasundharam, Logeswari Jayamani, Govind Rajkumar
- ❖ Anatomy of Maxillary Sinus *253*
- ❖ Development of Maxillary Sinus *255*
- ❖ Blood Supply and Nerve Supply *255*
- ❖ Microscopic Features *257*
- ❖ Functions *258*
- ❖ Clinical Considerations *258*

Chapter 17: Lymphatics of Orofacial Region 262

B Sivapathasundharam, Doddabasavaiah Basavapur Nandini
- ❖ Lymphatic Organs *262*
- ❖ Development of Lymphatic System *263*
- ❖ Lymph *264*

- Structure of Lymphatic System *264*
- Lymph Circulation *266*
- Lymphatics of the Head and Neck *267*
- Clinical Considerations *267*

Chapter 18: Age Changes in Oral Tissues   273

Einstein T Bertin A, B Sivapathasundharam

- Theories of Aging *273*
- The Cell Biology of Aging *274*
- Effects of Aging on the Human Body *276*
- Effects of Aging on the Oral and Circumoral Structures *277*
- Effect of Aging on the Dental Tissues *279*
- Forensic Implications of Age-related Changes of the Dental Tissues *283*

Chapter 19: Stem Cells   287

Shankaranarayanan S, Manimaran K, B Sivapathasundharam, Protyusha Guha Biswas

- History of Stem Cells *287*
- Classification of Stem Cells *288*
- Mechanism of Action of Stem Cells *289*
- Application of Stem Cells in Regenerative Medicine *290*
- Dental Stem Cells *290*
- Isolation of Dental Pulp Stem Cells *291*
- Applications of DPSCS in Regenerative Dentistry *292*

Chapter 20: Evolution of Jaws and Teeth   297

Mahesh Verma, Priya Kumar

- Agnathan to Gnathostome Transition *297*
- Hominid Jaw Evolution *298*
- Jaw Suspension *300*
- Theories of Evolution of Human Dentition *300*
- Theories of Cuspal Origin *302*
- Evolution of Periodontium *303*
- Trends in Evolution *304*

Chapter 21: Tissue Processing for Histological Examination   307

B Sivapathasundharam, Kavitha B, RJ Vijayashree

- Types of Preparation *308*
- Soft Tissue Processing *308*
- Tissue Sectioning *311*
- Frozen Sections *315*
- Digital Pathology *318*

Chapter 22: Histochemistry of Oral Tissues   322

Preethi Murali, B Sivapathasundharam

- Oral Tissues and their Chemical Composition *322*
- Epithelial Tissue and Derivatives *323*
- Connective Tissue *323*
- Cells and Fibers *323*
- Histochemical Techniques *324*
- Specific Histochemical Methods *324*
- Immunohistochemistry *326*
- Histochemistry of Oral Hard Tissues *326*
- Histochemistry of Oral Soft Tissues *326*
- Advanced Techniques *328*
- Clinical Considerations *330*

Appendices

Appendix 1: Oral Tissues: A Brief Description   335

Sabarinath B, Preethi S, Manoj Prabhakar, B Sivapathasundharam

- Comparison of Hard Tissues *335*
- Comparison of Hard Tissue Forming Cells *336*
- Comparison of Oral Mucosa *336*
- Comparison of Papillae of the Tongue *337*
- Comparison of Serous and Mucous Acini *337*
- Comparison of Major Salivary Glands *338*
- Classification of Cementum *338*
- Summary of Molecular Interplay in Tooth Development *338*
- Timeline of Tooth Eruption *339*
- Differences between Deciduous and Permanent Dentition *340*
- Effects of Aging on Oral and Circumoral Tissues *340*
- Abbreviations and Expansions *341*
- Glossary *343*

Appendix 2: Histologic Diagrams   357

B Sivapathasundharam, RJ Vijayashree

Index   373

CHAPTER 1

Overview of Oral Tissues

B Sivapathasundharam

Chapter Outline

- Enamel 3
- Dentin 3
- Pulp 3
- Cementum 3
- Periodontium 4
  » Periodontal Ligament 4
  » Alveolar Bone 4
- Maxillary Sinus 4
- Oral Mucous Membrane 4
- Salivary Gland 4
- Temporomandibular Joint 4
- Microscopic Structures of Oral Tissues 5
- Eruption and Shedding 5
- Cell Signaling 6

Mouth forms the lower one-third of the face and the upper end of the alimentary canal. It is an opening which helps in the intake of food and delivers sounds. It is bounded by lips, cheeks, palate, floor of the mouth, and pharynx. It is also called as oral cavity, buccal cavity or cavum oris **(Figure 1-1)**.

The oral cavity is formed by hard and soft tissues. Hard tissues are teeth and jaw bones namely—maxilla and mandible. The soft tissues include lips, cheek, floor of the mouth, and soft palate **(Figures 1-2A and B)**. However, the jaw bones are covered by soft tissues known as mucosa and are not exposed to the oral cavity or exterior. Unlike jaw bones, teeth are partly exposed to the oral cavity and the rest are embedded into the jaw bone.

The portion of tooth visible in the oral cavity is called crown (clinical crown), the remaining embedded portion is the root. The root is attached to the jaw bone by means of a soft connective tissue called periodontal ligament **(Figure 1-3)**. The junction between the crown and the root is called the cervical margin. The length of the crown and root varies from tooth to tooth.

The bulk of the tooth is made up of a hard tissue called dentin, which encloses a core of soft connective tissue known as pulp. Dentin is covered by the enamel, the hardest structure in the human body in the crown portion and cementum, another hard tissue in the root portion **(Figures 1-4A and B)**. The pulp contains various types of cells, fibers, nerves, blood vessels, and lymphatics. That portion of the tooth which is covered by the enamel is called as anatomical crown, and the portion covered by the cementum is the anatomical root.

Functions of teeth include mastication, speech, and providing the shape of the face. On occasions, it may act as a weapon or help in defense. Most mammals have two sets of teeth in their lifetime and are known as diphyodonts. In few vertebrates, teeth are replaced continuously during their lifetime and are called as polyphyodont. In humans, the first

Figure 1-1: Oral cavity and its parts.

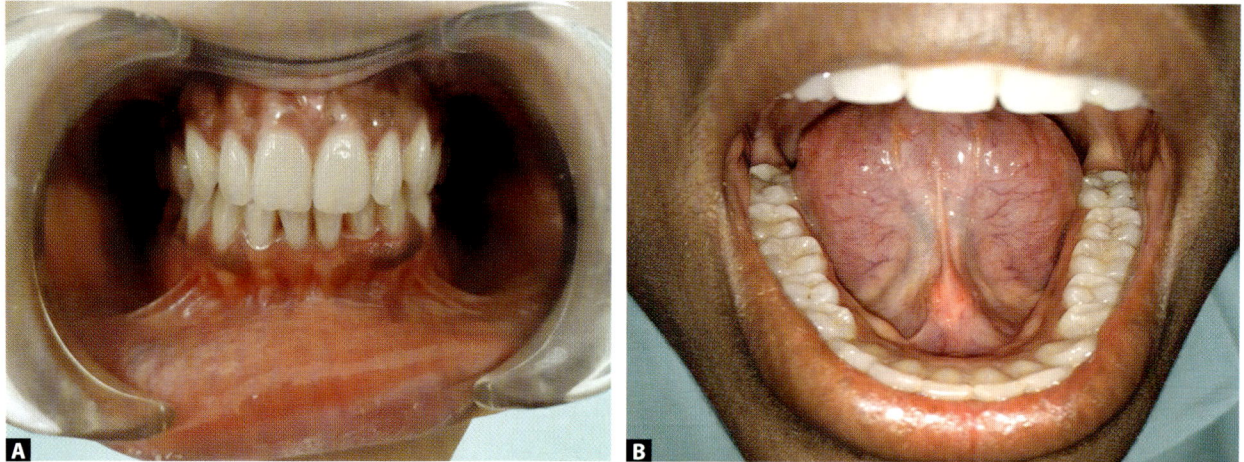

Figures 1-2A and B: (A) Vestibular cavity; (B) Floor of the mouth and ventral surface of the tongue.

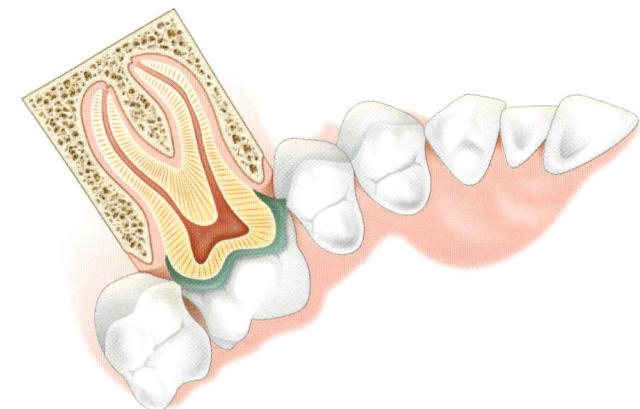

Figure 1-3: Crown, root, and supporting structures.

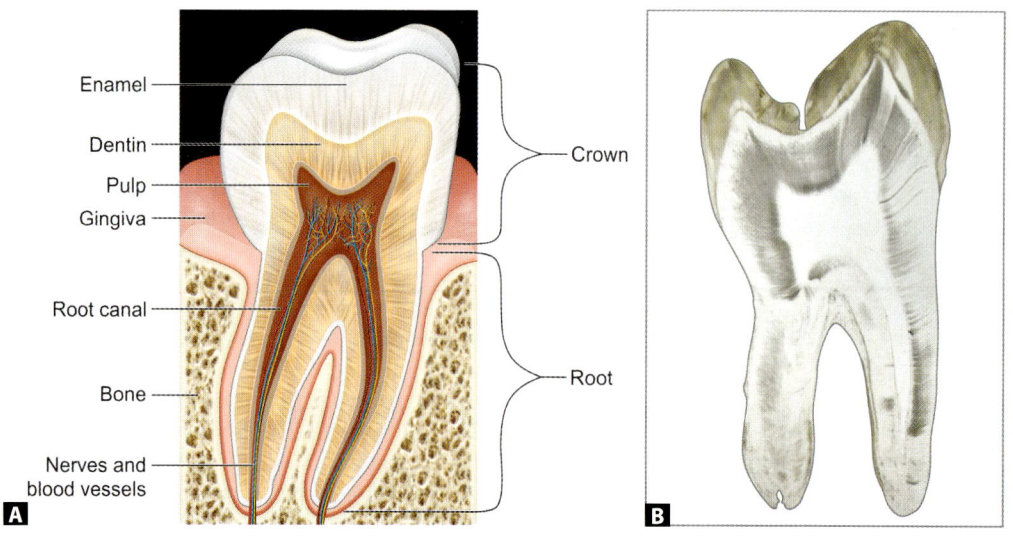

Figures 1-4A and B: (A) Diagrammatic representation of the anatomy of the tooth; (B) Ground section.

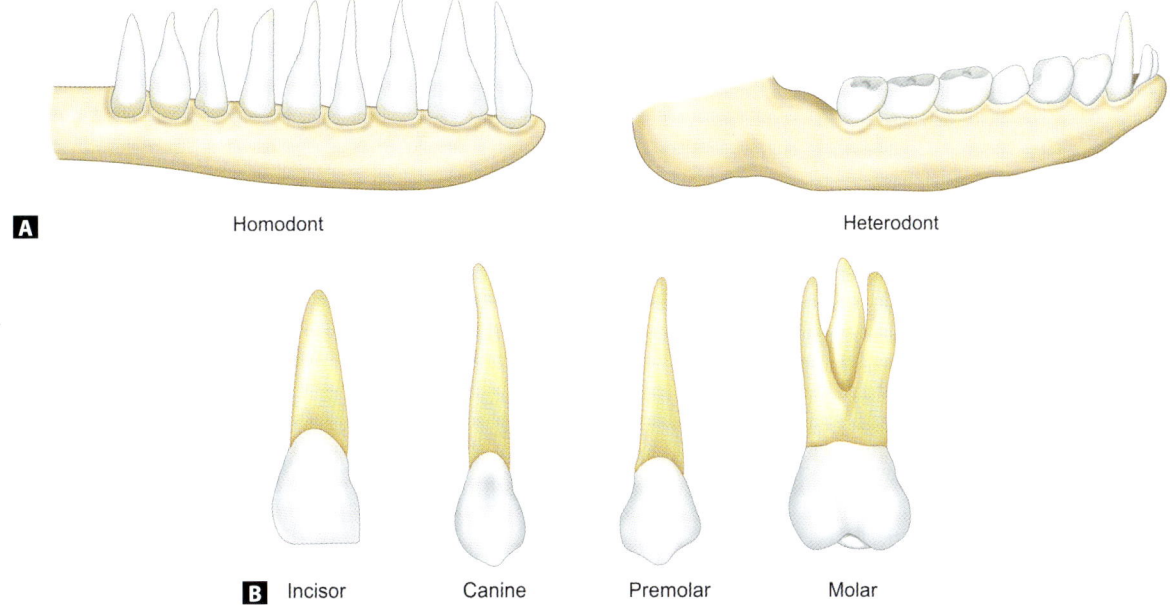

Figures 1-5A and B: (A) Showing differences between homodont and heterodont; (B) Different forms of teeth.

set of teeth is called deciduous (deciduous-falling off) teeth, milk teeth, or primary teeth. They are smaller in size and 20 in number. As the individual grows, there is increase in requirement of masticatory force. This is accomplished by increase in size of the jaw bones and masticatory muscles. Teeth once erupted will not become bigger, so the deciduous teeth are replaced by permanent dentition or secondary dentition, which is more in number, bigger in size, and relatively stronger.

In most of the vertebrates, except mammals, all the teeth are identical (homodonts), whereas mammals including human, possess more than one tooth type (incisors, canine, and molars) and are referred as heterodonts **(Figures 1-5A and B)**.

ENAMEL

Enamel, the lone ectodermal derivative of the tooth, is the hardest substance in the human body. It has the highest inorganic content of all the human hard tissues (96%) and is in the form of calcium phosphate hydroxyapatite crystals. It is acellular and does not contain blood vessels and nerve fibers, hence if damaged, it cannot heal or repair by itself. Color ranges from bluish white to yellowish white. Thickness of enamel varies from knife edge to 2.5 mm, depending on its location in the tooth. On microscopic examination, it is made up of enamel rods which are secreted by the cells called ameloblasts.

DENTIN

Dentin is the first formed hard tissue of the tooth. As said previously, dentin forms the bulk of the tooth. It is made up of dentinal tubules, which enclose the cytoplasmic process of the odontoblasts, the cells responsible for the formation of dentin. The number of tubules per unit area is more in the pulpal end than on the enamel or cemental end. After the formation of dentin, odontoblast moves toward the pulp and forms the part of the pulpal cells. Thus dentin and pulp are considered to be a single complex in terms of development and function. It is slight yellowish in color and becomes darker as age advances. Unlike enamel, dentin is considered to be a vital tissue. The physical and chemical properties of dentin are, to certain extent, similar to that of bone. The inorganic content is again made up of calcium phosphate hydroxyapatite crystals, which are smaller than the crystals of the enamel. The surface of dentin appears depressed like a saucer, which helps in mechanical retention of enamel. The dentin formation is continuous throughout the life and has reparative capacity to an extent.

PULP

Pulp is the only soft connective tissue present inside the tooth. It is a highly vascular tissue with undifferentiated and other cells to maintain the tooth vitality. The pulp resides in the space called pulp chamber in the crown and pulp canal or root canal in the root. It communicates with the periapical tissues through foramina in the apex. The sensory nerve fibers of the pulp respond to any stimuli only as pain irrespective of the type of stimuli. With increase in age, the volume of the pulp becomes reduced due to the continuous formation of dentin.

CEMENTUM

Cementum is another hard tissue of the tooth that covers the root portion and also acts as a medium for attachment of periodontal ligament fibers. Similar to the other hard tissues of tooth, cementum is also avascular and color is slightly yellower than the enamel. It remains thin at the cervical region and continues to increase in thickness at the apical region. The inorganic and organic content of the cementum is similar to that of the bone. Cells responsible for formation of cementum are cementoblasts, and with mineralization these cells get trapped into the cementum to become cementocytes.

■ PERIODONTIUM

The term *periodontium* includes the supporting structures of the tooth namely—cementum, gingiva, periodontal ligament, and alveolar bone.

Periodontal Ligament

The periodontal ligament attaches the tooth to the alveolar bone and distributes the masticatory forces applied to the tooth to the jaw bone. It is made up of collagen fibers as a major fiber component, and contains blood vessels, lymph vessels, nerves, various types of cells and intercellular ground substances.

The cells of the periodontal ligament include secretory cells, (*i.e.* cementoblasts, fibroblasts, and osteoblasts), resorptive cells (*i.e.* osteoclasts and cementoclasts), defense cells, and undifferentiated cells. It provides nutritional supply to the avascular cementum and provides tactile sensation by means of proprioceptive nerve endings. The embedded portion of the periodontal ligament fibers, with cementum on one end and bone on the other end, is known as Sharpey's fibers.

Alveolar Bone

It is that part of the maxilla or mandible, which gives attachment to the tooth by means of periodontal ligament. The inner aspects of the alveolar bone conforms the morphology of the root. Resorption of the alveolar bone occurs in periodontal diseases, and in some other pathological conditions which may lead to tooth loss. That part of the alveolar bone in which periodontal ligament fibers are inserted is known as bundle bone. Cells that are responsible for bone formation are osteoblasts, and they get entrapped within the formed bone as osteocytes. Osteoclasts, the multinucleated cells are responsible for bone resorption. Unlike cementum, bone undergoes constant resorption and deposition, depending on the forces applied on the tooth. This feature of alveolar bone is utilized for orthodontic tooth movement. The bone undergoes resorption when pressure is applied and deposition when there is a tension.

■ MAXILLARY SINUS

Maxillary sinus or antrum is a chamber/space present in the body of the maxilla. They are paired and the largest of all the paranasal sinuses. Along with other paranasal sinuses, it plays a role in lessening the weight of the skull, helps in increasing the resonance of voice, cools down the inhaled air to the body temperature, acts as a buffer against trauma to the face and the brain by serving as a mechanical shock absorber and plays a defensive role by filtering the air passage. All the paranasal sinuses open in the lateral wall of the nose through an opening called ostium. Maxillary sinuses are four-sided pyramidal in shape, located in the body of maxilla, with its base forming the lateral wall of the nasal cavity, and apex directed laterally toward the zygomatic process of the maxilla. The four sides are formed anteriorly by facial surface of maxilla, posteriorly by the infratemporal surface of maxilla, superiorly by the floor of the orbit and inferiorly related to the palate, alveolar process and posterior teeth of the maxilla. Maxillary sinuses are lined by pseudostratified ciliated columnar epithelium (respiratory epithelium), produce mucous, which keeps the sinus wet and moist.

■ ORAL MUCOUS MEMBRANE

The surface of the body is covered by skin and the body cavities are lined by the mucous membrane. Similarly the oral cavity is lined and protected by oral mucous membrane. Based on the functional adaptation, it is categorized into masticatory mucosa, lining mucosa, and specialized mucosa. Hard palate and alveolar bone is covered by masticatory mucosa, tongue by specialized mucosa, and remaining portion of the mouth are lined by lining mucosa. The masticatory mucosa is keratinized. The specialized mucosa of the tongue contains papilla and taste buds.

The mucous membrane comprises epithelium, which is avascular, however, it contains nerve endings and is supported by connective tissue. The epithelium and connective tissue are separated by basement membrane. The color of the oral mucosa varies among different areas of the oral cavity and depends on type of epithelium (keratinized, nonkeratinized), its thickness, the amount of melanin content, and vascularity and density of the connective tissue. The major and minor salivary glands discharge their secretions through ducts onto the surface of oral mucous membrane and keep the mucosa wet/moist always.

■ SALIVARY GLAND

The salivary glands are exocrine glands, which secrete saliva into the oral cavity and keep the oral cavity moist and wet. Saliva helps in mastication, deglutition, digestion, and the like. The secretory units of the glands are called acini. Secretions are expelled out via ducts. The saliva may be serous (watery) or mucus (thick and slimy). Accordingly, salivary glands are categorized into serous, mucous, and mixed glands. Depending on the size of the gland, they are typed into major (larger in size) and minor glands (smaller). Parotid, submandibular, and sublingual glands are paired major salivary glands **(Figures 1-6A and B)**. The minor glands are distributed throughout the oral cavity except in the gingiva and anterior part of the palate.

■ TEMPOROMANDIBULAR JOINT

The lower jaw or the mandible articulates with base of the skull by means of temporomandibular joint (TMJ), a synovial joint **(Figure 1-7)**. More precisely the joint is formed by the head of the condyle of the mandible and the glenoid fossa or mandibular fossa of temporal bone. The joint is separated into upper and lower compartment by means of interarticular disk

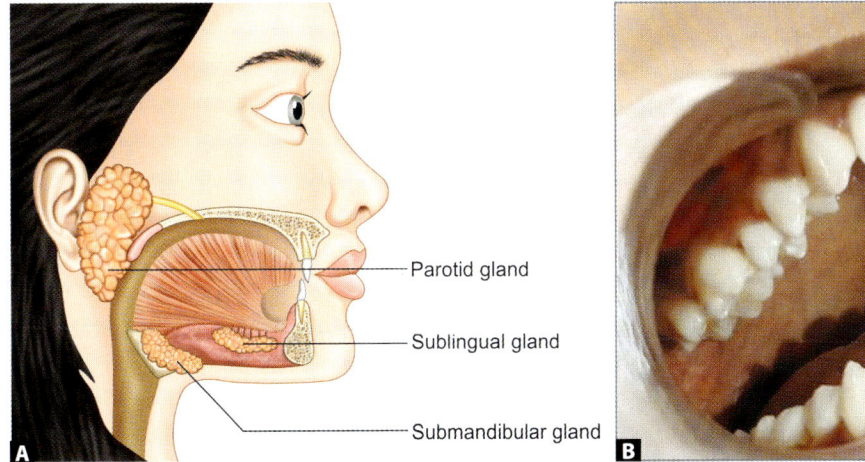

Figures 1-6A and B: (A) Major salivary glands; (B) Discharge of saliva via parotid duct.

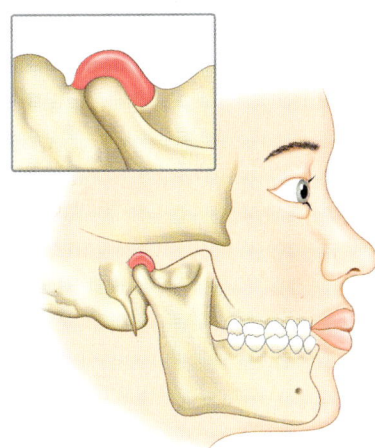

Figure 1-7: Schematic diagram of temporomandibular joint.

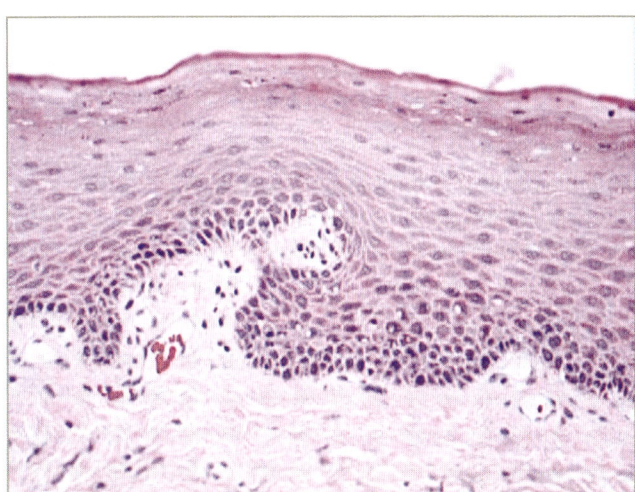

Figure 1-8: Photomicrograph of hematoxylin and eosin stained section showing epithelium and connective tissue of the oral mucous membrane.

known as meniscus. The articulating surfaces and the joint cavity are lined by synovial membrane supported by fibrous capsule and lubricated by synovial fluid. Though the TMJs are anatomically two separate joints, it is considered as single unit functionally. The movements are enabled by the muscles of mastication namely—masseter, temporalis, medial pterygoid, and lateral pterygoid.

MICROSCOPIC STRUCTURES OF ORAL TISSUES

Structure of the oral tissues can be better studied and appreciated by microscopic examination. To study the tissue under microscope, it has to be cut into thin slices, stained (hematoxylin and eosin are the stains commonly used), and fixed onto the glass slide **(Figure 1-8)**. A cutting instrument called microtome is used to section the specimen approximately 4–5 μ (μ - micron, which is one thousandth of a mm) thickness. This is called histological processing. This procedure is followed for all soft tissues. Hard tissues like teeth or bone cannot be cut by using a microtome like soft tissues because of its hardness due to the presence of calcium phosphate hydroxyapatite crystals. To make them soft, calcium has to be removed by the process known as decalcification. Usually mild acids are used for decalcification. After decalcification, the hard tissue becomes soft and can be treated like any other soft tissue for microscopic examination. Another method for preparation of hard tissue for microscopic examination is ground section. Here the tooth or the bone is initially cut into thin slices by using saw or abrasive disks and grind further to make it thinner approximately 50–80 μm thickness to make suitable for microscopic examination. Ground sections are not usually stained.

ERUPTION AND SHEDDING

Eruption is the process of movement of the tooth from the site of its development within the jaw bone to the site of its function in the occlusal plane. Eruption time may vary from tooth to tooth, gender, and race. The first teeth to erupt into the oral cavity are the deciduous mandibular central incisors and they erupt about six months after birth. Third molars, also called as wisdom teeth are the last teeth to erupt.

The process of falling or exfoliation of deciduous tooth to accommodate permanent tooth is called shedding. The jaws of the child can accommodate teeth, which are smaller in size and lesser in number. As stated previously, there is need for more masticatory force as the age advances, so the deciduous teeth are replaced by permanent teeth, which are larger in size and more in number. This is accomplished by shedding of the deciduous teeth by resorption of root. The cells which are responsible for tooth resorption are called odontoclasts, which are multinucleated cells analogous to osteoclasts of the bone.

■ CELL SIGNALING

Knowledge of growth factors and cell signaling is important to understand growth, development and function.

All living tissues are made up of cells, which are the structural and functional units. They communicate to the neighboring cells, distant cells, and to the intercellular substance by a process known as cell signaling. They send and receive numerous messages through chemicals known as signaling molecules. These signaling molecules are usually proteins, secreted by the specific cells, and released into the extracellular space. They travel through the intercellular matrix to the place, where it has to act on the target cells. In order to receive the appropriate signal, the target cell should possess the right receptor on its surface (cell surface receptors). Binding of a signaling molecule to its receptor, triggers a change inside the cell. Growth factors are also the signaling molecules (usually gene product) which are elaborated by the cells or group of cells and are responsible for cellular proliferation, growth, differentiation, and maturation **(Figure 1-9)**. There are different types of growth factors and each type of growth factor is specific for particular function.

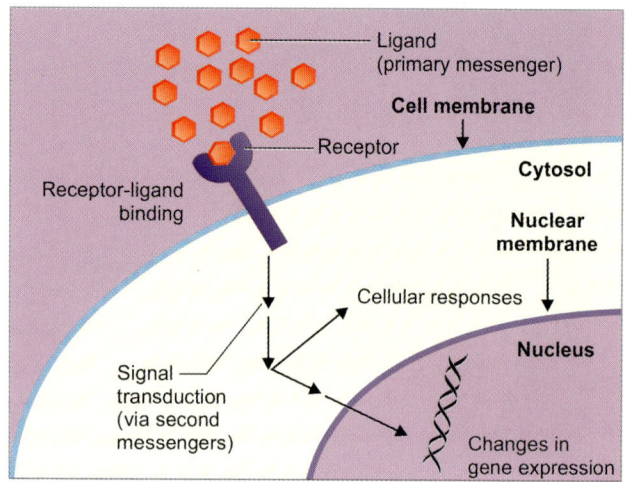

Figure 1-9: Cell signaling.

They exert their effect through endocrine, paracrine, and autocrine mechanisms. Each growth factor has a specific surface receptor on the target cells. The effect of growth factors on the target cells depends on concentration and binding ability of growth factors, type of receptors, number of target cells, and response of the target cells. The binding of growth factors to the receptors initiates the particular function. The examples of growth factors include fibroblastic growth factor, epidermal growth factor, transforming growth factor alpha, transforming growth factor beta, platelet-derived growth factors, etc.

Points to Remember

- Enamel, dentin and cementum are the hard tissues of the tooth.
- Enamel, dentin and cementum are avascular, whereas the pulp is vascular.
- Pulp is the only soft tissue present inside the tooth.
- Periodontal ligament attaches the tooth to the alveolar bone.
- Enamel is made up of enamel rods and dentin by dentinal tubules.
- Oral mucous membrane is of three types: masticatory mucosa, lining mucosa and specialized mucosa.
- Temporomandibular joint is formed by the head of the condyle of the mandible and the glenoid fossa of the temporal bone.
- Ground sections or decalcified sections are used to study the tooth under microscope.
- Signaling molecules are proteins secreted by the specific cells, and released into the extracellular space to act on the specific cell

PRACTICE QUESTIONS

1. What are all the soft tissues associated with the tooth?
2. What are all the muscles of mastication?
3. Write notes on tissues of periodontium.
4. Write a note on maxillary sinus.
5. How oral soft tissues are studied under microscope?
6. How tooth and bone are studied under microscope?
7. What is cell signaling?

MULTIPLE CHOICE QUESTIONS

1. **Enamel is**
   a. Endodermal in origin.
   b. Mesodermal in origin.
   c. Ectodermal in origin
   d. Ectomesenchymal in origin.

2. **The bulk of the tooth is made up of**
   a. Enamel
   b. Dentin
   c. Cementum
   d. Pulp
3. **Which one of the following is not a soft tissue?**
   a. Pulp
   b. Cementum
   c. Periodontal ligament
   d. Meniscus
4. **Which one of the following does not contain blood vessels?**
   a. Periodontal ligament
   b. Cementum
   c. Alveolar bone
   d. Pulp
5. **Cells responsible for the formation of enamel are called**
   a. Odontoblasts
   b. Cementoblasts
   c. Ameloblasts
   d. Osteoblasts
6. **Cells responsible for the resorption of tooth are called**
   a. Osteoclasts
   b. Osteoblasts
   c. Odontoblasts
   d. Odontoclasts
7. **Temporomandibular joint is lubricated by**
   a. Saliva
   b. Blood
   c. Synovial fluid
   d. Intercellular fluid
8. **Salivary glands are**
   a. Exocrine glands
   b. Endocrine glands
   c. Present in the anterior part of the hard palate
   d. Not seen in soft palate and buccal mucosa
9. **Muscles of mastication does not include**
   a. Temporalis
   b. Masseter
   c. Sternocleidomastoid
   d. Pterygoid

ANSWERS

1. c   2. b   3. b   4. b   5. c   6. d   7. c   8. a   9. c

BIBLIOGRAPHY

1. Ash MM. Wheeler's Dental Anatomy, Physiology, and Occlusion, 7th edition. Saunders: Philadelphia; 1993.
2. Avery JK. Oral Development and Histology, 3rd edition. Thieme: New York; 2002.
3. Berkovitz BKB, Holland GR, Moxham BJ. Oral Anatomy, Histology and Embryology, 4th edition. US: Elsevier; 2009.
4. Carlson BM. Human Embryology and Developmental Biology, 5th edition. Philadelphia: WB Saunders; 2014.
5. Chandra S, Chandra S, Chandra M, et al. Textbook of Dental and Oral Histology with Embryology & MCQ's, 2nd edition. India: Jaypee Brothers Medical Publishers (P) Ltd; 2010.
6. Chatterjee K. Essentials of Dental Anatomy and Oral Histology, 2nd edition. India: Jaypee Brothers Medical Publishers (P) Ltd; 2014.
7. Cohen B, Kramer IRH. Scientific Foundations of Dentistry, 1st edition. London: William Heinemann Medical Books Ltd; 1976.
8. Gaunt WA, Osborn JW, Ten Cate AR. Advanced Dental Histology, 2nd edition. Bristol: John Wright & Sons Ltd; 1971.
9. Kumar GS. Orban's Oral Histology and Embryology, 14th edition. India: Elsevier; 2015.
10. Nanci A. Ten Cate's Oral Histology: Development, Structure, and Functions, 8th edition. India: Elsevier; 2012.
11. Provenza VD, Seibel W. Oral Histology- Inheritance and Development, 2nd edition. USA: Lea & Febiger; 1986.
12. Schoenwolf GC, Bleyl S, Brauer P. Larsen's Human Embryology, 5th edition. US: Elsevier; 2015.
13. Schroeder HE. Oral Structural Biology, 4th edition. Thieme: New York; 1991.

CHAPTER 2

General Embryology

B Sivapathasundharam

Chapter Outline

- Fertilization   9
- Cleavage   9
- Formation of Bilaminar Germ Disk   9
- Prochordal Plate and Trilaminar Germ Disk Formation   9
- Formation of Neural Crest Cells   11
- Folding of the Embryo   13
- Development of Branchial Arches   13
- Fate of Pharyngeal Clefts   13

Embryology is the study of embryo and its development. It also includes the study of the prenatal development of gametes and fertilization. Human life begins as fertilized ovum. This single cell multiplies into millions of cells to form the human body. Human cell is made up of cytoplasm and a nucleus, which encloses the chromosomes. Chromosome contains genetic information in the form of deoxyribonucleic acid (DNA) and it can vary in number from species to species. Human somatic cells contain 46 chromosomes and are arranged in 23 pairs (diploid). Out of 46 chromosomes, 44 chromosomes (22 pairs) are similar and are called autosomes; the remaining two chromosomes may be similar or dissimilar and are called allosomes or sex chromosomes (X and Y chromosome, **Figure 2-1**).

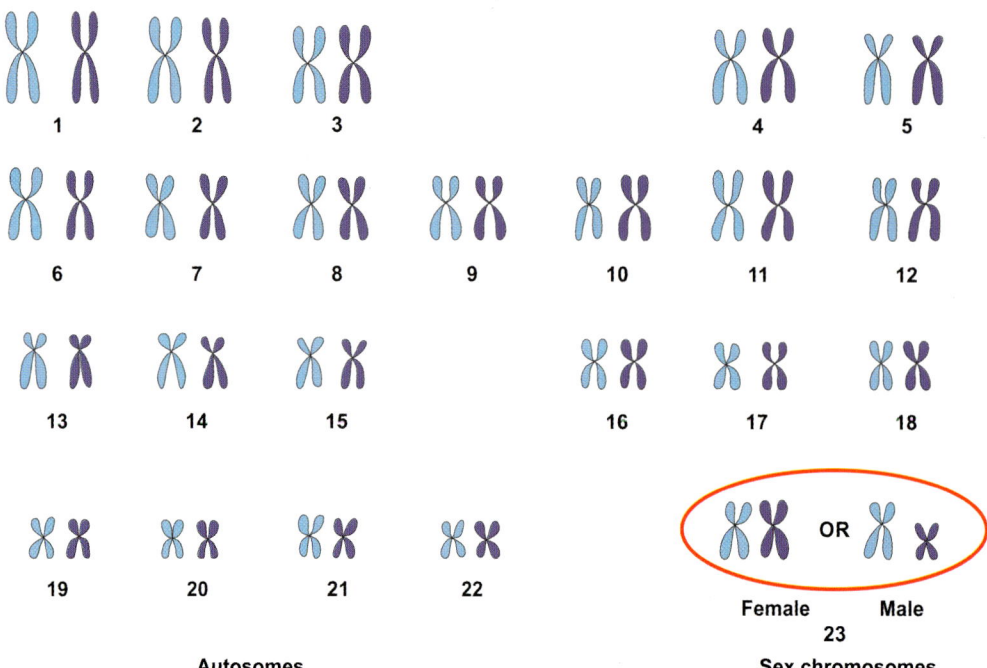

Figure 2-1: Diagrammatic representation of human chromosome showing 22 pairs of autosomes and one pair of sex chromosome.

> Apart from nucleus DNA is also found in mitochondria and is called mitochondrial DNA (mtDNA).

One chromosome of each pair is derived from father and the other from the mother. In contrast to somatic cells, the germ cells (sperm and ova, collectively called gametes) contain half the number of chromosomes (haploid). It is always 22 + X in case of females and it may be 22 + X or 22 + Y in case of males.

Cell multiplication is important for growth and replacement of dead cells. This is accomplished by cell division. When cells divide, the genetic information, which they contain is passed on to both the daughter cells, where the number of chromosomes and the genetic information are identical in both the daughter cells as of the mother cell. This process is known as mitosis and this occurs in somatic cell. In case of germ cells or gametes, this process is slightly different, called meiosis. Here the cell undergoes two successive divisions called first and second meiotic division, with the resultant daughter cells have half the number of chromosomes, genetic information that differs from one another.

■ FERTILIZATION

Fusion of sperm and ovum is called fertilization. This occurs in the ampulla of uterine tube, and results in formation of zygote **(Figure 2-2)**. Fertilization results in the following three events, namely—(A) Achievement of chromosomal diploidy, (B) Determination of sex of the embryo, and (C) Initiation of cleavage or cell division.

> A sperm surface protein called Fertilin plays an important role in fertilization. It is required for the migration of spermatozoa through the fallopian tube and adhesion of spermatozoa to the plasma membrane of the oocyte.

■ CLEAVAGE

The fertilized ovum is a large cell, which becomes smaller as it divides further. This zygote undergoes series of cell division to become two-cell stage, four-cell stage, eight-cell stage, and sixteen-cell stage. This process of cell division is known as cleavage. The sixteen-cell stage early embryo travels from the fallopian tube to the uterus in approximately three days after fertilization. During 16–32-cell stage, this clump of cells looks like mulberry and is called the morula. Fluid seeps into the morula and makes it into a fluid-filled sac known as blastocyst or blastocele **(Figure 2-3)**. The process of morula developing into blastula (blastocyst) is known as blastulation.

The fluid seepage into the blastocyst leads to realignment of the cells of the morula to form two distinct populations of cells. The lining of the blastocyst is formed by trophoblasts and the smaller inner cell mass is called embryoblast **(Figures 2-4A and B)**. Embryoblasts will form the embryo proper while trophoblasts form the supporting structures (placenta) and help in the implantation of the embryo.

From fertilization till the end of 8th week, it is called embryo; further from 8th week till birth, the fetus.

■ FORMATION OF BILAMINAR GERM DISK

After first week of intrauterine life, the embryoblasts differentiate themselves to form a two-layered circular structure known as bilaminar germ disk **(Figures 2-5A and B)**. The upper layer comprised of columnar cells is known as epiblasts (ectoderm) and the lower flattened cells, which become cuboidal later, are called hypoblasts (endoderm). This bilaminar germ disk divides the blastocyst cavity into two, the upper amniotic cavity and the lower yolk sac cavity.

At this stage, head or the tail end of the embryo is not determined. Soon, in a localized area near the periphery, the cuboidal cells of the endoderm become columnar and this region is known as prochordal plate also called prechordal plate, which determines the central axis of the embryo **(Figures 2-6A and B)**. This enables to distinguish the right and left halves and head and tail end of the future embryo. Prochordal plate sometimes referred to as head organizer and is the future site of the mouth.

■ PROCHORDAL PLATE AND TRILAMINAR GERM DISK FORMATION

During the third week, the ectodermal cells at the tail end proliferate to form a bulge, which proceeds as a linear structure toward the cranial end along the central axis to form primitive streak **(Figure 2-7A)**.

The cells alongside of primitive streak proliferate and migrate toward the lateral and cephalic direction in between ectoderm and endoderm sparing the prochordal plate to form mesoderm, the third germ layer **(Figure 2-7B)**. The prochordal plate, devoid of mesoderm, will form the future buccopharyngeal membrane, and give origin to the rostral cranial mesoderm. Thus, the bilaminar germ disk becomes trilaminar germ disk. The process of rearrangement of the blastula especially to form the trilaminar germ disk is called gastrulation. All the structures and organs of the body are derived from this trilaminar germ disk, through the processes of somitogenesis (Somites are bilaterally paired blocks of paraxial mesoderm that form along the anterior-posterior axis of the developing embryo), histogenesis and organogenesis.

These initial events are mainly concerned with cellular proliferation and migration. All these events concerned with cellular proliferation and migration occur continuously and on an inherent pattern.

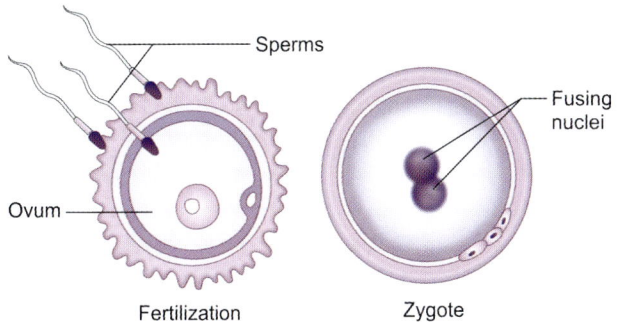

Figure 2-2: Fertilization and formation of zygote.

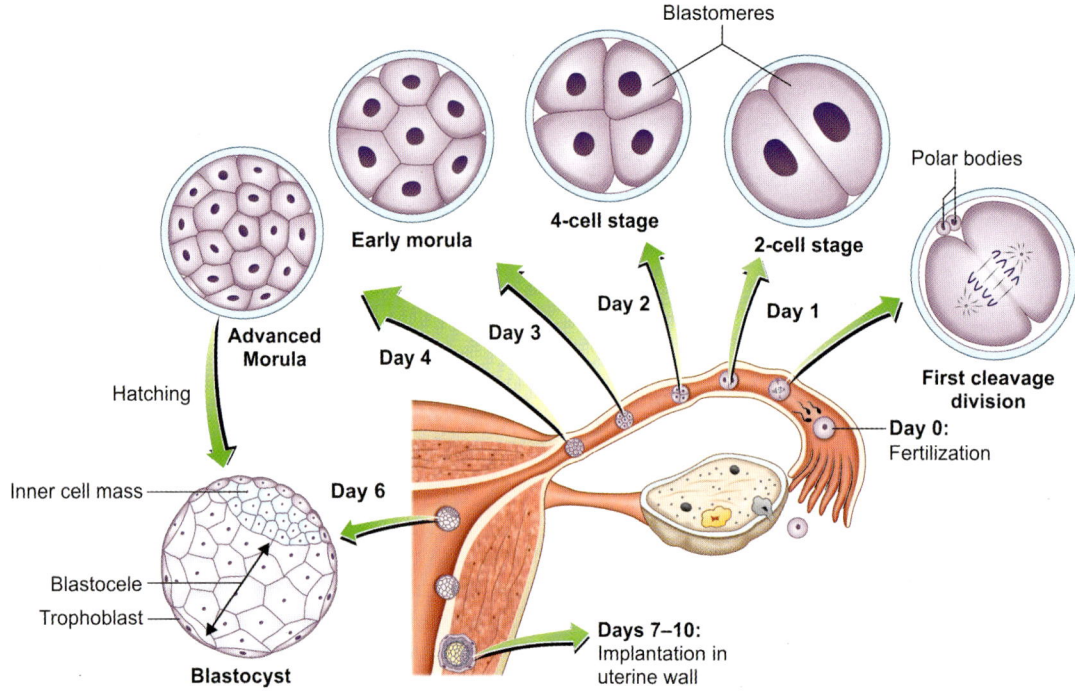

Figure 2-3: Cleavage or cell division from a zygote to blastocyst.

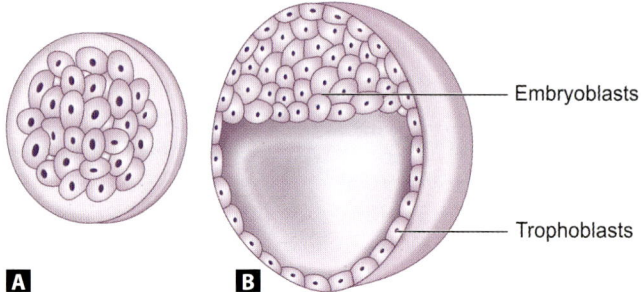

Figures 2-4A and B: (A) Morula; (B) Blastocyst containing inner cell mass, the embryoblast and an outer layer, the trophoblast.

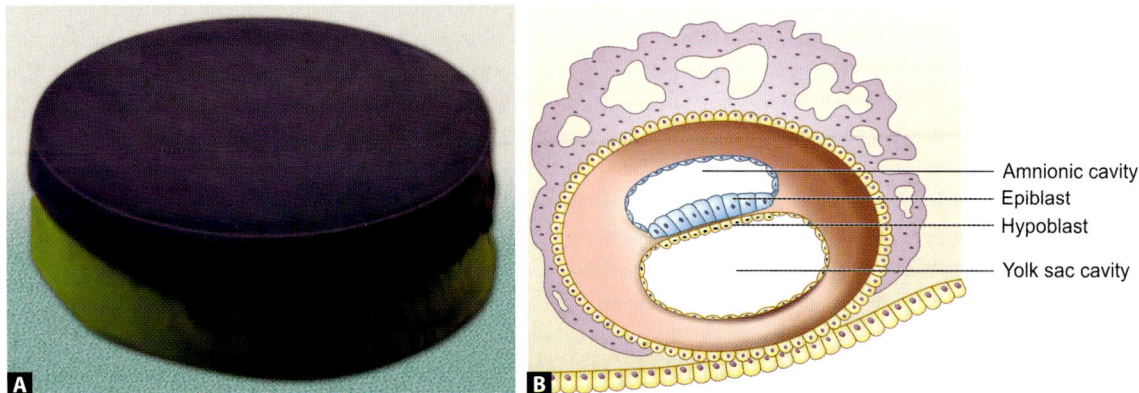

Figures 2-5A and B: Formation of bilaminar germ disk.

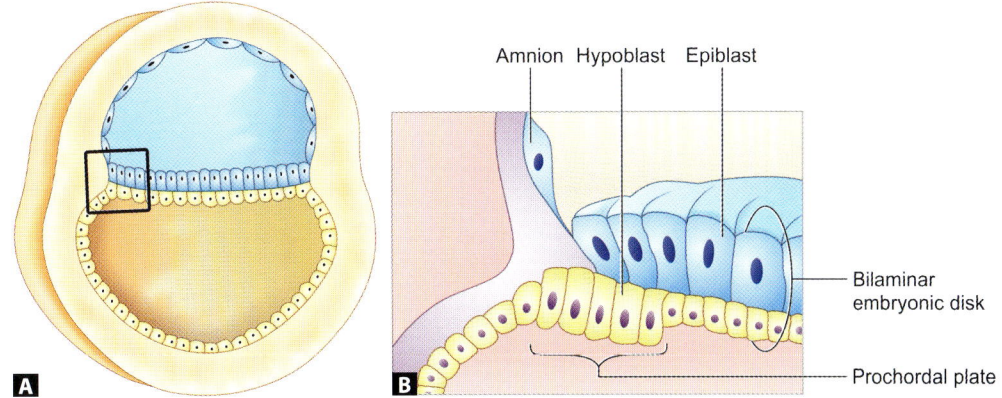

Figures 2-6A and B: (A) Transverse section showing prochordal plate formation; (B) Insert showing cells of the prochordal plate.

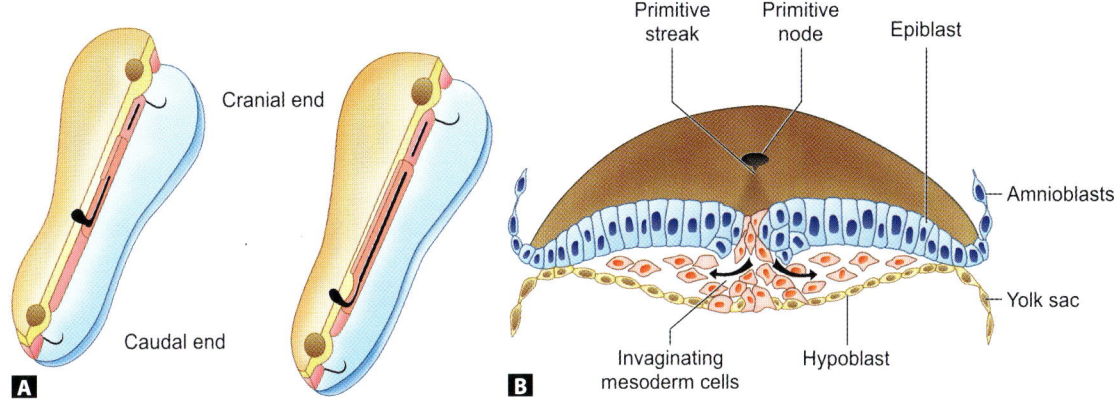

Figures 2-7A and B: (A) Primitive streak formation from the caudal end to the cranial end; (B) Proliferation of ectodermal cells from the primitive streak to form the mesoderm.

FORMATION OF NEURAL CREST CELLS

Notochord is the midline structure. It extends from the primitive streak and ends at the caudal end of prochordal plate **(Figures 2-8 and 2-9)**. Initially cranial end of the primitive streak thickens to form a primitive knot. The cells from the primitive knot proliferate and migrate cranially between the ectoderm and endoderm to form notochordal process. Later, this process gives rise to a solid rod-like structure known as notochord. Most of its part disappears later and only a small portion persists in the intervertebral disk as nucleus pulposus.

Nervous system develops from ectoderm. The ectoderm at the midline above the notochord thickens to form the neural plate. The margins of the neural plate rise to form a neural fold, this fold elongates and leaves a depression in the midline called neural groove. The folds grow further and fuse with each other converting the neural groove into neural tube **(Figures 2-10A to E)**. Soon this neural tube separates from the ectoderm. The cells which form the neural tube are called neuroectoderm. The cranial part of the neural tube forms brain and the caudal part forms the spinal cord.

A unique group of cells derived from the ectoderm along the lateral margins of the neural tube are called neural crest cells, which exist only in vertebrates. These cells are multipotent stem cells that migrate to various parts of the

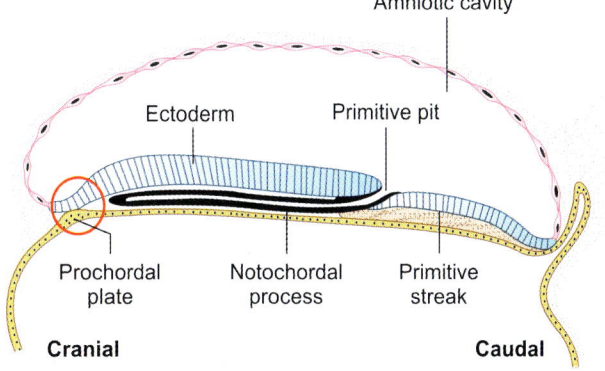

Figure 2-8: Primitive streak formation to form mesoderm excepting in the prochordal plate (circled).

embryo to generate broad array of cells and influence the other developing tissues. Because of this unique feature, it is also considered as fourth germ layer. They migrate beneath the surface ectoderm as sheet of cells. During differentiation, loss of cell adhesive properties and change in cytoskeletal organization occurs in neural crest cells, which lead to their delamination and migration. Bone morphogenetic protein, fibroblast growth factors, and some signaling molecules are responsible for this neural crest cascade.

CHAPTER 2: General Embryology

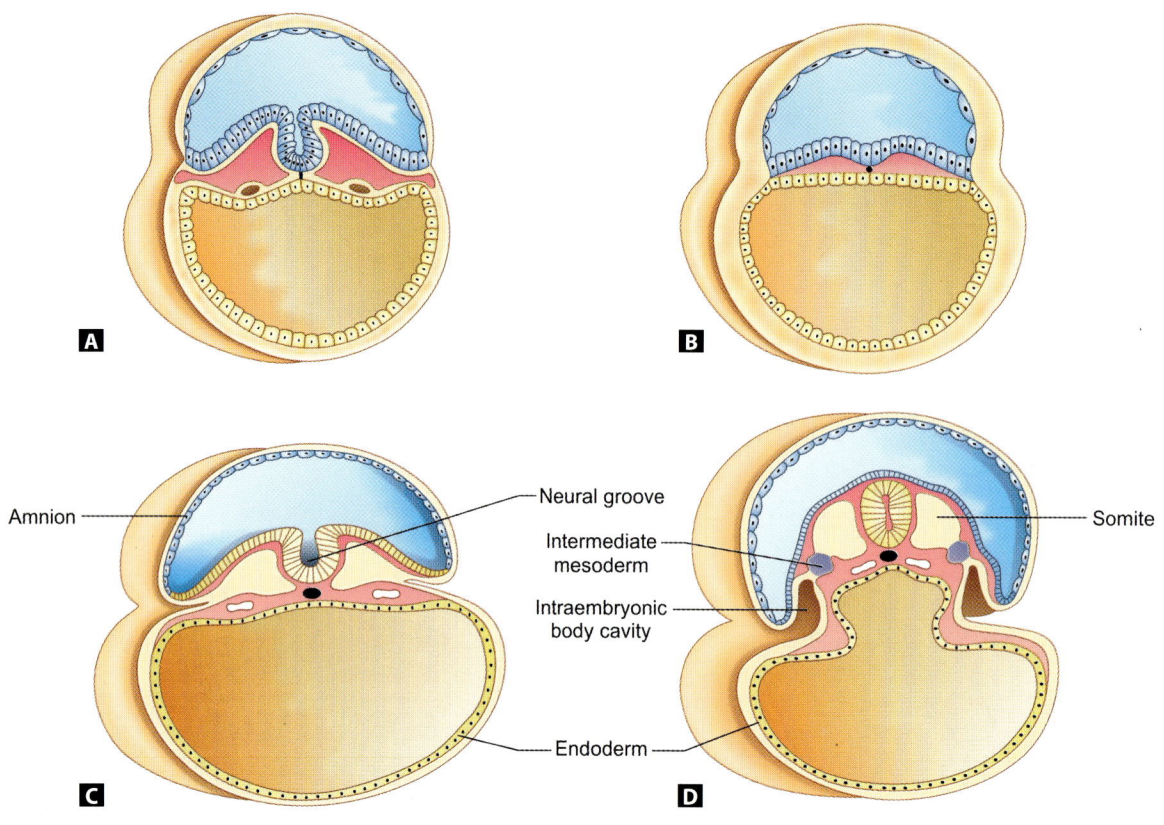

Figures 2-9A to D: Formation of neural tube.

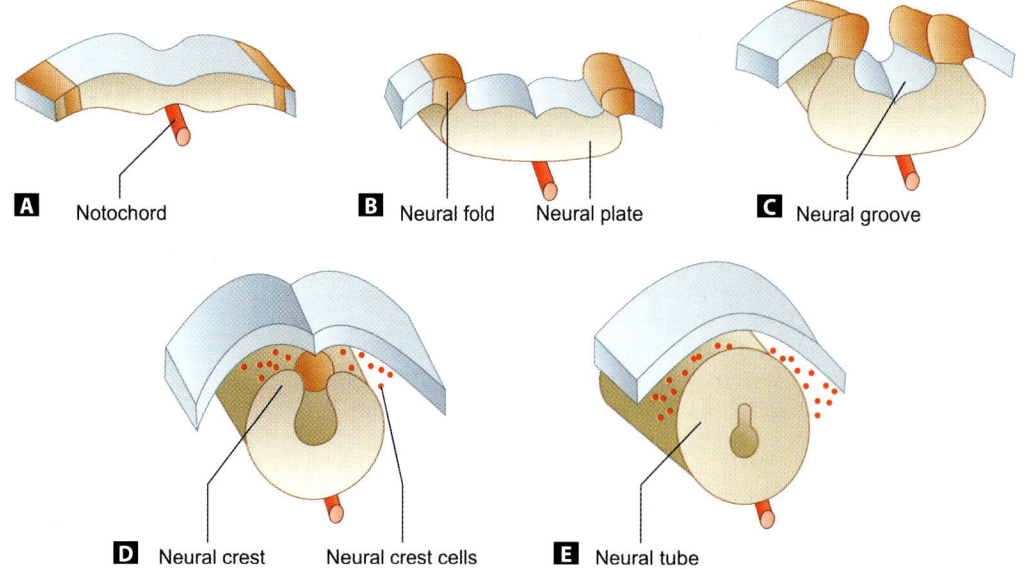

Figures 2-10A to E: Stages in the formation of neural tube.

For the neural crest cells to migrate, the tight binding between them has to be loosened. Slug protein activates the factors that dissociate the tight junctions between these cells. Another factor is the loss of N-cadherin, which bind the cells together. Further the extracellular matrices surrounding the neural tube control the path taken by the neural crest cells during their migration.

The mesenchyme of the upper facial region is derived from or influenced by the migrated neural crest cells and is known as *ectomesenchyme*. Elsewhere in the body the embryonic connective tissue is called mesenchyme. In the head and neck region, the neural crest cells contribute to development of skeletal and connective tissue, whereas in trunk region they form neural, endocrine, and pigment cells. Further in the trunk region the sensory ganglion, neuron, and Schwann cells are derived from neural crest cells. In the facial region, the epithelial portion of the tooth and the glands are derived from the ectoderm alone and the connective tissue components namely—osteoblasts, chondroblasts, odontoblasts, fibroblasts, adipocytes, smooth muscle cells, Schwann cells, pigment cells, and neurons are from ectomesenchyme.

FOLDING OF THE EMBRYO

Folding of the embryo is an important event in embryogenesis, which occurs as a result of embryonic growth, particularly the neural tube. Because of the folding, the ectoderm covers the body surfaces and the endoderm lines the body cavities. This occurs in both longitudinal (craniocaudal axis) and transverse axis (lateral), resulting in the transformation of the flat trilaminar germ disk into a three-dimensional cylindrical structure. This process separates the embryo from its embryonic membrane, which eventually becomes a thin stalk to form the umbilical cord. Since the distance between the head and tail ends of the embryonic germ disk remains unchanged, the dorsal region grows more rapidly than the ventral region. This causes the embryo to bulge dorsally. The longitudinal folding produces head and tail folds while the transverse folding results in left and right folds. This lateral folding toward the midline results in formation of cylindrical embryo. As a result of the formation of head and tail folds, the yolk sac is incorporated into the embryo to form the primitive gut **(Figure 2-11)**.

DEVELOPMENT OF BRANCHIAL ARCHES

The branchial apparatus consists of branchial arches, branchial grooves, pouches, and membranes, and contributes greatly to the formation of face, jaw, ear, and neck. These branchial arches also called pharyngeal arches or visceral arches are seen in vertebrates and begin to develop at the 4th week of the embryo. These pharyngeal arches are developed from all three germ layers. They are covered by ectoderm, lined by endoderm, and a mesodermal core consists of cartilaginous, muscular, vascular, and nerve component.

> Developmental genes such as homeobox genes like *Hox* and *Dlx* are crucial for patterning of branchial arches.

The developing heart descends downward to form the future neck; this is enabled mainly by the appearances of a series of bar-like thickenings. These bars grow ventrally in the floor of the pharynx and fuse with the opposing bar and form pharyngeal arches. The pharyngeal arches are six in number, out of which 5th one is rudimentary. The first arch is named as mandibular arch; second arch known as hyoid arch **(Figures 2-12A and B)**. Each arch mesoderm develops in the given order, *i.e.* artery, nerve, and cartilage. The cartilage of the first arch is called Meckel's cartilage, second arch known as Reichert's cartilage, and cartilages of the other arches do not have any specific names. The ectoderm in between two arches dip to form pharyngeal grooves or clefts and the analogous depression of the endodermal portion is called pharyngeal pouch.

First arch, the mandibular arch gives rise to maxilla and mandible, and the cartilage of this arch is known as Meckel's cartilage. It gives rise to incus, malleus, and squamous part of temporal bone, sphenomalleolar ligament, and sphenomandibular ligament. The external auditory meatus develops from the first pharyngeal groove. Tympanic membrane, tympanic cavity, maxillary antrum, and eustachian tube develops from the first pouch. The muscles that develop from the first arch include—muscles of mastication, anterior belly of digastric, tensor veli palatini, and tensor tympani. The nerve of the first arch is trigeminal nerve.

The second arch is known as hyoid arch and contributes to the formation of side of the neck. The cartilage of this arch is known as Reichert's cartilage, which gives rise to the formation of stapedius, superior part of greater horn of hyoid bone, lesser horn of hyoid bone, and styloid process of temporal bone. Muscles of facial expression, stylohyoid ligament, and posterior belly of digastric are muscles of this arch. The nerve of the second arch is facial nerve.

Contribution of other arches in the development of orofacial region is less, and hence not discussed in this chapter.

FATE OF PHARYNGEAL CLEFTS

The dorsal part of the first pharyngeal cleft gives rise to epithelial lining of external acoustic meatus. The external aspect of second arch grows faster compared to the existing arches and overlaps the external aspect of third, fourth, and sixth arch. The lower portion of the overhanging border of the second arch fuses with the tissues caudal to the 6th arch, to make the developing neck smoother. The space between the inner aspect of the overhanging second arch and external aspect of third, fourth, and sixth arch is called cervical sinus.

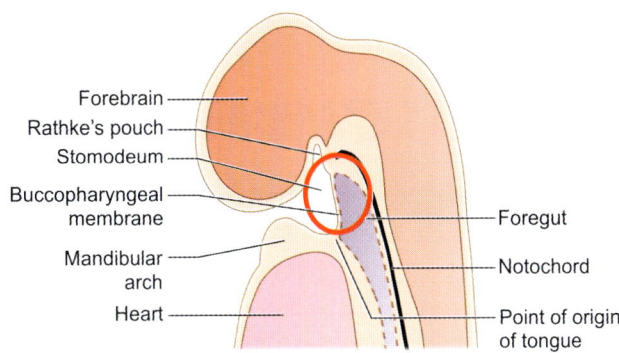

Figure 2-11: Folding of the embryo and formation of the primitive oral cavity and buccopharyngeal membrane (circled).

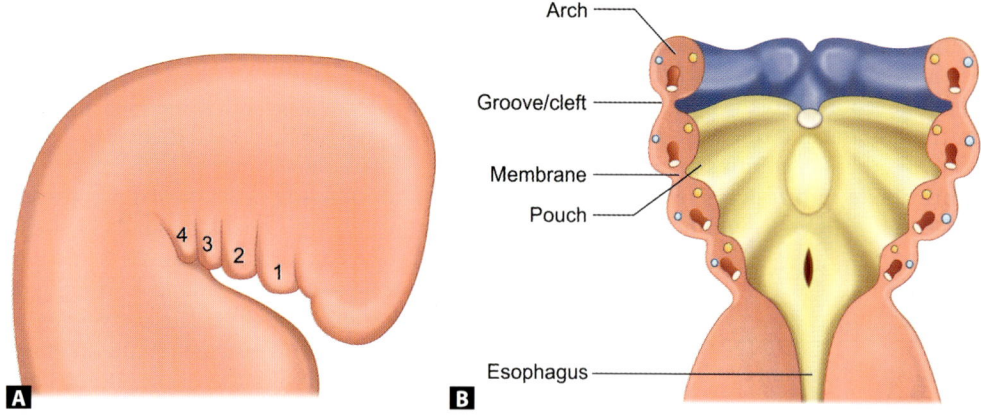

Figures 2-12A and B: (A) Pharyngeal arches; (B) Pharyngeal pouches and clefts with its contents.

Points to Remember

- Fusion of sperm and ovum is called fertilization.
- As a result of fertilisation the chromosomal diploidy is achieved, sex of the embryo is determined and cleavage or the cell division is started.
- Due to the cleavage the clump of cells will become morula. Fluid seeps inside the morula and it becomes blastocyt.
- The embryoblasts of the blastocyst arrange themselves to form bilaminar germ disk, which contain ectoderm and endoderm. In next stage this bilaminar germ disk is converted into trilaminar germ disk by the proliferation of cells in between them. The middle layer is called mesoderm.
- Neural crest and neural tube form from the ectoderm. Lateral to the neural tube a unique group of cells appear and are called neural crest cells, which migrate and influence the mesenchyme of the facial region.
- Folding of the embryo is an important event which converts the flat trilaminar germ disk into a three-dimensional structure and because of this folding the ectoderm covers the body surface and the endoderm covers the body cavities.
- Pharyngeal or branchial arches are bar-like thickenings that appear between the head bulge and the cardiac bulge. They are six in number, out of which 5th one is rudimentary.
- First arch is called mandibular arch and the second one is called hyoid arch.
- These pharyngeal arches are developed from all three germ layers. They are covered by ectoderm, lined by endoderm, and a mesodermal core consists of cartilaginous, muscular, vascular, and nerve component.
- First arch, the mandibular arch gives rise to maxilla and mandible, and the cartilage of this arch is known as Meckel's cartilage.
- The second arch is known as hyoid arch and contributes to the formation of side of the neck. The cartilage of this arch is known as Reichert's cartilage.

PRACTICE QUESTIONS

1. What is fertilization and the result of fertilization?
2. Write short notes on bilaminar germ disk.
3. Write short notes on folding of embryo.
4. Write short notes on neural crest cells.
5. Write short notes on pharyngeal arches.

MULTIPLE CHOICE QUESTIONS

1. **Fertilisation results in the following, *except***
   a. Chromosomal haploidy achieved
   b. Diploidy of chromosomes achieved
   c. Sex of the embryo is determined
   d. Cleavage starts
2. **Prochordal plate determines**
   a. Sex of the embryo
   b. Fate of the neural crest cells
   c. Head tail axis of the embryo
   d. Notochord formation
3. **Fourth germ layer is another name for**
   a. Ectoderm
   b. Neural crest cells
   c. Mesoderm
   d. Endoderm
4. **Trophoblasts form the**
   a. Embryo proper.
   b. Supporting structures of the embryo.
   c. Bilaminar germ disk.
   d. Notochord

5. Prochordal plate area will form the
   a. Notochord.
   b. Primitive knot.
   c. Neural crest.
   d. Buccopharyngeal membrane.
6. Prochordal plate contains
   a. Endoderm and mesoderm.
   b. Endoderm and ectoderm.
   c. Ectoderm and mesoderm.
   d. Only endoderm.
7. The inner cell mass of the blastocyst is called
   a. Trophoblasts.
   b. Amnioblasts.
   c. Embryoblasts.
   d. Neural crest cells.
8. Folding of the embryo results in
   a. The formation of neural tube.
   b. Conversion of flat trilaminar germ disk into a three-dimensional cylindrical structure.
   c. The formation of pharyngeal arches.
   d. The formation of neural crest cells.
9. The embryonic connective tissue influenced by the migrated neural crest cells is called
   a. Mesenchyme.
   b. Neuroectoderm.
   c. Ectomesenchyme.
   d. Neuromesenchyme.
10. Pharyngeal arches
    a. Are six in number.
    b. Contain rudimentary 5th arch.
    c. Develops from all three germ layers.
    d. All of the above.
11. Mandibular arch
    a. Is the first pharyngeal arch and forms maxilla alone.
    b. Forms the mandible.
    c. Forms maxilla and mandible.
    d. Contains Reichert's cartilage.
12. Cartilage of the hyoid arch is called
    a. Meckel's cartilage.
    b. Reichert's cartilage.
    c. Mandibular cartilage.
    d. Hyaline cartilage.

ANSWERS

1. a 2. c 3. b 4. b 5. d 6. b 7. c 8. b 9. c 10. d 11. c 12. b

BIBLIOGRAPHY

1. Alfarawati S, Goodall N, Gordon T, et al. Cytogenetic analysis of human blastocysts with the use of FISH, CGH and aCGH: scientific data and technical evaluation. Hum Reprod. 2011;26(2):480-90.
2. Avery JK, Chiego DJ. Essentials of Oral Histology and Embryology—A Clinical Approach, 3rd edition. US: Mosby; 2006.
3. Barnea ER, Hustin J, Jauniaux E (Eds). The first twelve weeks of gestation. Germany: Springer-Verlag Berlin Heidelberg; 1998.
4. Berkovitz BKB, Holland G, Moxham BJ. Oral anatomy, Histology and Embryology, 4th edition. US: Elsevier; 2009.
5. Blechschmidt E, Gasser RF. Biokinetics and biodynamics of human differentiation: principles and applications, reprint edition, Berkeley, California: North Atlantic Books; 2012.
6. Chen KG, Mallon BS, Mckay RD, et al. Human pluripotent stem cell culture: considerations for maintenance, expansion, and therapeutics. Cell Stem Cell. 2014;14:13-26.
7. Chiu PC, Lam KK, Wong RC, et al. The identity of zona pellucida receptor on spermatozoa: an unresolved issue in developmental biology. Semin Cell Dev Biol. 2014;30:86.
8. Cohen B, Kramer IRH. Scientific Foundations of Dentistry, 1st edition. London: William Heinmann Medical Books Ltd; 1976.
9. Cordero DR, Brugmann S, Chu Y, et al. Cranial neural crest cells on the move: their roles in craniofacial development. Am J Med Genet Part A. 2011;155:270.
10. Devi S. Inderbir Singh's Human Embryology, 11th edition. New Delhi: Jaypee Brothers Medical Publishers; 2017.
11. Dias AS, de Almeida I, Belmonte JM. Somites without a clock. Science. 2014;343:791-5.
12. Downs KM. The enigmatic primitive streak: prevailing notions and challenges concerning the body axis of mammals. Bioessays. 2009;31:892.
13. Fitz Patrick DR. Human embryogenesis. In: Magowan BA, Owen P, Thomson A (Eds). Clinical Obstetrics and Gynaecology, 3rd edition. Philadelphia: Saunders; 2014.
14. Gadella BM. Dynamic regulation of sperm interactions with the zona pellucida prior to and after fertilization. Reprod Fertil Dev. 2012;25:26.
15. Garg K. Chaurasia's Human Embryology, 2nd edition. India: CBS Publishers and Distributor Pvt Ltd; 2017.
16. Gasser RF, Cork RJ, Stillwell BJ, et al. Rebirth of human embryology. Dev Dyn. 2014;243:621.
17. Gibb S, Maroto M, Dale JK. The segmentation clock mechanism moves up a notch. Trends Cell Biol. 2010;20:593.
18. Gilbert SF. Developmental Biology. 6th edition. Sunderland (MA): Sinauer Associates; 2000. The Neural Crest. Available from: https://www.ncbi.nlm.nih.gov/books/NBK10065/
19. Khurana A, Khurana I. Human Embryology, 2nd edition. India: CBS Publishers and Distributor Pvt Ltd; 2012.
20. Kumar GS. Orban's Oral Histology and Embryology, 14th edition. India: Elsevier; 2015.
21. Lewis J, Hanisch A, Holder M. Notch signaling, the segmentation clock, and the patterning of vertebrate somites. J Biol. 2009;8:44.

22. Mayor R, Theveneau E. The neural crest. Development. 2013;140:2247-51.
23. Minoux M, Rijli FM. Molecular mechanism of cranial neural crest cell migration and patterning in craniofacial development. Development. 2010;137:2605.
24. Mio Y, Maeda K. Time-lapse cinematography of dynamic changes occurring during *in vitro* development of human embryos. Am J Obstet Gynecol. 2008;5:4.
25. Moore KL, Persaud TVN, Shiota K. Color Atlas of Clinical Embryology, 2nd edition. Philadelphia: Saunders; 2000.
26. Murillo-Gonzalés J. Evolution of embryology: a synthesis of classical, experimental, and molecular perspectives. Clin Anat. 2001;14:158.
27. Myers M, Pangas SA. Regulatory roles of transforming growth factor beta family members in folliculogenesis. WIREs Syst Biol Med. 2010;2:117.
28. Nanci A. Ten Cate's Oral Histology: Development, Structure, and Function. 8th edition. US: Elsevier; 2012.
29. Nusbaum RL, McInnes RR, Willard HF. Thompson and Thompson Genetics in Medicine, 7th edition. Philadelphia: Saunders; 2007.
30. Perris R, Perissinotto D. Role of the extracellular matrix during neural crest cell migration. Mech Dev. 2000;95:3-21.
31. Persaud TVN, Tubbs RS, Loukas M. A History of Human Anatomy, 2nd edition. Springfield, IL: Charles C. Thomas; 2014.
32. Piccolo S. Developmental biology: mechanics in the embryo. Nature. 2013;504:223.
33. Quenby S, Brosens JJ. Human implantation: a tale of mutual maternal and fetal attraction. Biol Reprod. 2013;88:81.
34. Rossant J, Tam PP. Blastocyst lineage formation, early embryonic asymmetries and axis patterning in the mouse. Development. 2009;136(5):701-13.
35. Simpson JL. Birth defects and assisted reproductive technology. Semin Fetal Neonatal Med. 2014;19:177.
36. Slack JMW. Essential Developmental Biology, 3rd edition. Hoboken, NJ: Wiley; 2012.
37. Steding G. The anatomy of the human embryo: a scanning electron microscopic atlas. Basel: Karger Publications; 2009.
38. Streit A, Berliner AJ, Papanayotou C, et al. Initiation of neural induction by FGF signalling before gastrulation. Nature. 2000;406:74-8.
39. Vasudeva N, Mishra S. Inderbir Singh's Textbook of Human Histology, 8th edition. New Delhi: Jaypee Brothers Medical Publishers; 2016.
40. Zorn AM, Wells JM. Vertebrate endoderm development and organ formation. Annu Rev Cell Dev Bio. 2009;25:221.

CHAPTER 3

Development of Face, Palate and Tongue

B Sivapathasundharam, Manoj Prabhakar

CHAPTER OUTLINE

- Development of Face 17
  » Development of Pharyngeal Arches 18
- Development of Palate 18
- Development of Tongue 21
- Clinical Considerations 21

DEVELOPMENT OF FACE

Development of face begins with the development of forebrain and prochordal plate mesoderm. The prochordal plate acts as an organizer for the development of face. The neural crest cell migration and its inductive influence in the mesenchyme plays a major role.

Development of face begins soon after the folding of the embryo during the 4th week of intrauterine life with the development of forebrain and prochordal plate mesoderm. After the formation of the head fold, the primitive oral cavity, also called stomodeum or stomatodeum is bounded above by the head bulge and below by the cardiac bulge. These two bulgings represent the developing brain cranially and pericardium caudally. The primitive oral cavity is separated from the foregut by buccopharyngeal membrane posteriorly **(Figure 3-1)**.

The cranial mesoderm proliferates in the midline to form a downward projection, superior to the stomodeum known as frontonasal process, which gives rise to forehead and later contributes to the formation of bridge of nose and part of palate known as premaxilla. Pharyngeal arches that are formed on the lateral and ventral surfaces of foregut, also lie in close vicinity to the stomatodeum, with the first arch lying on either side. The prochordal plate acts as an organizer for the development of face. The neural crest cell migration and its inductive influence in the mesenchyme plays a major role.

Between 4 and 10 weeks of intrauterine life, five facial prominences namely—one frontonasal, two maxillary, and two mandibular prominences appear to form the face **(Figure 3-2)**. These prominences or processes grow further and fuse to form the facial structures. These facial processes are actually swellings of mesenchyme with furrows in between; hence, the union involves elimination of furrow rather than fusion. Actual fusion occurs in certain instances, as in development of palate. These structures surrounding the stomatodeum namely, the unpaired frontonasal process from above, and paired first pharyngeal arch giving rise to two maxillary and

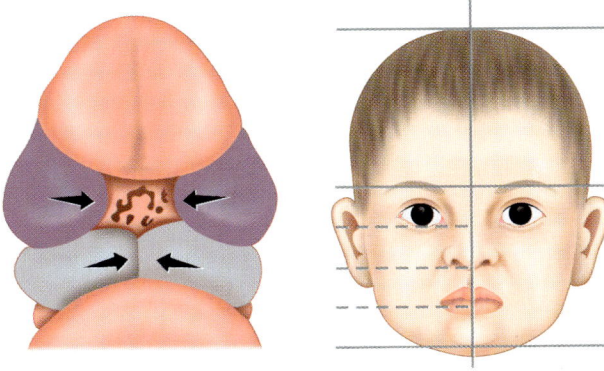

Figure 3-1: Development of face from the facial prominences.

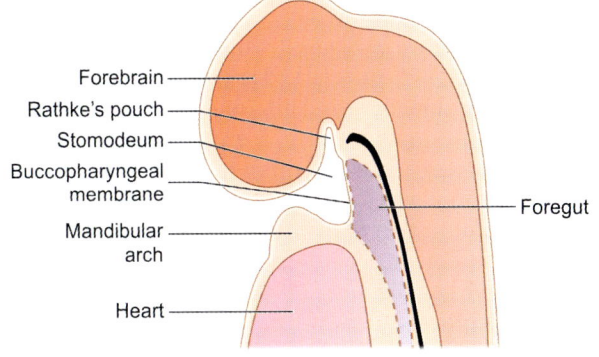

Figure 3-2: Folded embryo with primitive oral cavity bounded above by the head bulge and below by the cardiac bulge.

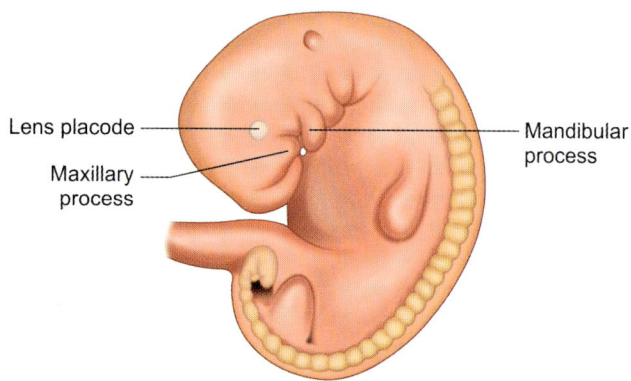

Figure 3-3: Lens placode in the lateral aspect of the developing head.

mandibular processes on each side, contributes majorly to the development of face.

> Growth factors including Shh (Sonic hedgehog) secreted by the prochordal plate, induce the development of forebrain which in turn signals the cranial mesoderm to induce the growth of the frontonasal prominence. The homeobox containing transcription factor Msx-1 is also important for the face development.

Bilateral localized horseshoe-shaped ectodermal thickenings of the frontonasal process induced by the forebrain appear just above the stomatodeum on either side of the midline. These thickenings are called as nasal placodes. These placodes sink at the center to form nasal pits, which are continuous with the stomodeum. The edges of the pits are raised, with the medial side called as medial nasal process and the lateral side as lateral nasal process. Similar thickening of the ectoderm appears lateral and cranial to nasal placodes. These are called as lens placodes, which lead to the formation of eye **(Figure 3-3)**.

Development of Pharyngeal Arches (Figures 3-4A to C)

Pharyngeal arches are the mesodermal thickenings that are present at the cranial most part of the foregut. The first pharyngeal arch, the mandibular arch, gives rise to two processes namely—maxillary process and mandibular process. The maxillary process grows medially and fuses with lateral nasal process first and medial nasal process next, to form the upper lip. This fusion is not restricted to the lip alone and includes the fusion of medial angle of the developing eye. This is initially marked by a linear depression called nasolacrimal furrow, and later, it is buried deeper to form the nasolacrimal duct. The medial and lateral nasal processes fuse together to separate the nasal pit from the stomodeum. The nasal pits at this stage are called as external nares.

The mesoderm and ectoderm of the lateral part of upper lip is derived from maxillary process; whereas, the mesoderm of the median portion of the upper lip, called philtrum, is derived from lower most portion of the enlarged medial nasal process, known as globular process of His. The ectoderm of the maxillary process grows over the mesoderm and meets the ectoderm of opposite maxillary process in the midline, which is the reason for the entire upper lip to get innervated by the maxillary nerves. The mandibular process on either side grows toward each other and fuses at the center to form the lower jaw and lower lip. The maxillary and mandibular processes later fuse with each other to form the cheek that makes the broad mouth opening into a narrow one **(Figure 3-5)**.

DEVELOPMENT OF PALATE

Development of palate starts at about 5th week of gestation. Initially there is a common oronasal cavity, which is occupied entirely by the developing tongue. The nasal cavity is separated from the oral cavity, after the formation of palate. Palate develops from two components, namely—primary palate (also known as primitive palate) and secondary palate **(Figures 3-6A and B)**. The primitive palate is formed from the frontonasal process and secondary palate from the palatine shelves of the maxillary process on either side. The maxillary process of the mandibular arch, apart from forming the upper lip, extends posteriorly and medially on either side of the stomodeum to form the palatal process or the palatine shelves. These palatine shelves of the maxillary process are positioned vertically on either side of the developing tongue **(Figures 3-7A to D)**. As the mandible grows, the developing tongue is moved forward and downward and allows the palatine shelves to snap up horizontally to form the secondary palate. The fusion occurs at the midline by merging of the ectomesenchyme. This actual fusion includes series of molecular, mechanical, and morphological events. Formation of permanent palate occurs by the fusion of palatal components. The palatal processes on either side will fuse with the primitive palate in a Y-shaped manner, at its posterior end. The medial portion of two palatal processes in turn fuses with each other horizontally to form the secondary palate. Further, it also fuses with the free lower border of the nasal septum, separating the two nasal cavities in the midline and from the oral cavity inferiorly.

> The contacting epithelium initially thins down due to cessation of cell division and apoptosis (programmed cell death). Thinned epithelium later breaks into islands. Soon these epithelial islands interact with ectomesenchyme and transform into cells resembling fibroblasts.
> This interaction and transition of the epithelial cells into mesenchymal cells is known as epithelial–mesenchymal transition. This is mediated by the production of extracellular surface substances like transforming growth factor-beta 3 (TGF-β3), fibroblast growth factor (FGF) signaling, and increase in cyclic adenosine monophosphate (cAMP) for the cessation of cell division.

Factors which facilitate the elevation of palatine shelves include differential growth of the palatine shelves, hydrostatic forces exerted by hyaluronic acid and other glycosaminoglycans (GAG), compressive forces from maxillary processes, descendance, and movement of tongue, and urge in mouth opening.

The anterior and mid part of the palate undergoes intramembranous ossification and forms the hard palate,

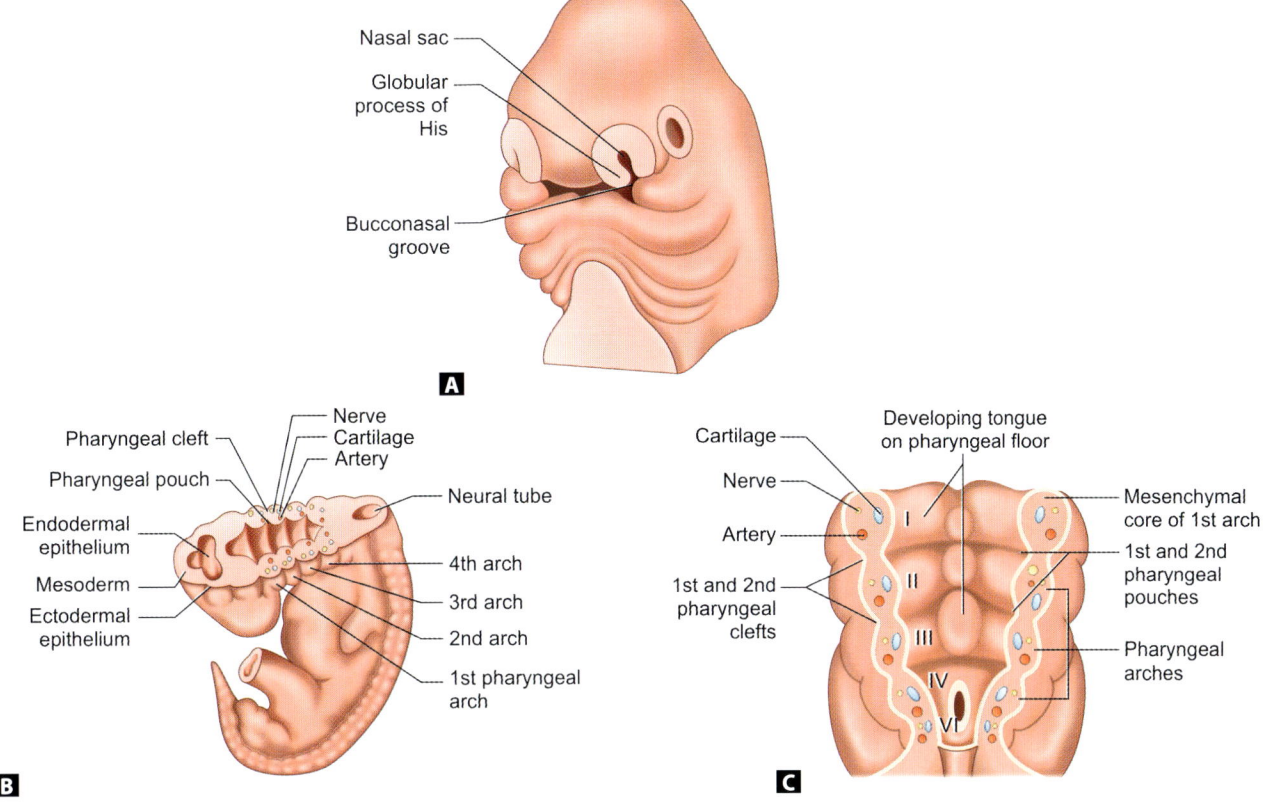

Figures 3-4A to C: Pharyngeal arches.

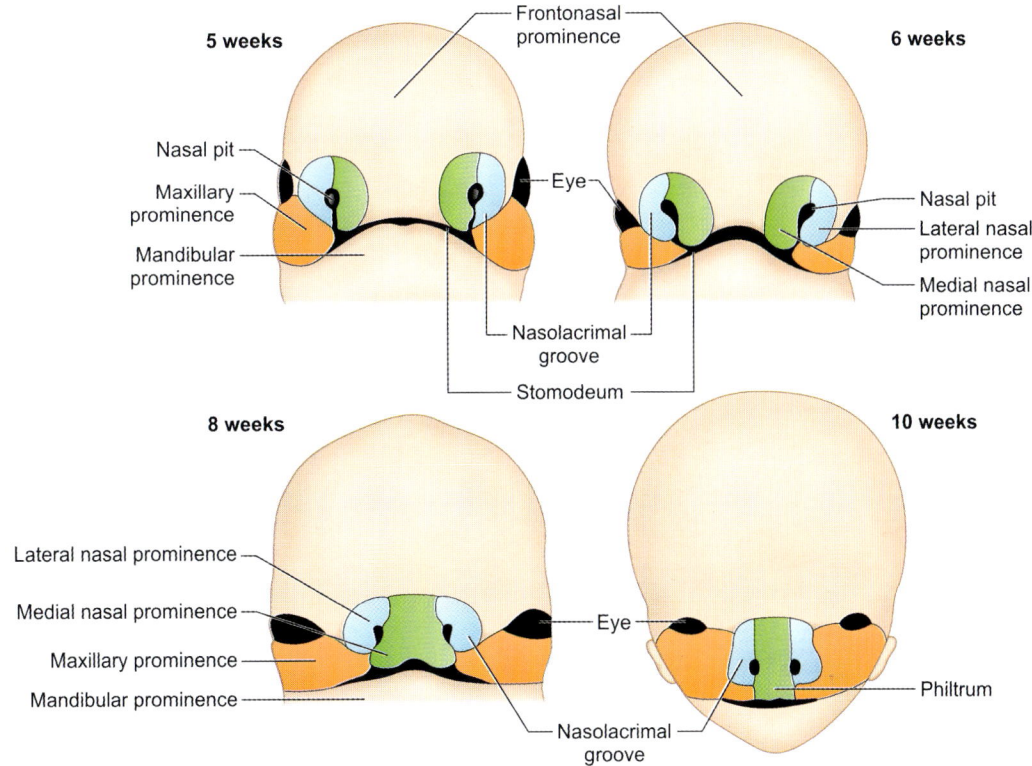

Figure 3-5: Development of face.

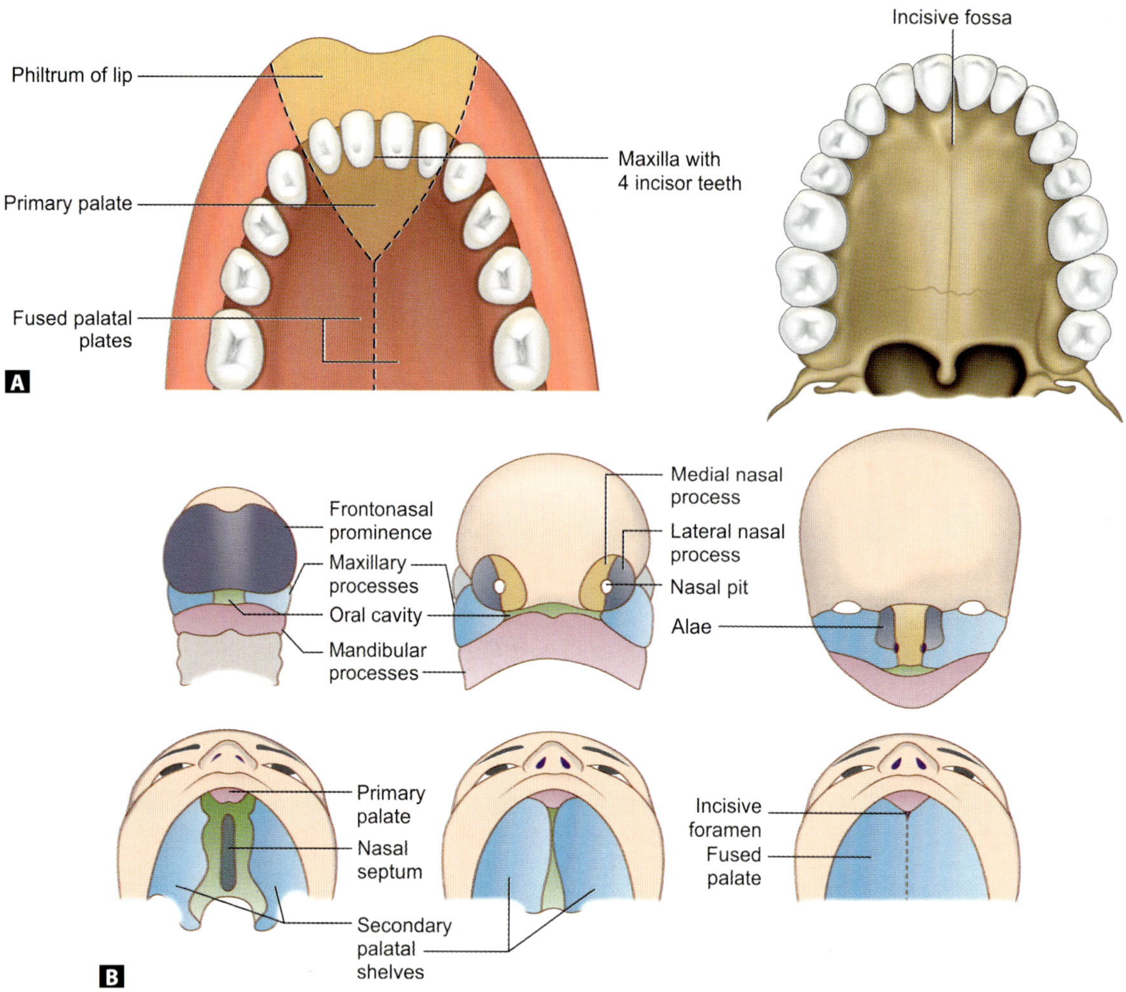

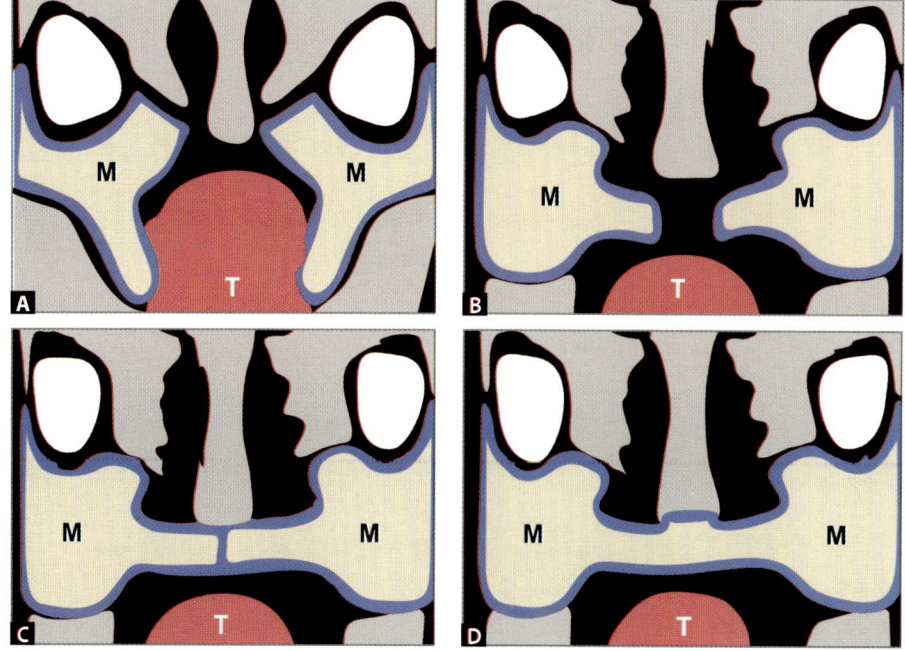

Figures 3-6A and B: (A) Primary and secondary palate; (B) Fusion of two palatine shelves to the primary palate.

Figures 3-7A to D: (A) Common oronasal cavity occupied by the developing tongue (T); (B) Horizontal snap-up of the palatine shelves from the vertical position due to the mandibular growth and descendance of the tongue; (C) Palatine shelves and nasal septum growing toward each other and fusing; (D) Oral cavity is separated from the nasal cavity by the palate (M—maxillary process).

while the posterior part does not ossify and is made up of muscles which forms the soft palate.

DEVELOPMENT OF TONGUE

The tongue is a muscular organ, which helps in mastication, deglutition, and speech. It is divided into two parts, namely anterior two-thirds (oral part) and posterior one-third (pharyngeal part), which is marked by a "V"-shaped faint groove called sulcus terminalis **(Figure 3-8)**.

Tongue develops at the same time as the palate develops at around 4th week of intrauterine life from the floor of the oral cavity. The pharyngeal arches contribute to the formation of anterior and posterior part of the tongue. Anterior part develops from three swellings namely—two lateral lingual swellings from the medial most part of the first pharyngeal arch and a midline swelling called tuberculum impar, from the same arch. The major portion of the anterior part of the tongue is thus formed by the fusion of two lateral lingual swellings and the rest is from tuberculum impar **(Figure 3-9A)**. Downward proliferation of the epithelium is noticed immediately behind the tuberculum impar, which contributes to the development of thyroid gland and is called as thyroglossal duct. This region is marked by a depression called foramen cecum. At about 5th to 6th week, another midline swelling called hypobranchial eminence (Copula of His) develops in relation to second, third and fourth arches, which has a cranial part and a caudal part. The cranial part, which is related to second and third arches is called copula, while the caudal part is related to the fourth arch. Copula forms the posterior part of the tongue and at this instance the mesoderm of the third arch overgrows the second arch to fuse with the first arch. The third arch endoderm thus forms the posterior part of the tongue, while the posterior most part is developed from the fourth arch. The mesenchymal contribution of the second arch in the development of the tongue is almost nil **(Figures 3-9B and C)**.

Innervation of tongue differs for anterior and posterior part as it involves multiple pharyngeal arches during development. The anterior part of the tongue is supplied by the lingual nerve and chorda tympani nerve. Lingual nerve is the branch of trigeminal nerve, which in turn is a nerve of first arch, while chorda tympani is the branch of facial nerve, which in turn is a pretrematic nerve of the first arch. The posterior one-third of the tongue is supplied by the nerve of third arch, the glossopharyngeal nerve and the posterior most part of the tongue is supplied by the superior laryngeal nerve, the nerve of the fourth arch. Taste buds, which are the specialized structures, are seen in relation to the terminal branches of the nerve fibers. The muscles of the tongue are developed from occipital myotomes and are supplied by the hypoglossal nerve.

CLINICAL CONSIDERATIONS

Development of face is a complex process, involving cellular proliferation, migration, interaction, differentiation, and organization. Disturbances in any of these events may result in developmental anomalies. These disturbances may be caused by environmental or genetic factors and may range from absence to deficiency and rarely an increase in size of the specific tissue or organ.

As formation of the face involves fusion of various components, any defect in failure or incomplete fusion may result in developmental anomalies particularly clefts. Several deformities associated with defective fusion have been reported, however, the frequent ones are given here.

Failure of fusion of facial prominences, results in various cleft anomalies in the face. Common cleft anomalies include cleft lip and cleft palate **(Figures 3-10 A to D)**.

Cleft lip is common in the upper lip, which results from the failure in fusion of maxillary process with the medial nasal process and can be unilateral or bilateral (hare lip). Cleft of the lower lip occurs due to the failure in fusion of mandibular process at the midline and is very rare.

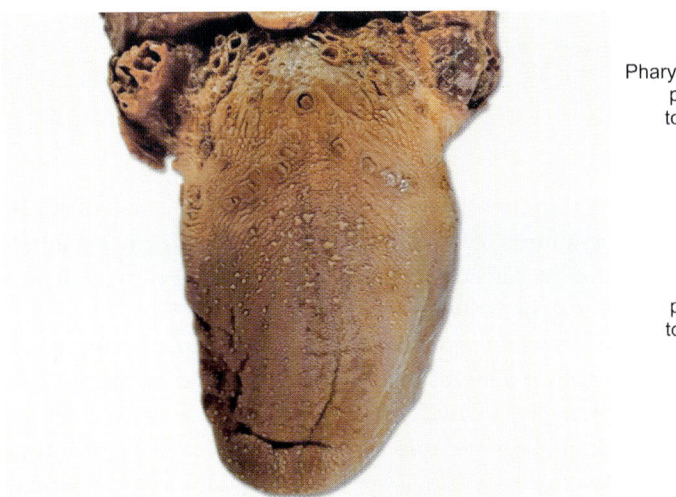
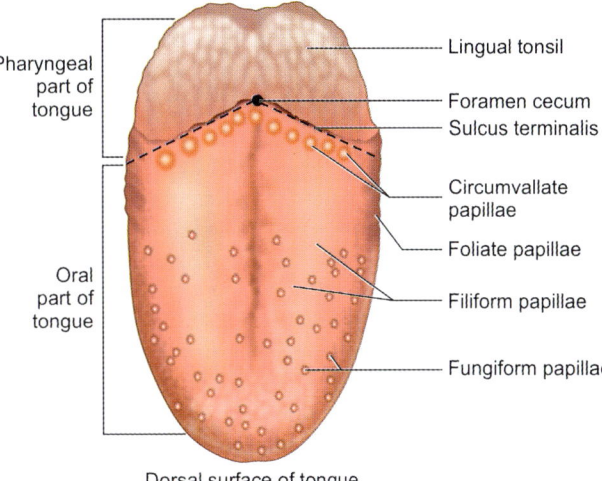

Figures 3-8: Anatomy of the dorsal portion of the tongue.

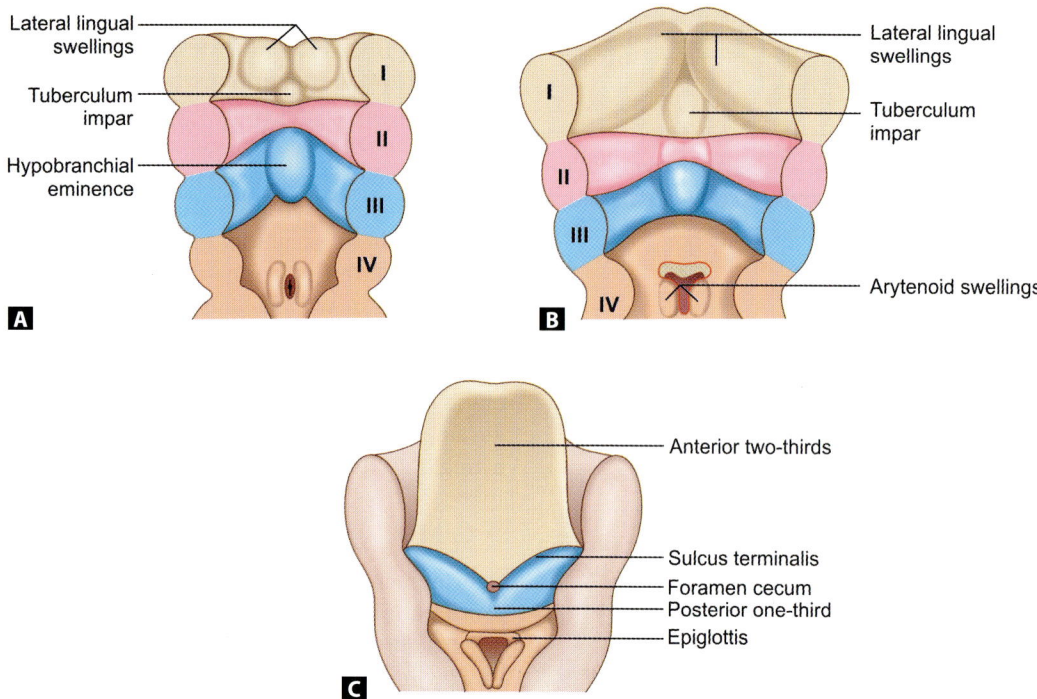

Figures 3-9A to C: (A) Three swellings from first arch giving rise to anterior tongue; (B) Fusion of two lateral lingual swellings and tuberculum impar to form the anterior portion of the tongue; (C) Overgrowth of hypobranchial eminence from the third arch to form the posterior portion of the tongue.

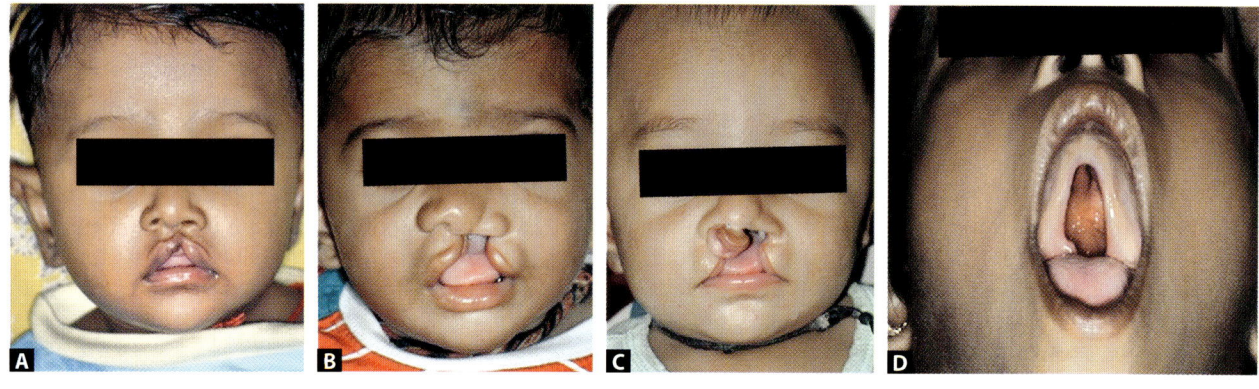

Figures 3-10A to D: (A) Incomplete or cleft lip; (B) Unilateral cleft lip and palate; (C) Bilateral cleft lip and palate; (D) Cleft palate.
Source: Dr Manikandhan R, Meenakshi Ammal Dental College, Chennai, India

Similar to cleft lip, cleft palate may form due to defective fusion of palatal components. It can be unilateral or bilateral, complete or incomplete, restricted to hard palate or extend to involve the soft palate.

Oblique facial cleft results from the non-fusion of maxillary and lateral nasal process. This cleft runs from medial canthus of the eye to the angle of the mouth, with the absence of nasolacrimal duct. Horizontal facial cleft results from incomplete fusion of maxillary and mandibular processes of the first arch. The milder form results in macrostomia (large mouth opening).

Genetically related anomalies like TreacherCollins syndrome or mandibulofacial dysostosis can occur when there is defect in the development of entire first arch on any one or both the sides.

Developmental deformity of tongue may be due to failure or incomplete fusion of two lateral lingual swellings resulting in median lingual cleft or cleft tongue. Other developmental anomalies include macroglossia (large-sized tongue), microglossia (small-sized tongue), and ankyloglossia (the apical portion attached to the floor of the mouth).

Points to Remember

- Buccopharyngeal membrane separates the primitive oral cavity from foregut.
- Face is formed majorly by frontonasal process, two maxillary and two mandibular processes.
- First pharyngeal arch gives rise to maxillary and mandibular process on each side.
- Maxillary process fuses with the lateral and medial nasal process to form the upper lip.
- Nasal placode and lens placode are ectodermal thickenings seen on the frontonasal process.
- Initially there is a common oronasal cavity that is occupied entirely by the developing tongue.
- Palate separates the nasal cavity from the oral cavity.
- Hard palate is formed by both primary and secondary palate.
- Secondary palate is formed by the fusion of two palatal processes of maxilla.
- Soft palate does not ossify and is formed by muscles.
- Tongue develops from the first, second, third and fourth pharyngeal arches, however, the mesenchymal contribution of the second arch in tongue development is almost nil.
- Anterior part of the tongue is formed by the fusion of two lateral swellings and tuberculum impar.
- The posterior part of the tongue is developed from hypobranchial eminence.
- Anterior two-thirds and posterior one third of the tongue is demarcated by 'V'-shaped faint groove called sulcus terminalis.
- Muscles of the tongue are developed from occipital myotomes.
- Failure in fusion of maxillary process with the medial nasal process results in the formation of cleft lip.

PRACTICE QUESTIONS

1. Explain the development of face.
2. Detail the events involved in the development of palate.
3. Briefly explain about the formation of tongue.
4. Write a short note on cleft lip and Cleft palate.
5. Describe the developmental anomalies of tongue.

MULTIPLE CHOICE QUESTIONS

1. **Stomatodeum is the other name for**
   a. Pharyngeal part of oral cavity.
   b. Primitive oral cavity.
   c. Anterior part of the oral cavity.
   d. Fully developed oral cavity.
2. **The primitive oral cavity is separated from the foregut by**
   a. Nasal placode.
   b. Palatal process of maxilla.
   c. Buccopharyngeal membrane.
   d. Soft palate.
3. **Maxillary and mandibular process is formed by**
   a. First arch.
   b. Second arch.
   c. Third arch.
   d. Fourth arch.
4. **Face develops from**
   a. Frontonasal process.
   b. Maxillary process.
   c. Mandibular process.
   d. All of the above.
5. **Maxillary process fuses with the lateral nasal process and then with the medial nasal process to form**
   a. Philtrum.
   b. Upper lip.
   c. Base of the nose.
   d. None of the above.
6. **The primitive palate is formed from**
   a. Lateral nasal process.
   b. Medial nasal process.
   c. Maxillary process.
   d. Frontonasal process.
7. **Secondary palate is formed by the**
   a. Fusion of primitive palate to nasal septum.
   b. Fusion of palatine shelves of maxillary process.
   c. Downward growth of tongue.
   d. Fusion of mandibular processes.
8. **Primary palate and secondary palate fuse to form**
   a. Anterior part of the hard palate.
   b. Posterior part of the hard palate.
   c. Soft palate.
   d. Both a and b.
9. **Which part of the palate does not ossify?**
   a. Primary palate.
   b. Secondary palate.
   c. Midline of palatine shelves.
   d. Soft palate.
10. **The anterior and posterior part of the tongue is demarcated by**
    a. Sulcus terminalis.
    b. Tuberculum impar.
    c. Epiglottis.
    d. Thyroglossal duct.
11. **Fusion of two lateral swellings and tuberculum impar forms**
    a. Posterior most part of the tongue.
    b. Anterior part of the tongue.
    c. Epiglottis.
    d. None of the above.
12. **The posterior part of tongue is formed from**
    a. First arch.
    b. Fifth arch.
    c. Hypobranchial eminence.
    d. Tuberculum impar.

13. **Which of the following arches contributes very minimally for the tongue development?**
    a. First arch.
    b. Second arch.
    c. Third arch.
    d. Fourth arch.
14. **Nerve of the first arch is**
    a. Facial nerve
    b. Trigeminal nerve
    c. Glossopharyngeal nerve
    d. Hypoglossal nerve
15. **Anterior part of the tongue is innervated by**
    a. Lingual nerve.
    b. Glossopharyngeal nerve.
    c. Vagus.
    d. Mental nerve.
16. **Hypobranchial eminence is otherwise called as**
    a. Tuberculum impar.
    b. Copula of His.
    c. Lateral swelling.
    d. Median swelling.
17. **Defective fusion of two palatal shelves result in**
    a. Unilateral cleft palate.
    b. Bilateral cleft palate.
    c. Midline cleft.
    d. Clefts of the soft palate.
18. **The condition where the apical portion the tongue is attached to the floor of mouth is called**
    a. Microglossia
    b. Macroglossia
    c. Aglossia
    d. Ankyloglossia
19. **Failure of fusion of maxillary process and lateral nasal process leads to the formation of**
    a. Cleft lip
    b. Oblique facial cleft
    c. Cleft of the lower lip
    d. Cleft palate
20. **Failure or incomplete fusion of two lateral lingual swellings result in**
    a. Cleft tongue.
    b. Bifid uvula.
    c. Ankyloglossia.
    d. Microglossia.

ANSWERS

1. b	2. c	3. a	4. d	5. b	6. d	7. b	8. d	9. d	10. a	11. b	12. c	13. b	14. b	15. a
16. b	17. c	18. d	19. a	20. a										

BIBLIOGRAPHY

1. Amano O, Doi T, Yamada T, et al. Meckel's cartilage: discovery, embryology and evolution—Overview of the specificity of Meckel's cartilage. J Oral Biosc. 2010;52:125-35.
2. Avery JK. Oral Development and Histology, 3rd edition. New York: Thieme; 2002.
3. Avery JK. Oral mucosa. In: Chiego DJ (Ed). Essentials of Oral Histology and Embryology, A Clinical Approach, 2nd edition. St. Louis: Mosby; 2000. pp. 165-82.
4. Berkovitz BK, Holland GH, Moxham BJ. Oral Anatomy, Histology and Embryology, 3rd edition. St Louis: Mosby; 2002.
5. Brinkley LL, Bookstein FL. Cell distribution during mouse secondary palate closure. II, Mesenchymal cells. J Embryol Exp Morpho. 1986;96:111-3.
6. Chai Y, Maxson RE. Recent advances in craniofacial morphogenesis. Dev Dyn. 2006;235:2353-75.
7. Chandra S, Chandra S, Chandra M, et al. Textbook of Dental and Oral Histology with Embryology and MCQ's, 2nd edition. New Delhi: Jaypee Brothers Medical Publishers (P) Ltd;2010.
8. Chatterjee K. Essentials of Dental Anatomy and Oral Histology, 2nd edition. New Delhi: Jaypee Brothers Medical Publishers (P) Ltd; 2014.
9. Creuzet S, Couly G, Le Douarin NM. Patterning the neural crest derivatives during development of the vertebrate head: insights from avian studies. J Anat. 2005;207:447.
10. Cuervo R, Covarrubias L. Death is the major fate of medial edge epithelial cells and the cause of basal lamina degradation during palatogenesis. Development. 2004;131:15-24.
11. Eames BF, Richard AS. The genesis of cartilage size and shape during development and evolution. Development. 2008;135:3947-58.
12. Fitchett JE, Hay ED. Medial edge epithelium transforms to mesenchyme after embryonic palatal shelves fuse. Dev Biol. 1989;131:455-74.
13. Gitton Y, Heude E, Vieux RM, et al. Evolving maps in craniofacial development. Semin Cell Dev Biol. 2010;21:301-8.
14. Hu D, Marcucio RS, Helms JA. A zone of frontonasal ectoderm regulates patterning and growth in the face. Development. 2003;130:1749-58.
15. Kumar GS. Orban's Oral Histology and Embryology, 14th edition. India: Elsevier; 2015.
16. Le Douarin NM, Dupin E. Multipotentiality of the neural crest. Curr Op Gen Dev. 2003;13:529-36.
17. Liu B, Rooker SM, Helms JA. Molecular control of facial morphology. Semin Cell Dev Biol. 2010;21:309-13.
18. Lundstrom A. Dental genetics. In: Dahlberg AA, Graber TM (Eds). Orofacial Growth and Development. The Hague: Mouton Publishers; 1977.
19. Moore KL, Persaud TV. The Developing Human: Clinically Orientated Embryology, 8th edition. Philadelphia: Saunders; 2007.
20. Nanci A. Tencate's Oral Histology, Development, Structure, and Functions, 8th edition. India: Elsevier; 2012.
21. Sadler TW (Ed). Langman's Essential Medical Embryology, Volume 1. Baltimore, Lippincott: Williams & Wilkins; 2005.
22. Sperber GH. Craniofacial Development and Growth. Toronto: B Decker Inc; 2000.
23. Szabo-Rogers HL, Smithers LE, Yakob W, et al. New directions in craniofacial morphogenesis. Dev Biol. 2010;341:84-94.
24. Vasudeva N, Mishra S. Inderbir Singh's Textbook of Human Histology, 8th edition. New Delhi: Jaypee Brothers Medical Publishers; 2016.
25. Vinvent D, Seibel W. Oral Histology- Inheritance and Development, 2nd edition. USA: Lea & Febiger; 1986.

CHAPTER 4

Development of Tooth

B Sivapathasundharam, Logeswari Jayamani

Chapter Outline

- Dental Lamina   26
- Vestibular Lamina   27
- Tooth Development   28
    » Initiation Stage (Bud Stage)   29
    » Proliferation Stage (Cap Stage)   31
    » Bell Stage   33
- Apposition and Hard Tissue Formation   36
- Root Formation   36
- Clinical Considerations   37
    » Defects at Initiation or Bud Stage   37
    » Defects at Proliferation or Cap Stage   37
    » Defects at Morphodifferentiation Stage   37
    » Defects at Histodifferentiation Stage   37

Odontogenesis or tooth development is a complex process that includes epithelial-mesenchymal interactions, morphogenesis, matrix formation, and mineralization. Development of all biological processes including tooth development is controlled by genetic and epigenetic factors. All teeth do not develop at the same time. Development of primary teeth starts between 6th and 8th week of intrauterine life, when the crown-rump length is around 7–19 mm and permanent teeth in 12th week. Due to the event called "folding of the embryo" the ectoderm covers the body surface and lines the primitive oral cavity, and endoderm lines the foregut. The ectoderm of the primitive oral cavity meets the endoderm of the foregut to form the buccopharyngeal membrane. This two-layered membrane separates the primitive oral cavity from the foregut and ruptures at around 26–27th day of intrauterine life. Thus the communication between the primitive oral cavity or the stomodeum and the foregut is established.

The connective tissue adjacent to the oral ectoderm is influenced by the migrated neural crest cells and is known as ectomesenchyme. This ectomesenchyme interacts with the overlying ectoderm to initiate tooth development **(Figure 4-1)**.

Tooth development begins at around 6th week of intrauterine life, with the appearance of primary epithelial band. This is nothing but a horse-shoe-shaped epithelial thickening in the location of the future dental arches. This thickening is formed by change in orientation of the mitotic spindles and cleavage planes of certain basal cells rather than the increase in proliferation of cells.

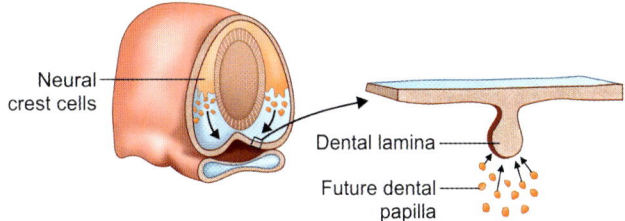

Figure 4-1: Schematic diagram showing influence of neural crest cells on the mesenchyme to form ectomesenchyme.

Molecular Insight
Like any other organ development, odontogenesis is a series of well-organized events, which include both morphological and genetic factors. The genetic events comprise sequential and reciprocal series of signals transmitted between the epithelium and neural crest influenced mesenchyme **(Table 4-1)**.

Morphological events are staged as—(A) bud stage; (B) cap stage; (C) early bell stage, and (D) advanced bell stage. Knowledge of cellular differentiation and molecular changes (*i.e.* interplay of inductive signals between epithelium and mesenchyme to form each component of tooth and its supporting structures) is essential for the better understanding of tooth development.

Organization of tissues and organs involve morphogenesis and differentiation, controlled by the gene expression. *Homeobox (HOX)* is a critical and a master gene involved in organ morphogenesis. The unique body pattern in every organism is determined by the different mode of action of this gene. *Homeobox* gene encodes a protein called homeodomain, which was first identified in

TABLE 4-1: Genes and signaling molecules involved in odontogenesis.

Stages of odontogenesis	Genes and signaling molecules
Tooth initiation	BMP4, Msx-1, FGF4, FGF8, and FGF9
Oral-aboral axis formation	FGF8, Lhx-6, Lhx7, and Gsc
Tooth germ positioning	BMP4, Pitx-2, FGF-8, Pax-9, Activin βA, and BMP2
Patterning of dentition	Barx-1, Dlx-1/2, Msx-1, Msx-2, and Alx-3
Regulation of ectodermal boundaries	Shh and Wnt-7b
Dental lamina stage	BMP-4, Msx-1, and Dlx
Bud stage	Wnt, Lef-1, Shh
Bud–cap transition	BMP4, Msx-1, Pax-9, Activin βA, and Shh
Enamel knot	BMP2, BMP4, BMP7, Wnt-10b, FGF4, FGF9, Slit-1, and Shh

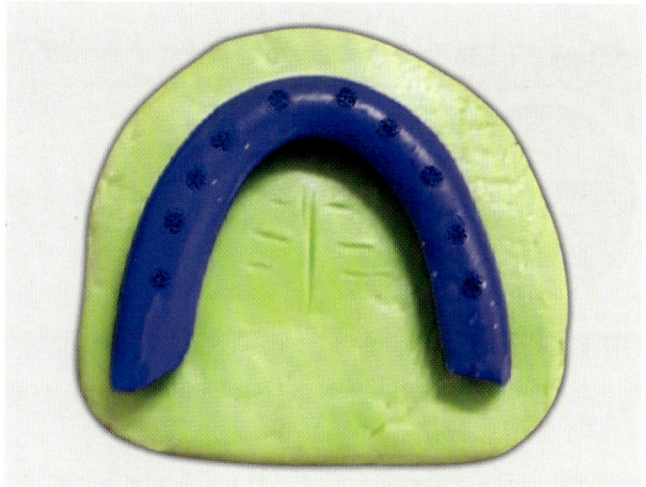

Figure 4-2: Horseshoe-shaped primary epithelial band on the oral ectoderm and localized thickenings denote the dental lamina

Drosophila (fruit fly). Around 300 genes and transcription factors that have homeodomain are found to play a vital role in different aspects of tooth development. This regulates other genes and growth factors, which determine the type, size, and position of each tooth organ. Further they also mediate the differentiation of enamel-secreting cells—the ameloblasts from the epithelium, and dentin-secreting cells—the odontoblasts from the ectomesenchyme by initiating the cascade of reciprocal signaling events between the epithelium and the connective tissue.

Signals are minute proteins secreted by one cell or tissue and transmitted to another. The cell interpretation of a received signal determines its growth, differentiation, gene expression, or cell death.

Among many other genes and pathways involved in regulation of tooth development, a fine balance between the four major signaling pathways, the *bone morphogenetic protein (BMP), fibroblast growth factor (FGF), sonic hedgehog (SHH),* and *WNT* ligands are crucial, which are frequently involved during the tooth development and regulate the epithelial–mesenchymal interactions. Any alteration in these genes can result in developmental disturbances in tooth formation, which may range from defective structure, altered density of the body part of the tooth, or phenotypic changes in patterning. Epithelial Wnt signaling is carefully regulated to control the number of teeth formed, while hyperactivating FGF and Wnt signaling leads to an increased number of tooth buds, leading to development of supernumerary tooth (Additional tooth), while mutations in *WNT10A* cause missing teeth in humans.

■ DENTAL LAMINA

The first evidence of tooth development is the occurrence of round to oval, localized epithelial thickenings in the primary epithelial band of both the arches, corresponding to the 10 deciduous teeth in each arch **(Figure 4-2)**. This is called the dental lamina and is the primordium for the developing teeth.

Molecular Insight
Tooth development is a complex process, which includes epithelial–mesenchymal interactions implicated by sophisticated molecular steps. To understand this exhaustive molecular genetics, various animal and human studies were employed as a tool in studying the role of genes at specific stages of tooth development, its regulations, patterning, and differentiation process. Most of the experimental studies on mammals were adopted in the mouse. In this chapter, the numbers following "E" indicate the embryonic day of the mouse.

The exceptional advances in genetics permit the isolation of epithelium from ectomesenchyme or recombine the epithelium or mesenchyme of one source with another in the tissue, organ, or cell culture to study the relationship or response of one to another. Various studies were carried out to establish the exact role played by transcription and growth factors in these tissues.

Establishment of Oral-Aboral Axis
The establishment of oral-aboral axis is an incipient event, where marked thickening of oral epithelium is secured on the surface of the first branchial arch, which later opens up the cascade of events to form the tooth. The expression of LIM *homeobox (Lhx)* domain genes, *Lhx-6* and *Lhx-7* genes in the first arch mesenchyme at E9 is an early sign to localize the oral epithelium on the first branchial arch. The expression of genes is evidenced adjacent to the epithelial thickening, which interacts with the ectomesenchyme to form the dental primordium. The restricted expression of fibroblast growth factor 8 *(FGF8)* in the confined site (anteroposterior expression) at a particular time in the first branchial arch, confirms the inductive role of *FGF8* in the epithelium and regulation of *Lhx* genes in the mesenchyme. Experiments from literatures are added below, to demonstrate that the signals originating from epithelium are responsible for induction of events in establishing oral and aboral axis.

Combining the second arch mesenchyme with first arch epithelium, evidenced the expression of *Lhx* genes, however, combining the second arch epithelium with first arch mesenchyme, failed to express the Lhx gene confirming the eminent role of signaling factors (FGF8) from first arch epithelium **(Figure 4-3)**.

Regionalization of Oral and Dental Ectoderm
The establishment of dental ectoderm from the oral ectoderm is determined by the expression of *Wnt-7b* and *Shh*. The expression of *Wnt-7b* is evidenced throughout the oral ectoderm except the presumptive dental arch. The expressions of *Wnt-7b* and *Shh* are

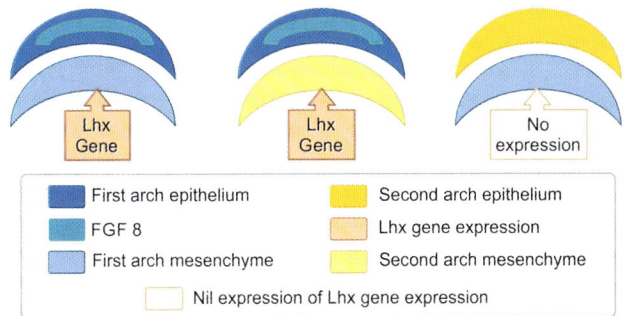

Figure 4-3: Schematic representation of the role of *FGF8* and *Lhx* in establishment of oral-aboral axis.

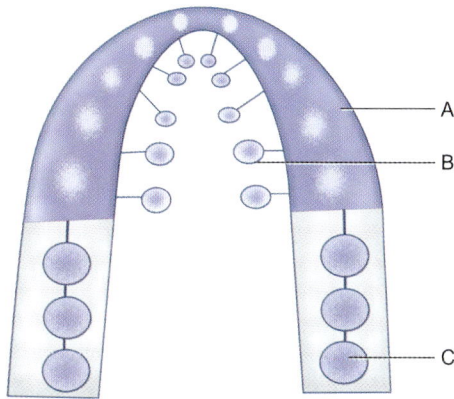

Figure 4-5: Diagram representing oral ectoderm with dental lamina A, successional lamina B, and accessional lamina C.

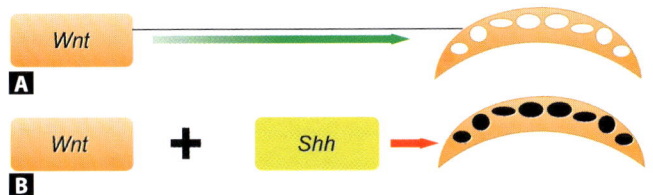

Figures 4-4A and B: (A) The expression of *Wnt* and suppression of the *Shh* expression proceeds to establishment of the dental arch; (B) The expression of *Wnt* and *Shh* results in failure of the dental arch establishment.

reciprocal; indented expression of *Wnt-7b* in presumptive dental ectoderm represses the expression of *Shh*, and leads to the failure of tooth development **(Figures 4-4A and B)**. The *Wnt* signals are mediated by Lef-1, and are found to be expressed in epithelium during bud formation and eventually shift to the condensing mesenchyme.

Dental lamina forms perpendicular to the oral ectoderm. It interacts with the underlying ectomesenchyme, which surrounds this epithelial ingrowth and forms the tooth bud (also called odontogenic apparatus or tooth germ) **(Figure 4-1)**. Each permanent tooth develops from the lingual extension of the dental lamina and is known as successional lamina. Since there are no predecessors for permanent molars, they develop directly from the distal extension of the dental lamina, called accessional lamina **(Figure 4-5)**.

As tooth development continues, the dental lamina loses its connection with the oral ectoderm and disintegrates with the invasion of surrounding mesenchyme. Thus dental lamina remains active only for 5 years. It begins to function from 6th prenatal week for primary teeth and continues to 15th year of birth for permanent third molar **(Table 4-2)**. In few areas, the remnants of dental lamina persist as cell rests or epithelial islands in the jaw bone or in the connective tissue of the gingiva. These remnants are known as epithelial pearls or cell rests of Serres.

VESTIBULAR LAMINA

Vestibular cavity is that part of the mouth which is situated between the lips and cheeks, and the teeth and alveolar bone when occluded. Initially there is no vestibular cavity or vestibular sulcus present. The oral vestibule is formed by labial or buccal extension of the primary epithelial band, called as vestibular lamina. The cells of the vestibular lamina enlarge and soon degenerate leaving a furrow between the lips and the buccal mucosa and alveolar portion of the jaw to form the labial and buccal vestibule **(Figures 4-6A to D)**.

TABLE 4-2: Timeline of tooth development.

Age	Stages in tooth development
6–7 weeks	Dental lamina formation
8th week	Bud stage for deciduous incisors, canines, and molars
14th week	Bell stage for deciduous teeth; bud stage for permanent teeth
18th week	Dentin formation and ameloblast differentiation for deciduous teeth
32nd week	Dentin formation and ameloblast differentiation for permanent first molars

Tooth Germ Positioning

The next important event in development of tooth is the appearance of epithelial thickening (tooth bud formation) at specific site in primary epithelial band. These sites are determined by stimulatory signals such as FGF and *Pax9* and inhibitory signals such as *BMP*. There is always an equilibrium that exists between these two and it is very important for the determination of the site.

The expression of *FGF* in the epithelium and paired box homeotic gene-9 (*Pax9*) in the mesenchyme defines the exact site for the tooth bud location. The *Pax9*, a member of *Pax* family, stimulated by *FGF8* proceeds toward tooth development. The expression of *FGF* and *Pax9* gene is known to be antagonized by the expression of *BMP2* in the mesenchyme and *BMP4* in the epithelium. Thus the field overlapping the expression of *FGF8* with *Pax9*, in the absence of *BMP* eventually proceeds toward tooth bud development, whereas the *FGF8*, *BMP2*, and *BMP4* extended area with lacking *Pax9* fail to form a tooth bud. In addition, *Pitx2*, potential regulator of the epithelium presses the *FGF8* and suppresses the expression of *BMP4*. The expression of other genes and regulatory factors like *Prx1* and *Prx2* are evidenced in the progression of tooth germ positioning **(Figures 4.7A and B)**.

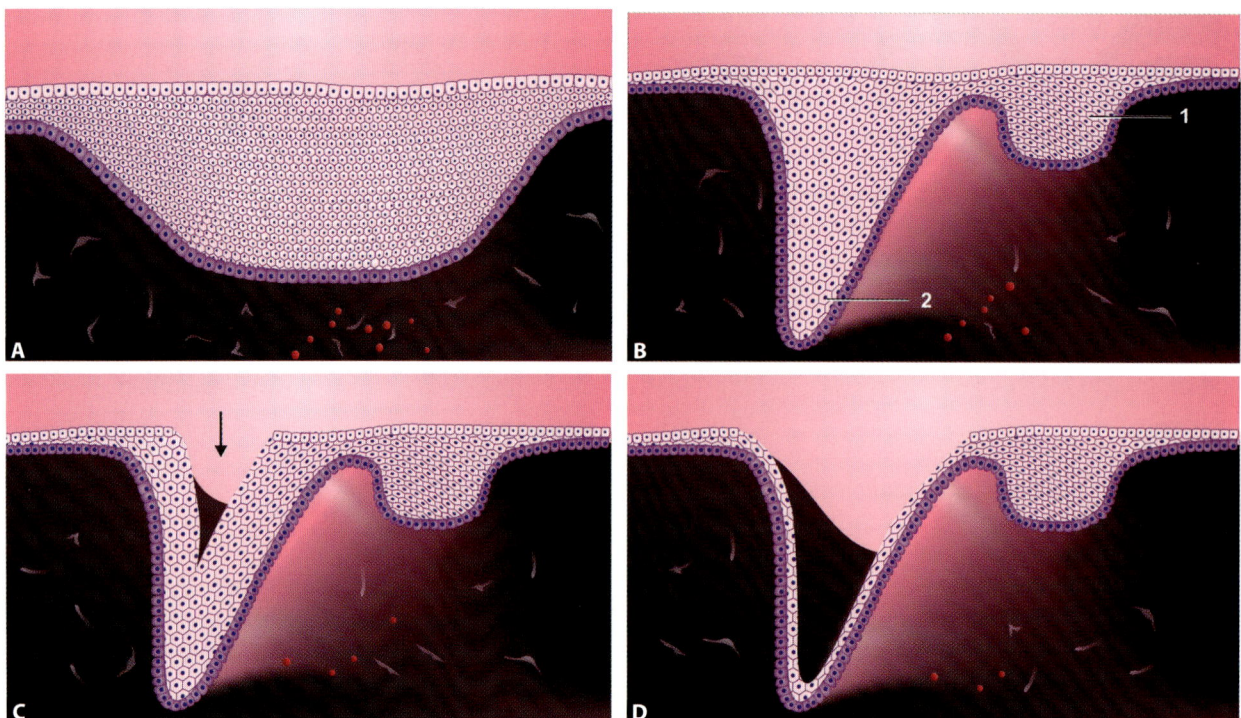

Figures 4-6A to D: Stages in development of dental lamina and vestibular lamina and vestibule: (A) Primary epithelial band; (B) 1: Lingually placed dental lamina, 2: Development of buccal extension called vestibular lamina; (C) Furrowing of vestibular lamina to form a vestibule (arrow); (D) Formation of buccal or labial vestibule.

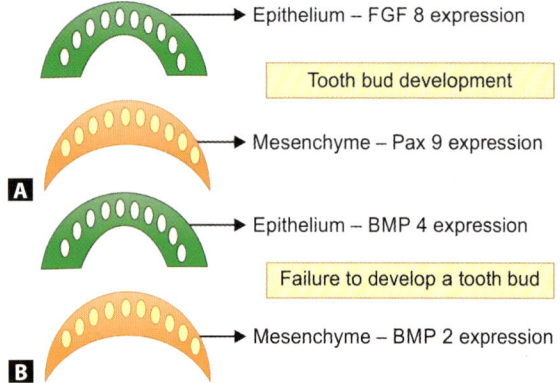

Figures 4-7A and B: Schematic representation representing together expression of *FGF8* in epithelium and *Pax9* in the mesenchyme with the absence of *BMP4* in the epithelium and *BMP2* in the mesenchyme along with regulatory factors like *Prx1*, *Prx2* and other genes promote tooth germ positioning and tooth bud development.

Various experimental animal studies have proved that disruption of genes, which are part of any of the signaling pathways, have resulted in aberrations of tooth development that may range from complete absence of tooth formation to malformed teeth depending on the severity of the aberration. For example conditional inactivation of *FGF8* in dental epithelium may result in arrest of tooth development at the dental lamina stage; similarly over-expression of *BMPR1A* may lead to arrest of tooth development.

TOOTH DEVELOPMENT

The development of tooth is composite and continuous process, which begins with 10 localized epithelial thickenings in the upper and lower jaw. These knobs-like swellings begin as an inward growth toward the ectomesenchyme, resembling a bud. This is called enamel organ. It was previously termed as dental organ, since it not only forms enamel but also plays an important role in the initiation of development of other tissues of the tooth as well as periodontal ligament and the alveolar bone. This bud-shaped enamel organ along with the ectomesenchyme undergoes morphological and physiological changes as it grows. This results in change in shape from bud to cap and then to bell **(Table 4-3)**.

The enamel organ proliferates unequally resulting in an increase in size, with central regression, allowing the condensed ectomesenchyme, now called as dental papilla, to occupy the central portion. This gives an appearance of a cap sitting on a ball. Further increase in size of the enamel organ due to proliferation, along with dental papilla in the deeper invagination, gives a bell-shaped appearance. The dental papilla eventually will form the dentin and pulp. The ectomesenchymal cells and fibers surrounding the dental organ condense to become dental sac or dental follicle, which will form the cementum, periodontal ligament, and alveolar bone.

Thus the enamel organ, dental papilla, and dental follicle undergo both morpho- and histodifferentiation and contribute to the components of the developing tooth **(Figure 4-8)**.

TABLE 4-3: Stages in tooth development.

Physiological stages	Morphological stages
Initiation	Bud stage
Proliferation	Cap stage
Histodifferentiation	Bell stage (Early)
Morphodifferentiation	Bell stage (Advanced)
Apposition	Formation of enamel and dentin

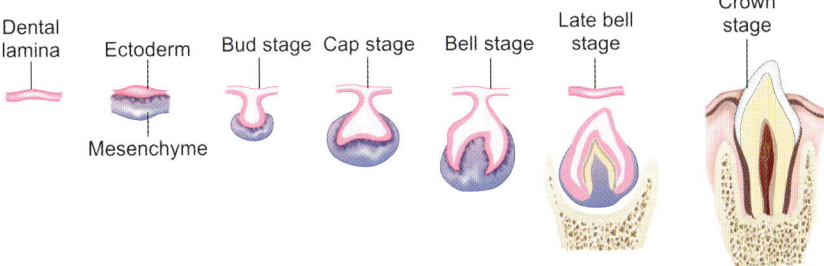

Figure 4-8: Stages of tooth development.

Tooth Initiation

Tooth development is a continuous process in which tooth initiation forms the elementary step. Various animal studies and examples have been considered from the literature to assess the tooth initiating potentiality either in the epithelium or in the dental mesenchyme.

When the first arch epithelium of murine is combined with the cranial or caudal neural crest cells in the anterior chamber of eye, it resulted in formation of tooth, wherein other combinations [neural crest cells either with limb epithelium or the second arch epithelium or the neural crest cells alone or the mandibular arch (first arch) epithelium alone], did not result in the same response, indicating the presence of tooth initiating potential within the epithelium and not in the mesenchyme.

Conversely in other studies, when the late first arch ectomesenchyme (after the day 12) is combined with the plantar (foot) epithelium, it formed the enamel organ, which suggested that the tooth initiating potential is in the ectomesenchyme and not within the epithelium. Similarly another experiment, where the dental epithelial organ is combined with the skin mesenchyme, witnessed the features of skin and not the tooth.

The above experiments evidenced that up to E9.5, the ectomesenchyme remains uncommitted and responds to epithelial signals regardless of their position. By E10.5, the spatial domain expression of genes and growth factors are established in ectomesenchyme, but depend on epithelium for signals (*FGF8* and *BMP4*) to stimulate the expression of numerous homeobox-like genes (*Msx- 1, Msx-2*) and distal-less gene (*Dlx*) in the mesenchyme and lose their competency to other signals from outside. Contrarily at E11, the gene expression domains are fixed in ectomesenchyme, independent of the signals from epithelium. Besides, these extensive signaling pathways with all the mentioned genes, other transcription factors, and growth factors, also seem to play a role in tooth initiation.

Collectively various studies carried out summarize the following: (A) Initially the factors initiating the odontogenesis reside in the first arch epithelium influencing the ectomesenchyme. (B) Over a period of time, once the initiating potential is achieved, the ectomesenchyme attains the dominant role in complex epithelial–mesenchymal interactions leading to tooth development **(Figure 4-9)**.

Initiation Stage (Bud Stage)

The dental lamina grows into the ectomesenchyme to form the bud-like epithelial enamel organ and initiates the tooth development. Bud stage of the deciduous anterior teeth is reached at 7th week of intrauterine life. Initially the dental lamina is shallow and is close to the surface epithelium. Growth of jaw causes displacement of the tooth germ into the deeper mesenchymal layer. Microscopically, enamel organ resembles the oral epithelium. It is made up of peripheral short columnar cells and central polygonal cells with slightly increased intercellular substances. There is increased mitotic activity seen within the epithelial enamel organ and the surrounding ectomesenchyme. Increased proliferation of the ectomesenchymal cells with little intercellular substance results in their dense grouping adjacent to the epithelial enamel organ and is henceforth known as dental papilla. Epithelial enamel organ is separated from the underlying ectomesenchyme by basement membrane, called membrana preformativa **(Figures 4-10A and B)**.

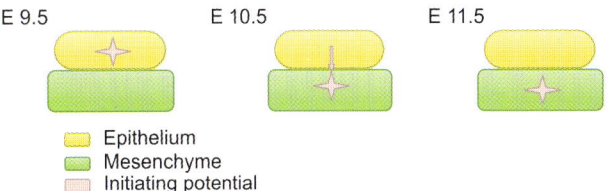

Figure 4-9: Schematic representation explaining signaling interdependence between epithelium and ectomesenchyme.

Molecular Events in Bud–Cap Stage

The localized growth in the form of bud protruding from the dental lamina into the mesenchyme is called the tooth bud (E11). The developing tooth bud expresses *BMP2, Shh, Wnt-10a, p21, Msx2,* and *Lef1* genes with the potential to initiate the tooth development.

The tooth inductive potential transfers from the epithelium to the mesenchyme, with the developing tooth bud and series of molecular events continue in this stage (E11.5–E-12). The expression of *BMP4* within the epithelium stimulates the expression of *BMP4* and *Msx*-1 in the mesenchyme, to restrict condensation of mesenchyme around the tooth bud. The epithelial expression of *Wnt*-10a and/or *Wnt*-10b mediated by *Lef-1* and β*-catenin* activates the expression of *FGF4* gene present within the epithelium. In turn the expression of *FGF4* induces the production of *FGF3* in the adjacent mesenchyme. Eventually the expression of *FGF3* together with other signals in the mesenchyme initiates the expression of *Shh* within the epithelium, which is essential for formation and growth of tooth bud and continues to play a role in determination of the morphology of the tooth **(Figure 4-11)**.

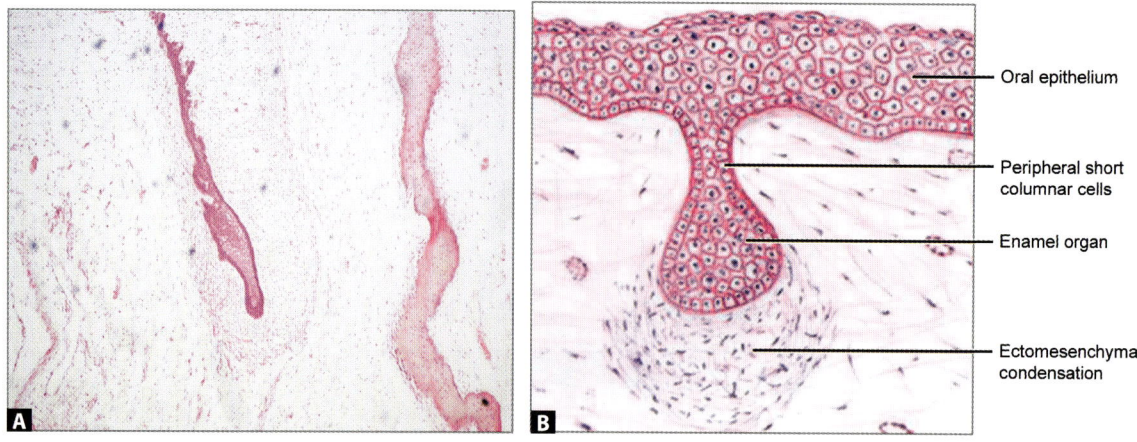

Figures 4-10A and B: (A) Photomicrography of bud stage; (B) Schematic representation.
Source: (B) Adapted from Oral Histology Diagrams in Oral Pathology India by Mandana Donoghue, http://www.oralpath.in

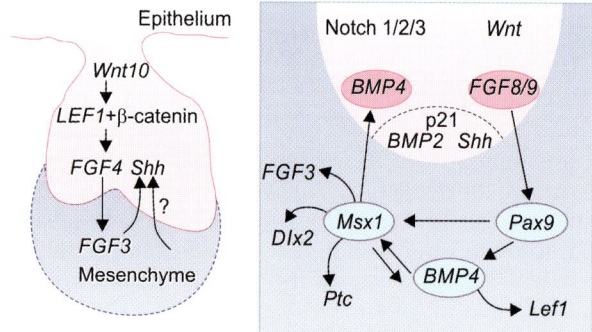

Figure 4-11: Representing the molecular interplay in the bud stage of tooth development.

Tooth Patterning

Tooth patterning describes the process and factors, which determine the shape and type of tooth. Tooth pattern varies in different living beings and generally is typed into two forms namely—homodont and heterodont. Homodont is a term used when all the teeth are of same shape as in case of some nonmammalian vertebrates like fish, lizards, frogs, and dolphins, while heterodonts possess more than one form of teeth, as seen in most of mammals like humans, dogs, and rabbits. The existence of different grades of teeth (incisiform, caniniform and molariform) is explained by two theories namely—field theory and clone theory.

Field theory as proposed by Butler (1967), suggested that within the graded field (expression of specified homeobox genes) all tooth primordia are analogous, and the altered shapes of teeth within the defined field are restrained by the substances and signals generated elsewhere within the jaw. Thus, the graded concentration of signals along the developing jaw, determines the shape of the tooth in different locations. The spatial and temporal expression of homeobox code gene (*Msx* gene and *Dlx* gene) within the first arch ectomesenchyme in each restricted field has been recognized, *i.e. Msx-*1, *Msx*-2, and *Alx*-3 are located in the anterior region (presumptive incisor region), while *Dlx-1,* *Dlx-2,* and *Barx*-1 in the proximal and posterior region (presumptive molar region) of the first arch. The area intersecting *Msx*-1, *Msx*-2, and *Dlx*-2 gene forms the canine region. Various recombination experiments quoted in literature reveal the presence of particular code with absence of other code, essential for the development of teeth with different morphology. For example, the expression of *Dlx-1* and *Dlx-2* (molar gene) with loss of *Msx-1* and *Msx-2* (incisor gene) in the defined field is required for the formation of molar. Further, the morphological differences among the multicuspid teeth or the incisors within the same field or in the different jaws are due to the variations in gene expression. For example, the expression of *Dlx-1* and *Dlx-2 is* evidenced in both maxillary and mandibular molars and *Dlx-5* and *Dlx-6* only in the mandibular primordium. Thus the tooth bud at the given location develops according to its position or field, expressing differing combination of patterning homeobox genes **(Figures 4-12A to C)**.

In contrast, Osborne (1978) suggested a clone model, whereby the ectomesenchymal cells are pre-programmed by the epithelium for different clone of teeth that further develop into specific tooth class, *i.e.* the shape of the tooth is determined from the moment the primordium is initiated. As each clone develops, the dental lamina grows both forward and backward. Once it attains its critical size, tooth development is initiated at the center with zone of inhibition expressed at the periphery. This zone of inhibition prevents the initiation of new tooth bud formation and allows to progress only after the escape from the zone of inhibition from the developing clone.

The various recombining experiments support the claims of both the theories and suggested the functional redundancy and their complexities. The mutations either in *Dlx-1* or *Dlx-2* in the proximal ends of first and second arch resulted in defects in the skeletal elements and not in the tooth formation. Conversely, the mutation of both *Dlx-1* and *Dlx-2* causes absence of upper molars. Thus the appropriate epithelial signals to ectomesenchyme initiate the type determination and eventually the ectomesenchyme takes the dominant role to produce teeth of a given pattern.

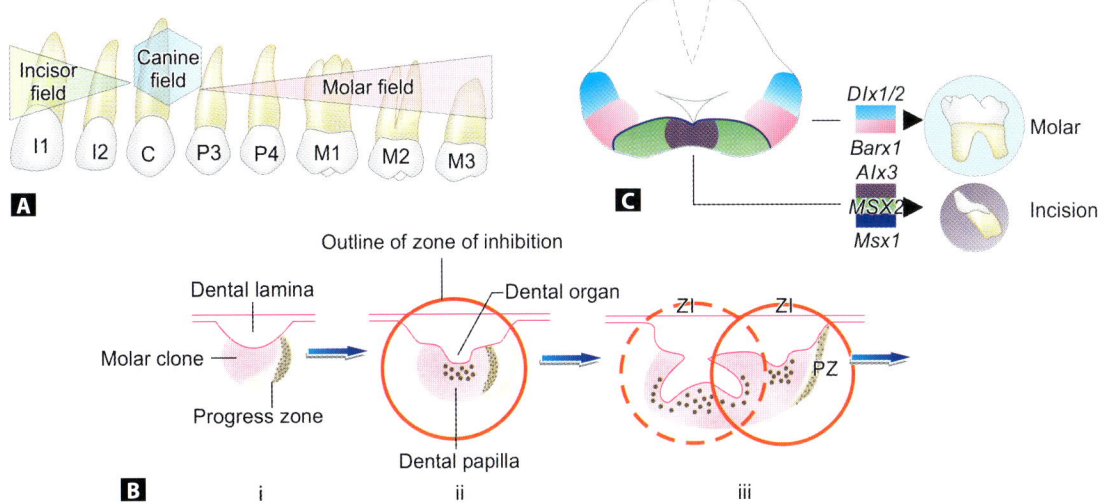

Figures 4-12A to C: Different theories for teeth patterning: (A) The field theory; (B) The clone model (ZI-Zone of inhibition, PZ- Progressive zone); (C) The molecular field or ontogenetic homeobox code model.

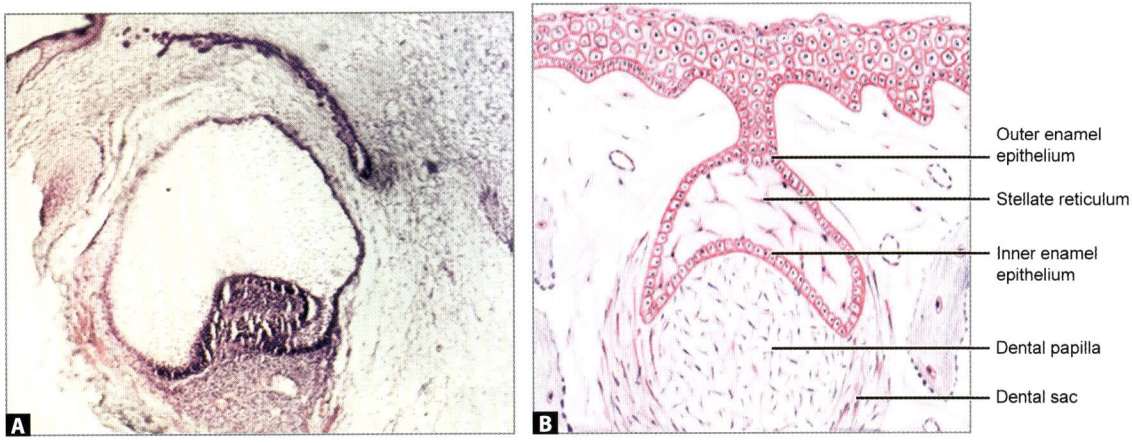

Figures 4-13A and B: (A) Photomicrography of cap stage; (B) Schematic representation.
Source: (B) Adapted from Oral Histology Diagrams in Oral Pathology India by Mandana Donoghue, http://www.oralpath.in

Proliferation Stage (Cap Stage)

In this stage, the shape of the epithelial enamel organ resembles a cap, and this stage is reached in 12th week of intrauterine life. The unequal and continuous proliferation of the epithelial enamel organ, particularly at the free end on the vestibular and lingual aspect, results in central invagination. This allows the enamel organ to change its shape from a bud to cap. Continuous proliferation of cells of the enamel organ and dental papilla results in cap sitting on a ball appearance. During this process, there is condensation of ectomesenchymal cells and fibers surrounding the enamel organ and the dental papilla and is known as dental follicle or dental sac.

The histodifferentiation begins at the end of the cap stage with differentiation of cells of enamel organ, which are transformed to both morphologically and functionally into distinct population of cells namely—outer enamel epithelium, inner enamel epithelium, and stellate reticulum **(Figures 4-13A and B)**.

Cell to cell and cell to extracellular matrix communications are important for the development, maintenance, and function of organs and tissues. The communication between the adjacent cells is enabled by specialized intercellular junctions, whereas the communication between the cells separated by certain distance is by the secretion of hormones, cytokines, and growth factors, etc. Cell surface receptors help to establish the communication between the cells and the matrix.

Most of the cells of the body are attached to each other and to the extracellular matrix by means of some kind of special contact sites called cell junctions. They are basically of three types namely—gap junction (communicating junction), occluding junction (tight junction), and adhering junction **(Figures 4-14A to C)**. Occluding junctions are seen only in epithelium in which the adjacent cells are fused to each other by means of anastomosing system of occluding ridges.

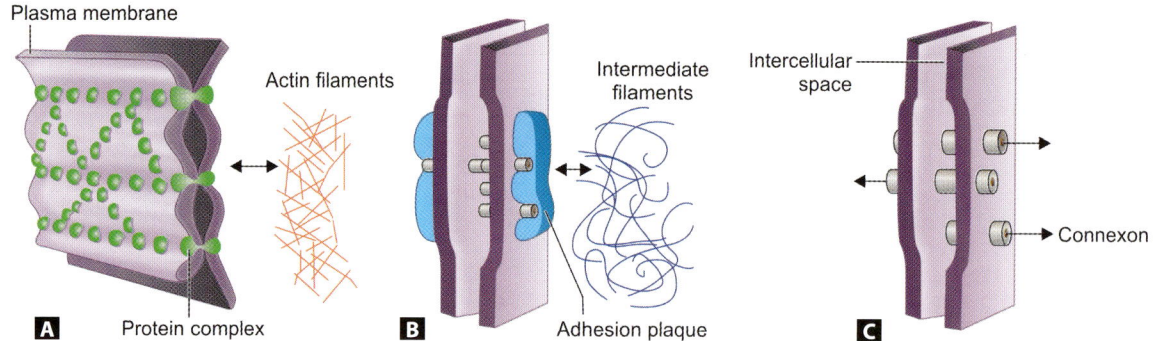

Figures 4-14A to C: (A) Tight junction; (B) Adhering junction; (C) Gap junction.

> Adhering junctions attach cells to one another and to the extracellular matrix. In contrast to the tight junction, there will be about 20 nm space between the cells. Desmosomes are one type of adhering junction, in which the cell is attached to the neighboring cells in a small spot (macula adherens). Hemidesmosomes attach cells to the basement membrane.
> Gap junctions will have narrow intercellular gap between the cells and are bridged by microchannels through which molecules are transported from one cell to another and to the extracellular matrix.

Outer enamel epithelium: The peripheral cells of the convexity of cap-shaped enamel organ form the outer enamel epithelium and are cuboidal in shape. It is separated from the dental follicle by means of a distinct basement membrane. These cells are attached to one another by desmosomes and to the basement membrane by hemidesmosomes.

Inner enamel epithelium: The short columnar cells lining the concavity of the enamel organ form the inner enamel epithelium, which eventually become tall columnar and will turn into an ameloblasts to form the enamel. These cells are attached to one another and to the basement membrane by desmosomes and hemidesmosomes, respectively. They are separated from the dental papilla cells by basement membrane. The avascular enamel organ particularly the inner enamel epithelial cells depend on the dental papilla for their nutrition.

Cervical loop: The junction between the outer enamel epithelium contributing the convexity and inner enamel epithelium contributing the concavity, at the rim of enamel organ forms the zone of reflexion or cervical loop. It plays a primary role in root formation.

Stellate reticulum: The central star-shaped cells of the enamel organ are called as stellate reticulum (stellate star-shaped, reticulum-network like). Central polygonal cells of the enamel organ secrete glycosaminoglycans (GAG) into the extracellular component, which are hydrophilic in nature and absorb water into the enamel organ. The increase in fluid into the enamel organ moves the cells apart; however the cells within this space grow longer and develop cytoplasmic extensions and remain in contact with one another by desmosomes. This gives the star-shaped appearance to the cells at the central portion of the enamel organ. Stellate reticulum provides cushion-like consistency, which protects and supports the inner enamel epithelial cells which are very frail.

The epithelial enamel organ is attached to the oral epithelium not by a cord of epithelial cells, but by sheet of cells with discontinuities. This discontinuous portion contains ectomesenchyme. Histologically this gives the appearance of double attachment made up of epithelial cells and appears like a niche and is known as *enamel niche*.

Enamel Knot and Cord

Cells at the central portion of the inner enamel epithelium clump and condense to form enamel knot. They also extend vertically from the inner enamel epithelium to the outer enamel epithelium to form enamel cord, which separates the enamel organ into two parts and is known as enamel septum.

Enamel knot and enamel cord are transient structures. They disappear (by a process called apoptosis) before the enamel formation. The cells of the enamel knot do not divide but they promote proliferation of neighboring epithelial cells and the ectomesenchymal cells. Their exact role in the development of tooth is unclear, however, may act as reservoir of proliferating cells of the enamel organ. According to the recent studies, they play an important role in determining the cuspal morphology by acting as signaling center and expressing growth factors. The reciprocal signaling of epithelium and the ectomesenchyme, and the role of enamel knot signaling according to the developmental stages of the tooth is depicted in **Figure 4-15A**. Recent animal studies believe these apoptotic cells develop as a small connective tissue band that connects the tooth germ and oral epithelium and called as dental stalk or gubernaculum. They are found to have role in tooth eruption.

Dental papilla: The ectomesenchymal cells in the center portion of invagination of epithelial enamel organ are called dental papilla cells which appear polygonal and display numerous cytoplasmic processes. They are separated from the inner enamel epithelium by means of the basement membrane. The dental papilla cells undergo active proliferation, which is exhibited by presence of mitotic and proliferating capillaries. These blood vessels course along with nerve fibers. More number of tiny capillaries is seen at the periphery. The dental papilla cells give rise to dentin and pulp.

Dental sac: The condensation of ectomesenchymal cells and fibers around the dental papilla and the cervical portion of the enamel organ is called dental sac. The dental sac plays an important role in development of cementum, periodontal ligament, and alveolar bone proper.

Enamel Knot—Signaling Center for Tooth Formation
The transient epithelial structure in the center of the enamel organ called the enamel knot, plays an important role in the control of growth and patterning of tooth cusps. The development of enamel knot is regulated by signals derived from mesenchyme and it also expresses several signaling molecules like *BMP2, BMP4, BMP7, Wnt-10b, FGF4, FGF9, Slit-1*, and *Shh* whose exact role remains uncertain. Shortly after the expression of *Shh* within the epithelium, *p21* gene can be detected among the enamel knot precursor cells at the tip of tooth buds. *p21* gene expression existence is known to localize until they disappear by apoptotic pathway. *BMP4* is a potent inducer of *p21* gene where the expression of *BMP2* is presumed to induce enamel knot formation. Role of *FGF's* expression within the enamel knot is to stimulate cell division in the enamel epithelium and in the dental papilla **(Figures 4-15A and B)**. The receptors of *FGFs* are missing within the enamel knot, excepting the *FGF4* in primary and secondary enamel knots, preventing the response to the mitogenic stimulus. *Msx-2* is involved in regulating *FGF4* and/or genes responsible for cessation of proliferation in enamel knot. *Slit-1* and *FGF4* are the only markers localized within both the primary and secondary enamel knots (future cuspal tips in molars).

Bell Stage

The continued growth of the epithelial enamel organ along with the dental papilla deepens the central invagination and leads to the change in its shape from a cap to bell. In this stage of tooth development, the tooth-forming cells acquire their distinct phenotype (*i.e.* inner enamel epithelial cells will become ameloblasts, the enamel-forming cells). This process is known as histodifferentiation and this occurs at early bell stage. The morphology of the tooth is determined in the later part of the bell stage and is called stage of morphodifferentiation. Another important event that occurs in this stage is the separation of tooth germ from the oral epithelium by the fragmentation of dental lamina. The fragmented cells of the dental lamina exist as discrete clusters of epithelial cells. These cell rests degenerate usually and some remain as cell rests of Serres and are seen in gingiva and jaw bone.

Histodifferentiation Stage (Early Bell Stage)

At this stage, four distinct cell populations can be discerned in the epithelial enamel organ. They are inner enamel epithelium, stratum intermedium, stellate reticulum, and outer enamel epithelium **(Figures 4-16A and B)**.

Inner enamel epithelium: The short columnar cells lining the concavity of the enamel organ eventually become tall columnar cells, the preameloblasts. These cells are attached to their neighboring cells by means of junctional complexes and to the cells of stratum intermedium by desmosomes. The inner enamel epithelial cells contain large oval nuclei at

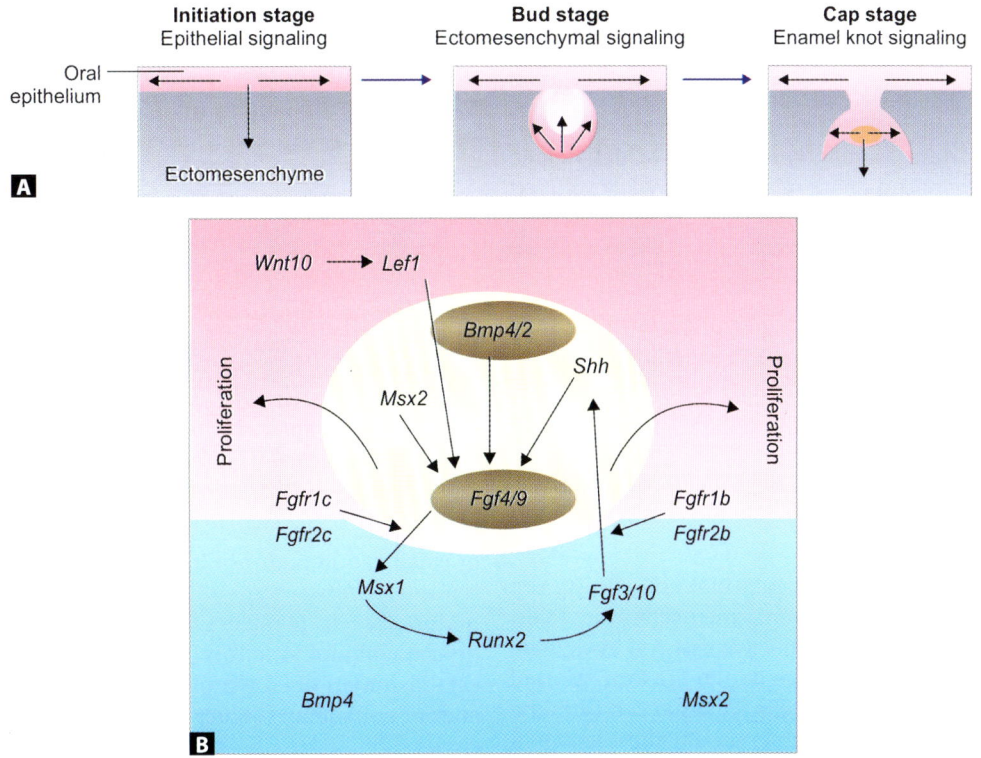

Figures 4-15A and B: Interplay of growth factors of the enamel knot to enamel organ and to the dental papilla.

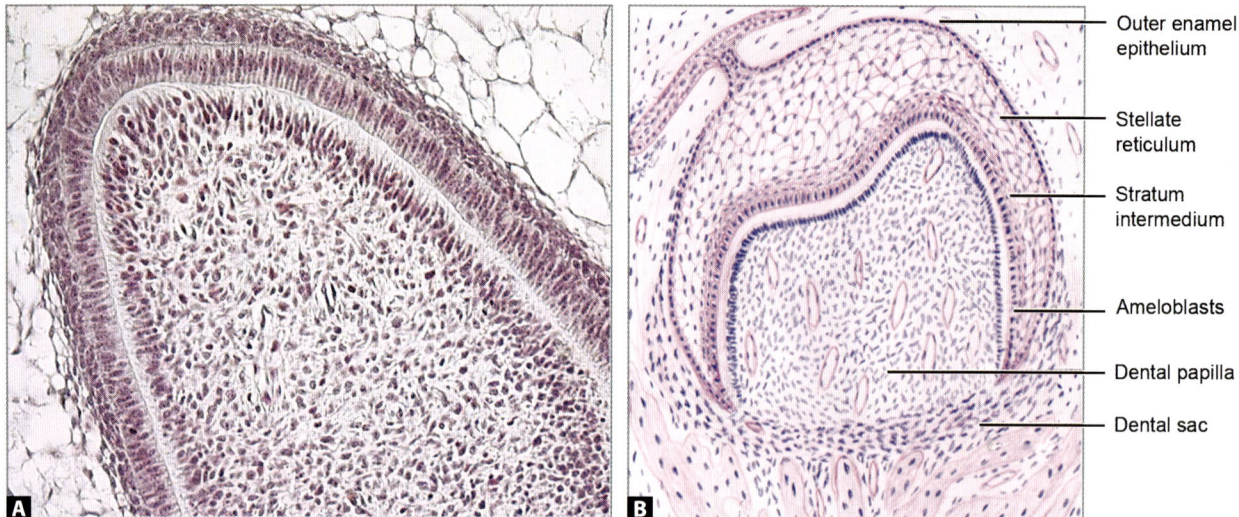

Figures 4-16A and B: (A) Photomicrography of early bell stage; (B) Schematic representation.
Source: (A) Dr Nandini DB, Dr Ngairangbam Sanjeeta, Dr Sumitha Banerjee, Dr P Aparnadevi, Dental College, RIMS, Imphal, Manipur, India (B) Adapted from Oral Histology Diagrams in Oral Pathology India by Mandana Donoghue, http://www.oralpath.in

their center. Mitochondria are evenly distributed throughout the cells. Rough endoplasmic reticulum is few and Golgi complex is not well-developed. Glycogen content of the cell is increased.

The expanding cell organelles reflect the intense synthesis and secretory stage of the preameloblasts, which later become ameloblasts and secrete enamel. Further these cells influence the dental papilla cells by expressing and secreting several growth factors to differentiate into odontoblasts, the dentin-forming cells.

Stratum intermedium: Few layers of cells, that lie between stellate reticulum and inner enamel epithelium, are squamous cells and form the stratum intermedium (stratum-layer, intermedium-in between). They are attached to one another and cells of inner enamel epithelium and stellate reticulum cells by means of desmosomes. These cells have high degree of metabolic activity and this is reflected by well-developed cellular organelles, acid mucopolysaccharides, and glycogen content. This layer is very important for enamel formation. This layer is absent in cervical loop, which forms the root.

Stellate reticulum: Cells of stellate reticulum form the bulk of the enamel organ and this expands further by increase in the amount of intercellular fluid. Soon the cells of stellate reticulum collapse before the formation of enamel and result in reduction of the distance between the ameloblasts and nutrient capillaries near the outer enamel epithelium. Thus these cells are no longer distinguishable from stratum intermedium.

Outer enamel epithelium: The cuboidal cells lining the convexity of the enamel organ arrange themselves into folds. This allows the surrounding connective tissue to invaginate into these folds. In the later stage due to the formation of dentin, inner enamel epithelial cells are distanced from the dental papilla cells and nutritional supply. But the nutritional source is re-established from the surrounding connective tissue by the folding of the outer enamel epithelium.

Dental papilla: The peripheral cells of the dental papilla differentiate into cuboidal cells and later columnar cells to become odontoblasts. This event occurs under the organizing influence of inner enamel epithelial cells. The dental papilla cells, after the set number of cell division become competent, to express the cell surface receptors, to receive the growth signals to become the odontoblasts. During this differentiation, changes also occur in the extracellular portion of the dental papilla. These include synthesis and clustering of fine fibrils, increase in basophilic staining of the interstitial space, capillary ingrowth that will form peripheral subodontoblastic plexus, and ingrowth of nerve fibers. The odontoblasts form dentin, which is the first hard tissue to be formed in the tooth. Presence of dentin is essential for the formation of enamel. In the late bell stage, shortly before the dentin formation, the basement membrane of the inner enamel epithelium becomes thicker with a mass of fine aperiodic fibrils and is known as membrana preformativa.

Dental sac: Dental sac separates the dental papilla from the surrounding ectomesenchyme of the jaw; the cells of the dental sac appear like fibroblasts. In addition to these numerous fibroblast-like cells, the dental sac contains increased amount of collagen fibrils oriented parallel to the surface of the tooth germ.

Morphodifferentiation Stage (Advanced Bell Stage)

In advanced bell stage or late bell stage, the morphology of the tooth is determined and is characterized by initiation of calcification and root formation. During this stage, the boundary between the inner enamel epithelium and the peripheral cells of the dental papilla will become the future dentinoenamel junction (DEJ). This will be preceded by establishment of crown patterning by folding of the inner enamel epithelium **(Figure 4-17)** into the shape of the future crown.

Odontoblasts differentiate from the peripheral cells of the dental papilla and form a layer of dentin. As soon

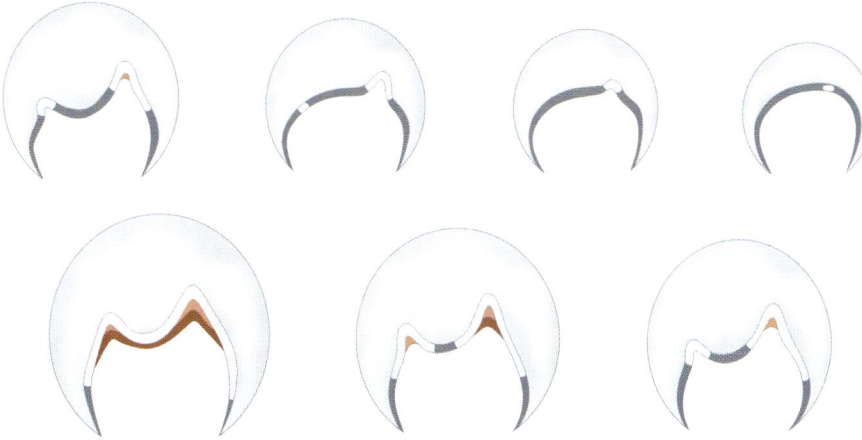

Figure 4-17: Infolding of the inner enamel epithelium in accordance to the crown pattern.

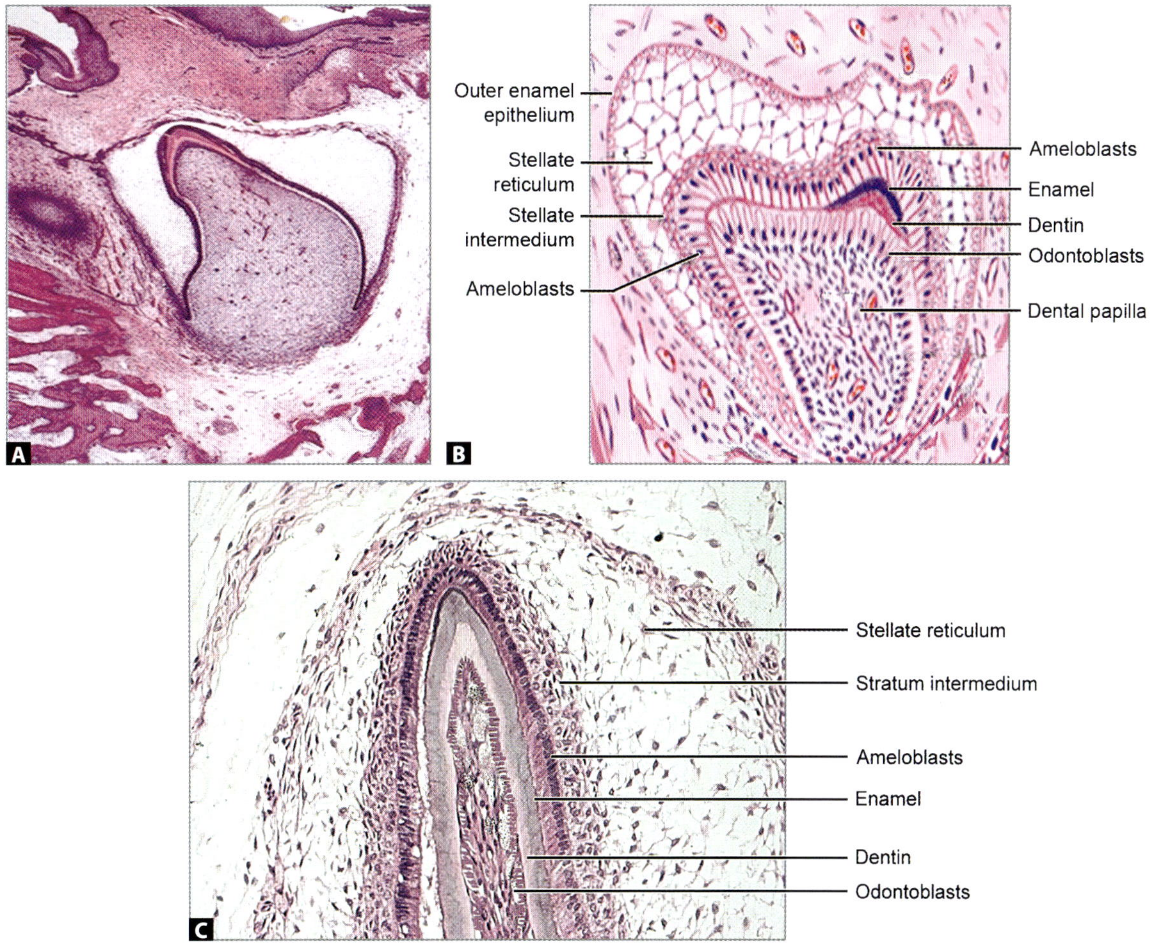

Figures 4-18A to C: (A) Photomicrography of late bell stage; Ameloblasts secreting enamel matrix; (B) Schematic presentation; and (C) Photomicrograph.
Source: (A) Dr Pratibha Ramani, Saveetha Dental College, Chennai, India; (B) adapted from Oral Histology Diagrams in Oral Pathology India by Mandana Donoghue, http://www.oralpath.in; (C) Dr Nandini DB, Dr Ngairangbam Sanjeeta, Dr Sumitha Banerjee, Dr P Aparnadevi, Dental College, RIMS, Imphal, Manipur, India

as the dentin is formed, the inner enamel epithelial cells (preameloblasts) differentiate into ameloblasts and lay down a layer of enamel over the dentin. The formation of enamel begins at the DEJ and elaborates toward the surface, since the ameloblasts move away from DEJ as they secrete enamel matrix **(Figures 4-18A to C)**. Deposition of enamel occurs initially at the cusp tip and progresses cervically. Enamel and dentin formation occurs in two stages, namely matrix deposition and mineralization similar to the other hard tissue formation. Further the cervical portion of the epithelial enamel organ gives rise to formation of Hertwig's epithelial root sheath to form the root.

APPOSITION AND HARD TISSUE FORMATION

Hard tissues such as enamel, dentin, cementum, and bone are formed in two stages, namely—matrix formation and mineralization. The matrix of all the hard tissues, except enamel, consists of collagen fibers and ground substance. The hardness of the mineralized tissue is determined by the amount of the inorganic substances present. The percentage of the inorganic content varies from one tissue to another and is in the form of calcium phosphate hydroxyapatite crystals and other minerals and elements in traces. Hard tissue formation occurs in intervals, wherein period of active deposition followed by period of rest, in a rhythmic manner, which is reflected by formation of incremental or resting lines.

As odontoblast secretes the dentin matrix, it moves away from the matrix, (toward the dental papilla) and leaves the cytoplasmic extensions called odontoblastic process within the matrix. The first formed dentin is known as mantle dentin. As the ameloblast secretes the enamel matrix over the mantle dentin it moves away and ultimately participates in the formation of reduced enamel epithelium. In contrast cementoblasts and osteoblasts get entrapped in their respective matrix to become cementocytes and osteocytes.

Thus deposition of dental hard tissue occurs by apposition/reciprocal induction where elongation of inner enamel epithelium inducts the peripheral cells of dental papilla to differentiate into odontoblasts and secretes dentin matrix, which in turn inducts the differentiation of ameloblasts which secrete enamel matrix **(Figure 4-19)**.

ROOT FORMATION

Root development begins by the proliferation of Hertwig's epithelial root sheath from the cervical loop **(Figures 4-20A to E)**

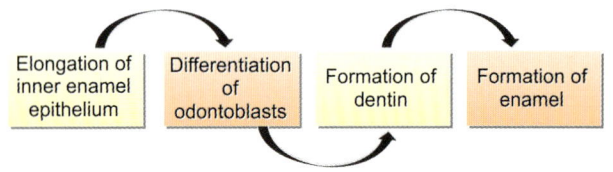

Figure 4-19: Reciprocal induction in tooth development

after the crown is formed. Hertwig's epithelial root sheath is a bilayered structure, devoid of stellate reticulum and stratum intermedium and consists only of inner and outer enamel epithelium. This root sheath serves as a mold and aids in determining the shape, size, and number of the roots. The rim of the Hertwig's epithelial root sheath bends more or less horizontally at the future cementoenamel junction to form the epithelial diaphragm. With the proliferation of the root sheath, the dental papilla continues to be enclosed by the root sheath and separated from the dental sac. The inner enamel epithelial cells of the Hertwig's epithelial root sheath induce the dental papilla cells, close to them to differentiate into odontoblasts. These odontoblasts lay down first layer of root dentin. As soon as the root dentin is formed, the Hertwig's epithelial root sheath breaks down to expose the newly formed dentin to the dental sac cells. These dental sac cells comprise undifferentiated ectomesenchymal cells. Upon contact with the newly formed root dentin, the dental sac cells differentiate into cementoblasts, osteoblasts, and fibroblasts to form cementum, alveolar bone, and periodontal ligament, respectively. The cementum is incrementally deposited over the root dentin. The fragmented epithelial cells of the root sheath remain as clumps or network of cords and move away from the surface of the root dentin. These are known as cell rests of Malassez and are included in the periodontal ligament during the development of periodontium.

The plane or the position of the epithelial diaphragm is relatively fixed in its horizontal position during the further development of the root. The root lengthens by the occlusal movement of the tooth germ, allowing the Hertwig's epithelial root sheath to proliferate vertically. Thus the coronal free end of the diaphragm proliferates to contribute for the lengthening of the root.

The wide diaphragmatic opening forms the primary apical foramen. It will be narrowed down further by the root dentin formation, which continues to become a tiny opening called apical foramen.

Multirooted tooth is also formed in the similar way, except that the single diaphragmatic opening is divided into two or three, depending on the number of roots, by the formation of a tongue-like extension toward each other **(Figures 4-21A to C)**.

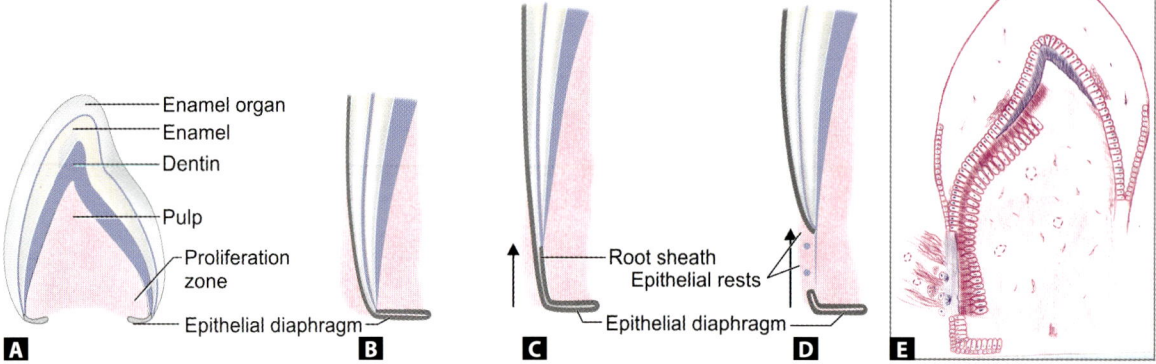

Figures 4-20A to E: Root development.

CHAPTER 4: Development of Tooth

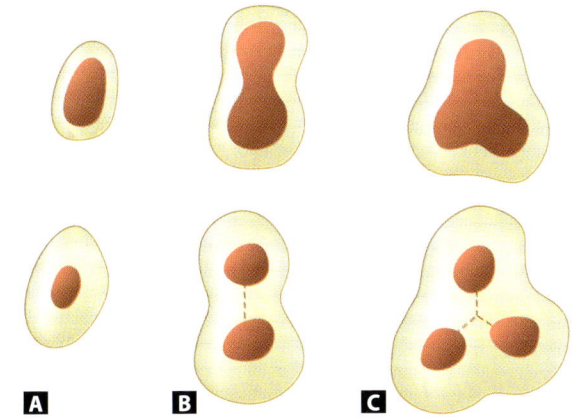

Figures 4-21A to C: (A) Root formation in single-rooted tooth; (B) Tongue-like extension developing to form a two-rooted tooth; (c) Tongue-like extension developing to form a three-rooted tooth.

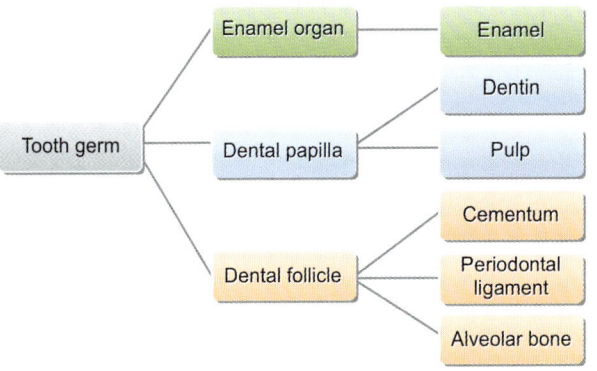

Figure 4-22: Schematic diagram representing tooth germ and its derivatives.

To summarize the tooth germ comprises of epithelial enamel organ, which gives rise to enamel, the dental papilla, which gives rise to dentin and pulp and dental sac or dental follicle, which gives rise to cementum, periodontal ligament and alveolar bone **(Figure 4-22)**.

Genes in Tooth Development
Barx: BarH1 homolog
BMP: Bone morphogenetic proteins
Dlx: Distal-less homolog
FGF: Fibroblast growth factor (SP)
Hgf: Hepatic growth factor
Lef: Lymphoid enhancer-binding factor (TF)
Lhx: LIM homeobox domain GENe
LIM: Lin11/Isl1/Mec3.
Msx: Msh-like genes in vertebrates (TF)
Pax: Paired box homeotic gene (TF)
Shh: Sonic hedgehog
Wnt: Wingless homolog

SP: Signaling Protein TF: Transcription Factor

CLINICAL CONSIDERATIONS

Defects at Initiation or Bud Stage

Lack of initiation or an arrest in the proliferation of cells results in complete absence of tooth development called total anodontia, while one or two teeth are missing it is called as partial anodontia **(Figures 4-23 and 4.24)**. Abnormal initiation or continued budding of the dental organ causes development of extra teeth known as supernumerary teeth **(Figure 4-25)**.

Defects at Proliferation or Cap Stage

Dens in dente: Accidental invagination of enamel organ into the dental papilla, gives tooth within a tooth appearance. Permanent maxillary incisors are commonly affected teeth.

Dens evaginatus: A localized area of proliferation and evagination of the inner enamel epithelium and the subjacent ectomesenchyme results in the formation of an accessory cusp or a globule of enamel at the occlusal surface, usually between the buccal and lingual cusp of the premolars **(Figure 4-26)**.

Gemination: Attempted division of single tooth germ into two, resulting in the formation of two completely or incompletely separated crowns with single root **(Figures 4-27A and B)**.

Fusion: Union of two adjacent tooth germs. Depending on the stage of development, fusion may be complete or incomplete **(Figures 4-28A and B)**.

Defects at Morphodifferentiation Stage

Disturbances and aberrations in morphodifferentiation lead to the formation of tooth with abnormal size and shape.

For example, peg-shaped tooth **(Figure 4-29)**, microdontia—small tooth, macrodontia—large tooth, and odontome.

Defects at Histodifferentiation Stage

Disturbances in the differentiation of the formative cells of the tooth germ result in abnormal structure of the enamel or dentin leading to the conditions called amelogenesis imperfecta **(Figures 4-30A and B)** or dentinogenesis imperfecta. Epithelial cell rests of the tooth development may give rise to the formation of odontogenic cysts and tumors.

Molar incisor hypomineralization (MIH), described as a qualitative defects of enamel that appears as yellow/brown defects in one to four permanent molars with incisors commonly involved **(Figures 4-31A and B)**. These teeth with defective enamel areas are believed to be less resistant to mechanical forces and have a higher degree of porosity, thereby resulting in increased likelihood of dental caries and also increased sensitivity to temperatures.

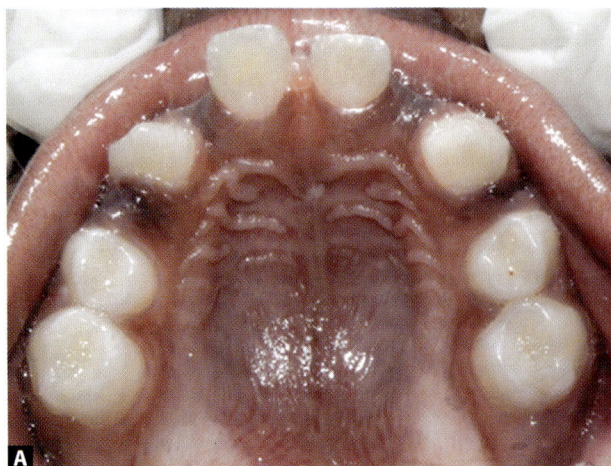
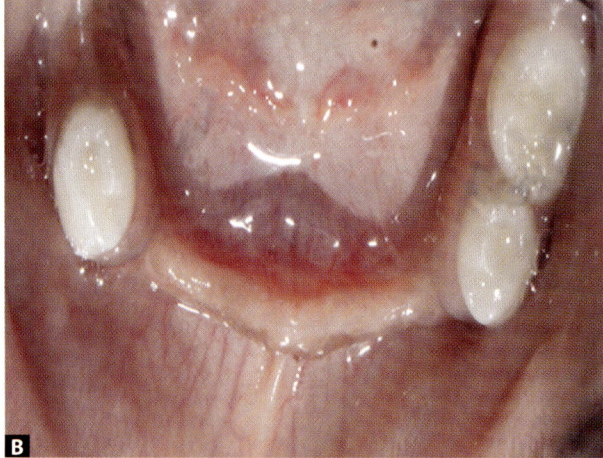

Figures 4-23A and B: Presence of multiple missing deciduous teeth in upper and lower jaw.

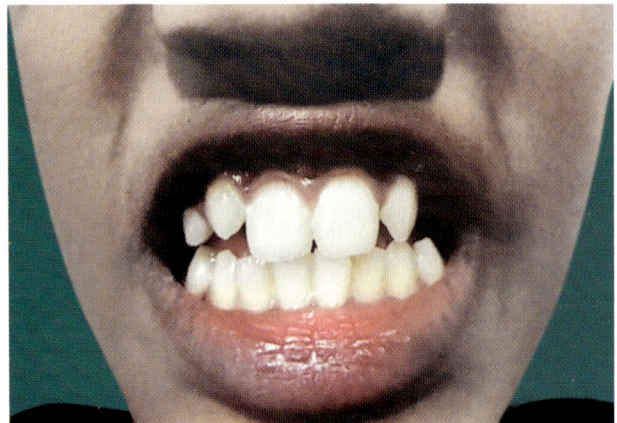

Figure 4-24: Partial anodontia. Missing permanent lateral incisors.
Source: Dr S Rohini, GRM Dental Clinic, Ambattur, Chennai, India

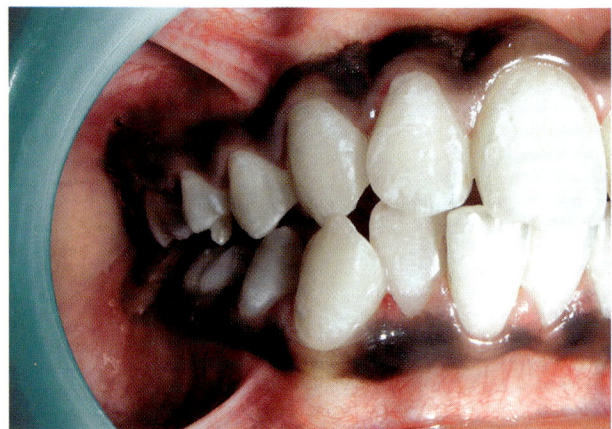

Figure 4-26: Dens evaginatus in second premolars.
Source: Dr Priya, Department of Pedodontics, Meenakshi Ammal Dental College, Chennai, India

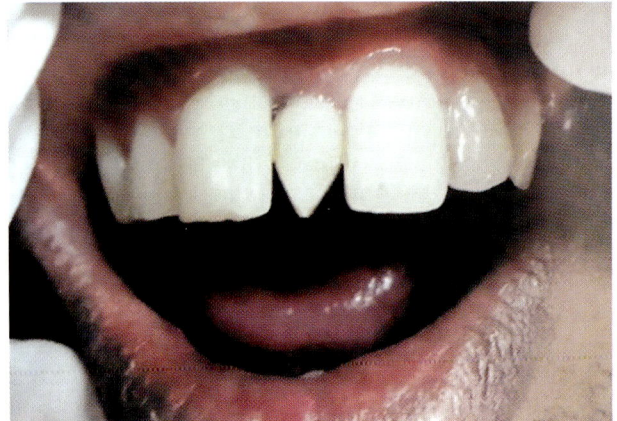

Figure 4-25: Mesiodens. Supernumerary tooth in between permanent central incisors.
Source: Dr S Rohini, GRM Dental Clinic, Ambattur, Chennai, India

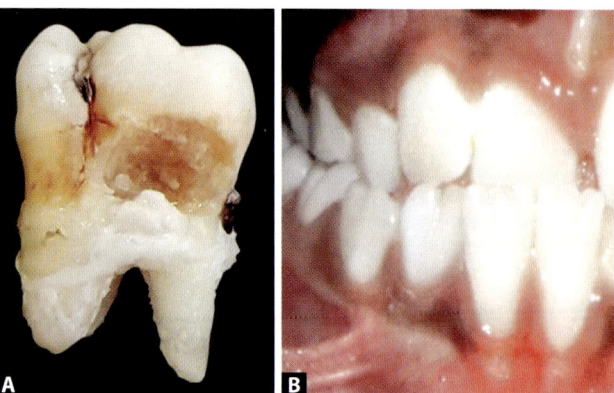

Figures 4-27A and B: (A) Gemination in maxillary first molar; (B) Gemination in mandibular lateral incisor
Source: Dr S Rohini, GRM Dental Clinic, Ambattur, Chennai, India

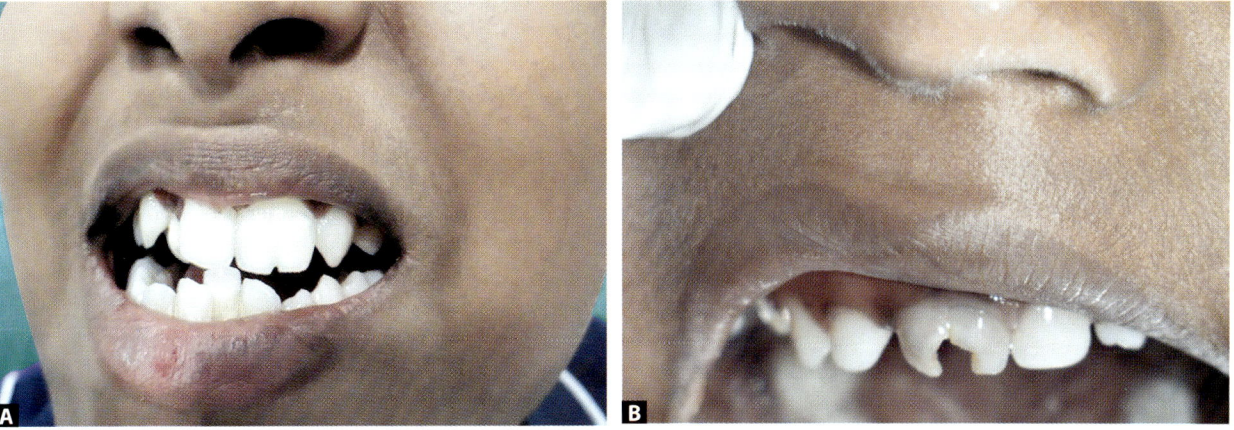

Figures 4-28A and B: (A) Fusion of permanent central and lateral incisors; (B) Fusion of Deciduous central and lateral incisors.
Source: Dr S Rohini, GRM Dental Clinic, Ambattur, Chennai, India

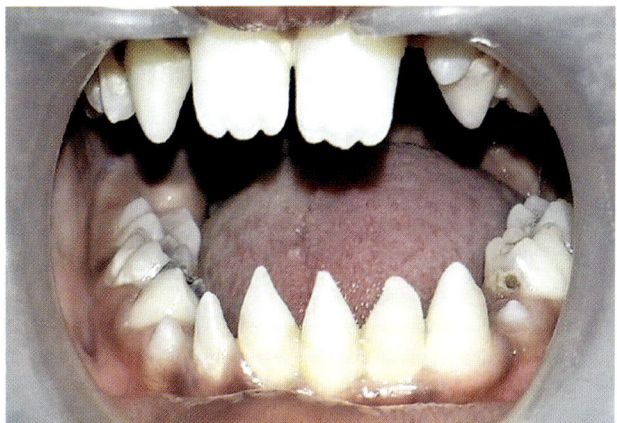

Figure 4-29: Peg-shaped mandibular incisors.
Source: Dr Aswin Devasya and Dr Mytthri Sapangala, Department of Pedodontics and Preventive Dentistry, Kannur Dental College, Kannur, India

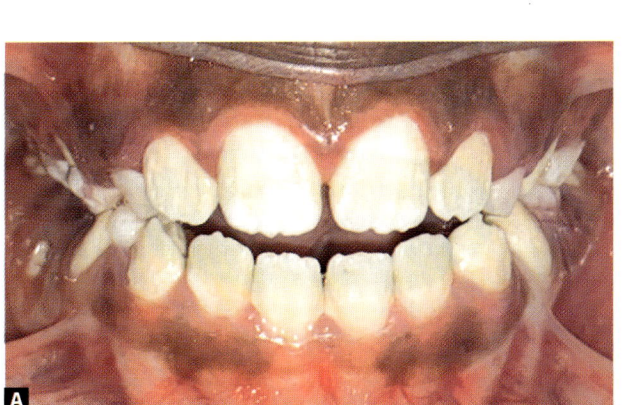
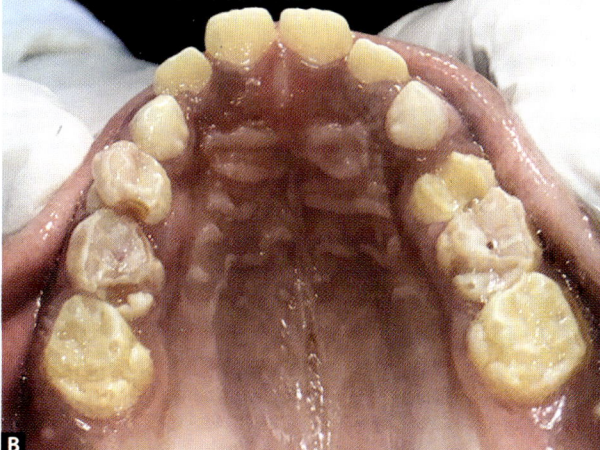

Figures 4-30A and B: Amelogenesis imperfecta, generalized defective enamel formation.

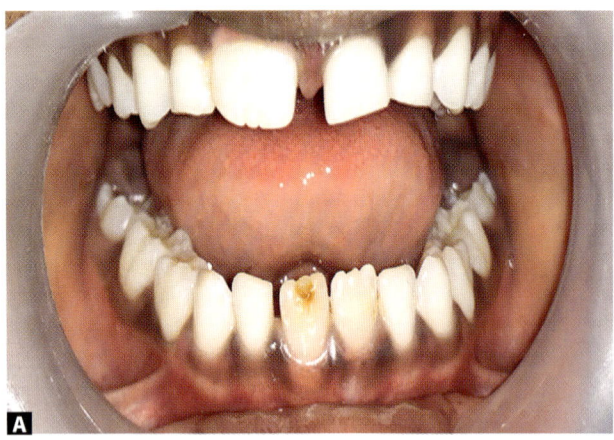 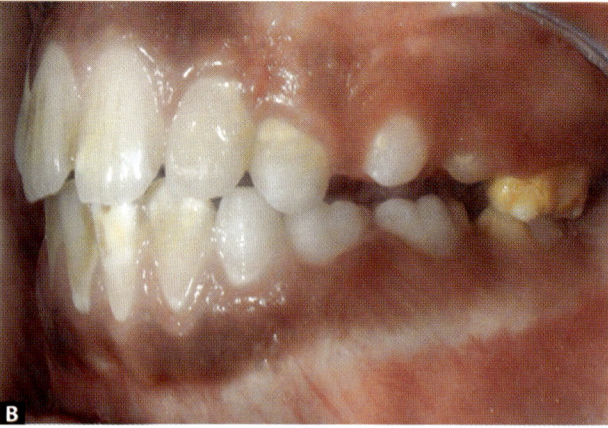

Figures 4-31A and B: Localized yellow to brown defects of enamel in incisors and molars.

Points to Remember

- Tooth development is a complex process that includes well-organized series of events, which include morphological and genetic factors. Development of primary teeth starts between 6th and 8th week of intrauterine life and permanent teeth in 12th week. Tooth development begins with the appearance of horseshoe-shaped epithelial thickening in the location of the future dental arches called **primary epithelial band**.
- The first evidence of tooth development, the primordia of developing teeth begins to develop as 10 round to oval, localized epithelial thickenings in the primary epithelial band, corresponding to the 10 deciduous teeth in each arch and are called as **dental lamina** while permanent tooth develops from the lingual extension of the dental lamina and is known as **successional lamina.**
- Dental lamina forms perpendicular to the oral ectoderm and interacts with the underlying ectomesenchyme. Thus, the tooth development comprises sequential and reciprocal series of morphological and genetic influences between the epithelium and ectomesenchyme.
- These knob-like swellings begin as an inward growth toward the ectomesenchyme, resembling a bud. This is called epithelial enamel organ and also plays an important role in the initiation of development of tooth and its supporting structures. This bud-shaped enamel organ along with the ectomesenchyme undergoes series of morphological and physiological changes and results in change in shape from bud to cap and then to bell. Accordingly the morphological events are staged as—(A) budstage; (B) cap stage; (C) early bell stage, and (D) advanced bell stage based on their shape.
- **Bud stage:** The dental lamina grows into the ectomesenchyme to form the bud-like growth called enamel organ. Microscopically, this consists of peripheral short columnar cells and central polygonal cells. Increased proliferation of the ectomesenchymal cells with little intercellular substance results in their dense grouping adjacent to the epithelial enamel organ and is known as dental papilla. Epithelial enamel organ is separated from the dental papilla by basement membrane, called membrana preformativa. The ectomesenchymal cells and fibers surrounding the dental organ condense to form dental sac or dental follicle.
- **Cap stage:** The unequal and continuous proliferation of the epithelial enamel organ with central invagination changes the shape of the enamel organ from a bud to cap, while continuous proliferation of cells of the dental papilla results in cap sitting on a ball appearance.
- During this process, there is condensation of ectomesenchymal cells and fibers surrounding the enamel organ. Thus at the end of the cap stage with differentiation of cells of enamel organ, distinct population of cells namely outer enamel epithelium, inner enamel epithelium, and stellate reticulum will be evident. The peripheral cells of the convexity of cap-shaped enamel organ form the ***outer enamel epithelium*** and are cuboidal in shape. The short columnar cells lining the concavity of the enamel organ form the ***inner enamel epithelium***, which eventually will turn into an ameloblasts to form the enamel. The junction between the outer enamel epithelium contributing the convexity and inner enamel epithelium contributing the concavity, at the rim of enamel organ forms **cervical loop** and plays a primary role in root formation. The central star-shaped cells of the enamel organ are called as ***stellate reticulum***. These cells secrete glycosaminoglycans into the extracellular component, which are hydrophilic in nature and absorb water into the enamel organ. The increase in fluid into the enamel organ moves the cells apart; however, the cells remain in contact with one another by desmosomes. This gives the star-shaped appearance to the cells at the central portion of the enamel organ, which provides cushion-like consistency, to protect and support the inner enamel epithelial cells.
- The epithelial enamel organ is attached to the oral epithelium not by a cord of epithelial cells, appears like a niche and is known as ***enamel niche***. Cells at the central portion of the inner enamel epithelium clump and condense to form ***enamel knot***. They also extend vertically from the inner enamel epithelium to the outer enamel epithelium to form ***enamel cord***, which separates the enamel organ into two parts and is known as ***enamel septum***. Their exact role in the development of tooth is unclear, however may act as reservoir of proliferating cells of the enamel organ.
- **Bell stage**: The continued growth of the epithelial enamel organ along with the dental papilla deepens the central invagination and leads to the change in its shape from a cap to bell. In the early bell stage four distinct cell populations can be discerned in the epithelial enamel organ. They are inner enamel epithelium, stratum intermedium, stellate reticulum, and outer enamel epithelium. *Inner enamel epithelium*. The short columnar cells lining the concavity of the enamel organ eventually become tall columnar cells, the preameloblasts. The expanding cell organelles in these cells reflect the intense synthesis and secretory stage of the preameloblasts, which later become ameloblasts and secrete enamel. Further these cells influence the peripheral cells of dental papilla to differentiate into odontoblasts, the dentin-forming cells. Few layers of cells that lie between stellate reticulum and inner enamel epithelium, are squamous cells and form the *stratum intermedium*. This layer is very important for enamel formation. This layer is absent in cervical loop. The cells of stellate reticulum which was forming the bulk of the enamel organ soon collapse at this stage before the formation of enamel and result in reduction of the distance between the ameloblasts and nutrient capillaries near the outer enamel epithelium. Thus these cells are no longer distinguishable from stratum intermedium. *Outer enamel epithelium*, the cuboidal cells lining the convexity of the enamel organ arrange themselves into folds. This allows the surrounding connective tissue to invaginate into these folds.

- **Dental papilla:** The peripheral cells of the dental papilla differentiate into cuboidal cells and later columnar cells to become odontoblasts. This event occurs under the organizing influence of inner enamel epithelial cells. Presence of dentin is essential for the formation of enamel.
- **Advanced bell stage or late bell stage:** The morphology of the tooth is determined in this stage; this will be preceded by establishment of crown patterning by folding of the inner enamel epithelium into the shape of the future crown. Odontoblasts differentiate from the peripheral cells of the dental papilla and form a layer of dentin. As soon as the dentin is formed, the inner enamel epithelial cells differentiate into ameloblasts and lay down a layer of enamel over the dentin. Enamel and dentin formation occurs in two stages, namely matrix formation and mineralization similar to the other hard tissue formation. Further the cervical portion of the epithelial enamel organ gives rise to formation of Hertwig's epithelial root sheath to form the root.
- Thus the enamel organ, dental papilla, and dental follicle undergo both morpho and histodifferentiation and contribute to the components of the developing tooth, while enamel organ deposits enamel, the dental papilla eventually will form the dentin and pulp. The ectomesenchymal cells and fibers surrounding the dental organ condense to become dental sac, which will form the cementum, periodontal ligament, and alveolar bone.
- After the tooth development, the dental lamina loses its connection with the oral ectoderm and disintegrates with the invasion of surrounding mesenchyme. The fragmented cells of the dental lamina exist as discrete clusters of epithelial cells. These cell rests degenerate usually and some remain as cell rests of Serres.
- Root development begins after the crown is formed by the proliferation of Hertwig's epithelial root sheath from the cervical loop. Hertwig's epithelial root sheath is a bilayered structure, devoid of stellate reticulum and stratum intermedium and consists only of inner and outer enamel epithelium. This root sheath serves as a mold and aids in determining the shape, size, and number of the roots.
- The inner enamel epithelial cells of the Hertwig's epithelial root sheath induce the dental papilla cells to differentiate into odontoblasts to lay down first layer of root dentin. As soon as the root dentin is formed, the Hertwig's epithelial root sheath breaks down to expose the newly formed dentin to the dental sac cells. Upon contact with dental sac cells, with the newly formed root dentin they differentiate into cementoblasts, osteoblasts, and fibroblasts to form cementum, alveolar bone, and periodontal ligament, respectively. Multirooted tooth is also formed in the similar way, except by the formation of a tongue-like extension toward each other. After the root completion, the sheath fragments, remains as clumps or network of cords and moves away from the surface of the root dentin. These are known as cell rests of Malassez.
- To summarize, the tooth germ comprises epithelial enamel organ, which gives rise to enamel; the dental papilla, which gives rise to dentin and pulp; and dental sac or follicle, which gives rise to cementum, periodontal ligament and alveolar bone.

PRACTICE QUESTIONS

1. List the stages in tooth development and write in detail about bell stage.
2. Write notes on Hertwig's epithelial root sheath and root development.
3. Write notes on enamel knot, cord and septum.
4. Write notes on reciprocal induction.
5. Cell rests in tooth development.

MULTIPLE CHOICE QUESTIONS

1. **The process of tooth development is called as**
   a. Odontogenesis
   b. Dentinogenesis
   c. Matrix formation
   d. Eruption
2. **Following are derivatives of dental papilla**
   a. Enamel, dentin and pulp
   b. Enamel
   c. Dentin and pulp
   d. Enamel, dentin, pulp and cementum
3. **Cells responsible for the formation of enamel are called**
   a. Odontoblasts
   b. Ameloblasts
   c. Preameloblasts
   d. Enamel organ
4. **Cells responsible for the formation of dentin are called**
   a. Preameloblasts
   b. Odontoblasts
   c. Pulp
   d. Dental papilla
5. **Dental lamina is active upto**
   a. 5 years
   b. 2 years
   c. 10 years
   d. 18 years
6. **Permanent tooth develops from the lingual extension of dental lamina and are called as**
   a. Primary epithelial band
   b. Successional lamina
   c. Dental placodes
   d. Vestibular band
7. **At 6th week of intrauterine life, horseshoe-shaped epithelial thickenings appear in the future dental arches are called as**
   a. Dental lamina
   b. Primary epithelial band
   c. Vestibular lamina
   d. Stomodeum
8. **Stages of tooth development namely bud, cap and bell stage is based on the**
   a. Shape of dental sac
   b. Shape of the tooth formed
   c. Shape of the epithelial enamel organ
   d. Shape of the dental papilla
9. **Stage of histodifferentiation in tooth development is also called**
   a. Bud stage
   b. Cap stage
   c. Early bell stage
   d. Advance bell stage

10. **The term odontogenic apparatus includes**
    a. Only enamel organ
    b. Enamel organ and dental papilla
    c. Enamel organ, dental papilla and dental sac
    d. Dental papilla and sac
11. **The remnants of dental lamina is called as**
    a. Hertwig's epithelial root sheath
    b. Cell rest of Serres
    c. Cell rest of Malassez
    d. Dental rests
12. **Bilayered Hertwig's epithelial root sheath is made up of**
    a. Stellate reticulum and stratum intermedium
    b. Stratum intermedium and inner enamel epithelium
    c. Inner and outer enamel epithelium
    d. Inner enamel epithelium and stellate reticulum
13. **Cell rests rests of Malassez are**
    a. Remnants of dental lamina
    b. Remnants of dental sac
    c. Remnants of Hertwig's epithelial root sheath
    d. Remnants of enamel organ
14. **Transient structure in enamel organ includes**
    a. Enamel knot and enamel cord
    b. Stratum intermedium and stellate reticulum
    c. Ameloblasts and odontoblasts
    d. Inner enamel epithelium
15. **Developing tooth bud is separated from the underlying dental papilla by basement membrane, called**
    a. Dental follicle
    b. Cervical loop
    c. Enamel niche
    d. Membrana performative
16. **The below statements are true about Hertwig's epithelial root sheath, except**
    a. Bilayered epithelium
    b. Remnant are called as cell rest of Malassez
    c. Acts as a mould for the root formation only for single rooted tooth
    d. Induce the dental papilla cells to differentiate into odontoblasts
17. **The peripheral cells of dental papilla differentiate into cuboidal cells and later to columnar cells under the influence of inner enamel epithelium to become**
    a. Cementoblasts
    b. Odontoblasts
    c. Ameloblasts and odontoblasts
    d. Preameloblats
18. **First formed dental hard tissue is**
    a. Enamel
    b. Dentin
    c. Cementum
    d. Alveolar bone
19. **Dental sac gives rise to**
    a. Enamel
    b. Dentin
    c. Cementum, periodontal ligament and alveolar bone
    d. Pulp
20. **Union of two adjacent tooth bud is called as**
    a. Germination
    b. Fusion
    c. Supernumerary tooth
    d. Odontoma
21. **The star-shaped appearance of stellate reticulum cells, located at the central portion of the enamel organ is due to the secretion of**
    a. Albumin
    b. Enamel matrix
    c. Glycosaminoglycans
    d. Proteoglycans
22. **Desmosomes are**
    a. Macula adherens
    b. Gap junctions
    c. Occluding junctions
    d. Connection between cells and the extracellular matrix
23. **Amelogenesis imperfecta is an enamel defect that occurs due to the disturbances in**
    a. Proliferation stage
    b. Morphodifferentiation stage
    c. Histodifferentiation stage
    d. None of the above
24. **Overactivity of dental lamina results in**
    a. Anodontia
    b. Supernumerary tooth
    c. Dens in dente
    d. Dens evaginatus

ANSWERS

| 1. a | 2. c | 3. b | 4. b | 5. a | 6. b | 7. b | 8. c | 9. c | 10. c | 11. b | 12. c | 13. c | 14. a | 15. d |
| 16. c | 17. b | 18. b | 19. c | 20. b | 21. c | 22. a | 23. c | 24. b | | | | | | |

BIBLIOGRAPHY

1. Avery JK, Chiego DJ. Essentials of Oral Histology and Embryology- A Clinical Approach, 3rd edition. US: Mosby; 2006.
2. Avery JK. Oral Development and Histology, 3rd edition. New York: Thieme; 2002.
3. Berkovitz BKB, Holland GR, Moxham BJ. Oral Anatomy, Histology and Embryology, 4th edition. US: Elsevier; 2009.
4. Bloch-Zupan A, Sedano H, Scully C. Dento/Oro/Craniofacial Anomalies and Genetics. Elsevier; 2012.
5. Bruce M Carlson: Human Embryology and Developmental Biology, 5th edition. Philadelphia: W.B. Saunders; 2014.
6. Catón J, Tucker AS. Current knowledge of tooth development: patterning and mineralization of the murine dentition. J Anat. 2009;214(4):502-15.

7. Chatterjee K. Essentials of Dental Anatomy and Oral Histology, 2nd edition. New Delhi: Jaypee Brothers Medical Publishers (P) Ltd; 2014.
8. Cobourne MT, Sharpe PT. Making up the numbers: The molecular control of mammalian dental formula. Semin Cell Dev Biol. 2010;21:314-24.
9. Davidovich Z (Ed). The biological mechanisms of tooth eruption and root resorption. Birmingham: EBSCO Information Services; 1988.
10. Eversole LR, Leider AS. Maxillary Intraosseous neuroepithelial structures resembling those seen in the Organ of Chievitz. Oral Surg. 1978;46:58.
11. Gaunt WA, Osborn JW, Ten Cate AR. Advanced Dental Histology, 2nd edition. Bristol: John Wright & Sons Ltd; 1971.
12. Harris EF. Odontogenesis- A Companion to Dental Anthropology. New Jersey: John Wiley & Sons, Inc; 2016.
13. Hillson S. Development, Function, and Evolution of Teeth (review). Human Biol. 2001;73:903-4.
14. Hodson JJ. Epithelial residues of the jaw with special reference to the edentulous jaw. J Anat. 1962;96:16-24.
15. Jingyuan Li, Carolina Parada, Yang Chai. Cellular and molecular mechanism of tooth root development. Development 2017;144(3): 374–84.
16. John Abramyan, Poongodi Geetha-Loganathan, Marie Šulcová and Marcela Buchtová. Role of Cell Death in Cellular Processes During Odontogenesis Cell Dev. Biol. 9:671475. doi: 10.3389/fcell.2021.671475
17. Kallenbach E, Piesco NP. The changing morphology of the epithelium-mesenchyme interface in the differentiation of growing teeth of selected vertebrates and its relationship to possible mechanisms of differentiation. Bioi Buccale. 1978;6:229-40.
18. Khurana A, Khurana I. Human Embryology, 2nd edition. India: CBS Publishers and Distributor Pvt Ltd; 2012.
19. Kumar GS. Orban's Oral Histology and Embryology, 14th edition. India: Elsevier; 2015.
20. Lisi S, Peterková R, Peterka M, et al. Tooth morphogenesis and pattern of odontoblast differentiation. Connect Tissue Res. 2003;44(1):167-70.
21. McClatchey KD. Tumors of the dental lamina: a selective review. Semin Diagn Pathol. 1987;4:200-4.
22. Mitsiadis TA, Graf D. Cell fate determination during tooth development and regeneration. Birth Defects Res C Embryo Today. 2009;87:199.
23. Mitsiadis TA, Luder H. Genetic basis for tooth malformations: from mice to men and back again. Clin Genet. 2011;80:319-29.
24. Mitsiadis TA, Smith MM. How do genes make teeth to order through development? J Exp Zool B Mol Dev Evol. 2006;306(3):177-82.
25. Mjör IA, Fejerskov O. Histology of the Human Tooth, 2nd edition. Copenhagen: Munksgaard; 1979.
26. Nanci A. Ten Cate's Oral Histology, Development, Structure, and Functions, 8th edition. India: Elsevier; 2012.
27. Ooe T. Development of human first and second permanent molar, with special reference to the distal portion of the dental lamina. Anat Embryol Berl. 1979;155:221-40.
28. Ooe T. On the early development of human dental lamina. Okajimas Folia Anat Jpn. 1959;32:97-108.
29. Ophir D Klein, Snehlata Oberoi, Ann Huysseune, Maria Hovorakova, Miroslav Peterka, Renata Peterkova. Developmental disorders of the dentition: an update. Am J Med Genet C Semin Med Genet. 2013 November; 163(4)
30. Osborn JW. Relationship between Growth and the Pattern of Tooth Initiation in Alligator Embryos J Dent Res. 1998;77:1730.
31. Robinson C, Kirkham J. Dynamics of amelogenesis as revealed by protein compositional studies. In: Butler WT (Ed). The Chemistry and Biology of Mineralized Tissues. Birmingham, Alabama: EBSCO Media; 1985. pp. 248-63.
32. Schoenwolf G, Bleyl SB, Brauer P. Larsen's Human Embryology, 5th edition. US: Elsevier; 2015.
33. Simpson HE. The degeneration of the rests of malassez with age as observed by the apoxestic technique. J Periodontal. 1965;36:288-91.
34. Thesleff I, Vaahtokari A. The role of growth factors in the determination of odontoblastic cell lineage. Proc Finn Dent Soc. 1992;88:357-68.
35. Trainor PA. Neural Crest Cells. US: Academic Press; 2014.
36. Valderhaug JP, Nylen MU. Function of epithelial rests as suggested by their ultrastructure. J Periodontal Res. 1966;1: 69-78.
37. Warshawsky H, Josephsen K, Thylstrup A, et al. The development of enamel structure in the rat incisor as compared to the teeth of monkey and man. Anat Rec. 1981;200(4):371-99.
38. Wise GE, Marks SC Jr, Cahill DR. Ultrastructural features of the dental follicle associated with the eruption pathway in the dog. Oral Pathol. 1985;14:15-26.

CHAPTER 5

Enamel

Mandana Darafsh Donoghue, B Sivapathasundharam, RJ Vijayashree

Chapter Outline

- ◆ Physical Properties 44
- ◆ Chemical Composition 45
  - » Enamel Proteins 46
- ◆ Structure of Enamel 46
  - » Enamel Rods 46
  - » Dentinoenamel Junction (Amelodentinal Junction) 47
  - » Incremental Lines of Retzius 49
  - » Hunter-Schreger Bands 49
  - » Gnarled Enamel 49
- ◆ Hypomineralized Structures of Enamel 49
  - » Enamel Spindles 49
  - » Enamel Lamellae 50
  - » Enamel Tufts 51
- ◆ Surface Structures of Enamel 51
  - » Enamel Cuticle 51
  - » Aprismatic Enamel 51
  - » Enamel Rod End 51
  - » Surface Defects 52
  - » Perikymata (Imbrication Lines of Pickerill) 52
  - » Acquired Enamel Pellicle 52
- ◆ Amelogenesis 52
- ◆ Age Changes 59
- ◆ Clinical Considerations 59

The tooth is made up of dentin and the projected portion in the oral cavity is covered by the enamel (**Figures 5-1A and B**). Enamel is the hardest substance in the human body and covers the anatomical crown of the tooth. It is the only ectodermal derivative of the tooth, and is formed by the cells called ameloblasts. Also, it is the only epithelial-derived calcified tissue in vertebrates and also the only tissue exposed to mineralization in spite of the absence of blood vessels. Unlike the other hard tissues, the cells responsible for the formation of enamel, the ameloblasts, are lost after amelogenesis (enamel formation). They either die by apoptosis or ultimately become the part of junctional epithelial cells. Similar to other dental hard tissues, enamel is also avascular but does not have collagen fibers in its matrix like other hard tissues.

Increasing hardness equates brittleness, and yet a relatively thin layer of very hard enamel is sufficiently elastic to withstand the impact of the massive forces, encountered during chewing. Ensuring that enamel can withstand great forces is achieved by the inorganic contents and organizational arrangement of the enamel matrix proteins and crystals.

■ PHYSICAL PROPERTIES

The major function of the tooth is mastication and the projected part of the tooth, the crown, takes care of it.

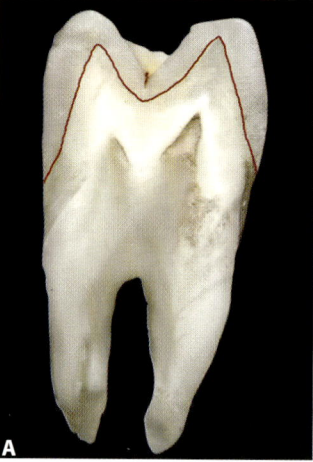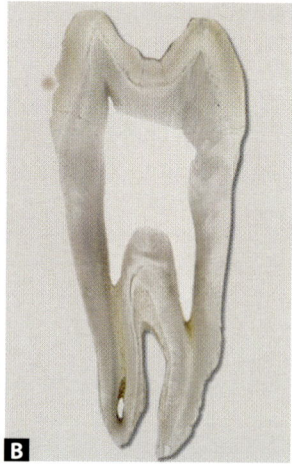

Figures 5-1A and B: (A) Section of a molar to show the enamel; (B) Ground section showing enamel, dentin, and cementum.

The enamel, by having unique physical properties and chemical composition, protects the tooth and bears the masticatory load and transfers it to the underlying resilient dentin. It is translucent and the color ranges from yellowish white to grayish or bluish white. Color of the tooth crown depends on the translucency and thickness of the enamel and

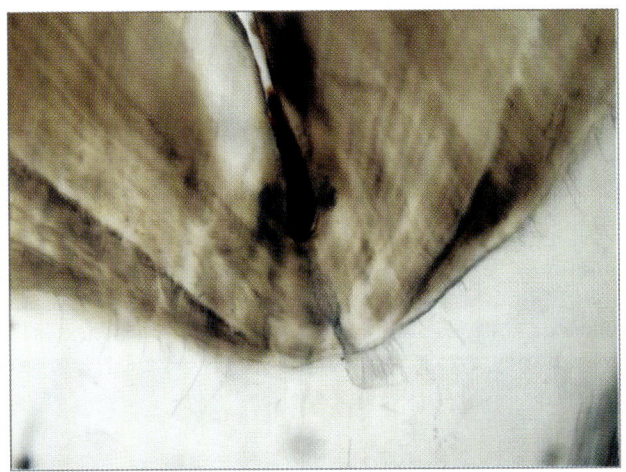

Figure 5-2: Base of a deep fissure having thin enamel.

the color of the underlying dentin. Tooth appears yellowish when the enamel is more translucent, since the underlying dentin is visible through the enamel and grayish in case of opaque enamel. Incisal edges do not contain dentin and have only enamel, which gives them a bluish tinge. Enamel translucency depends on the degree of calcification and homogeneity.

Thickness of enamel varies between persons and between teeth. It even varies from one region of the tooth to the other region. It is thickest at the cusp tips (about 2–2.5 mm) and thinned down to a knife edge at the cervical margin. The occlusal surface of the posterior teeth is not smooth. They have imperfections called pits and fissures. Pit is a pointed depression and fissure is a narrow groove. The enamel may be very thin or even absent at the base of the pits or fissures **(Figure 5-2)**. The specific gravity of enamel is 2.8. The refractive index is 1.62.

CHEMICAL COMPOSITION

Enamel is the highly mineralized hard tissue in the human body. It consists of 96% of inorganic material and 4% of organic material and water **(Flowchart 5-1)**. The inorganic content increases from the dentinoenamel junction (DEJ) to the enamel surface and is in the form of calcium phosphate hydroxyapatite crystal $[Ca_{10}(PO_4)_6(OH)_2]$. These crystals are extremely large, well-oriented, and packed into a rod-like structure. Enamel crystallites, similar to those in other mineralized tissues have a short a-axis and a long c-axis.

The crystal has a central core, the c-axis formed by the hydroxyl ion, around which calcium and phosphorus ions are arranged in the form of triangles **(Figure 5-3)**. This crystal may contain impurities such as carbonate, which replaces phosphate or hydroxyl ion, magnesium can replace calcium, and fluoride may substitute for hydroxyl ion in the crystal lattice. Other ions such as chloride, strontium, lead, zinc, and aluminum if present during amelogenesis, will also be incorporated into the crystals. Hydroxyapatite crystals are hexagonal in cross section. The width of the crystal is about 70 nm and the thickness is about 26 nm **(Figure 5-4)**. The length of the crystals is considered to be very long and some authors believe that the length extends about the entire thickness of the enamel. It is suggested that a minor quantity of non-apatite minerals may also be present in mature enamel. The high mineral content makes the enamel extremely hard and brittle.

The water content of the enamel is about 2% by weight. Water molecules are present between the crystals and surround the organic material. Porosity of the enamel is implicated with its water content.

Organic matrix of the enamel is amorphous and gel-like and occupies 1–2% by weight. It is made up of noncollagenous enamel proteins and proteolytic enzymes. The enamel proteins are divided into two groups, namely amelogenins and non-amelogenins. Amelogenins form 90% of the organic content, while non-amelogenins such as ameloblastin, enamelin, amelotin, and tuftelin form the remaining 10%. In general, the lipid content is meager than the proteins and it resides at striae of Retzius, Hunter-Schreger bands, prism sheath, and core in mature enamel. Lipids of the enamel are

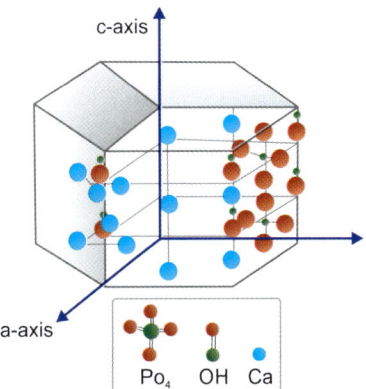

Figure 5-3: Calcium phosphate hydroxyapatite crystal.

Flowchart 5-1: Chemical composition of enamel.

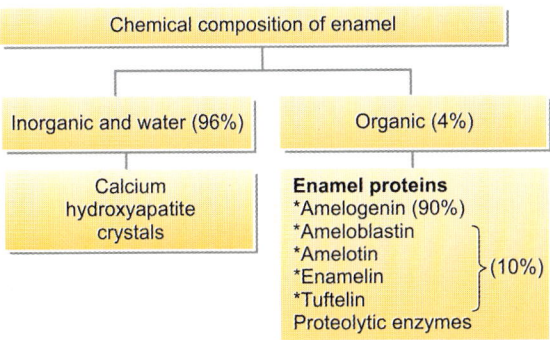

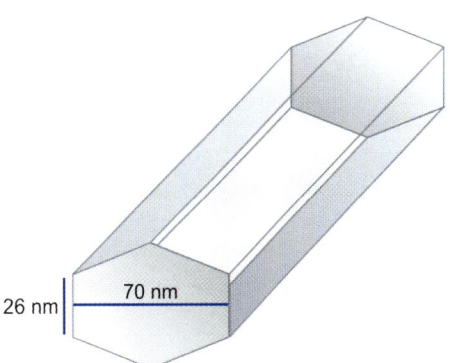

Figure 5-4: Dimension of a calcium phosphate hydroxyapatite crystal of enamel.

thought to be membranous remnants pinched-off from the Tomes' process during amelogenesis. Besides, the proteolytic enzymes of the enamel that break down the proteins are matrix metalloproteinase-20 (MMP-20 or enamelysin) and kallikrein-related peptidase-4 (KLK-4).

Enamel Proteins

The extracellular matrix of enamel contains different proteins and proteolytic enzymes. The main structural proteins include amelogenin, ameloblastin, enamelin, amelotin, and tuftelin. The proteinases that break down the proteins are MMP-20 (or enamelysin) and KLK-4.

Amelogenin and its cleavage products are the major structural protein in enamel constituting 90% of the enamel organic matrix and are rich in proline, histidine, and glutamine. These proteins are low-molecular-weight (20–25 kDa) proteins that are critical for orderly enamel formation by controlling the organization and growth of enamel crystals. Most isoforms of amelogenin can self- assemble into nanospheres that consist of approximately 100 amelogenin molecules and are about 20 nm in diameter. These nanospheres are believed to maintain spaces between the forming and growing crystals of secretory stage enamel. It is also proposed that amelogenin forms a mold in which the initiated crystals elongate.

Ameloblastin (also called sheathlin or amelin) is the second most abundant protein in enamel. It constitutes 5% of the total protein. It is a proline-rich protein of 65 kDa molecular weight. Ameloblastin is believed to have a role in ameloblast differentiation and mineralization because of its adhesion and affinity for calcium. An absence of ameloblastin will lead to detachment of enamel layer and failure of mineralization. Ameloblastin is secreted throughout amelogenesis but is highest in volume during enamel secretion. It is rapidly broken down after secretion and is therefore not found in the older enamel near DEJ.

Enamelin is the largest enamel protein. Nearly one-third of its molecular weight (180–190 kDa) comes from glycosylation. It is rapidly cleaved by proteases post secretion. Since most of the cleavage products are also rapidly broken down, enamelin constitutes only 3–5% of the enamel protein matrix. Intact enamelin is restricted to the mineralization front while the 32 kDa cleavage product is the only form found in the deeper more matured enamel. Enamelin is critical to crystal nucleation and growth; no enamel crystals will form in its absence.

Amelotin is expressed in the maturative stage of amelogenesis. It is a promoter of calcium phosphate mineralization. It plays a critical role in the formation of compact mineralized, aprismatic enamel surface layer during the maturation stage.

Tuftelin is an acidic enamel protein that is thought to play an important role in enamel mineralization during amelogenesis and implicated in dental caries susceptibility. It is also believed to be present in various other soft tissues such as the brain, kidney, eyes, testis, liver, lung and stomach. Therefore, tuftelin is thought to have a wide tissue distribution and to be multifunctional.

Proteases

Matrix metalloproteinase-20, is the protease that cleaves enamel matrix proteins. The cleavage enables the products to move to different areas of the forming enamel, which gives sufficient space for the elongation of the enamel crystallites. MMP-20 is present in the secretory stage of amelogenesis. KLK4 cleaves amelogenin after completion of secretory stage. KLK4 is essential to cleave the amelogenin mold so that it can be removed and the maturing crystallites can interlock and form a cohesive rod structure. KLK4 is present in the maturation stage of amelogenesis.

STRUCTURE OF ENAMEL

Enamel Rods

The structural unit of the enamel is enamel rod or prism and interrod or interprismatic substance. The number of enamel rods per tooth ranges from 5 million to 12 million. It is roughly hexagonal in outline and composed of millions of calcium phosphate hydroxyapatite crystals (**Figures 5-5A and B**). The enamel rods are cylindrical and the long axis of the packed apatite crystals is generally parallel to the long axis of the enamel rods (**Figure 5-5C**). Enamel rods are not very closely packed. There is a space in between the adjacent rods and is known as interrod substance. In this portion the apatite crystals are oriented in such a way that they deviate 40–60° from those in the rod. Each enamel rod is covered by an organic material called rod sheath (**Figure 5-6**).

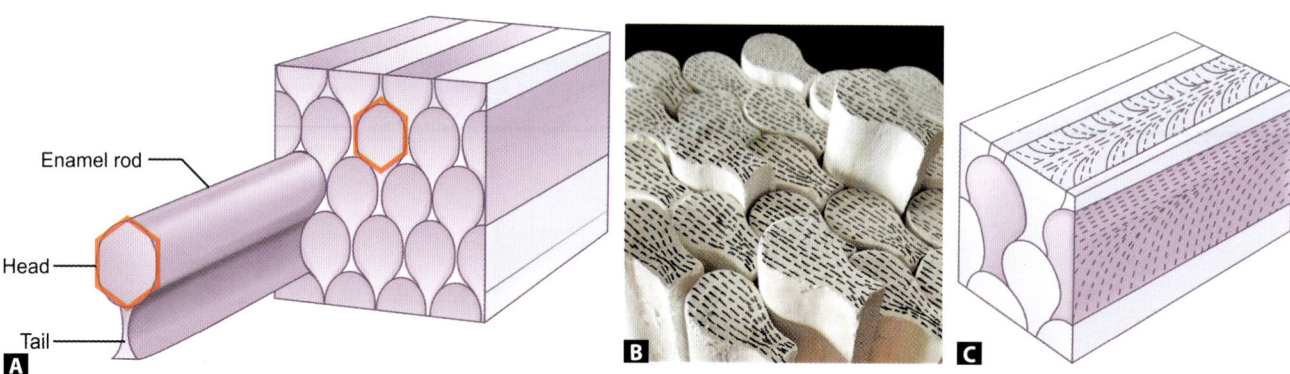

Figures 5-5A and B: (A and B) Roughly hexagonal enamel rods packed with hydroxyapatite crystals; (C) Long axis of the crystals is parallel to the long axis of the enamel rods.

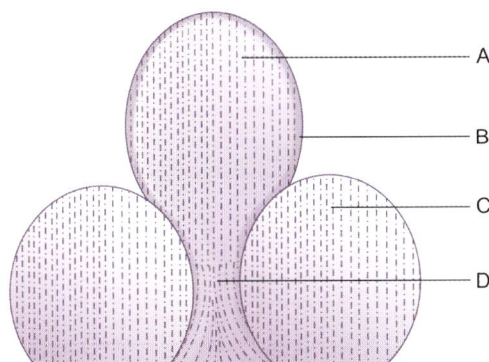

Figure 5-6: Enamel rods: A. Hydroxyapatite crystals; B. Rod sheath; C. Head portion; and D. Tail portion. Tail portion is otherwise called interrod substance, in which the apatite crystals fan out at 40–60°.

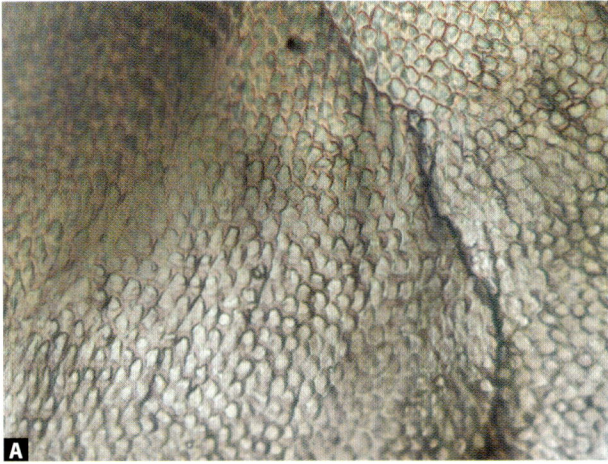
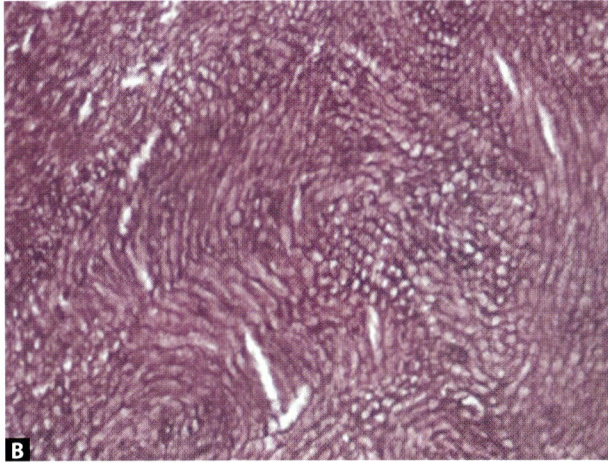

Figures 5-7A and B: Paddle-shaped and fish scale appearance of enamel rods in cross section: (A) Ground section; (B) Decalcified section.

Enamel rods run from DEJ to the surface. The diameter of the enamel rod is about 5–6 μm and the height is about 9 μm. In cross section, enamel rods appear as circular, oval, fish scale, key-hole or paddle-shaped pattern **(Figures 5-7A and B)**. It has a head and tail portion. Head is formed by the enamel rod and the tail portion is by the interrod substance **(Figure 5-6)**. Head of the rod is oriented towards the cuspal or incisal surface and the tail towards the cervical or apical direction **(Figure 5-8)**.

Direction of Enamel Rods

The course of the enamel rods is not straight. They have a wavy or sinusoidal course. The tortuous course of the enamel rods represents the mineralized trail taken by the ameloblast and its Tomes' process as it migrates outward from the DEJ. The length of the enamel rod is more than the thickness of the enamel, since they are obliquely placed **(Figures 5-9A and B)**. They meet the enamel surface at an angle and that may vary depending on the region. In cervical region, they meet the surface at right angle. In occlusal surface, the angle will be around 60°. In the pits or fissures, they form about 20° with the surface.

The surface area of the enamel at the occlusal surface or incisal edge is more than the surface area at the DEJ, but the number of rods is equal in both regions. This is accomplished by the increase in the thickness of the rods from the DEJ towards the surface. They are roughly twice bigger at the enamel surface than at the DEJ.

Cross Striations or Rod Segments

Lines that are present at right angle to the long axis of the enamel rod at about 3–6 μm intervals are called cross striations or rod segmentations **(Figures 5-10A and B)**. There are various views regarding this appearance.

Few believe that this appearance may be due to the variation in the thickness of the rods or a change in the organic matrix or crystal orientation.

Alternate view is that this is an apparent optical phenomenon. When the roughly cylindrical rods are sectioned, the interrod substance region where the apatite crystals are oriented at different fashions, appear like the border between the two adjacent segments. Actually a cross section is misinterpreted as longitudinal section with segmented enamel rods.

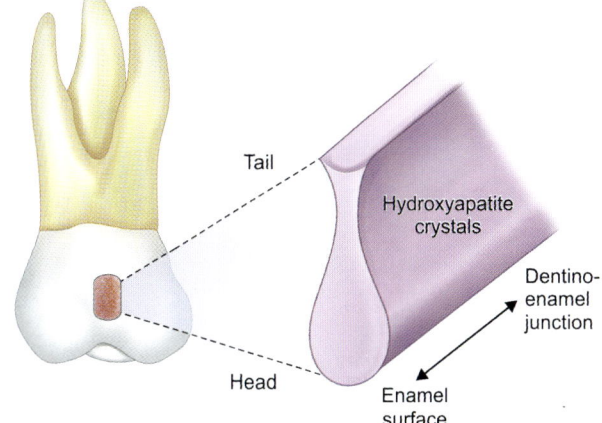

Figure 5-8: Head of the enamel rod facing towards the occlusal aspect and the tail towards the cervical portion of the tooth.

Dentinoenamel Junction (Amelodentinal Junction)

The borderline between enamel and dentin is known as dentinoenamel junction (DEJ). In sections, it appears scalloped with the concavities facing the enamel

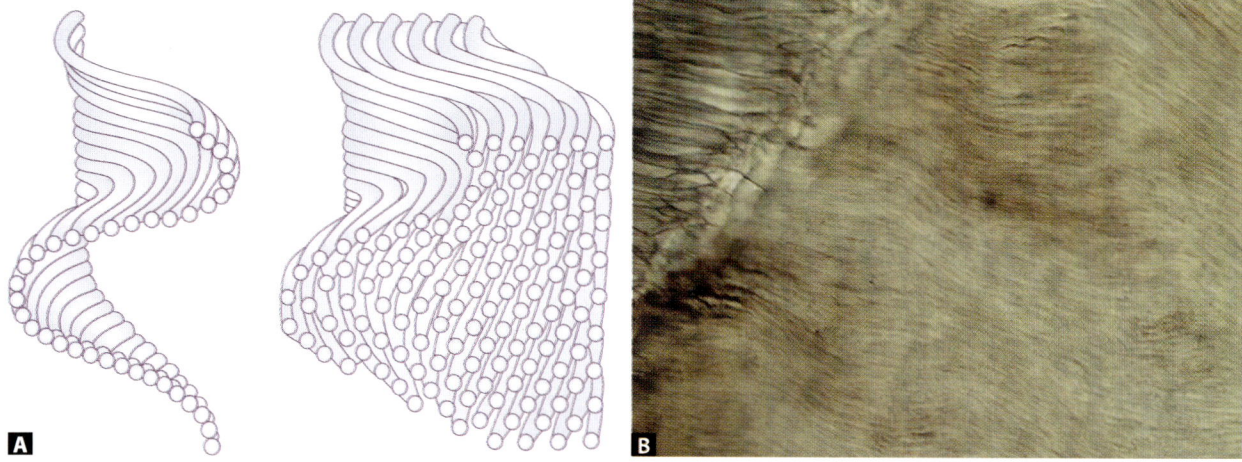

Figures 5-9A and B: Wavy and tortuous course of enamel rods: (A) Schematic representation; (B) Ground section.

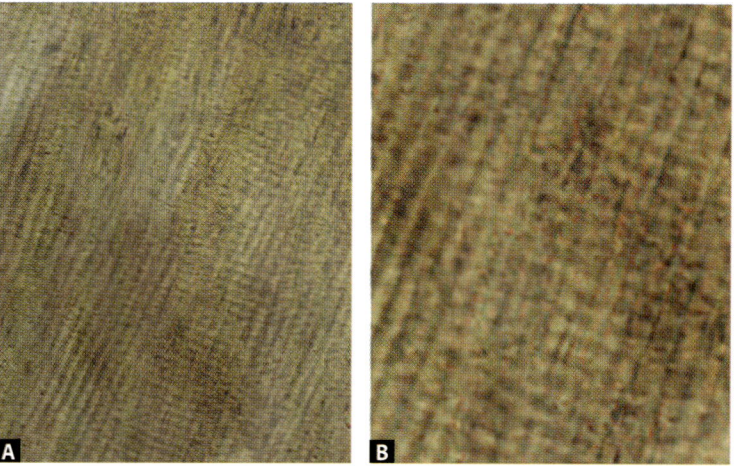

Figures 5-10A and B: Cross striations or segmented appearance of the enamel rods in ground section.

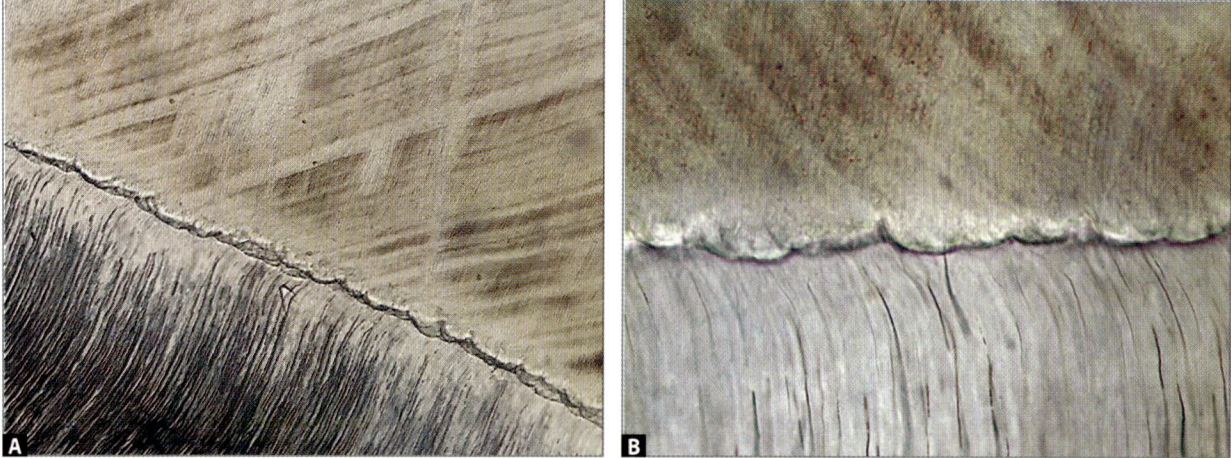

Figures 5-11A and B: Scalloped dentinoenamel junction. Ground section: (A) Low power; and (B) High power.

(**Figures 5-11A and B**). This is more pronounced in the crown. This reflects the fact that the dentinal surface is pitted not smooth, onto which the enamel cap is tightly bound. The dentinal surface of the enamel has rounded projections. These projections fit into the shallow depressions on the dentinal surface. On electron microscopy, the dentinal surface appears to have ridges rather than pits and this arrangement increases the surface area for the firm attachment of the enamel over the dentin and withstands the masticatory stress. Further this prevents the propagation of cracks. In DEJ, the hydroxyapatite crystals of the enamel and dentin intermingle. The DEJ is less mineralized than the rest of the enamel and dentin.

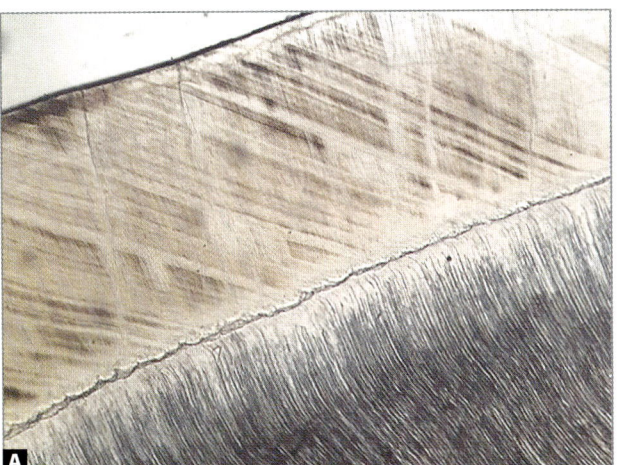
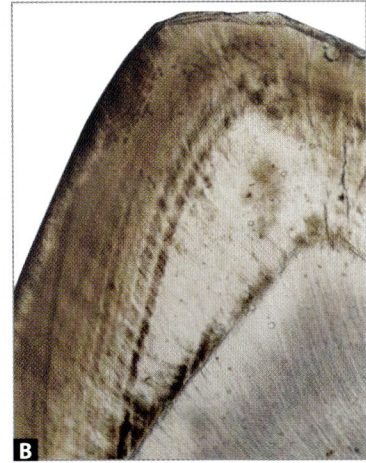

Figures 5-12A and B: (A) Incremental lines of Retzius, running oblique to the dentinoenamel junction in the middle portion of the crown; (B) Concentric circle around the cusp tip.

Incremental Lines of Retzius

Incremental lines are the growth lines that represent a quasi rhythmical deposition pattern of any hard tissue like enamel, dentin, cementum or bone. Incremental lines of enamel were first observed by Dr Retzius and termed them as striae of Retzius. These growth lines run oblique to the DEJ and reflect the enamel deposition at a particular point during amelogenesis **(Figures 5-12A and B)**. These lines are also frequently accredited for the rest period in between two active secretory phases during amelogenesis. This period is not uniform and accounts up to 4–16 days approximately, that attributes to the varying thickness of the lines or bands from 4 μm to 150 μm.

The incremental lines extend throughout the enamel and taper as they move occlusally. In ground sections, under transmitted light, these lines appear brownish and parallel over the dentinal core, and appear bluish white in reflected light. In cross sections, they display a concentric ring pattern closely resembling the annual rings of a tree. These lines may reflect variation in structure and mineralization.

Striae of Retzius have been variously ascribed to, the coinciding of the minute undulations of the enamel rods and variation in organic component or reflecting the physiologic calcification rhythm. The incremental lines are clinically viewed as wavy bands separated by fine furrows on the surface of the enamel, called perikymata in the newly erupted teeth.

Neonatal lines, noticed in deciduous teeth, are the accentuated incremental lines that demarcate the enamel deposited before and after birth. Microscopically both the prenatal and postnatal enamel vary in structure due to the abrupt change in nutrition and environment. Apparently the prenatal enamel is known to have fewer defects compared to the postnatal enamel in general.

Hunter-Schreger Bands

This is an optical effect of enamel and can be appreciated in longitudinal sections under reflected light. These are alternating dark and light bands of varying widths (approximate width 50 μm), produced by the change in orientation or direction between adjacent group of enamel rods, *i.e.* groups of rods bend left or right at a slightly different angle than the adjacent group of rods. They reflect the wavy course of the enamel rods in three-dimensional space for functional adaptation. The groups of rods which are sectioned longitudinally produce the dark band are called as parazones and those groups sectioned transversely to produce the light band are called diazones. These parazones and diazones give the appearance for the bands. Hunter-Schreger bands extend from the DEJ to one-half to two-thirds of the thickness of the enamel **(Figures 5-13A and B)**. In outer quarter of enamel the rods run in same direction, so these bands are not present. In cross section they appear as circular structures. The alternate views regarding the formation of Hunter-Schreger bands are that they occur due to the difference in the permeability and organic content.

Gnarled Enamel

In the cuspal regions, the enamel rods twist around one another to withstand the masticatory load, particularly the shearing force. This arrangement is referred to as gnarled enamel. In histologic sections, they appear to be in a disordered fashion, but this is an apparent one due to the artifact of sectioning **(Figures 5-14A and B)**. In cuspal regions, the enamel rods are in spiral arrangement and appear as intertwined bundles. Another view for the appearance of gnarled enamel is that during the secretory stage the ameloblasts move away from the dentin. They tend to move in groups that slide by one another, resulting in gnarled prism pattern in the molars.

■ HYPOMINERALIZED STRUCTURES OF ENAMEL

Though enamel is a highly mineralized tissue of the tooth, it has inherent hypomineralized areas, namely—enamel spindles, enamel tufts, and enamel lamellae.

Enamel Spindles (Figures 5-15A and B)

They are dark spindle or club-shaped structures of varying length starting from the DEJ perpendicularly and extending

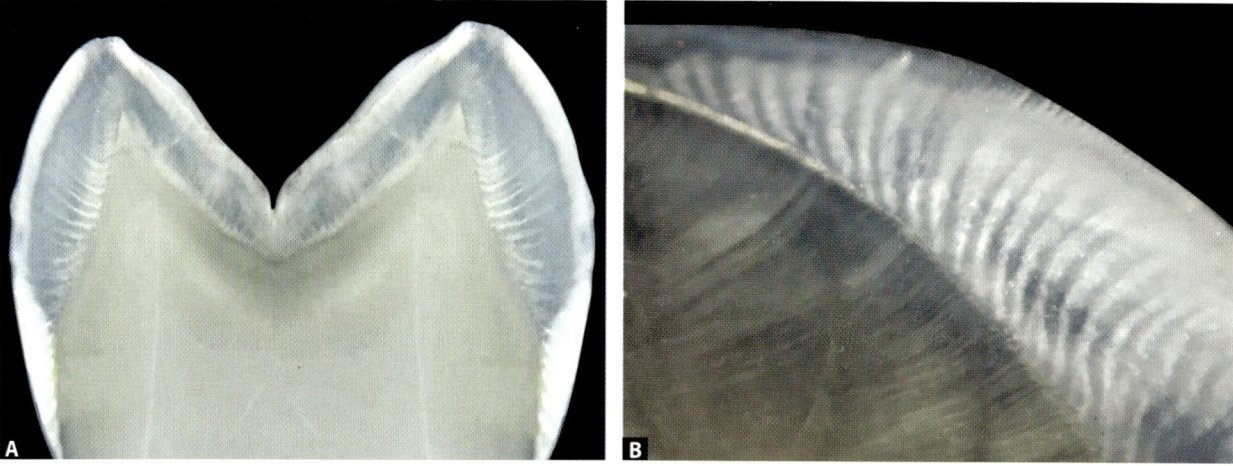

Figures 5-13A and B: Hunter-Schreger bands of enamel in reflected light: (A) Low power; (B) High power.

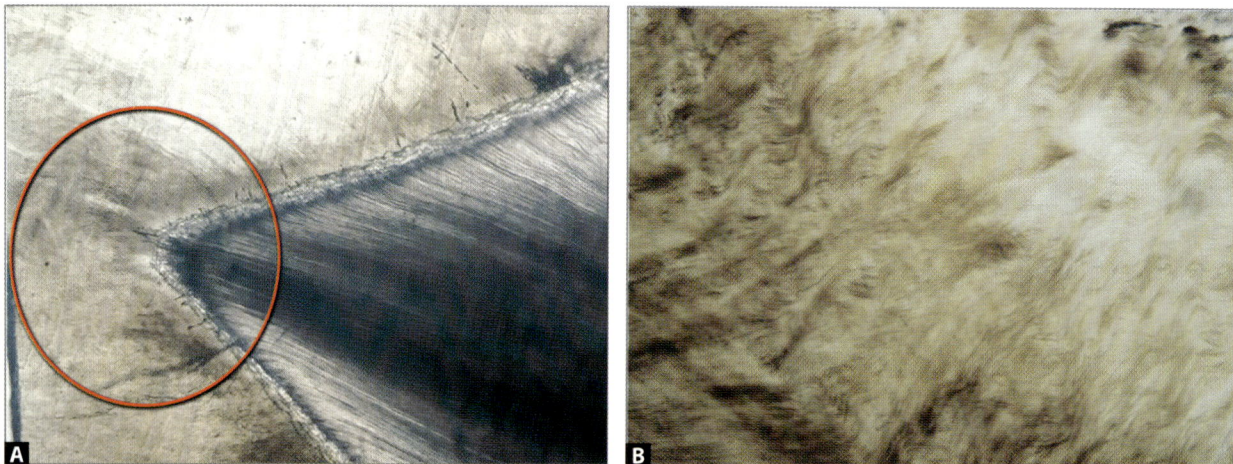

Figures 5-14A and B: Gnarled enamel made up of intertwined enamel rods at the cusp tips: (A) Low power; and (B) High power.

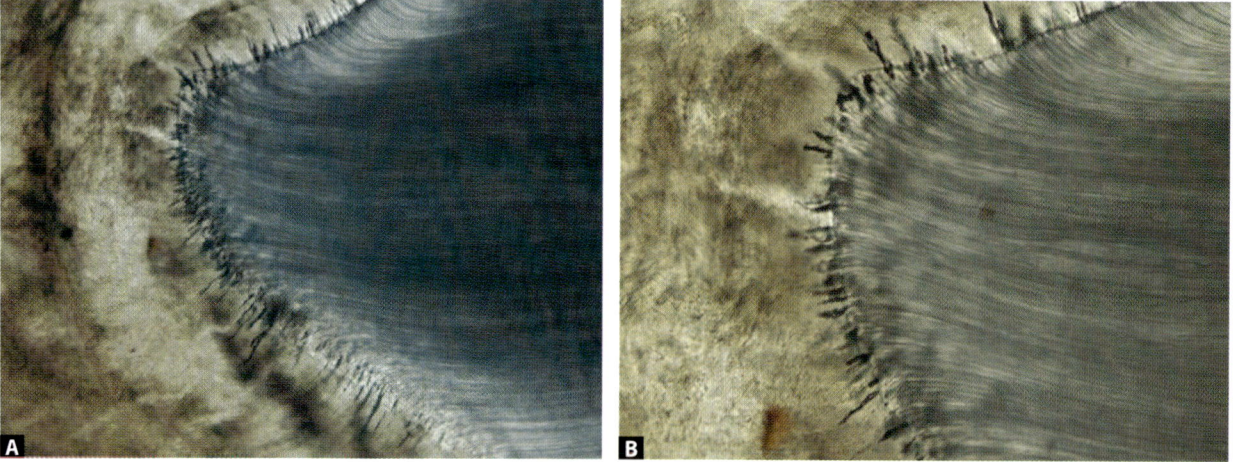

Figures 5-15A and B: Enamel spindles in ground sections: (A) Low power; and (B) High power.

into the enamel (up to 25 μm). Their course may not coincide with the direction of enamel rods and are partially mineralized. They are more at the cuspal region and may be continuous with the dentinal tubules. They are formed by the extension of odontoblastic process before the formation of enamel. Enamel forms around this odontoblastic process and leaves a tubular space. The odontoblastic process within the space may be viable and may contribute to the sensitivity at the DEJ.

Enamel Lamellae

They are thin leaf-like hypomineralized structures that extend from the enamel surface toward the DEJ and sometimes cross the DEJ **(Figures 5-16A and B)**. They were considered to be cracks present in enamel. They are linear longitudinal defects filled with organic material. This organic material is derived from organic

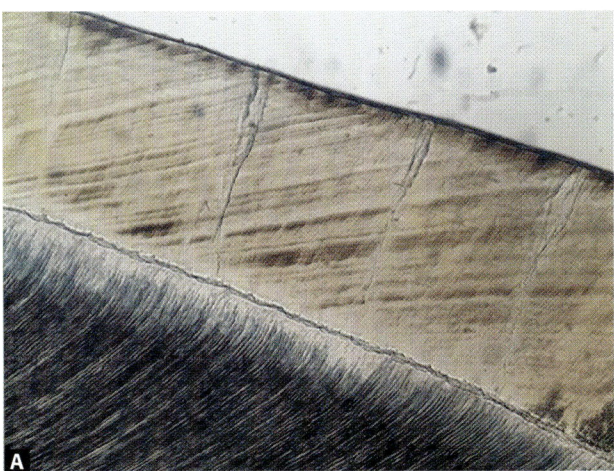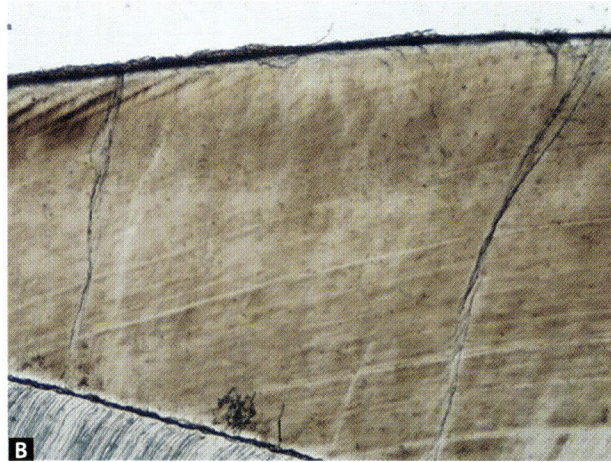

Figures 5-16A and B: Enamel lamellae running from the surface toward the dentinoenamel junction.

substances from the oral cavity in case of erupted tooth and trapped enamel organ component or connective tissue cells surrounding the dental organ in unerupted tooth. They are less common than the enamel tufts and are best visualized in transverse ground sections. Cracks produced during section preparation may resemble enamel lamellae at times. Cracks disappear when the section is decalcified, while the lamellae remain. There are different views regarding the development of enamel lamellae. They are thought to be formed either due to incomplete maturation of enamel rod groups or at areas of tension due to loading of enamel. These may provide pathway for the microbial invasion during the development of dental caries. Three types of enamel lamellae are described as Type A, Type B and Type C. Type A is made up of poorly calcified rod segments and is confined only to the enamel. Type B consists of degenerated cells and type C made up of mucoproteins from the oral cavity. Type B and C extend into the dentin.

Enamel Tufts

They are hypomineralized structures that originate at the DEJ, and resemble a tuft of grass in ground sections **(Figures 5-17A and B)**. They extend approximately up to the inner one-third to one-fifth of the enamel. They are best visualized in transverse sections. Their formation has been attributed to stress and is considered to be a form of defect. These defects in enamel are filled with organic material. They are twisted ribbon-like defects or imperfections. The appearance of the tuft is an apparent one as the defect does not start from a single point; rather the imperfections lie in more than one plane and heading toward different directions, which give the tuft-like appearance in thick sections. Enamel tufts are made up of hypomineralized enamel rods and interrod substance. On electron microscopy they exhibit tubular structures with cross striations. The spaces are filled with organic material termed enamelin. According to one view, the major organic substance of the enamel tuft is sheathlin, a 13–17 kDa sheath protein.

SURFACE STRUCTURES OF ENAMEL

Enamel Cuticle

Primary enamel cuticle of approximately 30 nm thickness is the basal lamina interposed between the reduced enamel epithelium and the enamel. This basal lamina is the end product of ameloblasts and enables the attachment of the reduced enamel epithelium to the formed enamel. The reduced enamel epithelium and the basal lamina together constitute the Nasmyth's membrane. This will be lost as tooth erupts by the degeneration of the epithelial cells. It is also lost due to attrition and abrasion.

Surface enamel physically and chemically differs from the subsurface enamel. Surface enamel is harder, less permeable, less soluble, and more radiopaque than the subsurface enamel.

Aprismatic Enamel

The enamel surface of approximately 30 μm, near the cervical region does not contain usual enamel rods, instead is made up of rodless enamel otherwise known as aprismatic or prismless enamel. This is the final product of the ameloblasts, formed after the loss of the distal portion of Tomes' process (a cone-shaped cytoplasmic extension of ameloblast through which the enamel matrix is discharged) and is more mineralized than the rest of the enamel. Here the calcium phosphate hydroxyapatite crystals do not form the typical enamel rods. The apatite crystals are parallel to each other and perpendicular to the incremental lines of Retzius. This aprismatic enamel is seen in all deciduous teeth and 70% of the permanent teeth.

Enamel Rod End

The enamel rod ends at the surface appear concave. The depth of the concavity varies from region to region. They are deeper at the incisal edges and occlusal surfaces and shallower in the cervical region. Indentations with a diameter of about 6 μm are considered to be the incomplete enamel rods formation caused by the premature retraction of the Tomes' processes

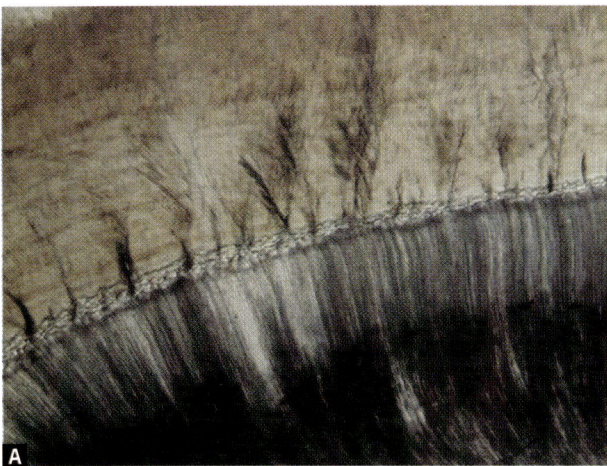
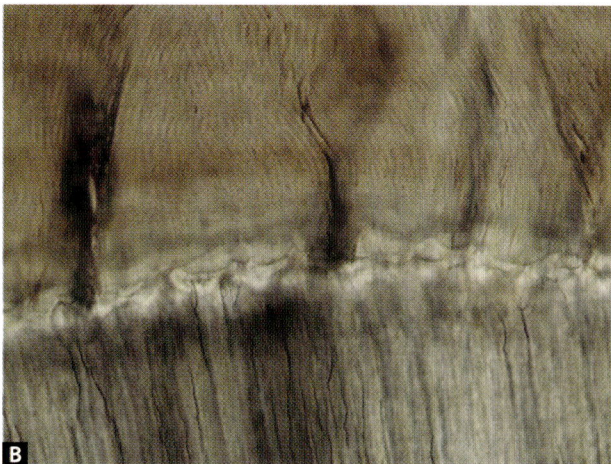

Figures 5-17A and B: Enamel tufts in: (A) Low power; and (B) High power.

(they were the space occupied by the Tomes' process of the ameloblast).

Surface Defects

The surface enamel of unerupted and newly erupted teeth exhibits many irregularities, which can be well appreciated by scanning electron microscopy. These include fine fissures, tiny pits, and micro craters. These are caused by local disturbances during amelogenesis and are more common in the central portion of the smooth surface of the crown.

Surface elevations with a diameter of about 10–15 µm are formed by the enamel deposition over a non-mineralizable debris during development. These are called enamel caps. These may be lost by attrition or abrasion and expose the depressions called "focal holes". Larger elevations with the diameter of about 30–50 µm may be seen in premolars. They are called enamel broaches **(Figure 5-17C)**. They are made up of radiating groups of hydroxyapatite crystals. Minute surface cracks found on the enamel represent the areas of weakness. The extension of the cracks depends on the orientation of the enamel rods to the surface. If the rods form acute angle with the surface, the cracks do not progress further. The cracks are also considered to be the outer edges of enamel lamellae.

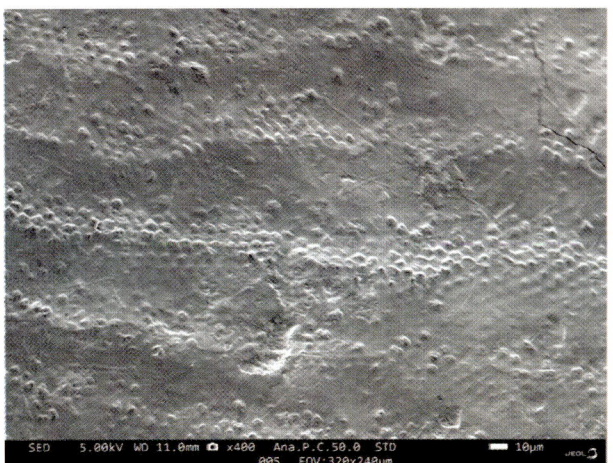

Figure 5-17C: Scanning electron microscopic appearance of enamel broach.

Perikymata (Imbrication Lines of Pickerill)

They are closely packed wavy, transverse ridges separated by fine grooves present in the surface of the enamel and are parallel to the cementoenamel junction. They can be appreciated by the naked eye and are more prominent in newly erupted teeth **(Figure 5-18A)**. They form a complete circle around the crown except near the cervical portion as they are interrupted by cementoenamel junction, and are considered to be the external manifestation of incremental lines of Retzius **(Figure 5-18B and C)**. The grooves correspond to the intersection of lines of Retzius with the surface of the enamel. Near the occlusal region they are less in number due to the wide space between them and are closely packed near the cervical region (approximately 30 per mm). Further the width of the ridges decreases from occlusal to cervical. They may be removed in course of time due to attrition and abrasion.

Acquired Enamel Pellicle

It is a thin film of organic material covering the erupted teeth. This is derived from the salivary proteins **(Flowchart 5-2)**.

AMELOGENESIS

Formation of enamel is called amelogenesis. A complex series of coordinated cellular, morphological, and functional changes and movements is involved in the production of enamel.

The cells that form enamel are called ameloblasts. These cells are of epithelial origin and differentiate from the inner enamel epithelium of the enamel organ during the late bell stage **(Figures 5-19A and B)**. In humans, the formation of enamel starts in the third trimester at the cusp tip or incisal edge of developing teeth. Enamel formation occurs one layer at a time in an apical and outward direction **(Figure 5-20)**. The ameloblasts follow a path that is outward and sideways sliding by each other as they move away from the dentin, producing the characteristic intertwined pattern.

The process of amelogenesis broadly involves a secretory stage where ameloblasts secrete and partly mineralize the

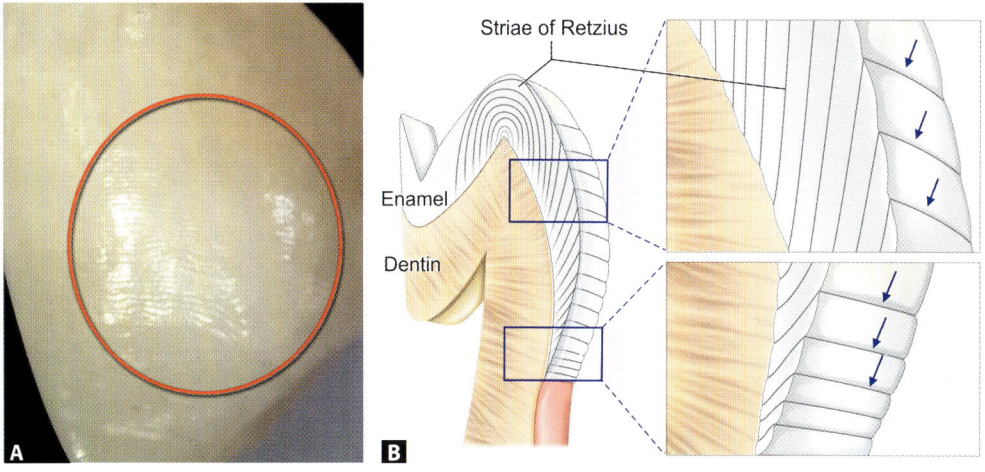

Figures 5-18A and B: Perikymata on labial surface of canine.

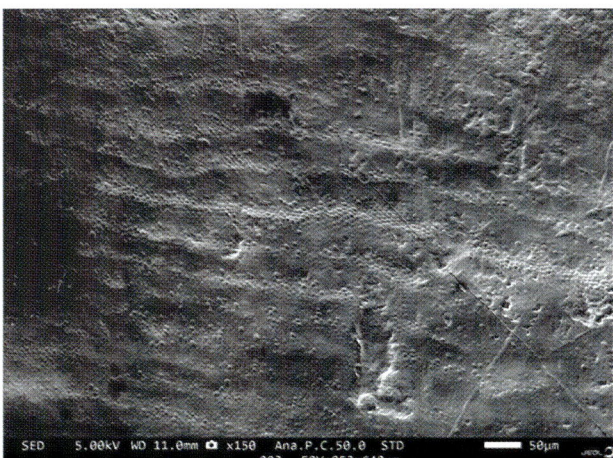

Figure 5-18C: Scanning electron microscopic appearance of perikymata.

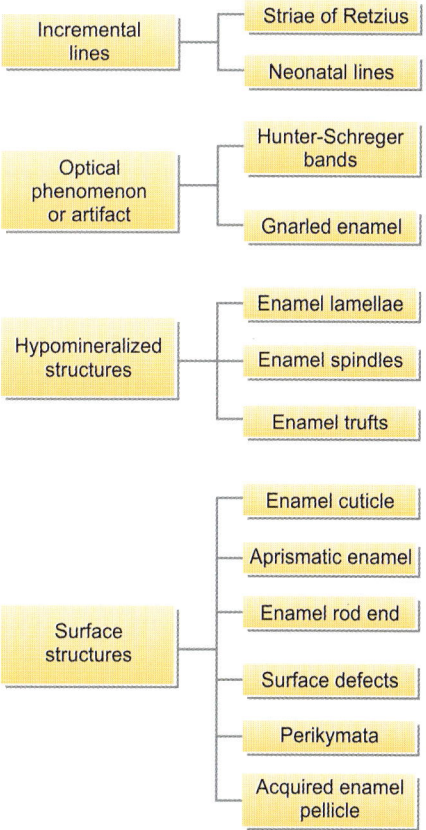

Flowchart 5-2: Summary of enamel structure.

enamel and a maturation stage, where proteins and water are removed from the matrix and replaced by minerals to produce the hardest substance in the human body. A short pre-secretory stage prepares the cells for their specialized role through final differentiation of inner enamel epithelial cells to pre-ameloblasts and ameloblasts, and a transition stage prepares the cells for the maturative role. The complete formation and mineralization of enamel which is approximately 2.5 mm thick, can take up to 6 years.

The process that brings about this level of mineralization is achieved through a series of cellular, physiologic, and chemical processes that are reflected in the life cycle of the ameloblasts.

Ameloblast Life Cycle and Amelogenesis

Presecretory stage	Morphogenetic stage
	Differentiation stage
Secretory stage	Aprismatic enamel secretion
	Prismatic enamel secretion
Transitional stage	
Maturation stage	
Post- maturation stage	Protective stage
Desmolytic stage	

Presecretory Stage (Morphogenetic and Differentiation Stage)

This is a short yet essential stage that makes amelogenesis possible through two distinct phases. The first phase is the morphogenic phase. During the bell stage, the crown shape of the tooth is determined by the growth and infolding of the inner enamel epithelial cells based on their interactions with the dental papilla cells derived from ectomesenchyme. The finalization of the tooth morphology prepares the template upon which hard tissues of the crown namely— dentin and enamel will be formed.

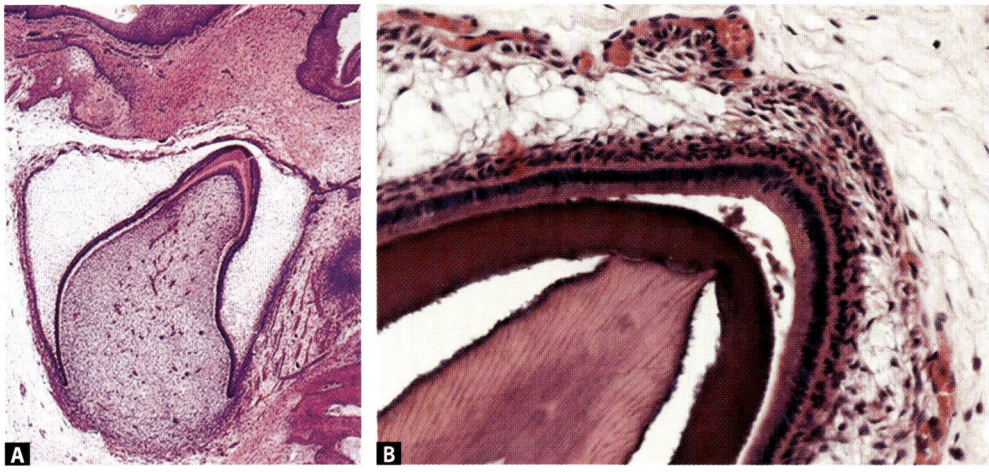

Figures 5-19A and B: Late bell stage.
Source: (A) Dr Pratibha Ramani, Saveetha Dental College, Chennai, India; (B) Adapted from Oral Pathology India by Mandana Donoghue, http://www.oralpath.in.

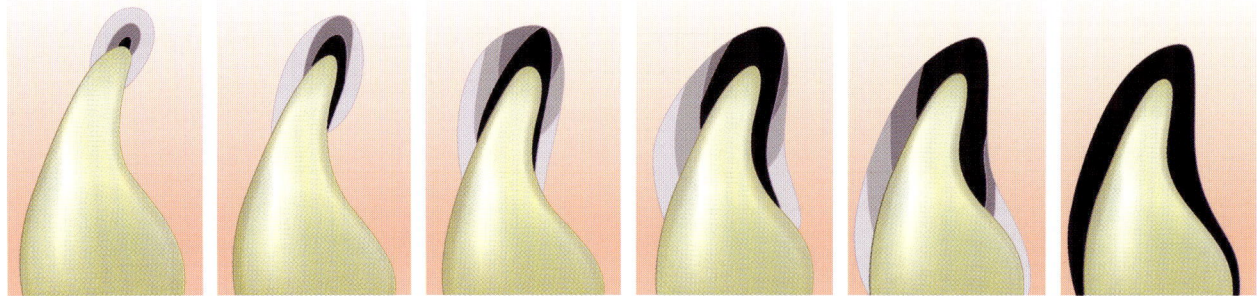

Figure 5-20: Enamel matrix formation and mineralization starts from the tip of the cusp and progresses cervically.

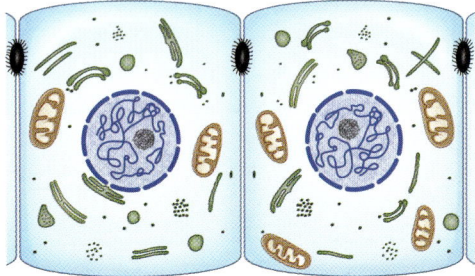

Figure 5-21: Ameloblasts in presecretory stage.

At this point, the inner enamel epithelial cells, which take an active part in the morphogenic phase are undifferentiated and can undergo mitosis. The cells are cuboidal to low columnar with large central nuclei, poorly developed Golgi apparatus, and a junctional complex at the proximal end of the cell towards the stratum intermedium **(Figure 5-21)**.

The second phase is the differentiation phase, which begins after dentin formation commences. Reacting to stimuli produced by the differentiated odontoblasts, the inner enamel epithelial cells stop multiplying and undergo a series of morphologic and functional changes that lead to their differentiation into pre-ameloblasts. Polarization is essential for an epithelial cell to perform its function. Therefore, ameloblasts also undergo polarization in the presecretory stage.

Cell polarization is a complex process, in which there is interaction between the cytoskeletal components of the cells particularly microfilaments and microtubules, extra- and intracellular signals and organelles. This makes the cells to perform specialized functions by distinct structural orientations or protein localization.

Polarization of the amelolasts is mediated by *AT-rich sequence-binding protein-1 (STAB1)* gene. Amelogenin, ameloblastin and *shh* signaling are also vital for polarization.

The inner enamel epithelial cells elongate to accommodate increasing amount of Golgi apparatus and rough endoplasmic reticulum (rER), in preparation for enamel secretion and partial mineralization. The nuclei and mitochondria of these pre-ameloblasts move to the proximal end of the cells toward stratum intermedium. The Golgi apparatus moves close to the nucleus and an additional junctional complex develops at the distal end of the cells **(Figure 5-22)**. The distal junctional complex divides the cell into a body containing the organelles and a secreting end. The junctional complexes which encircle the cells hold the cells tightly together and determine what passes between the cells. Proximal end of the pre-ameloblasts are attached by the desmosomes to the stellate reticulum. Apical end is attached by hemidesmosomes to the basal lamina.

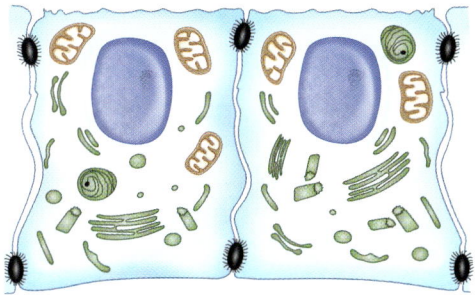

Figure 5-22: Ameloblasts in differentiation stage.

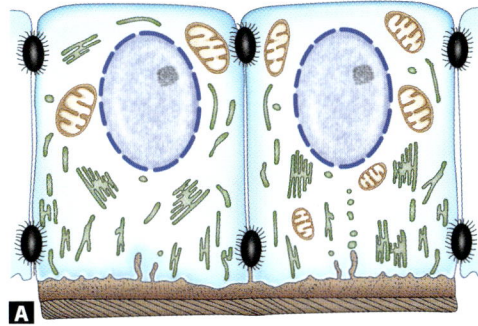

By the late bell stage, odontoblasts have laid down the first layer of dentin; pre-ameloblasts secrete proteins that include dentin sialophosphoprotein (DSPP) on this matrix.

Just before the mineralization begins, pre-ameloblasts breakdown the basal lamina separating them from the predentin and thereby establish the future DEJ.

Secretory Stage (Formative Stage)

Preameloblasts undergo final differentiation to enamel-secreting ameloblasts as soon as the basal lamina separating them from predentin is lost. The formation and mineralization of the first layer of dentin cut off the nutritional supply of the differentiated ameloblasts from the blood vessels of the dental papilla. The enamel organ is altered to receive nutrition from the blood vessels in the dental sac in a process referred to as reversal of nutrition. Further compensation is achieved by the collapse of the stellate reticulum, which reduces the distance between the blood vessels invaginating the outer enamel epithelium and the ameloblasts.

The secretory ameloblast increases markedly in length to accommodate the increasing volume of endoplasmic reticulum, Golgi apparatus, and mitochondria required for the proteosecretory and mineral transportation role of the secretory cell.

The ameloblast at this stage is a tall columnar cell, approximately 40 μm in length and 4 μm in diameter. The cell reverses its polarity with the nucleus moving to the proximal end of the cell near the stratum intermedium. The Golgi apparatus moves around the nucleus to take a supranuclear position and mitochondria are scattered in the cell with a higher concentration at the poles, especially the proximal pole. Proximal and distal cell junctions connect the cells to each other **(Figures 5-23A and B)**.

The first layer of enamel is secreted rapidly from the functional end at the distal extremity of the cell. The ameloblasts secrete large amounts of enamel matrix proteins namely—amelogenin, ameloblastin, enamelin, and enamelysin into irregularities on the predentin surface. Secretory stage enamel is rich in proteins and has a cheese-like consistency. Enamel mineralization begins within these irregularities by heterogeneous or epitactic nucleation (mineral crystal formation due to seeding by some other substances, which is similar to hydroxyl apatite) and progresses as long thin ribbons of enamel mineral that are formed almost immediately as the ameloblast lays down enamel matrix. The first mineral is an amorphous calcium phosphate, which later

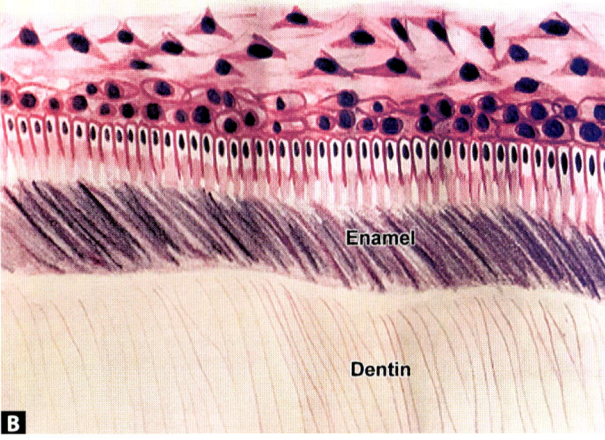

Figures 5-23A and B: Ameloblasts in secretory stage become elongated with nucleus moves proximally (toward stratum intermedium).

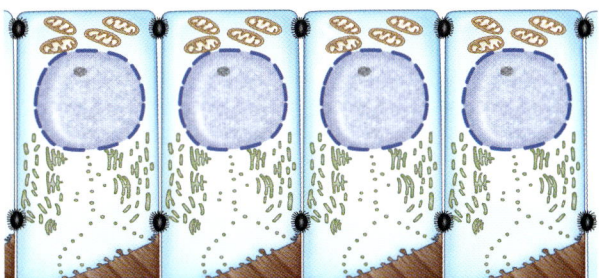

Figure 5-24: Ameloblasts with Tomes' process.

becomes crystalline apatite. Hydroxyapatite crystals grow perpendicular to the secreting face of the ameloblast forming structureless aprismatic enamel with parallel crystals that are not uniform or well-arranged.

After the aprismatic or rodless enamel has been laid down, the ameloblasts begin their synchronized movement away from the dentin. As the cells migrate, they develop a cytoplasmic projection called the Tomes' process, which is responsible for the unique prismatic structure of enamel with a discernible rod and interrod architecture and the indentation of the enamel surface **(Figure 5-24)**. Initially, the Tomes' process has only a proximal portion extending from the distal junctional complex to the surface of the enamel; later as the cells move, the proximal portion lengthens to form the distal portion of Tomes' process. The Tomes' process organizes the enamel crystals into rod and interrod by a two-compartment protein secretion and mineralization fronts that are angled in relation to each other.

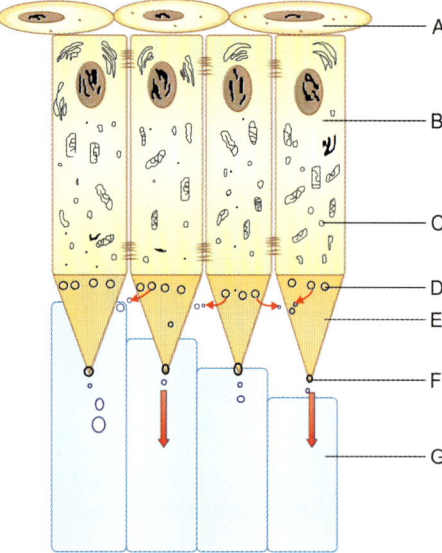

Figure 5-25: Ameloblasts with Tomes' process, A. Stratum intermedium; B. Ameloblast; C. Secretory granule; D. Proximal secretory site; E. Tomes' process; F. Distal secretory site, and G. Enamel.

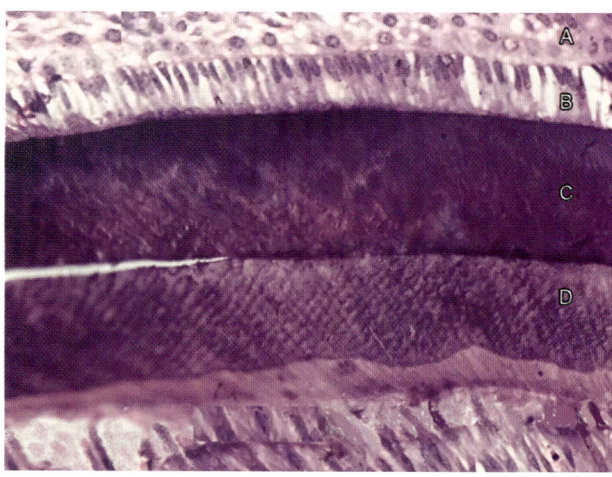

Figure 5-26: Ameloblasts at an angle to the secreted enamel. A. Stratum intermedium; B. Ameloblasts; C. Enamel, and D. Dentin.

Protein and minerals intended to form the interrod enamel exit the ameloblast near the base of the Tomes' process, called proximal secretory sites. Those involved in the rod formation exit the cell near the tip (distal secretory site) at the secretory face of the Tomes' process **(Figure 5-25)**.

> Tomes' process is a six-sided pyramid or cone-shaped projection extending from the secretory or distal end of the ameloblast **(Figure 5-24)**. These asymmetric cellular projections have two parts, a proximal portion and a distal portion. The proximal portion of Tomes' process is the shoulder that is created by the meeting of the cell walls at the distal junctional attachments while the distal portion is the angled pyramidal or cone-shaped extension that protrudes past the proximal portion creating a picket fence-like appearance.
>
> Only one surface of each cell's distal portion of Tomes' process is the secretory surface and rows of neighboring ameloblasts secrete enamel matrix and mineral from the same side of the process. The Tomes' processes arrange the enamel into rod and interrod by sequential formation of enamel and differential orientation of the secreting surface. Enamel secretion occurs first at proximal portion of Tomes' process perpendicular to the cell, thereby making a crypt or wall at the shoulder between the projections with crystals that are perpendicular to the secreting surface; this interconnected framework becomes the interrod enamel. Next the crypts are filled by enamel secretion from the angular distal portion of Tomes' process forming the rod enamel. The secretory surface of the distal portion is at an angle to the proximal portion and therefore enamel matrix formed in this part although perpendicular to the secretory surface, is at an angle to the enamel formed by the proximal portion **(Figure 5-26)**. This variation in the enamel rod arrangement brings about the rod–interrod or prismatic–interprismatic arrangement of enamel.

Each rod is the product of a single ameloblast while three ameloblasts form the interrod substance or the tail portion of the enamel rod **(Figure 5-27)**. The crystals continue to grow as long, thin, and parallel ribbons until the entire thickness of enamel has been formed. Secretory enamel is mineralized

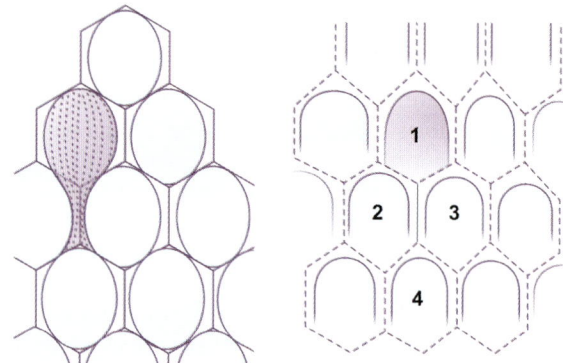

Figure 5-27: Head of the rod is formed by one ameloblasts while the tail portion is contributed by three ameloblasts.

to a level of 10–20% mineral by volume. The mineral is added by daily increments of 4 μm. Structurally the daily increments can be recognized as cross-striations and the more prominent weekly increments are seen as incremental lines of Retzius.

As the distal portion of Tomes' process secretes enamel matrix proteins into the cavity created by the proximal portion of Tomes' process and the cells move away, the process becomes longer and progressively thinner until it is completely lost. The space it leaves behind is filled with organic matter seen as the rod sheath that separates the rod and interrod enamel along the nonsecretory surface of Tomes' process.

The breakdown products of proteins removed for partial mineralization of the secretory stage enamel will either accumulate in the enamel or is reabsorbed by the ameloblasts.

Transitional Stage

As the enamel nears its full thickness, the secretory stage of the ameloblast cell ends while, cells prepare for their maturative or mineralization role. The transition stage ameloblasts stop moving and lose their Tomes' processes. These cells form the final layer of enamel from the same part of the cell surface that formed the initial aprismatic layer. The final layer is also aprismatic and smoothens the outer surface of the rods and forms a continuum with the initial aprismatic layer and the inter-prismatic enamel.

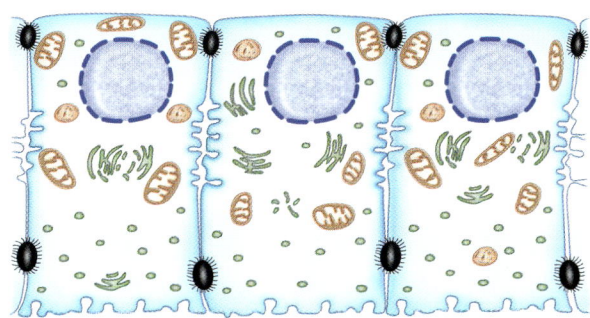

Figure 5-28: Ameloblasts in transitional stage.

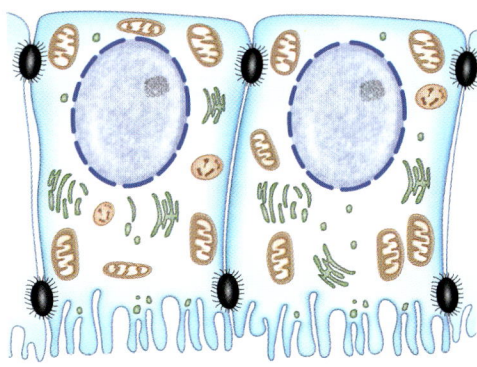

Figure 5-29: Ameloblasts with ruffled border.

Transitional ameloblasts secrete a basal lamina on the enamel that is similar to other basal lamina with the difference that it contains the molecular components amelotin and odontogenic ameloblast-associated protein (ODAM). This structurally and functionally unique glycoconjugate-rich basal lamina is attached to the ameloblasts via hemidesmosomes. It has special adhesive and charge-selective functions and regulates the movement of materials and relays information about the enamel to the cells. Further it provides firm attachment between the ameloblasts and the enamel, which will form dentogingival junction in future.

The transitional ameloblast reduces in height and increases in width **(Figure 5-28)**. Additionally, up to 25% of ameloblasts die during the transition stage, reducing the secretory stage 1:1 ratio between the ameloblasts and rods to 1:1.3 by the end of the transition stage. Reduced number of ameloblasts causes the remaining cells to spread out over the surface slowly. This causes loss of row organization with cells shifting to a polygonal shape. Simultaneously the stratum intermedium becomes a single layer along with the previously collapsed stellate reticulum and the outer enamel epithelium. Capillaries from the dental sac form a layer called the papillary layer because of similarity to histological appearance of papillae.

Maturation Stage

After completion of prismatic enamel and formation of the aprismatic surface layer by transitional stage ameloblasts, the enamel crystals stop growing in length.

At this point, mineral content of enamel is 10–20% by volume; further, increase to over 95% occurs by progressive replacement of matrix proteins and water with calcium phosphate.

The maturation process is directed by ameloblasts, which go through cycles of morphologic and functional changes called modulation. During the cycles, ameloblasts periodically produce and then shed ruffled apical membranes **(Figure 5-29)**. The ruffle-ended cell has infolded membrane with irregular cytoplasmic extensions. The ruffle-ended cell supports electrolyte exchange and mineralization while the smooth-ended cell's function is protein absorption, water removal, and cell recovery.

The smooth-ended ameloblasts secrete kallikrein-related peptidase-4 (KLK4) to breakdown the remaining enamel protein matrix. KLK4 helps the ameloblasts to reabsorb the water and peptides hydrolyzed from enamel matrix proteins. Endocytosis removes the protein fragments and the space that is freed up is used for increased mineral deposition by the growth of rod and interrod crystals in width and thickness. The ruffle-ended ameloblasts move calcium, phosphate, and bicarbonate ions into the matrix to enable the crystal growth. The developing crystals are not homogeneous, with some crystals such as those containing bicarbonate are less acid-resistant than others. Significantly the maturation stage modulations cause the pH of the fluid surrounding the crystals to cycle from less than 6 during the ruffle-ended part of the cycle to 7.2 during the smooth-ended part. The less acid-resistant high carbonate containing crystals are selectively dissolved and replaced during the low pH part of the cycle. On the other hand, the near neutral pH during the smooth-ended cycle stabilizes the crystals and prevents reverse demineralization of crystals.

Post-maturation (Protective Stage)

Ameloblasts undergo further changes in morphology and function after enamel maturation **(Figure 5-30)**. They become flattened and together with the shrunken remnants of the enamel organ called the reduced enamel epithelium, which along with the basal lamina form the Nasmyth's membrane. This membrane covers the tooth crown until eruption, at

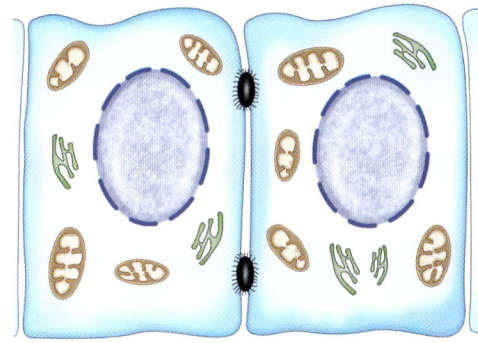

Figure 5-30: Ameloblasts in maturation stage.

which point it undergoes another change and becomes the junctional epithelium. The function of Nasmyth's membrane is to prevent enamel surface exposure to dental sac cells, which would bring about the formation of a layer of cementum on the enamel. Additionally, the Nasmyth's membrane and the papillary layer formed by the dental sac are responsible for the inflectionless eruption of teeth.

Desmolytic Stage

The reduced enamel epithelium produces proteases and other desmolytic enzymes, which degrade the connective tissue between the erupting tooth and the oral epithelium. The broken down products are phagocytosed by the epithelial cells.

Mineralization

The mineral phase of enamel like the other mineralized tissues (bone, dentin, and cementum) is a crystal similar to calcium apatite. Enamel differs significantly from the other mineralized tissues by being the only epithelium produced hard tissue and by mineralization level of above 96%.

The enamel mineral that is mostly carbonated hydroxyapatite nucleates by heterogeneous nucleation in a tissue-specific microenvironment from crystals initiated in dentin. The degree of mineralization is dependent on the supersaturation of the surrounding fluid with calcium and phosphate, which is under the influence of a large number of matrix proteins. The mineral supersaturation is achieved by active transport, cell membrane carrier proteins, and movement of minerals across concentration gradients.

Crystallites are initially flat and ribbon-like but become hexagonal or rhomboidal after maturation.

> The smallest unit of apatite in enamel is a crystallite with submicroscopic size. Enamel crystallites like those in other mineralized tissues have a short a-axis and a long c-axis however unlike other mineralized tissue, the enamel crystallites are very long ranging up to 100 μm in length. Up to 10,000 crystallites coalesce to make a single prism.

Crystals in first formed aprismatic enamel are irregular in size, shape, and organization. These crystals grow in length under the control of amelogenin nanospheres. These protein nanospheres maintain spaces between growing crystals and prevent their fusion during the secretory stage mineralization.

By the time maturation is taking place, the matrix proteins do not have an essential role since they are degraded long before crystal growth ends.

> ### Ameloblast Life Cycle and Amelogenesis
>
> *Morphogenetic stage*: Ameloblasts originate from the inner enamel epithelium (**Figure 5-31A**).
>
> *Differentiation stage*: Inner enamel epithelial cells differentiate to preameloblasts by increase in height to accommodate increase in synthetic organelles. The cells develop distal junctional attachments, and reverse their polarity. The position of DEJ is determined with formation of first layer of dentin. The basal lamina begins to break down (**Figure 5-31B**).
>
> *Secretory stage (aprismatic enamel)*: Complete breakdown of the basal lamina and contact with the mineralizing dentin marks the beginning of the secretory stage and conversion of preameloblasts to secretory ameloblasts that secrete the initial aprismatic or rodless enamel into uneven surface of the freshly laid dentin (**Figure 5-31C**).
>
> *Secretory stage (prismatic enamel)*: Ameloblasts develop an asymmetric conical projection at their distal end called the Tomes' process with proximal and distal secretory sites. The differences in the heights and angulation of the secretory surface of the proximal and distal extensions of the Tomes' process create the prismatic arrangement that characterizes enamel (**Figure 5-31D**).
>
> *Transitional stage*: As enamel thickness nears completion, the cells lose the Tomes' process, reduce in height and synthetic organelles, and produce a specialized basal lamina. The final aprismatic layer of enamel is formed and the enamel crystals stop growing in length (**Figure 5-31E**).
>
> *Maturation stage*: After completion of the full thickness of the enamel, maturation begins by a cell-controlled process of water and protein removal and mineral addition. The ameloblast achieves this dual function by a process called modulation in which the cell goes from being smooth-ended ameloblast involved in the removal of water and protein, to being ruffle-ended ameloblast and increasingly mineralizing the enamel. The cycles continue until the mineral content reaches 95% (**Figure 5-31F**).
>
> *Protective stage*: Post-maturation ameloblasts reduce in numbers, height, and amount of organelles. These cells become a part of the reduced enamel epithelium and form a protective layer on the newly formed enamel surface (**Figure 5-31G**).
>
> *Desmolytic stage*: Reduced enamel epithelium, which contains ameloblasts, secretes desmolytic enzymes, degrades the connective tissue between the formed tooth and the oral epithelium, and helps in the eruption.

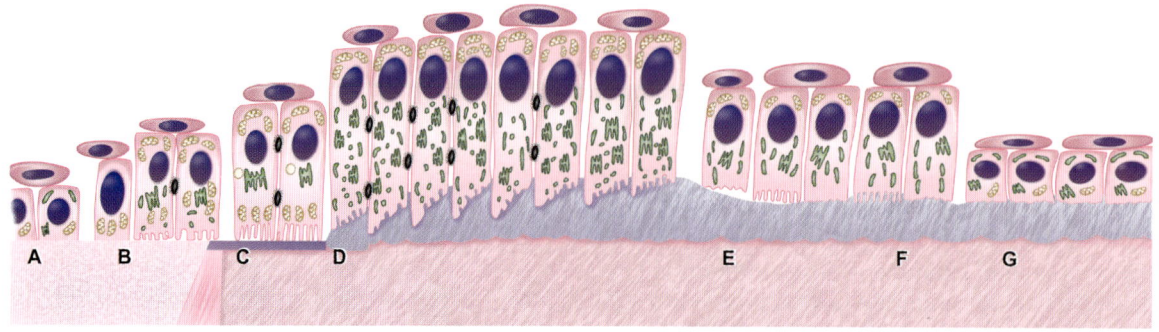

Figures 5-31A to G: Life cycle of ameloblasts.

Genetic Control of Enamel Formation

The genetic control over enamel formation is evident from the preservation of enamel form and organization through generations and its involvement ranging from total absence to localized defects in a number of genetic conditions. Thousands of genes are involved in the regulation of enamel formation. Various genes are expressed as the ameloblasts pass through the different stages of their life cycle and associated enamel-forming activities. The genes involved in enamel formation, code for a variety of proteins including enamel matrix proteins, enzymes, transmembrane proteins, transcription factors, regulatory proteins and other functions.

Early enamel formation is dependent upon the four secreted proteins namely enamelin (ENAM), ameloblastin (AMBN), amelogenin (AMELX) and matrix metalloproteinase 20 (or enamelysin). ENAM and AMBN are specialized proteins essential for enamel formation and preserved across all enamel forming species while AMELX and enamelysin are essential for continued normal formation and maturation of enamel.

The genes that encode for amelogenin, enamelin, and ameloblastin are a part of the secretory calcium-binding phosphoprotein (SCPP) gene family. *AMTN*, which encodes amelotin is derived from ENAM. These genes are all located on the q arm of the chromosome 4 (q421) except the amelogenin gene which is located on both X and Y sex chromosomes. The *AMELX* gene located on the X chromosome produces the required amelogenin with minimal or no contribution from the *AMELY* gene on the Y chromosome. Tuftelin is encoded by the TUFT1 gene.

Nearly 908 genes are expressed by the presecretory ameloblasts and 1203 genes by the secretory ameloblasts. The genes involved with cell adhesion, ion transport, biomineralized tissue development, epithelial appendage development, transcriptional regulation and neuron differentiation are upregulated in both the stages. The genes involved with cell motility, cell cycle, cellular component organization and cellular catabolism regulation are downregulated.

■ AGE CHANGES

Enamel gets attrited due to aging. Attrition is defined as wearing away of tooth substance due to tooth-to-tooth contact as in mastication **(Figure 5-32)**. Enamel is the first hard tissue to get affected by the continuous masticatory force and it cannot repair such loss by itself. Attrition also results in loss of perikymata, flattening of the cusps and subsequent reduction in vertical dimension, elimination of shallow grooves and pits and reduction in the dental arch length due to flattening of the proximal contact areas. It also leads to exposure of the dentin, which results in sensitivity.

Inorganic content of the enamel becomes increased. There will be increase in the size of the apatite crystals. Permeability is decreased. Enamel becomes harder and more brittle. The color becomes darker due to the addition of organic material from the environment. Continuous ion exchange with the oral environment results in alteration in the composition of the surface enamel.

■ CLINICAL CONSIDERATIONS

Any alteration in the quantity, quality of the mineral or morphology of the outer surface of enamel has consequences

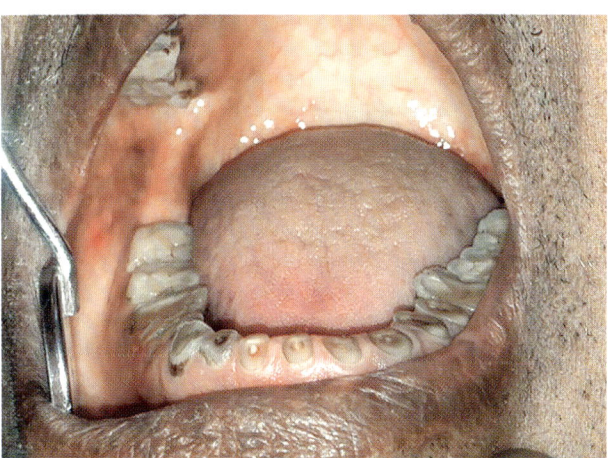

Figure 5-32: Severe attrition exposing the dentin and pulp.
Source: Dr S Rohini, GRM Dental Clinic, Ambattur, Chennai, India.

in the clinical care of the affected individual. The clinical outcome of various disturbances of amelogenesis depends on the timing and stage of the development of enamel at the time of occurrence. The manifestations therefore range from hypoplasia with disturbances of the secretory stage, hypocalcification with disturbances of the maturation stage, and very rarely to the extent of altered tooth or enamel morphology with disturbances of morphogenesis.

Although generally well-preserved, enamel is at times affected by hereditary conditions. The most common among these genetic conditions are those that affect the coding of the enamel proteins leading to a group of conditions called amelogenesis imperfecta (AI). This group of conditions is caused by the mutations in the X-chromosome amelogenin gene and mutations in the enamelin gene that are inherited as X-linked, autosomal dominant or recessive traits.

> AI is also rarely caused by mutations of non-enamel protein genes. Autosomal dominant AI is caused by mutation of *FAM83H* and *LAMB3* and autosomal recessive AI is caused by mutations in *WRD72*, *C4 or f26*, and *SCLA24A4*.

It may be of hypoplastic type (affects the enamel matrix formation), hypocalcified (affects the mineralization of the enamel matrix) or hypomaturative (affects the maturation of the mineralized enamel matrix). Clinically the teeth appear discolored, pitted or grooved and prone for rapid wear and fracture. Enamel may be soft and even absent in some areas.

Mutations of some nonenamel protein genes can also cause both nonsyndromic and syndromic enamel defects.

As quoted by Smith BH, every individual's enamel is a record of the first 8 or 9 years of their life when the crowns are formed. Disturbances caused by the environmental factors also affect the enamel formation as ameloblasts are the most sensitive group of cells in terms of their function.

Environmental factors like nutritional deficiency, exanthematous diseases, congenital syphilis, hypocalcemia, birth injury, local infection, trauma, and ingestion of chemicals like fluoride and tetracycline may cause enamel hypoplasia.

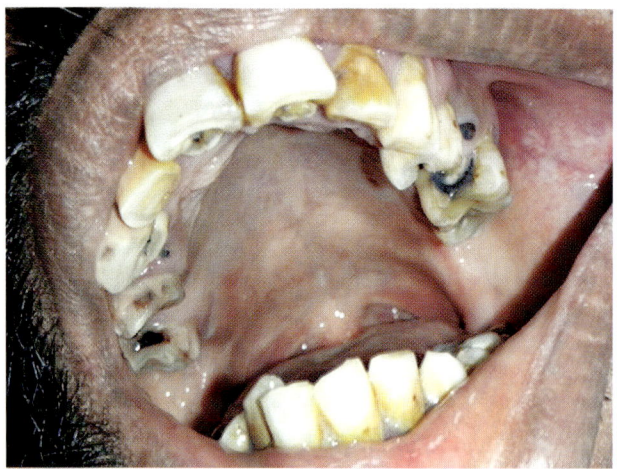

Figure 5-33: Discolored teeth in dental fluorosis.

Chronic fluoride (above 5 ppm) ingestion during tooth development causes *dental fluorosis*. Fluoride ion interferes with the function of the ameloblasts, which results in the formation of mottled enamel. In dental fluorosis, the appearance of teeth ranges from very mild change such as small opaque spots to highly discolored teeth with corroded appearance **(Figure 5-33)**. Ingestion of tetracycline during tooth development causes brown pigmentation.

Molar incisor hypomineralization: It is defined as hypomineralization of systemic origin affecting one or all first permanent molars and the permanent incisors **(Figures 5-34A to C)**. It is the result of a variety of environmental factors affecting the developing enamel, with an underlying genetic predisposition. The affected tooth has white opaque spots or the affected portion appears soft and porous.

Enamel pearl: A small nodule of enamel formed at the cervical or root portion of the tooth is called enamel pearl or enamel drop **(Figure 5-35)**. This is formed by the misplaced ameloblasts.

Abrasion: Wearing away of tooth substance due to mechanical means. For example, in case of faulty tooth brushing technique, a V-shaped groove is produced in the cervical third of the buccal surface of the posterior teeth.

Abfraction is the loss of tooth substance caused by occlusal loading causing flexure and ultimate fatigue.

Erosion is wearing away of tooth surface caused by acids. The source may be dietary (consumption of frequent and long-term acidic beverages/food substances) or increased salivary acids level. The affected surface appears as rounded depression with discoloration.

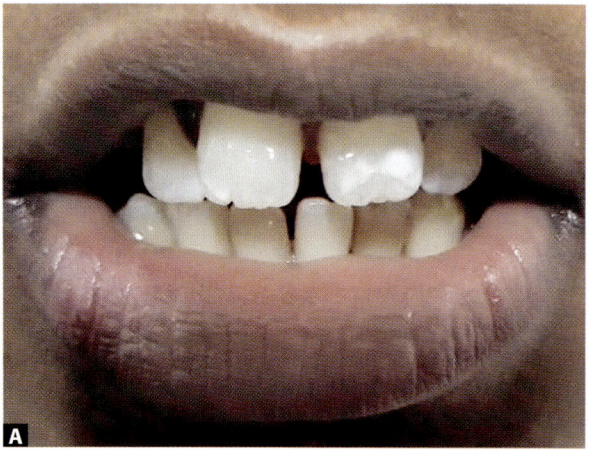
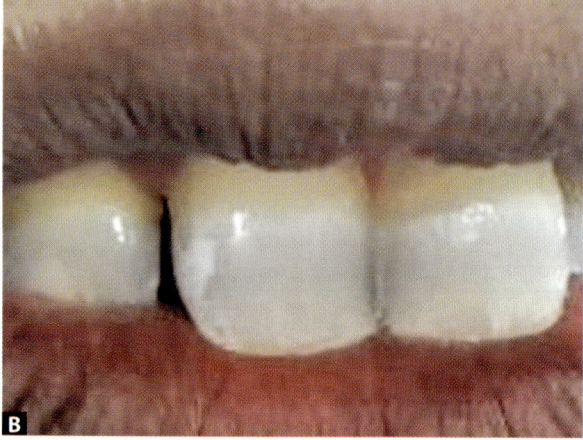
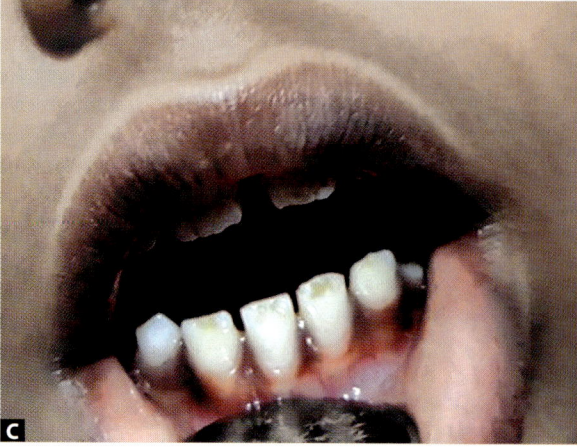

Figures 5-34A to C: Hypomineralized area in the central incisor appears as white spots and pitted appearance clinically.
Source: Dr S Rohini, GRM Dental Clinic, Ambattur, India.

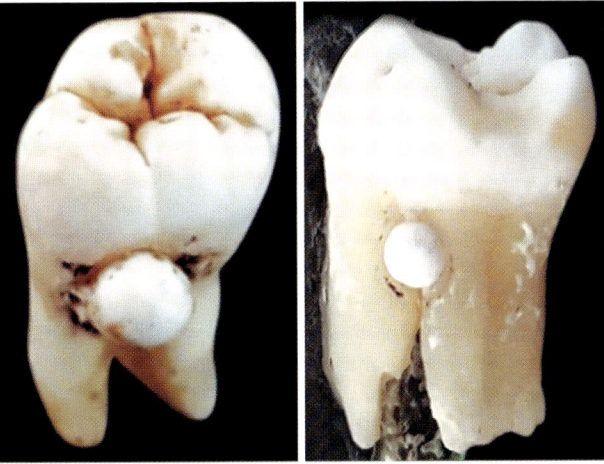

Figure 5-35: Enamel pearl in the furcation area of molar.

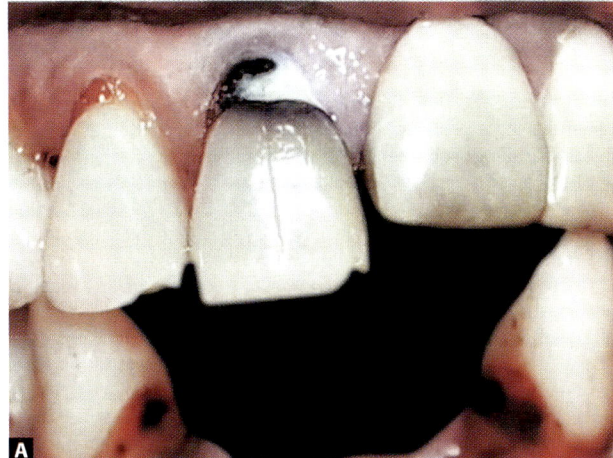

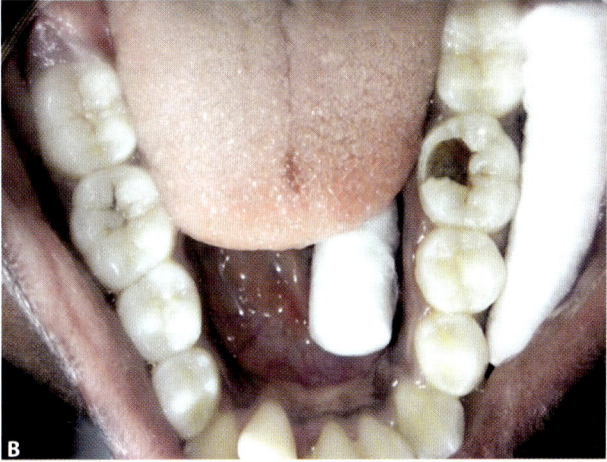

Figures 5-36A and B: Dental caries in upper central incisor and lower molar.
Source: Dr R Preethi, Meenakshi Ammal Dental College, Chennai, India

Dental caries: It is the most common microbial disease affecting the hard tissues of the tooth. In this disease, the cariogenic bacteria act on the refined carbohydrates, which are lodged on the retentive areas of the enamel (pit and deep fissures usually on the occlusal surface) and produce acids which decalcify the enamel. This decalcification results in cavity formation **(Figures 5-36A and B)**.

Acid etching: It is an important step in restoring the tooth with composite resins, sealing pit and fissures, and cementing orthodontic brackets. In this procedure, 30–40% phosphoric acid is applied and is left on the tooth's surface for about 20 seconds. This causes roughening of the enamel surface by selective dissolution of the crystals and creates minute pores, which provides better bonding of the composite resin to the tooth surface.

Paleoproteomics

It is the study of ancient proteins preserved in fossils. Tooth enamel can be used as a record of ontogeny. It can be a useful tool in archeological research and forensic studies. The proteins in this highly mineralized structure can remain well preserved for even millions of years, compared to the proteins preserved in the more porous mineralized structures like the bones. They are preserved longer than the nucleic acids.

Sex Determination

The genomic sequences of the protein amelogenin can be used in sex determination, when DNA and bone preservation is either compromised or contaminated. The variations in the sequence of the *AMELX* and *AMELY* genes on the X and Y chromosome, respectively, allow for the sex determination.

Age Estimation

Perikymata are the external manifestations of the incremental lines of Retzius. They can be used in forensics for age estimation of the fossils. They also help in determining the age at which growth alterations have occurred.

Points to Remember

- Enamel is the hardest substance in the human body and covers the anatomical crown of the tooth. It is formed by the cells called ameloblasts and the formation of enamel is called amelogenesis. Enamel is translucent and color ranges from yellowish white to grayish or bluish white. Color of the tooth crown depends on the translucency and thickness of the enamel and the color of the underlying dentin.
- Enamel consists of 96% of inorganic material and 4% of organic material and water. The enamel proteins are divided into two groups, namely amelogenins and non-amelogenins. Amelogenins form 90% of the organic content, while non-amelogenins such as ameloblastin, enamelin, amelotin, and tuftelin form the remaining 10%.

- Enamel is made up of enamel rods or prisms and interrod or interprismatic substance. The number of enamel rods per tooth ranges from 5 million to 12 million. Lines that are present at right angle to the long axis of the enamel rod at about 3–6 µm intervals are called cross striations or rod segmentations.
- The borderline between enamel and dentin is known as dentinoenamel junction (DEJ), which is scalloped with the concavities facing the enamel and is more pronounced in the crown. Incremental lines of Retzius run oblique to the DEJ and reflect the enamel deposition at a particular point during amelogenesis.
- Perikymata are closely packed wavy, transverse ridges separated by fine grooves present in the surface of the enamel and are parallel to the cementoenamel junction. They are considered to be external manifestations of striae of Retzius.
- Neonatal lines, noticed in deciduous teeth, are the accentuated incremental lines that demarcate the enamel deposited before and after birth.
- Hunter Schreger bands are dark and light band of varying widths (approximate width 50 µm), produced by the change in orientation or direction between adjacent groups of enamel rods and can be appreciated in longitudinal sections under reflected light.
- The intertwined enamel rods at cuspal regions in spiral arrangement are called gnarled enamel.
- Enamel spindles are dark spindle or club-shaped structures of varying length starting from the DEJ perpendicularly and extending into the enamel. They are formed by the extension of the odontoblastic process in between the inner enamel epithelial cells before the formation of enamel.
- Enamel lamellae are thin leaf-like hypomineralized structures that extend from the enamel surface toward the DEJ and sometimes cross the DEJ.
- Enamel tufts are hypomineralized structures that originate at the DEJ, and resemble a tuft of grass in ground sections. This appearance is due to lying of imperfections in more than one plane and heading toward different directions.
- Primary enamel cuticle is the basal lamina interposed between the reduced enamel epithelium and the enamel. This is the end product of ameloblasts.
- Aprismatic enamel is the final product of the ameloblasts, formed after the loss of the distal portion of Tomes' process and is more mineralized than the rest of the enamel.
- The process of amelogenesis broadly involves a secretory stage where ameloblasts secrete and partly mineralize the enamel and a maturation stage, where proteins and water are removed from the matrix and replaced by minerals to produce the hardest substance in the human body.
- A short pre-secretory stage prepares the cells for their specialized role through final differentiation of inner enamel epithelial cells to pre-ameloblasts and ameloblasts, and a transition stage prepares the cells for the maturative role.
- The complete formation and mineralization of enamel which is approximately 2.5 mm thick, can take up to 6 years.
- Tomes' process is a six-sided pyramid or cone-shaped projection extending from the secretory or distal end of the ameloblast. These asymmetric cellular projections have two parts, a proximal portion and a distal portion.
- Attrition is defined as wearing away of tooth substance due to tooth to tooth contact as in mastication. *Abrasin is w*earing away of tooth substance due to mechanical means. Wearing away of tooth surface caused by acids is *known as erosion*.
- Amelogenesis imperfecta may be of hypoplastic type (affects the enamel matrix formation), hypocalcified (affects the mineralization of the enamel matrix) or hypomaturative (affects the maturation of the mineralized enamel matrix).
- Molar incisor hypomineralization is defined as hypomineralization of systemic origin affecting one or all first permanent molars and the permanent incisors.
- A small nodule of enamel formed at the cervical or root portion of the tooth is called enamel pearl or enamel drop.

PRACTICE QUESTIONS

1. Explain the physical and chemical properties of enamel.
2. Structure of enamel rods with diagrammatic representation.
3. Write in detail about the hypocalcified areas of enamel.
4. Write short notes on incremental lines of Retzius.
5. Write in brief about perikymata.
6. What are Hunter-Schreger bands?
7. Write in detail about amelogenesis and life cycle of ameloblasts.
8. Age changes of enamel.
9. What are the clinical considerations with respect to enamel?

MULTIPLE CHOICE QUESTIONS

1. **The hardest substance in the human body is**
   a. Dentin
   b. Enamel
   c. Cementum
   d. Pulp
2. **Specific gravity of enamel is**
   a. 3.8
   b. 2.8
   c. 4.8
   d. 45.8
3. **The percentage of inorganic matter in fully mature enamel is**
   a. 98%
   b. 95%
   c. 96%
   d. 99%
4. **The major structural protein in enamel is**
   a. Amelotin
   b. amelogenin
   c. enamelin
   d. tuftelin

5. **The key hole pattern appearance in the cross section is a feature of**
   a. Prismatic enamel
   b. Aprismatic enamel
   c. Interglobular dentin
   d. Enamel spindle
6. **Dentinoenamel junction is**
   a. Flat and smooth
   b. Scalloped with convexities towards the enamel
   c. Scalloped with concavities towards the enamel
   d. Similar to cementodentinal junction in permanent tooth
7. **Externalization of incremental lines of Retzius is called**
   a. Enamel lamellae
   b. Enamel spindles
   c. Perikymata
   d. Tomes' process
8. **Which of the following is an optical phenomenon?**
   a. Striae of Retzius
   b. Enamel lamellae
   c. Enamel cuticle
   d. Hunter-Schreger bands
9. **Thin leaf-like hypomineralized structures that extend from the enamel surface toward the DEJ are called**
   a. Enamel spindles
   b. Enamel lamellae
   c. Enamel tuft
   d. Perikymata
10. **Which type of lamellae is confined to the enamel?**
    a. Both A and C
    b. Type A
    c. Type B
    d. Type C
11. **All are hypomineralized structures seen in enamel, except**
    a. Enamel tufts
    b. Enamel spindles
    c. Enamel rods
    d. Enamel lamellae
12. **Dark spindle or club-shaped structures of varying length starting from the DEJ perpendicularly and extending into the enamel are called as**
    a. Enamel tufts
    b. Enamel spindles
    c. Enamel rods
    d. Enamel lamellae
13. **Gnarled enamel is seen at the**
    a. DEJ
    b. Cervical region
    c. Cusp tips
    d. Below deep fissures in the enamel
14. **Thickness of aprismatic enamel is approximately**
    a. 20 μ
    b. 30 μ
    c. 3 μ
    d. 2 μ
15. **The formation and mineralization of full thickness of enamel of approximately 2.5 mm, takes how many years to complete?**
    a. 6
    b. 2
    c. 4
    d. 8
16. **Enamel formation starts at**
    a. DEJ
    b. Cusp tip
    c. Middle third of the crown
    d. Proximal region
17. **The formative cells of which of the following tissues is lost once tissue is formed?**
    a. Dentin
    b. Cementum
    c. Enamel
    d. Pulp
18. **Enamel forming cells are called as the**
    a. Odontoblasts
    b. Ameloblasts
    c. Osteoblasts
    d. Osteocytes
19. **Ameloblasts are derived from the cells of the**
    a. Dental papilla
    b. Dental sac
    c. Inner enamel epithelium
    d. Hertwig's epithelial root sheath
20. **Daily increments of 4 μm of enamel is seen as**
    a. Cross striations
    b. Enamel cuticle
    c. Enamel lamellae
    d. Enamel tuft
21. **Ruffled border develops in which stage of amelogenesis?**
    a. Presecretory
    b. Secretory
    c. Transitional
    d. Maturation
22. **Reversal of nutrition and reversal of polarity occurs in which stage of amelogenesis?**
    a. Pre-secretory
    b. Secretory
    c. Maturation
    d. Transition
23. **Nutritional supply of ameloblasts during most of their cell cycle is from**
    a. Dental papilla
    b. Dental sac
    c. Enamel organ
    d. Dental pulp
24. **Metalloproteinases are used in which stage of amelogenesis?**
    a. Pre-secretory
    b. Secretory
    c. Maturation
    d. Transition
25. **Modulation process happens in which stage of amelogenesis?**
    a. Desmolytic
    b. Transitional
    c. Maturation
    d. Secretory
26. **Wearing away of tooth structure due to tooth contact during mastication is**
    a. Attrition
    b. Abrasion
    c. Abfraction
    d. Erosion

27. **The type of amelogenesis imperfecta that affects the mineralization of the enamel matrix is**
   a. Hypocalcified
   b. Hypomaturative
   c. Hypoplastic
   d. Hypodontic

ANSWERS

1. b	2. b	3. c	4. b	5. a	6. c	7. c	8. d	9. b	10. b	11. c	12. b	13. c	14. b	15. a
16. b	17. c	18. b	19. c	20. a	21. d	22. a	23. b	24. b	25. c	26. a	27. a			

BIBLIOGRAPHY

1. Aghanashini S, Puvvalla B, Mundinamane DB, Apoorva SM, Bhat D, Lalwani M. A Comprehensive Review on Dental Calculus. J Health Sci Resc. 2016;7(2):42-50.
2. Amizuka N, Uchida T, Fukae M, et al. Ultrastructural and immunocytochemical studies of enamel tufts in human permanent teeth. Arch Histol Cytol. 1992;55:179-90.
3. Amizuka N, Uchida T, Nozawa-Inoue K, et al. Ultrastructural images of enamel tufts in human permanent teeth. J Oral Biosc. 2005;47:33-41.
4. Aoba T, Komatsu H, Shimazu Y, et al. Enamel mineralization and an initial crystalline phase. Connect Tissue Res. 1998;39:129.
5. Athanassiou PM, Kim D, Harbron L, et al. Molecular and circadian controls of ameloblasts. Eur J Oral Sci. 2011;119(suppl 1): 35-40.
6. Avery JK, Chiego DJ. Essentials of oral histology and embryology—a clinical approach, 3rd edition. US: Mosby; 2006.
7. Bajaj D, Arola DD. On the R-curve behavior of human tooth enamel. Biomaterials. 2009;30(23–24):4037–46.
8. Bartlett JD, Beniash E, Lee DH, et al. Decreased mineral content in MMP-20 null mouse enamel is prominent during the maturation stage. J Dent Res. 2004;83:909-13.
9. Bartlett JD, Ganss B, Goldberg M, et al. Protein C-protein interactions of the developing enamel matrix. Curr Top Dev Biol. 2006;74:57.
10. Bartlett JD, Ganss B, Goldberg M, et al. Protein–protein interactions of the developing enamel matrix. Curr Top Dev Biol. 2006;74:57-115.
11. Bartlett JD, Simmer JP. Proteinases in developing dental enamel. Crit Rev Oral Biol Med. 1999;10:425-41.
12. Bartlett JD, Skobe Z, Nanci A, et al. Matrix metalloproteinase 20 promotes a smooth enamel surface, a strong dentino-enamel junction, and a decussating enamel rod pattern. Eur J Oral Sci. 2011;119:199-205.
13. Bartlett JD, Yamakoshi Y, Simmer JP, et al. MMP20 cleaves E-cadherin and influences ameloblast development. Cells Tissues Organs. 2011;194:222-6.
14. Bartlett JD. Dental Enamel Development: Proteinases and Their Enamel Matrix Substrates. ISRN Dent. 2013;2013:1-24.
15. Begue CK, Krebsbach PH, Bartlett JD, et al. Dentin sialoprotein, dentin phosphoprotein, enamelysin and ameloblastin: tooth-specific molecules that are distinctively expressed during murine dental differentiation. Eur J Oral Sci. 1998;106:963-70.
16. Beniash E, Stifler CA, Sun CY, Jung GS, Qin Z, Buehler MJ, et al. The hidden structure of human enamel. Nat Commun. 2019;10(1):1-13.
17. Berkovitz BKB, Holland GR, Moxham BJ. Oral Anatomy, Histology & Embryology, 4th edition. US: Elsevier; 2009.
18. Beust TB. Occurrence of enamel tufts. J Dent Res. 1932;12:601-8.
19. Bodecker CF. The Illusory Sheath of Neumann. J Dent Res. 1947;26:53-66.
20. Boyde A. Amelogenesis and the structure of enamel. In: Cohen B, Kramer IR (Eds). Scientific Foundations of Dentistry. London: William Heinemann Medical Books Ltd; 1976. pp. 341-3.
21. Boyde A. Microstructure of enamel. In: Chadwick DJ, Cardew G (Eds). Dental Enamel: Ciba Foundation Symposium 205. New York: John Wiley & Sons; 1997. pp. 18-31.
22. Deutsch D, Palmon A, Young MF, et al. Mapping of the human tuftelin (TUFT1) gene to chromosome 1 by fluorescence in situ hybridization. Mamm Genome. 1994;5:461-2.
23. Dunglas C, Septier D, Carreau J-P, et al. Developmentally regulated changes in phospholipid composition in murine molar tooth. Histochem J. 1999;31:535-40.
24. Fincham AG, Moradain-Oldak J, Simmer JP. The structural biology of the developing dental enamel matrix. J Struct Bio. 1999;126:270-99.
25. Fukumoto S, Kiba T, Hall B, et al. Ameloblastin is a cell adhesion molecule required for maintaining the differentiation state of ameloblasts. J Cell Biol. 2004;167:973-83.
26. Gibson CW, Yuan ZA, Hall B, et al. Amelogenin-deficient mice display an amelogenesis imperfecta phenotype. J Biol Chem. 2001;276:31871-5.
27. Gil-Bona A, Bidlack FB. Tooth enamel and its dynamic protein matrix. Int J Mol Sci. 2020;21(12):1-25.
28. Goldberg M, Septier D. Phospholipids in amelogenesis and dentinogenesis. Crit Rev Oral Biol Med. 2002;13:276-90.
29. Hartsock A, Nelson WJ. Adherens and tight junctions: structure, function and connections to the actin cytoskeleton. Biochimica et Biophysica Acta. 2008;1778:660-9.
30. Hodson JJ. Micro-dissection and other techniques for the investigation of human enamel. Brit D J. 1952;92:195-203.
31. Hu JCC, Chun YHP, Al Hazzazzi, et al. Enamel formation and amelogenesis imperfecta. Cells Tissues Organs. 2007;186: 78-85.
32. Hu JCC, Hu Y, Smith CE, et al. Enamel defects and ameloblast- specific expression in Enam knock-out/lacZ knockin mice. J Biol Chem. 2008;283:10858-71.
33. Hu JCC, Sun X, Zhang C, et al. Enamelysin and kallikrein-4 mRNA expression in developing mouse molars. Eur J Oral Sci. 2002;110:307-15.
34. Hubbard MJ. Calcium transport across the dental enamel epithelium. Crit Rev Oral Biol Med. 2000;11:437.
35. Kierdorf H, Kierdorf U, Richards A, et al. Fluoride-induced alterations of enamel structure: an experimental study in the miniature pig. Anat Embryol. 2004;207:463-74.

36. Kierdorf H, Witzel C, Upex B, et al. Enamel hypoplasia in molars of sheep and goats, and its relationship to the pattern of tooth crown growth. J Anat. 2012;220:484-95.
37. Kim JW, Seymen F, Lee KE, et al. lamb3 mutations causing autosomal-dominant amelogenesis imperfecta. J Dent Res. 2013;92(10):899-904.
38. Kumar GS. Orban's Oral Histology and Embryology, 14th edition. India: Elsevier; 2015.
39. Kunin AA, Evdokimova AY, Moiseeva NS. Age-related differences of tooth enamel morphochemistry in health and dental caries. EPMA J. 2015;6(1):1-11.
40. Lacruz RS, Nanci A, Kurtz I, et al. Regulation of pH during amelogenesis. Calcif Tissue Int. 2010;86:91-103.
41. Li S, Risnes S. SEM observations of Retzius lines and prism cross-striations in human dental enamel after different acid etching regimes. Arch Oral Biol. 2004;49:45-52.
42. Manjunath K, Sriram G, Saraswathi TR, et al. Enamel rod end patterns: A preliminary study using acetate peel technique and automated biometrics. J Forensic Odontology. 2008;1:33-6.
43. Margolis HC, Beniash E, Fowler CE. Role of macromolecular assembly of enamel matrix proteins in enamel formation. J Dent Res. 2006;85:775.
44. Moffatt P, Smith CE, St-Arnaud R, et al. Characterization of Apin, a secreted protein highly expressed in tooth-associated epithelial. J Cell Biochem. 2008;103:941.
45. Moffatt P, Smith CE, St-Arnaud R, et al. Cloning of rat amelotin and localization of the protein to the basal lamina of maturation stage ameloblasts and junctional epithelium. Biochem J. 2006;399:37.
46. Nanci A, Smith CE. Matrix-mediated mineralization in enamel and the collagen-based hard tissues. In: Goldberg M, Boskey A, Robinson C (Eds). Chemistry and biology of mineralized tissues, Rosemont, IL: American Academy of Orthopaedic Surgeons; 1999.
47. Nanci A. Ten Cate's Oral Histology, 9th edition. US: Elsevier; 2018.
48. Nishikawa S. Cytoskeleton, intercellular junctions, planar cell polarity, and cell movement in amelogenesis. J Oral Biosci. 2017;59(4):197-204.
49. Osborn JW. Directions and interrelationships of enamel prisms from the sides of human teeth. J Dent Res. 1968;47:223-32.
50. Osborn JW. Evaluation of previous assessments of prism directions in human enamel. J Dent Res. 1968;47:217-22.
51. Osborn JW. The mechanism of prism formation in teeth: a hypothesis. Calcif Tissue Res. 1970;5:115-32.
52. Paulson RB. Scanning electron microscopy of enamel tuft development in human deciduous teeth. Arch Oral Biol. 1981;26:103-9.
53. Provenza VD, Seibel W. Oral Histology- Inheritance and Development, 2nd edition. USA: Lea & Febiger; 1986.
54. Reid DJ, Ferrell RJ. The relationship between number of striae of Retzius and their periodicity in imbricational enamel formation. J Hum E. 2006;50:195-202.
55. Reith EJ. The ultrastructure of ameloblasts from the growing end of rat incisors. Arch Oral Biol. 1960;2:253-62.
56. Reith EJ. The ultrastructure of ameloblasts during matrix formation and the maturation of enamel. J Biophys Biochem Cytol. 1961;9:825-39.
57. Risnes S. Growth tracks in dental enamel. J Hum E. 1998;35: 331-50.
58. Risnes S. Mature enamel morphology and forming enamel dynamics: crystal orientation, crystal continuity, prism diameter, Retzius lines, and prism cross striations. In: Mayhall JT, Heikkinen T (Eds). Proceedings of the 11th International Symposium on Dental Morphology. Oulu: Oulu University Press; 1999. pp. 312-22.
59. Roa I, del-Sol M. Perikymata: A Non-existent Term. A Scientific Literature Invention? Terminology Analysis and Proposal. Int J Morphol. 2017;35(4):1230-2.
60. Robinson C, Brookes SJ, Shore RC, et al. The developing enamel matrix: nature and function. Eur J Oral Sci. 1998;106:282-91.
61. Robinson C, Hudson J. Tuft protein: protein cross-linking in enamel development. Eur J Oral Sci. 2011;119:50-4.
62. Shapiro IM, Wuthier RE, Irving JT. A study of phospholipids of bovine dental tissues—I. Enamel matrix and dentine. Arch Oral Biol. 1966;176:167-80.
63. Simmer JP, Fincham AG. Molecular mechanisms of dental enamel formation. Crit Rev Oral Biol Med. 1995;6(2):84–108.
64. Simmer JP, Hu JC. Expression, structure, and function of enamel proteinases. Connect Tissue Res. 2002;43:441.
65. Simmer JP, Hu Y, Lertlam R, et al. Hypomaturation enamel defects in Klk4 knockout/LacZ knock in mice. J Biol Chem. 2009;284:19110-21.
66. Simmer JP, Papagerakis P, Smith CE, et al. Regulation of dental shape and hardness. J Dent Res. 2010;89:1024.
67. Smith BH. Standards of human tooth formation and dental age assessment. In: Kelley MA, Larsen CS (Eds). Advances in Dental Anthropology. New York: Wiley-Liss; 1991. pp. 143-68.
68. Smith CE, Chong DL, Bartlett JD, et al. Mineral acquisition rates in developing enamel on maxillary and mandibular incisors of rats and mice: implications to extracellular acid loading as apatite crystals mature. J Bone Miner Res. 2005;20:240-9.
69. Smith CE. Cellular and chemical events during enamel maturation. Crit Rev Oral Biol Med. 1998;9:128-61.
70. Tabata MJ, Matsumura T, Fujii T, et al. Fibronectin accelerates the growth and differentiation of ameloblast lineage cells in vitro. J Histochem Cytochem. 2004;51:1673-79.
71. Thesleff I, Vaahtokari A, Kettunen P, et al. Epithelial- mesenchymal signaling during tooth development. Connect Tissue Res. 1995;32:9-15.
72. Tucker A, Sharpe P. The cutting-edge of mammalian development; how the embryo makes teeth. Nat Rev Genet. 2004;5:499-508.
73. Vaananen A, Tjaderhane L, Eklund L, et al. Expression of collagen XVIII and MMP-20 in developing teeth and odontogenic tumors. Matrix Biology. 2004;23:153-61.
74. Willmott NS, Bryan RA, Duggal MS. Molar- incisor hypomineralisation: A literature review. Eur Arch Paediatr Dent. 2008;9:172-9.
75. Walker BN, Makinson OF, Peters MGRB. Enamel cracks. The role of enamel lamellae in caries initiation. Aust Dent J. 1998;43(2):110–6.
76. Witzel C, Kierdorf U, Schultz M, et al. Insights from the inside: Histological analysis of abnormal enamel microstructure associated with hypoplastic enamel defects in human teeth. Am J Phys Anthropol. 2008;136:400-14.
77. Zhang Y, Zheng L, Le M, Nakano Y, Chan B, Huang Y, et al. SATB1 establishes ameloblast cell polarity and regulates directional amelogenin secretion for enamel formation. BMC Biol. 2019;17(1):1–16.

CHAPTER 6

Dentin

B Sivapathasundharam

Chapter Outline

- Physical Properties 66
- Chemical Composition 67
- Histology of Dentin 68
  - Dentinal Tubules 68
  - Peritubular Dentin (Intratubular Dentin) 69
  - Intertubular Dentin 70
  - Odontoblastic Process 70
  - Dentinal Fluid 71
  - Dentin Innervation 72
  - Predentin 72
- Structural Patterns of Dentin 72
  - Primary Dentin 72
  - Secondary Dentin 73
  - Interglobular Dentin 73
  - Tomes' Granular Layer 73
  - Incremental Lines 74
  - Contour Lines of Owen 75
  - Sclerotic Dentin 75
  - Reparative Dentin 76
  - Dead Tracts 76
- Dentin Sensitivity 76
- Dentinogenesis 77
  - Mineralization of Dentin 77
  - Odontoblasts Differentiation and Matrix Formation 78
- Clinical Considerations 79

Dentin is a living, hard, avascular connective tissue and forms the bulk of the tooth. Normally, it is not exposed to the oral environment. It is covered by enamel (the hardest substance in the human body) in the crown and cementum in the root. It encloses the soft tissue called the pulp. Dentin is considered to be a living tissue since it contains cytoplasmic extension of the odontoblasts, the cells responsible for the formation of dentin. Since dentin formation starts before the formation of enamel, it determines the morphology of the tooth.

The portion of the dentin, which forms the crown is called the coronal dentin, whereas the dentin of the root is known as radicular dentin.

Physical and chemical properties of dentin are almost similar to that of bone, however dentin is slightly harder than bone, avascular, and normally do not contain any cells within them. Unlike enamel, dentin is porous with numerous closely packed minute canals known as dentinal tubules. These tubules extend from the periphery of the pulp toward enamel and cementum, and house the odontoblastic process, which is bathed in tissue fluid called dentinal lymph.

PHYSICAL PROPERTIES

The color of the dentin is light yellowish. It gives the color to the tooth; however it is modified by the nature of enamel. The tooth appears whitish if the enamel is opaque and yellowish in translucent enamel. The color of the dentin darkens with age. Nonvital or endodontically treated tooth appears grayish black because of the entrapment of necrotic debris and/or blood products within the dentinal tubules. It is harder than the bone and cementum and softer than enamel. Vicker's hardness number of dentin ranges from 50 to 60 and the hardness is not uniform throughout the tooth. It is harder in the center than near the pulp (circumpulpal) or near the dentinoenamel or cementodentinal junctions. The circumpulpal dentin is found to be 30% less hard than the hardest dentinal portion of the tooth. The hardness also varies from tooth to tooth. Dentin of the permanent teeth is harder than the deciduous teeth.

Dentin is permeable and permeability decreases with age. Its permeability is more near the pulp chamber because of the increased diameter and number of the tubules per unit area.

Dentin is elastic. This gives the flexibility, which prevents the fracture of the brittle enamel cap during function. Enamel is tightly attached to the dentin at the dentinoenamel junction **(Figure 6-1)**. The surface of the dentin at this junction contains many saucer-shaped depressions and appears scalloped in sections **(Figures 6-2A and B)**. This provides firm mechanical retention, whereas the cementodentinal

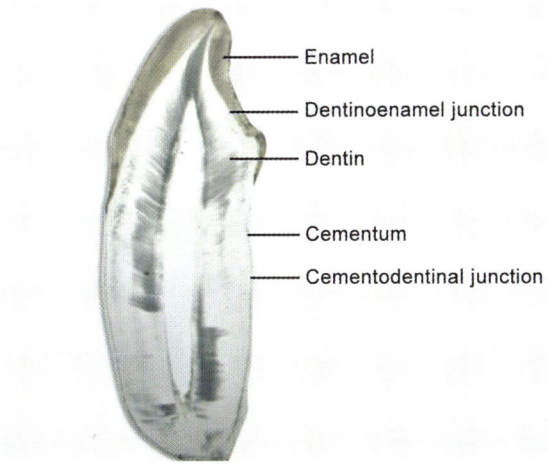

Figure 6-1: Ground section of the tooth showing enamel, dentin, cementum, and dentinoenamel and cementodentinal junction.

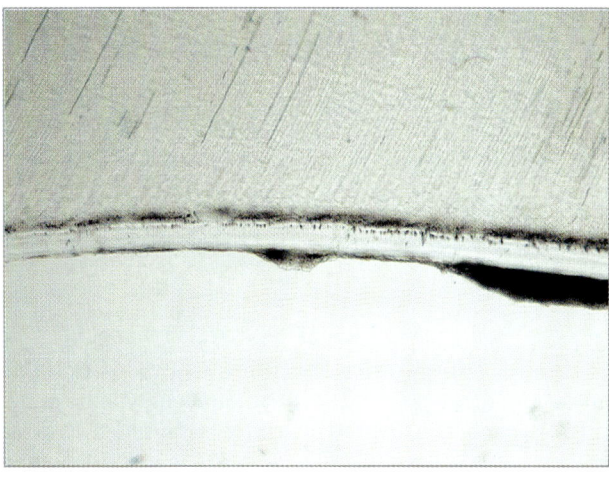

Figure 6-3: Ground section showing flat cementodentinal junction.

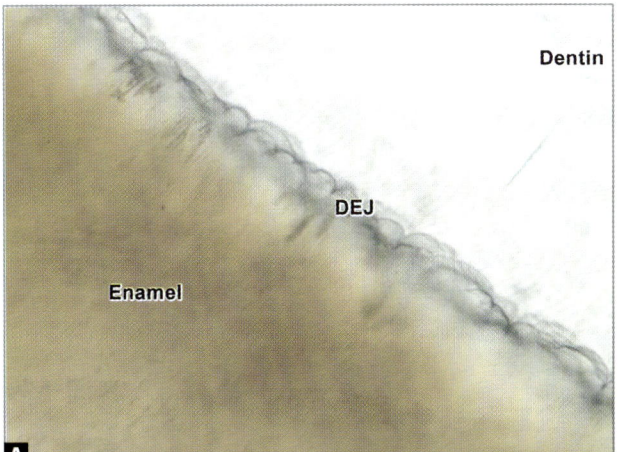

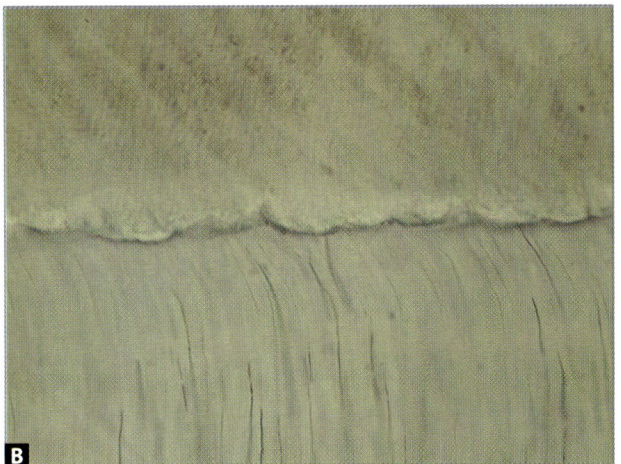

Figures 6-2A and B: Ground sections showing scalloped dentinoenamel junction.

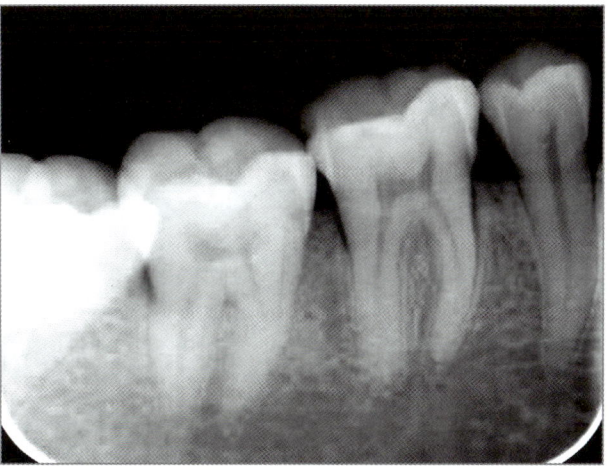

Figure 6-4: Periapical view radiograph of mandibular molars and premolars reveals descending degree of radiopacity in the order of enamel, dentin, and cementum with radiolucent pulp at the center.

junction is relatively flat and the collagen fibers of the both tissues intermingle with each other **(Figure 6-3)**. However in deciduous teeth the cementodentinal is scalloped.

Mineralized tissue does not allow the X-ray photons to pass through and appears white in radiographs. This is called radiopacity. In contrast, the unmineralized tissue allows the X-rays to penetrate and appears black in radiographs and called as radiolucency. In between these two extremes, lie varying shades of gray depending on the degree of mineralization of the tissue to be radiographed.

In radiographs, enamel appears radiopaque because of its high inorganic content; dentin and cementum appear relatively less radiopaque and indistinguishable from each other. The pulp and periodontal ligament appear radiolucent **(Figure 6-4)**.

CHEMICAL COMPOSITION

Dentin is made up of 65% inorganic and 35% of organic material and water **(Flowchart 6-1)**. The mineral components of the dentin are calcium and phosphate in the form of hydroxyapatite crystals. These crystals are about 60–70 nm in length and 20–35 nm in width with 3–4 nm thickness. These crystals are plate-shaped, smaller than the hydroxyapatite crystals of the enamel. Apart from this, dentin also contains small amounts of carbonates, magnesium, and varying concentrations of fluoride. Trace elements present in the dentin include lead, zinc, potassium, and copper.

Flowchart 6-1: Chemical composition of dentin.

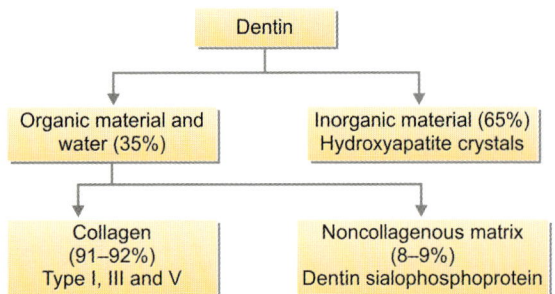

Organic components include 91–92% of collagen (predominantly type I and small amounts of type III and V) and 8–9% of noncollagenous matrix (glycosaminoglycans and proteoglycans) or ground substances. The noncollagenous matrix proteins regulate mineralization and can act as inhibitors, promoters, and/or stabilizers; these proteins include dentin phosphoprotein/phosphophoryn (DPP), dentin sialoprotein (DSP), dentin glycol protein (DGP), and dentin matrix protein-1 (DMP 1), which are combined together and typed as dentin sialophosphoprotein, with small amounts of citrate, chondroitin sulfate, insoluble proteins, and lipids.

HISTOLOGY OF DENTIN

The dentin is made up of closely packed microchannels called dentinal tubules. This encloses cytoplasmic process of odontoblasts and contains dentinal fluid. The rim of dentinal tubule is slightly more mineralized and is called as peritubular dentin. That portion of dentin that lies in between the tubules is called intertubular dentin **(Figures 6-5A and B)**.

Dentinal Tubules

The dentinal tubules are the spaces or voids formed during the movement of odontoblasts toward the pulp during dentinogenesis. They occupy 20–30% of the volume. Dentinal tubules start from peripheral portion of the pulp and end at dentinoenamel junction and dentinocemental junction. The dentinal tubules start perpendicular from the pulpal surface. In transverse sections, they appear to radiate from the pulp; however course of dentinal tubules is not straight. In longitudinal sections they show a gentle "s"-shaped curvature known as primary curvature **(Figures 6-6A and B)**.

The first convexity of this curvature is facing toward the root. Primary curvature is more pronounced in the coronal dentin and it is relatively straight in radicular dentin, incisal edges, and cusp tips **(Figure 6-6B)**. Secondary curvatures are mild undulations present in each dentinal tubule depicting the course taken by the odontoblasts during the formation of dentin **(Figures 6-7A to C)**.

The average number of dentinal tubules per square millimeter ranges from 40,000 to 80,000. The outline of the dentinal tubule is usually circular and the density of the tubules is more in crown compared to the root and it is least in the apical thirds **(Figures 6-8 and 6-9)**. The number of tubules per unit area in pulpal surface is more than the other

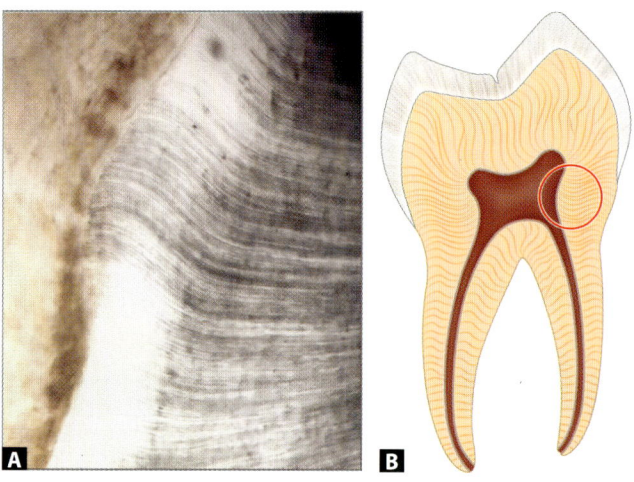

Figures 6-6A and B: (A) Ground section showing the primary curvature of the dentinal tubules; (B) Primary curvature is more pronounced in the crown.

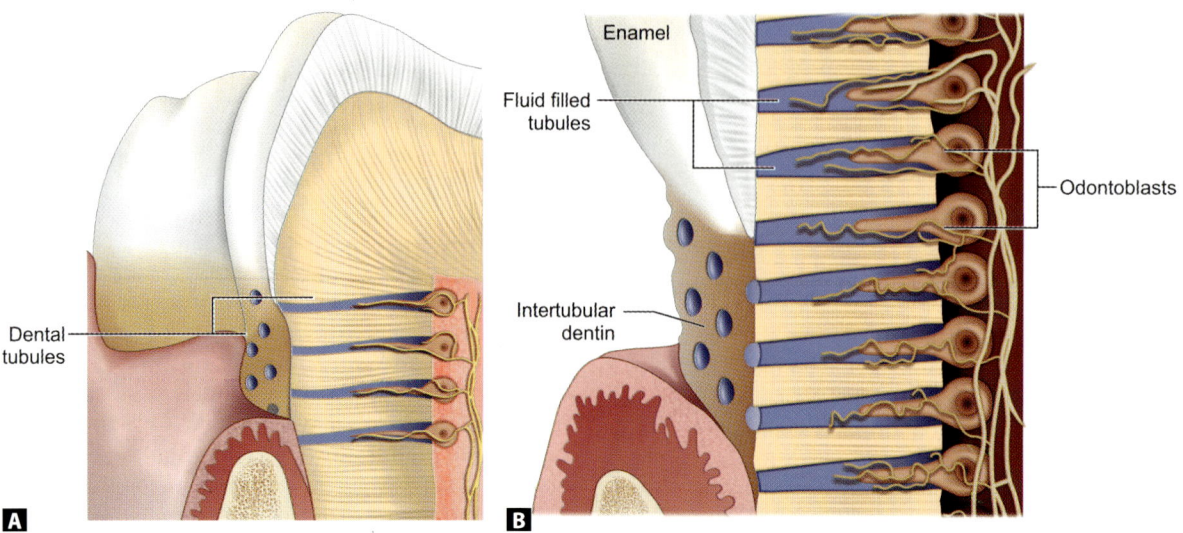

Figures 6-5A and B: (A) Course of the dentinal tubules with its content; (B) Closer view showing odontoblastic process and dentinal fluid.

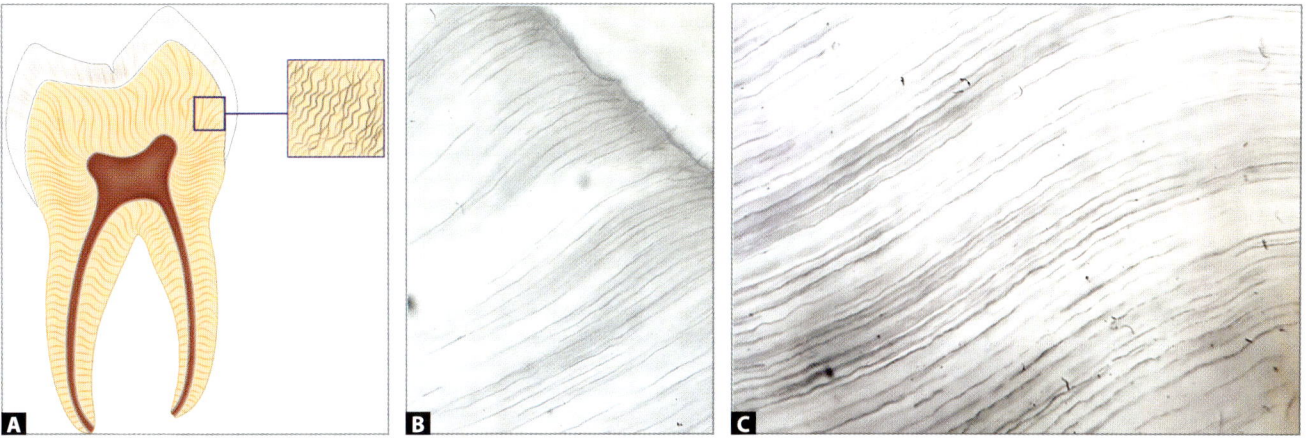

Figures 6-7A to C: Illustration of secondary curvatures in the insert (A) and secondary curvatures in ground section (B and C).

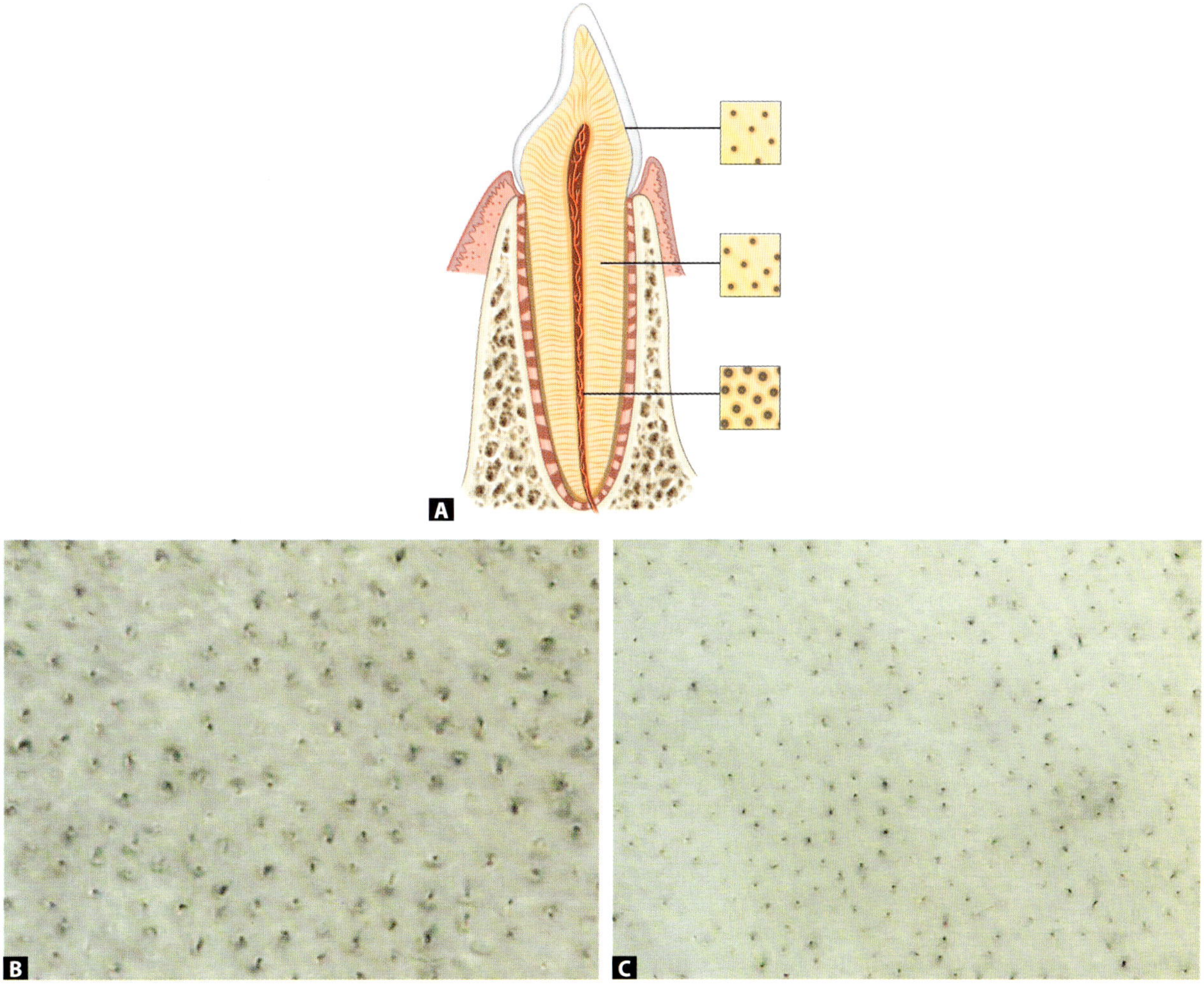

Figures 6-8A to C: (A) Image showing varying sizes and numbers of the dentinal tubules in different locations; (B and C) Cross section of dentinal tubules in ground section.

areas. Similarly, the diameter of each tubule is also more in this region (3–4 µm). The diameter of tubule towards the cementum and enamel is about 1 µm.

The dentinal tubules branch periodically (for every 1–2 µm) and these lateral branches are called as canaliculi. They start approximately perpendicular to the main tubule. The diameter of each canaliculus is about 1 µm. These lateral ramifications anastomose with the neighboring ones and are more pronounced in the root near the cementum.

Peritubular Dentin (Intratubular Dentin)

This forms the inner rim of the dentinal tubule (**Figure 6-10**). Ideally, it should be called intratubular dentin and it

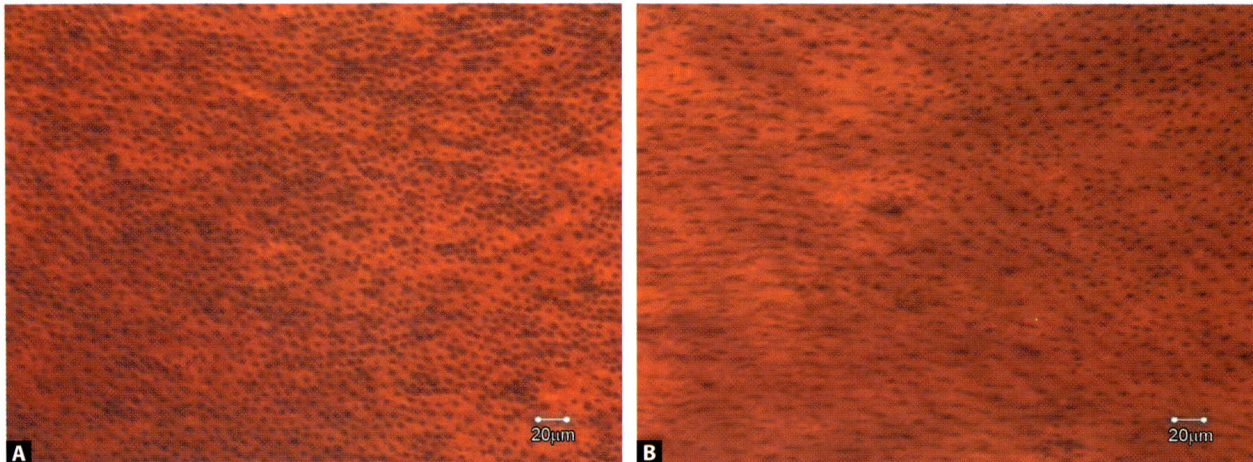

Figures 6-9A and B: Cross section of dentinal tubules in decalcified section under confocal microscope.
Source: Dr N Malathi, Department of Oral Pathology, Sri Ramachandra Dental College, Chennai, India, and Dr J Logeswari, Department of Oral Pathology, Meenakshi Ammal Dental College, Chennai India

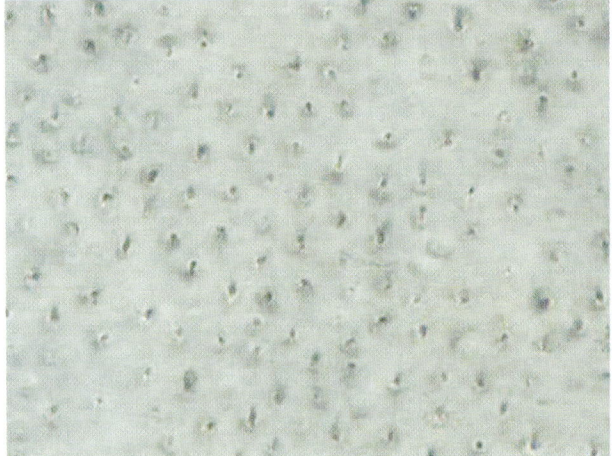

Figure 6-10: Peritubular dentin in ground section.

was called so, since it lines the dentinal tubules. It is dense, uniformly mineralized (about 10% more mineralized than that of the intertubular dentin), and slightly more radiopaque. Its matrix composition and the shape of the hydroxyapatite crystals are different from that of the intertubular dentin. The organic matrix of the peritubular dentin contains less amount of collagen fibers and more amount of noncollagenous proteins like DSP and DMP, which is secreted by the odontoblasts and deposited onto the already mineralized wall of the dentinal tubule through the odontoblastic process. It was also postulated that the mineralization of intratubular dentin occurs by precipitation of calcium from the dentinal fluid. The thickness of the peritubular dentin varies from one location to another location, more at the outer portion and less near the inner dentin. It is absent in predentin (unmineralized dentin matrix).

> Peritubular dentin does not result from such transformation of predentin into dentin, but rather from the adsorption along the lumen of the tubules of an amorphous matrix, may be secreted by the odontoblastic processes within dentin, or taking origin from the serum (dentinal lymph).

A thin organic membrane high in glycosaminoglycans lines the intratubular dentin and is known as lamina limitans. This is considered by some as the plasma membrane of the odontoblastic process. This is actually a hypomineralized intratubular dentin.

Intertubular Dentin

The intertubular dentin forms the core component of the dentin by occupying 50% of its volume. It is present in between the peritubular dentin and the dentinal tubules. The volume of the intertubular dentin is less near the pulp than the dentinoenamel and cementodentinal junction because the number and the diameter of dentinal tubules are more and the surface area of the dentin is less in the circumpulpal dentin.

Intertubular dentin is less mineralized than the peritubular dentin; however the organic content is more and predominately composed of collagen fibers. These collagen fibers are oriented randomly in the crisscross pattern with size of each fibril ranges from 0.2 μm to 0.5 μm and exhibits 64 nm periodicity. The organic components, namely proline and hydroxyproline are comparatively more. The collagen fibers of the intertubular dentin are arranged randomly and are more or less perpendicular to the dentinal tubules. The hydroxyapatite crystals of the intertubular dentin are smaller than the apatite crystals of the enamel and the average length is about 40 nm. The crystals are needle-shaped and laid over the collagen fibers with their long axis parallel to the fibrils. The crystals, when deposited, grow on the surface of the collagen fibrils and later into the fibrils and eventually obscuring them.

Odontoblastic Process

Odontoblastic process, also called as Tomes' fiber, is the cytoplasmic extension of the odontoblast and occupies the dentinal tubule. As the odontoblasts secrete predentin (dentin matrix), they move away from the basement membrane which separates them from the inner enamel epithelial cells (*i.e.* toward the pulp), leaving many small cytoplasmic extensions.

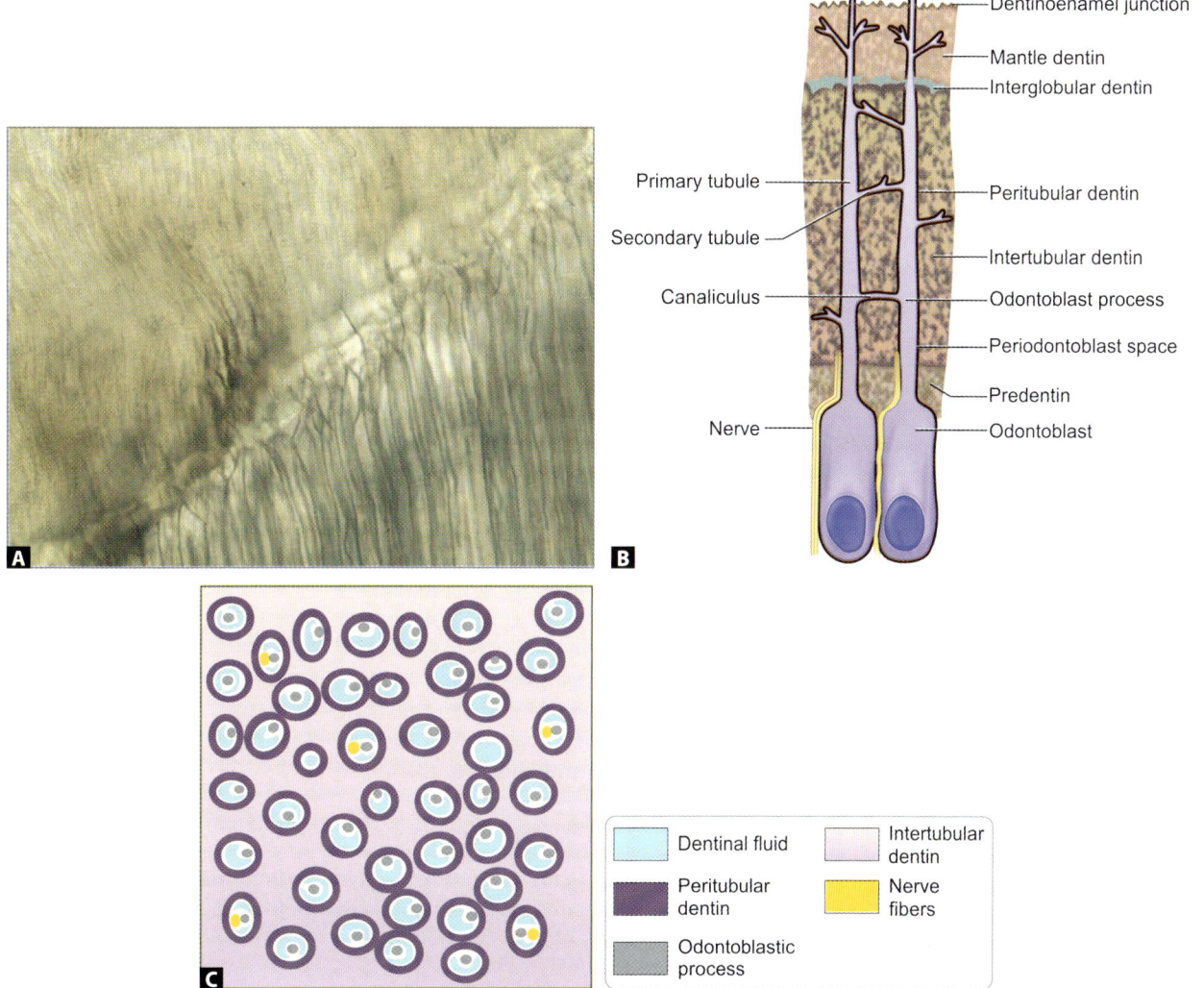

Figures 6-11A to C: (A) Ground section showing terminal branching of odontoblastic process; (B) Schematic representation showing the odontoblastic process; and (C) The content of the dentinal tubules.

These extensions join to form one process. Ultimately each dentinal tubule is occupied by one odontoblastic process with its lateral branches entering into the canaliculi (**Figures 6-11B**). The diameter of the odontoblastic process is large (3–5 µm) near the pulp and it diminishes gradually. Usually, odontoblastic process starts from the neck of the odontoblasts and extends till the dentinoenamel junction (**Figures 6-11A to C**). This is proved by the demonstration of "tubulin", an intracellular protein of microtubules in entire thickness of the dentin. Rarely odontoblastic process crosses the basement membrane and placed between the ameloblasts. Enamel forms surrounding this process and is called as **enamel spindle**. Few odontoblastic processes may be shorter and do not traverse the entire thickness of the dentin. The remaining unoccupied portion of these dentinal tubules is filled with tissue fluid, organic debris or may be obliterated by mineral deposits. These are devoid of major cellular organelles. They contain predominantly microtubules and microfilaments. Mitochondria, lysosomes, and coated and pinocytic vesicles are also seen to an extent. During the formation of dentin, secretory granules are transported toward the odontoblastic process for their discharge. They also mediate the formation of the peritubular dentin.

Dentinal Fluid

Dentinal fluid, also called dental lymph, is present inside the dentinal tubules, a reason for relatively high water content. It can be demonstrated on the surface of the freshly cut dentin. It is the ultrafiltrate of pulpal capillary blood. So it is considered to be the transudate and it occupies 22% of the dentin volume. It is not considered to be derived from odontoblastic process, since the sodium–potassium ratio of this is closer to the interstitial fluid. It is an important component of the pulp-dentin complex and acts as a medium for dentin and pulp communication. Rapid movement of this fluid within the dentin causes dentin sensitivity.

> Molecular markers present in dentinal fluid can be used to study the nature of pulpal inflammation. Recent researches show that the dentinal fluid penetrates the dentin and alter the dental caries biofilm. It is also demonstrated that the MMP-9 level in the dentinal fluid correlates with the depth of dental caries penetration.

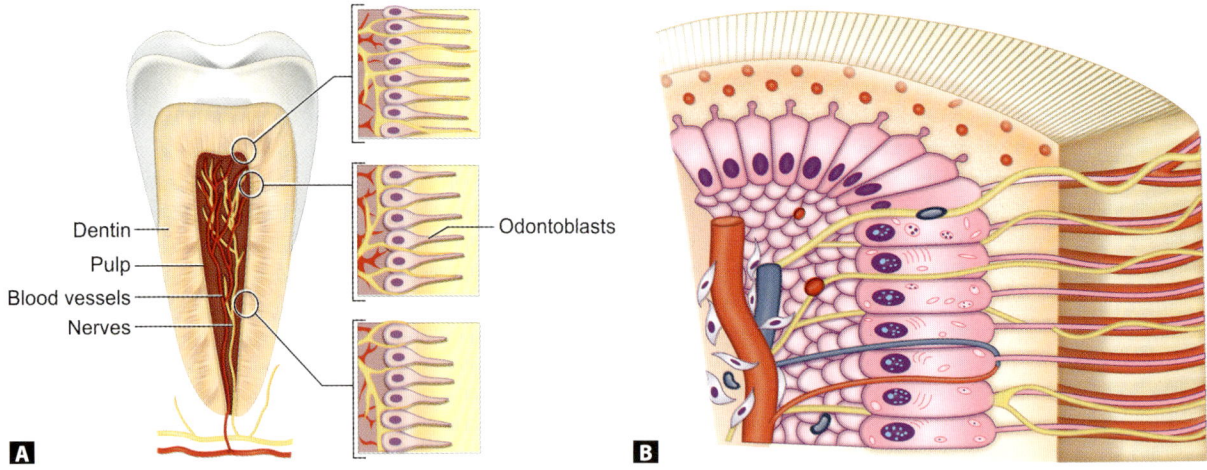

Figures 6-12A and B: (A) Dentin innervations; (B) Closer view showing the odontoblasts bordering the pulp.

Dentin Innervation

Few dentinal tubules containing nerve fibers and nerve endings are a variable feature. Nerves arrive at the dentinal tubules from the Raschkow plexus of pulp through predentin **(Figures 6-12A and B)**. They run parallel to the odontoblastic process and may partially encircle the odontoblastic process; however they do not form any discernible junction or synopsis with it. On occasions, they travel till the dentinoenamel junction.

Predentin

Unmineralized dentin matrix is called predentin, comparable to the osteoid of the bone, and it forms the boundary between the odontoblastic layer of the pulp and the dentin. Thickness of the predentin is about 10–20 μm in the crown. The thickness becomes minimal in resting period. As the dentin matrix gets mineralized to become the circumpulpal dentin, a new layer of predentin forms around the pulp **(Figure 6-13)**. So there is always presence of a layer of predentin at the proximal portion of the odontoblasts. It is mainly composed of collagen fibers and ground substances secreted by the odontoblasts.

STRUCTURAL PATTERNS OF DENTIN

Dentin which is formed before the root completion is known as primary dentin and the one which is formed after the root completion is known as secondary dentin **(Flowchart 6-2 and Figure 6-14)**.

Primary Dentin

Primary dentin is of two types namely, mantle dentin and circumpulpal dentin **(Figure 6-14)**.

Mantle Dentin

Mantle dentin, the first formed dentin presents parallel to the dentinoenamel junction and is a product of not fully differentiated odontoblasts. It occupies the space of the basement membrane, which separates the inner enamel epithelium from the odontoblastic layer of the pulp. Mantle dentin and the first formed enamel interdigitate to form the dentinoenamel junction and gives the scalloped appearance. It is about 20 μm in thickness. It is composed of large collagen fibers, which run roughly perpendicular to the dentinoenamel junction. The fibrillar component of the

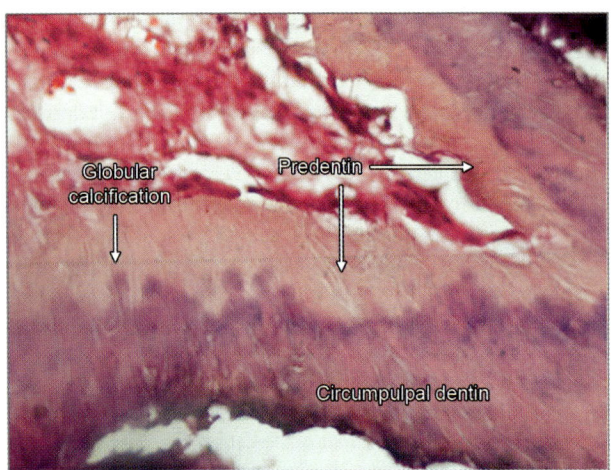

Figure 6-13: Hematoxylin and eosin-stained section showing pulp, predentin, and circumpulpal dentin.

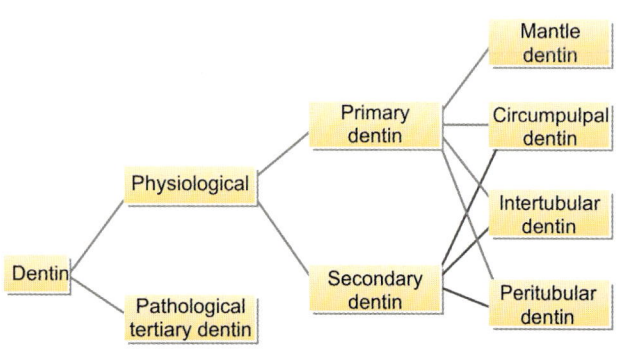

Flowchart 6-2: Structure of dentin.

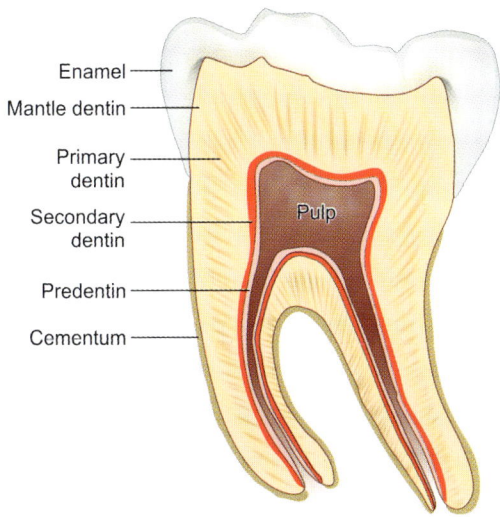

Figure 6-14: Structural pattern of dentin.

mantle dentin includes aperiodic collagen fibers, von Korff fibers, and collagen fibers. von Korff fibers run parallel to the odontoblasts and they fan out at the dentinoenamel junction. According to some workers, Korff fibers are large diameter fibers (100 μm–200 μm) and made up of type III collagen. Others believed that they are not actual fibers and are made up of glycosaminoglycans and glycoprotein, which take up the silver stain and appear as fibers. Their existence is still controversial. Mantle dentin is hypomineralized with more profusely branched tubules, compared to the circumpulpal dentin.

Circumpulpal Dentin

It is seen adjacent to the mantle dentin and forms the bulk of the primary dentin. The junction between the mantle dentin and circumpulpal dentin is demarcated by the occurrence of increased hypomineralized areas (interglobular dentin). Circumpulpal dentin is formed by the fully differentiated odontoblasts and made up of collagen fibers secreted by the odontoblasts. It is always bounded by a layer of predentin at the pulpal side. The collagen fibers of the circumpulpal dentin are smaller, dense, interwoven, parallel to the plane of apposition and roughly perpendicular to the direction of odontoblastic process. It is slightly more mineralized than the mantle dentin.

Secondary Dentin

Formation of dentin is a process that occurs throughout the life as long as the pulp is viable. Dentin, which is formed after root completion is known as secondary dentin and is in continuity with the primary dentin; however there will be an abrupt bending of the dentinal tubules in the primary dentin–secondary dentin interface. Course of the tubules in secondary dentin is irregular. This is a physiologic process and occurs at a slower rate. Continuous formation of secondary dentin results in the reduction of the pulp volume. Secondary dentin is not deposited evenly around the pulp and it is deposited at a slower rate. It is formed more in roof and floor of the pulp chamber and in teeth which are subjected to increased masticatory stress.

> Secondary dentin deposition results in the alteration of the size and shape of the pulp chamber and pulp canals. Since the volume of the dentin increases with age due to the deposition of secondary dentin, the color of the tooth becomes more yellowish. As secondary dentin formation continues and the odontoblasts move toward pulp, they become crowded. This is due to the reduction in the pulpal volume, which causes an increase in the number of odontoblasts per unit area. This crowding of odontoblasts leads to the death of few due to apoptosis. The corresponding dentinal tubules become empty or get mineralized and occluded.

Interglobular Dentin

As mentioned previously, it is more commonly seen adjacent to the junction between the mantle dentin and circumpulpal dentin. These are hypomineralized areas (**Figures 6-15A to D**).

Mineralization of dentin occurs in two patterns, *i.e.* globular and linear. The spherical foci of hydroxyapatite are formed from calcium phosphate nucleating sites and this is called calcospherites or calcifying globules. These calcifying globules enlarge and fuse with adjacent globules. Often they fail to fuse completely and the spaces between these globules are hypomineralized or unmineralized. These areas are called interglobular dentin.

In interglobular dentin, the course of the dentinal tubules is uninterrupted, denoting the defect in the mineralization and not in the matrix formation. Intratubular dentin (peritubular dentin) is absent in this region. In ground sections, interglobular dentin appears dark under transmitted light and is characterized by scalloped outline of nonfused calcifying globules. Usually they occur more in crown, at the junction of the mantle dentin and circumpulpal dentin, however on occasions they can be seen in the cervical one-third of the radicular dentin.

Tomes' Granular Layer

Radicular dentin adjacent to cementum exhibits granular appearance and is known as Tomes' granular layer (**Figures 6-16A and B**). This is composed of numerous closely packed minute areas of hypomineralized dentin. It extends from the cervical portion of the root to the apex and its thickness increases toward the apex. This is another structural defect like interglobular dentin. It can be seen only in ground section and appears as dark granules in the transmitted light. Various views regarding the occurrence of Tomes' granular layer have been put forth namely—(1) coalescing and looping of the dentinal tubules, (2) considered to be the true spaces, (3) miniature of interglobular dentin, and (4) peculiar arrangement of collagen and noncollagenous matrix proteins at dentinocemental junction. These areas are hypomineralized or unmineralized. Calcium and phosphate concentrations are more in Tomes' granular layer when compared to other hypomineralized areas of the tooth.

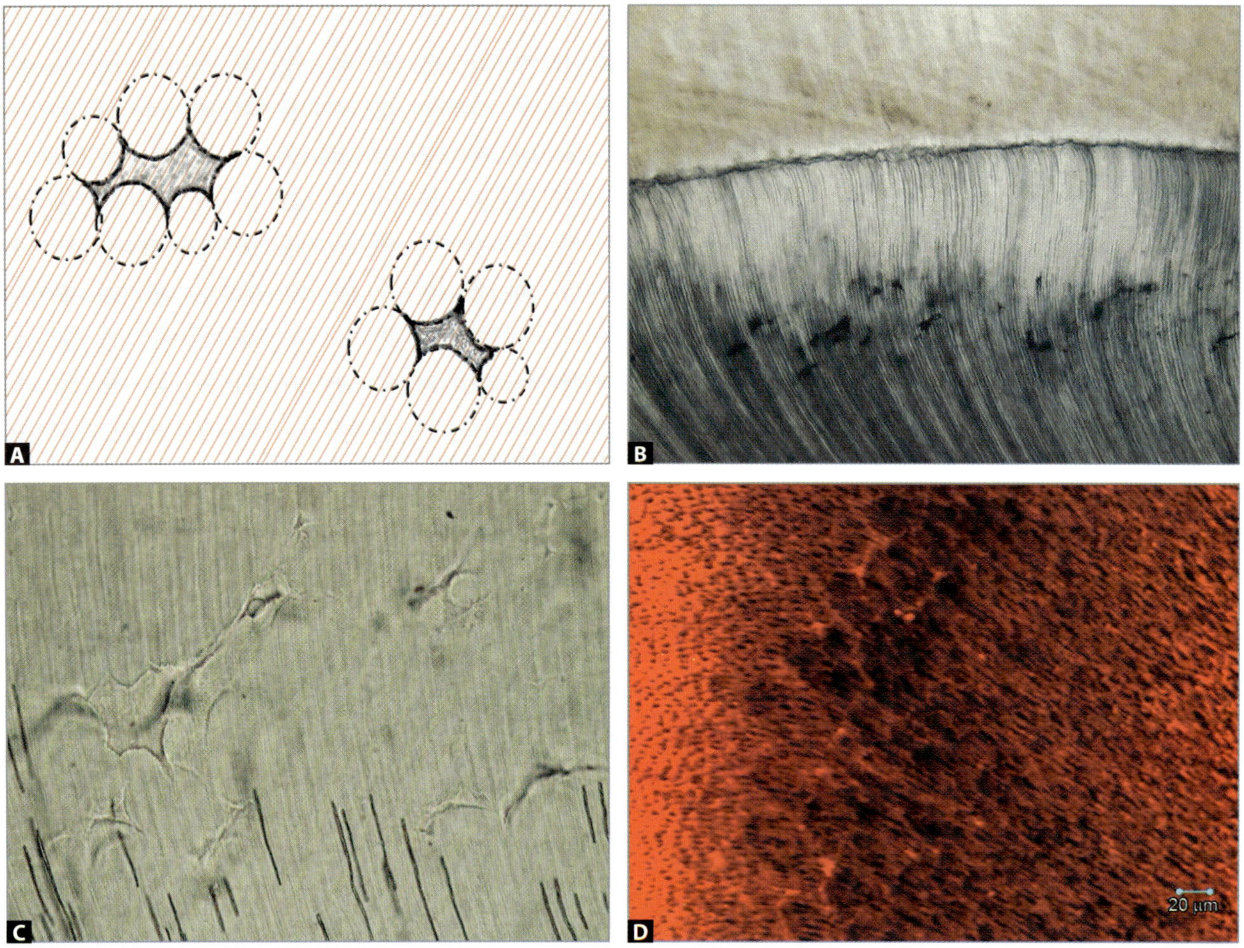

Figures 6-15A to D: (A) Formation of interglobular dentin; (B) Ground section of interglobular dentin in low power; (C) High power; and (D) Decalcified section under confocal microscope.

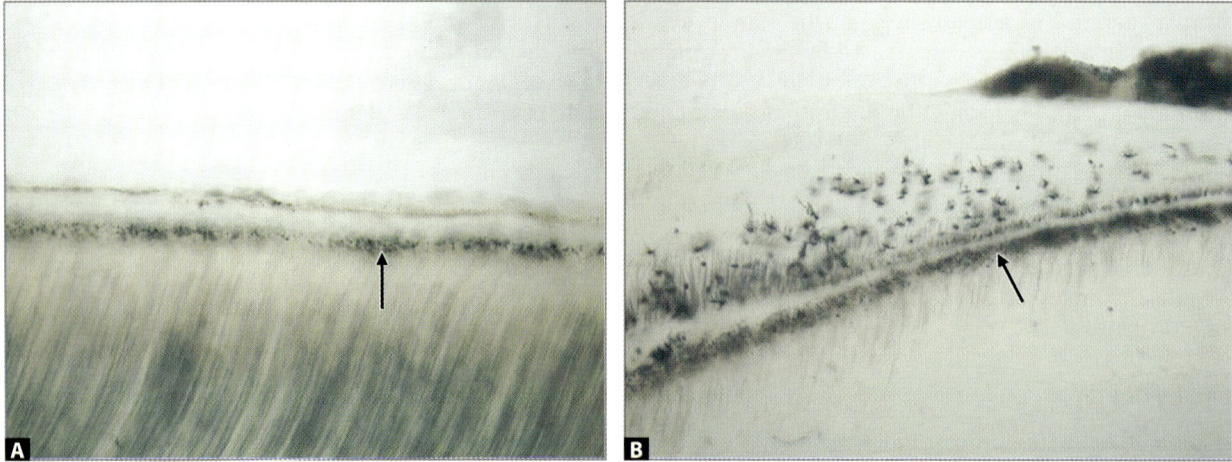

Figures 6-16A and B: Ground sections showing Tomes' granular layer.

Incremental Lines

Similar to the formation of other hard tissue, dentin formation occurs in rhythmic pattern. There is a period of activity followed by period of rest and is reflected by the occurrence of incremental lines **(Figure 6-17)**. They are also known as "imbrication lines of von Ebner". They appear as fine lines or striations with 20 μm intervals and run perpendicular to the dentinal tubules. About 4–8 μm thickness of dentin is formed everyday during dentin development. Between each increment there is a minute change in orientation of the collagen fibers. The change in the collagen fiber orientation is more exaggerated at five days interval, which is indicated by an incremental line.

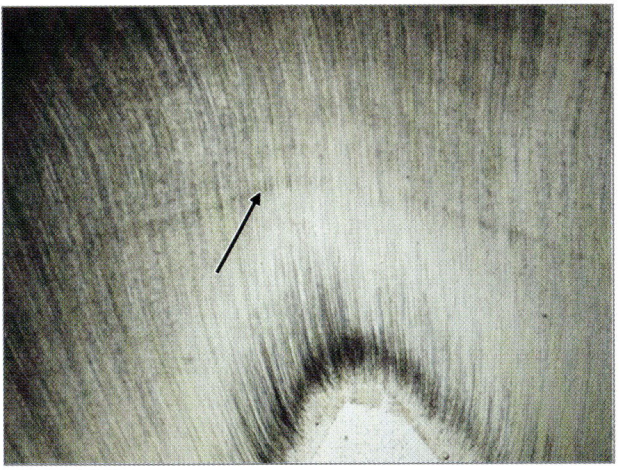

Figure 6-17: Ground section showing incremental line of von Ebner.

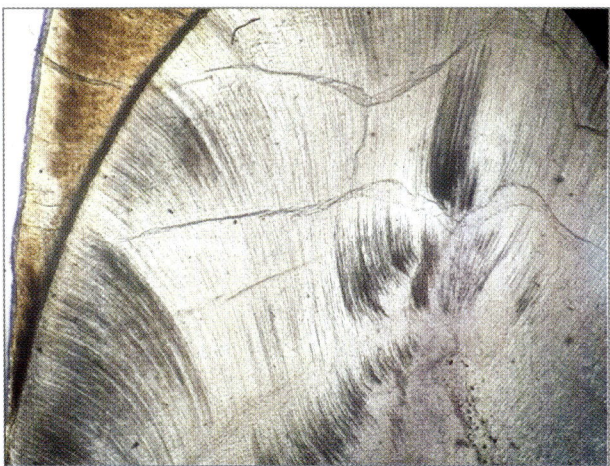

Figure 6-18: Contour lines of Owen.

Contour Lines of Owen

Accentuated incremental lines are called contour lines of Owen. They represent the normal physiologic change in the pattern of mineralization. Alternate view regarding the formation of these lines is the coincidence of secondary curvature of the dentinal tubules. These lines are hypomineralized. They are present at irregular intervals and in variable numbers **(Figure 6-18)**. *Neonatal line* demarcates the dentin developed before birth and after birth. It is nothing but the exaggerated contour lines of Owen and typifies the environmental changes namely nutritional, hormonal, etc. that occur at the time of birth. They are usually seen in deciduous teeth and permanent first molars.

Sclerotic Dentin

This is also known as transparent dentin. The mineral content and hardness of the sclerotic dentin is more while the permeability is lesser than the rest of the dentin. This occurs due to the occlusion of dentinal tubule by mineralization of the dentinal tubules, which results in change in the refractory index of the dentin, the reason for being transparent or glass-like **(Figure 6-19)**.

Dentinal sclerosis increases with advancing of age. It most commonly occurs in the apical third of the root and midway between the dentinoenamel junction and pulpal wall in crown. Dentinal sclerosis may be physiologic or stimulated. Continuous formation of intratubular dentin resulting in dentinal sclerosis is physiologic.

Stimuli such as caries, attrition, abrasion, erosion, and cavity preparation also induce the formation of sclerotic dentin. Collagen fibers and apatite crystals appear in the dentinal tubules and gradually the lumen of the tubules will be filled with dentin similar to the formation of intertubular dentin. Alternatively calcium salts are precipitated within the tubule and cause occlusion of the dentinal tubules.

When odontoblast is dead or their process is retracted, the tubules become empty. These are called *dead tracts* **(Figure 6-20)**. Further, damaged or dead and dying odontoblastic process induces or enhances mineralization. Blocking of the dentinal tubule is considered as a defense mechanism by which the permeability of the dentin is reduced and pulp is protected.

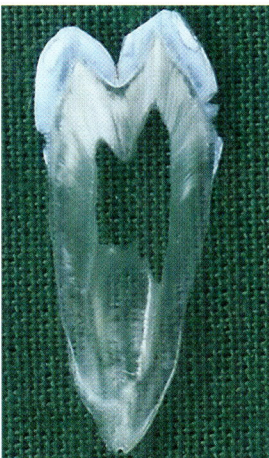

Figure 6-19: Sclerotic or transparent dentin.

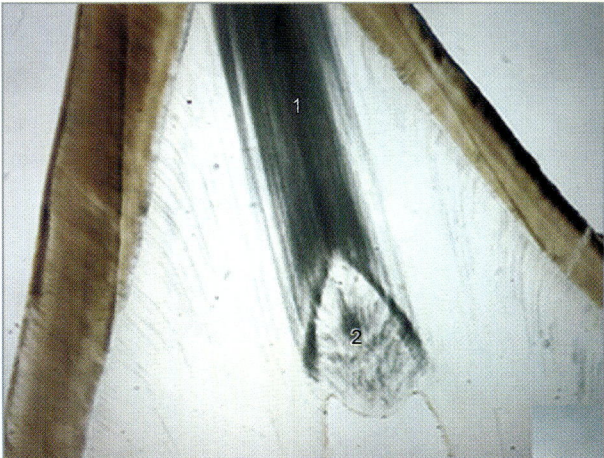

Figure 6-20: Ground section showing: (1) Dead tracts; and (2) Sclerotic dentin.

Reparative Dentin

(Tertiary dentin, Irregular secondary dentin, Response dentin, Reactive dentin)

Enamel once damaged cannot be repaired by itself, since the enamel-forming cells, the ameloblasts, do not exist after the formation of enamel. But dentin has the reparative capacity as long as the odontoblasts are viable in the pulp.

Reparative or tertiary dentin is formed in response to a number of pathological stimuli such as caries, attrition, abrasion, erosion or restorative procedures, unlike secondary dentin, which is a physiologic process. It is a defensive reaction of the pulp–dentin complex.

Tertiary dentin formed by injured, damaged or normal odontoblasts of the odontoblastic layer of the pulp is known as reactionary or regenerated dentin. If the dentin is formed by newly differentiated odontoblasts from the cells of the subodontoblastic layer to replace the dead odontoblasts, it is called *reparative dentin* **(Figure 6-21)**.

Reparative dentin differs from the secondary dentin by having fewer, irregular, and more twisted dentinal tubules. It is more mineralized and localized to the area of injury. It is demarcated from the secondary dentin by a line called calciotraumatic line.

> Growth factors such as bone morphogenetic protein (BMP), insulin-like growth factor (IGF), and fibroblast growth factor (FGF) from the dentin matrix act as inductive stimuli for the cell proliferation and differentiation of odontoblasts to form the tertiary dentin.
>
> On occasions, rate of tertiary dentin deposition is rapid. During this process, the odontoblasts get entrapped in the dentin matrix and the formed dentin resembles bone **(Figures 6-22A to D)**. This is known as osteodentin and formation of which is implicated with BMP. Sometimes vascular inclusions result in the formation of vasodentin. Formation of atubular fibrodentin is also not uncommon. During reparative dentin formation, nestin and notch protein along with other growth factors are re-expressed, while they are absent in matured odontoblasts.

Dead Tracts

When odontoblastic process is retracted or degenerated, or odontoblast is dead, the dentinal tubules become empty

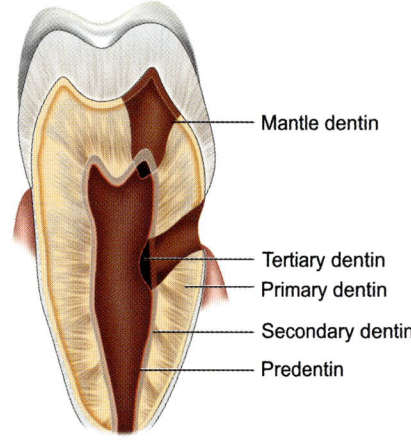

Figure 6-21: Different types of dentin present in the tooth.

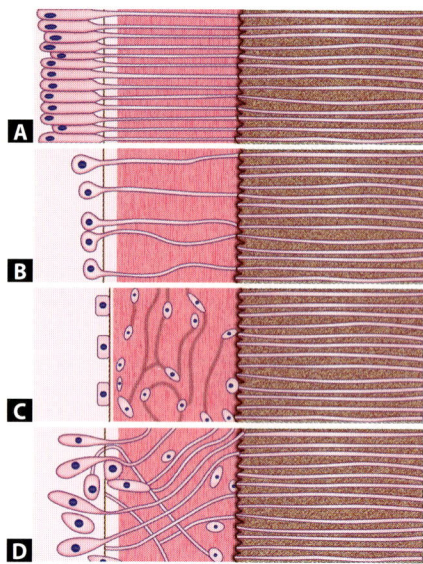

Figures 6-22A to D: Schematic diagram of reparative dentin: (A) Normal; (B) Few tubules; (C) Osteodentin; (D) Irregular.

and they appear dark in transmitted light. This may be due to caries, attrition, and abrasion or as a physiologic process. Dead tracts extend from dentinoenamel or dentinocemental junction to the pulp and are often bounded by a band of sclerotic dentin **(Figure 6-20)**.

In the region of narrow pulp horns, there is crowding of the odontoblasts within the pulp. This results in death of some of them. This may cause the formation of dead tracts in the pulp horn region, which is physiologic.

DENTIN SENSITIVITY

Dentin is a sensitive tissue. When dentin is exposed during restorative procedure or due to wearing off, the tooth becomes extremely sensitive. Also the dentin becomes sensitive in gingival recessions exposing the radicular dentin. Enamel and cementum meets at the cervical portion of the tooth and is known as cementoenamel junction. Enamel may meet the cementum at a sharp line or cementum may overlap enamel. In small percentages of cases, cementum and enamel do not meet (*i.e* there is no cementoenamel junction) and the radicular dentin is exposed. In such cases, when the gingiva is receded, tooth becomes sensitive.

There are three theories put forward to explain the dentin sensitivity, namely—(1) direct neural theory, (2) transduction theory, and (3) hydrodynamic theory **(Figure 6-23)**.

Direct neural theory: Terminal nerve fibers from the pulp accompany the odontoblastic process within the dentinal tubules. These intratubular nerves are seen in 30–70% of the tubules. In occlusal dentin especially over the pulp horn, almost every other dentinal tubule will have a nerve fiber. These are somatosensory unmyelinated nerve fibers and pass between the odontoblasts to extend into the predentin and dentinal tubules. Some of the nerve fibers exhibit dendritic ramifications in predentin.

Vesiculated nerve endings are more common in pulp horn region (extension of coronal pulp corresponds to the abolish sensitivity. Also this theory does not explain why dentinoenamel junction is more sensitive than rest of the dentin.

Transduction theory: According to this theory, odontoblast with its process acts as a receptor cell and it converts the stimuli into an impulse and propagates it. This is based on the fact that odontoblasts are of neural crest origin and they retain the capacity to do so. But there is no synoptic relationship between the odontoblast—axon was demonstrated. Membrane potential of the odontoblasts is too low to permit transduction and also no neurotransmitters seem to exist in the odontoblastic process.

Hydrodynamic theory: This is the most accepted and popular theory. As per this theory, transmission of stimuli is aided by the movement of dentinal fluid that excites the nerves closely associated with the odontoblastic process. Thermal, mechanical or osmotic change commonly causes the movement or displacement of the dentinal fluid. This movement causes mechanical disturbance of the intratubular nerve endings. This explains why the air desiccation or consumption of sweets causes sensitivity or pain when dentin is exposed.

DENTINOGENESIS

Formation of dentin is called dentinogenesis. Dentin is the first hard tissue to be formed in the tooth. Cells responsible for the formation of dentin are called odontoblasts. These cells are differentiated from the ectomesenchymal cells (dental papilla cells) of the dental organ by the organizing influence of the inner enamel epithelial cells.

Odontoblasts are biologically related to osteoblasts of the bone. Dentin formation starts first at the bell stage of tooth development, at the cusp tips. There are multiple formation sites for multicusped teeth. Adjacent formative sites fuse gradually. Coronal dentin forms at a rate of 4 μm per day initially. Radicular dentin forms at a slightly slower rate. It further slows down to approximately 1 μm per day after the eruption. The rate of dentin deposition formed in reaction to any insult (reparative dentin *q.v.*) is again about 4 μm per day. As stated previously, formation of dentin is a constant process and occurs throughout the life as long as the pulp is viable.

Similar to the formation of other hard tissues, dentin formation also occurs in two stages, namely—matrix (predentin) formation and mineralization.

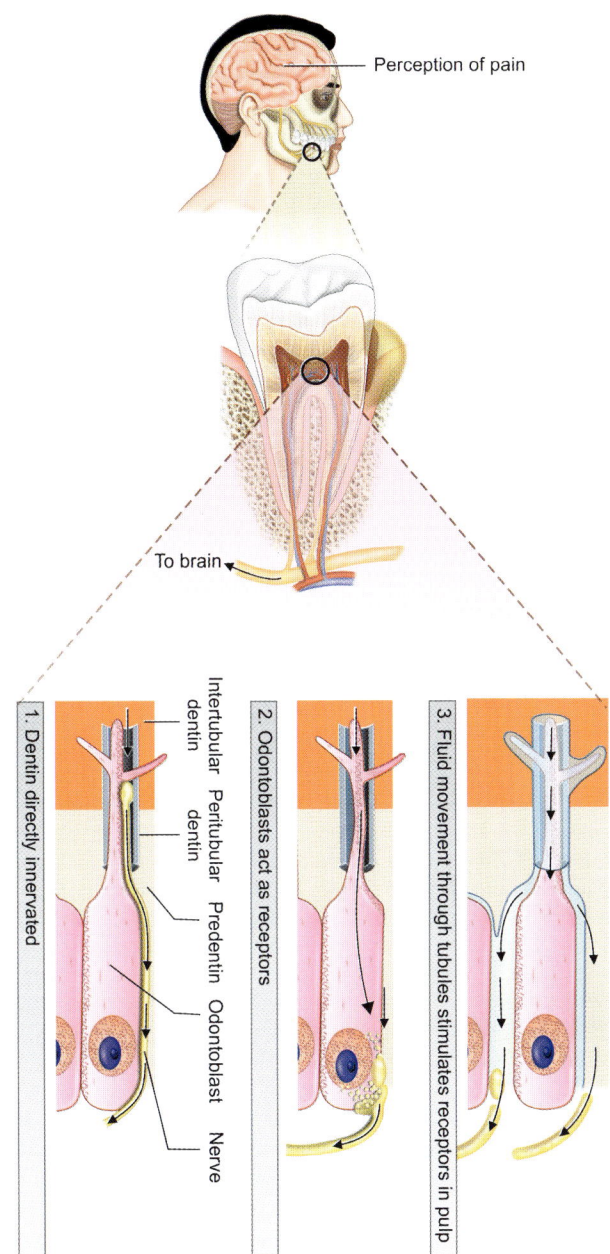

Figure 6-23: Schematic diagram representing the three theories of dentin sensitivity.

cusp of the tooth). The nerve endings within the tubules in proximity to the pulp were described electron microscopically being round to oval in outline and seemed to contain few mitochondria and minute vesicles. Existence of junctions or synopsis between the odontoblastic process and the intratubular nerves is a subject of controversy. According to few, there exists gap junction or synoptic contact between the odontoblastic process and the nerves but others refute this.

According to the direct neural theory, pain perception or dentin sensitivity is due to the direct stimulation of intratubular nerves. But this is not accepted by the majority, since pain producing substances like histamine, 5-hydroxytryptamine or prostaglandin fail to produce pain when applied on the dentin. Further, application of topical anesthetic does not

Mineralization of Dentin

Mineralization of the matrix results from a complex series of well-coordinated events that require optimal function of numerous genes and their products. Enamel, dentin and bone are major tissues that develop through matrix-mediated mineralization processes.

Matrix of the mantle dentin gets mineralized before enamel is secreted by ameloblasts. Matrix vesicles from odontoblasts provide nucleation sites for mineralization of the mantle dentin to form the outer layer. In contrast, mineralization of the inner layer of dentin, *i.e.* circumpulpal dentin proceeds via spreading of mineral deposition from the preexisting mineralized dentin matrix.

Organic components of the dentin matrix are degraded when mineralization occurs. Enzymes such as matrix metalloproteinases (MMPs) expressed and secreted by odontoblasts degrade organic components such as proteoglycans to allow the mineral crystals composed of poorly crystalline hydroxyapatite to grow and concentrate.

> Though the term "calcification" is generally used synonymously with mineralization, it is usually not a physiologic event. But mineralization is generally physiologic.
> Biomineralization is the deposition of minerals orchestrated by the cells. It is a cell-mediated process by which hydroxyapatite crystals are deposited in the extracellular matrix (ECM) of skeletal structures. Structural molecules of the ECM and a series of enzymes direct the entry and fixation of mineral salts exclusively in bone and mineralized dental tissues.
> During dentin formation, three different types of mineralization occur namely, the cell-derived matrix vesicles-driven mineralization occurring in the mantle dentin, the extracellular matrix molecules-derived mineralization in circumpulpal dentin accounting for the majority of dentin formation, and the serum-derived precipitation occurring in the peritubular dentin. Dentin phosphophoryn (DPP) are implicated in intertubular dentin mineralization. There are evidences to suggest that the collagen can act as the inducer or nucleating substance.

Mineralization of dentin (except intratubular dentin) occurs in two patterns namely, linear and globular. In the linear pattern of mineralization, very fine plate of hydroxyapatite crystals are deposited initially on the surface of the collagen fibers and in the ground substance. It is followed by the laying down of crystals within the fibrils.

The long axis of the crystals is parallel to the long axis of the collagen fibrils and arranged in an orderly fashion.

In globular pattern of mineralization, also known as spherulitic calcification, there is formation of calcifying globules called calcospherites. Globular calcification begins at a point in several discrete areas. The center of mineralization slowly enlarges radially to fuse with the adjacent ones. Failure of complete fusion the adjacent globules result in the formation of hypomineralized or unmineralized areas in between them and are known as interglobular dentin **(Figures 6-15A to D)**.

> Core-binding factor α (Cbfa1) is an important transcription factor for osteoblastic differentiation and osteogenesis. Odontoblasts and osteoblasts are similar to certain extent at molecular level. Cbfa1 also influence odontoblast differentiation.
> There are two views regarding the action of Cbfa1. According to the first view, the inductive signals are turned on in dental epithelium by a Cbfa1-dependent pathway and that these molecules then act back upon the mesenchyme to stimulate odontoblast differentiation. The other view is that the Cbfa1 may regulate the expression of other inductive molecules in the mesenchyme that directly influence odontoblast differentiation.

Odontoblasts Differentiation and Matrix Formation

Dentin matrix (predentin) formation begins at early bell stage, wherein the star-shaped peripheral cells of the dental papilla differentiate into odontoblasts, the dentin-secreting cells.

Differentiation of ectomesenchymal cells into odontoblasts involves many molecular mechanisms, which are still not clear. Various morphogens, cytokines, extracellular matrix molecules, and cell–cell interactions have been implicated in the differentiation of odontoblasts.

Signaling molecules and growth factors like fibronectin, decorin, laminin, and chondroitin sulfate in the dental papilla are responsible for odontoblast differentiation.

> Studies have also included the role of laminin α2, a laminin subunit for matrix secretion. Similarly growth factors like transforming growth factor (TGF), IGF, and BMP present at the inner enamel epithelium have an inducting influence on the peripheral cells of the dental papilla (preodontoblasts). These factors also have influence on the cytoskeleton of the preodontoblasts for the relocation of nucleus and other cellular organelles, which occur during odontoblastic differentiation.

Dental papilla cells undergo certain number of mitosis to differentiate into odontoblasts. Odontoblastic differentiation is characterized by cessation of cell division, changes in the cell size and shape, polarization of nuclei, and increase in the organelle content.

> The peripheral cells of the dental papilla, adjacent to the basement membrane, undergo mitosis. During mitosis, the mitotic spindle of some cells may be perpendicular to the basement membrane. In such cells, the daughter cell, one which is close to the basement membrane, becomes the odontoblasts. The other cell, which partially receives the inductive influence from the inner enamel epithelial cells, remains in the subodontoblastic layer **(Figure 6-24)**. When necessity comes, the cells of the subodontoblastic layer differentiate into odontoblasts as in case of reparative dentin.

At initial stages, the star-shaped dental papilla cells contain large circular nuclei and minimal amount of cytoplasm with few indistinct organelles and numerous free ribosomes. In between the basement membrane and dental papilla cells, there exists a narrow band of tissue, devoid of cells. It is called acellular zone and this zone contains fine fibrils.

As these cells differentiate into preodontoblasts, they become short columnar with increase in cytoplasmic volume and organelles. Nucleus gradually migrates toward the basal end with increase in the amount of synthetic organelles. The shape of these cells changes from a short columnar to tall columnar to become fully differentiated young odontoblasts. As they differentiate into tall columnar cells, they develop one or more apical process, later they unite to form a single odontoblastic process. The acellular zone between the basal membrane and preodontoblasts disappears due to the lengthening of the odontoblast.

When the odontoblasts are ready for secretion of dentin matrix, they become large plump cells (with about 40–50 μm length, with 7 μm width) with open-faced nucleus situated basely. The apical end of the cell consists of full complement of secretory organelles in their cytoplasm. This includes large cisternae of rough endoplasmic reticulum arranged parallel

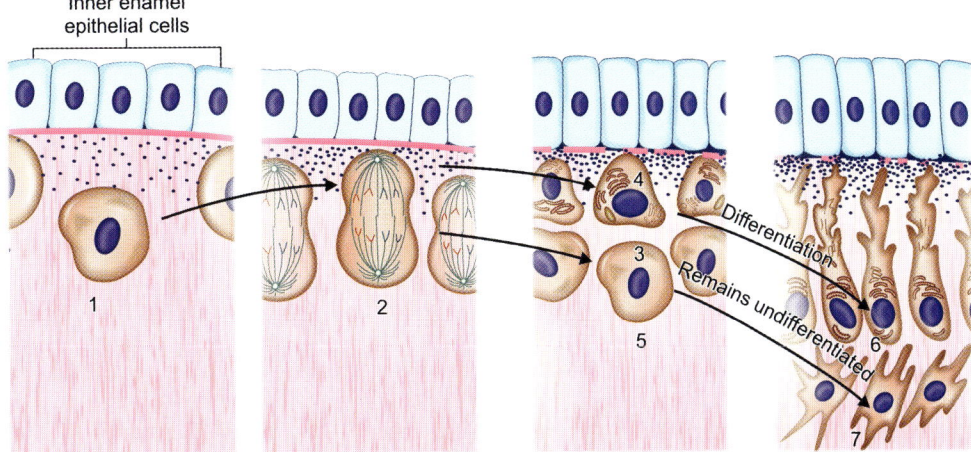

Figure 6-24: Differentiation of odontoblasts. 1. Undifferentiated dental papilla cell; 2. Mitotic spindle; 3. and 4. daughter cells; 5. Pulp; 6. Odontoblast; 7. Cell of the subodontoblastic layer.

to the long axis of the cell, large amount of Golgi apparatus, and secretory granules. They also exhibit alkaline phosphatase activity. The odontoblasts arrange themselves in a row with extensive junctional complexes and gap junctions between them.

After the differentiation of odontoblasts, the next step is to form the organic matrix of the dentin, which consists of collagen (type I and III) fibers and the ground substance. Ground substance consists of glycosaminoglycans, glycoproteins, and phosphoproteins. Procollagen, the precursor for the dentin collagen is synthesized in the rough endoplasmic reticulum and gets concentrated in Golgi apparatus. Further these molecules combine with the carbohydrates to form glycoproteins and are packed within the Golgi vesicles as carbohydrate–protein complexes, and are called as presecretory granules. These granules mature into secretory granules as they move toward the odontoblastic process and discharge as collagen of predentin through exocytosis. These procollagen building blocks polymerize extracellularly, that is, within the predentin, into collagen fibrils.

All of these substances are secreted at the distal cell poles of the odontoblasts, mainly around the odontoblastic process, where they form the predentin, which accumulates distal to the odontoblastic layer (against the ameloblasts). As the odontoblasts secrete dentin matrix they move toward the center portion of the dental organ.

Later this dentin matrix mineralizes at a distinct distance from the odontoblastic layer. Predentin is laid down first near the future incisal edges and the cusps tips and progresses toward the cervical region **(Figure 6-25)**. Predentin remains unmineralized for a day and till the next layer of predentin is formed. So there will be always a layer of unmineralized dentin matrix present at the pulpal border, like osteoid of the bone.

Radicular dentin formation differs from the coronal dentin in the following aspects. It is formed at a slower rate. Collagen fibers are laid down parallel to the cementodentinal junction and fibers intermingle with the fibers of the cementum. Radicular dentin is slightly less mineralized than the coronal dentin.

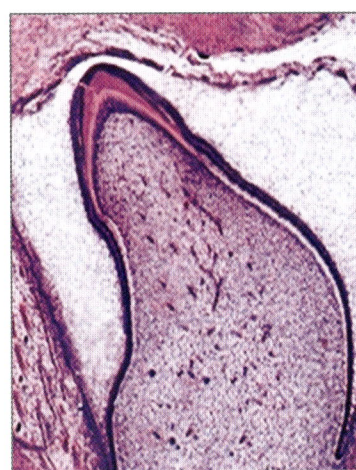

Figure 6-25: Late bell stage in tooth development with dentin secreted by odontoblasts and enamel by ameloblasts.

CLINICAL CONSIDERATIONS

Formation of dentin is affected in dentinogenesis imperfecta, dentin dysplasia, and regional odontodysplasia. These are hereditary diseases.

In dentinogenesis imperfecta, the affected teeth appear gray to yellowish-brown in color. Crown is bulbous with exaggerated cervical constriction. This condition is caused by mutation in gene encoding dentin sialophosphoprotein. Dentin dysplasia may affect crown or root. Clinically tooth appears normal. In this condition, enamel is normal, dentin is dysplastic, and pulpal morphology is abnormal.

Roots are malformed and may be short and blunt.

Regional odontodysplasia, also called as ghost tooth, affects maxillary anterior teeth. Radiographically enamel and dentin appears thin and pulp chamber is exceedingly large.

As stated previously, dentin is a vital tissue though avascular. Tooth preparation is routine in dental practice for any restorative procedures. When one square millimeter of dentin is exposed, there is exposure of about 40,000 dentinal tubules along with odontoblastic process.

Since dentinal tubules act as pathways for the spread of microorganisms, rate of caries spread towards the pulp is more rapid when it reaches dentin. Further when the dental caries process reaches the dentinoenamel junction it spreads laterally. Lateral branching of the dentinal tubules paves way for the spread of caries in lateral aspect when it reaches the dentin.

Tooth sensitivity in patients with dentin exposure when taking sweets can be explained by the hydrodynamic theory (the osmotic effect).

The thickness of dentin left between the pulp and the floor or wall of the prepared tooth is known as "remaining dentin thickness (RDT)". When RDT is above 2 mm, there is no requirement of any lining material and the pulp is relatively safe. If it is less than 2 mm, the pulp is at a risk of chemical, thermal, and microbial injury and a protective lining or base is mandatory.

When there is severe trauma to the tooth, the blood supply to the pulp is severed and the tooth becomes nonvital. A nonvital tooth usually appears gray. This is due to the entry of the products of hemolysis into the dentinal tubules.

In restorations involving direct bonding composite resin, the tooth substance is etched with 37% phosphoric acid. This procedure creates micropores in the enamel. In dentin, acid etching causes decalcification of intratubular dentin, and the dentinal tubules become wider. Also, it exposes the collagen fibers. Bonding material is attached to the collagen fibers thereby enhancing the retention of the composite resin to the dentin.

Points to Remember

- Formation of dentin is called dentinogenesis. Cells responsible for the formation of dentin are called odontoblasts.
- Similar to the other hard tissues dentin formation occurs in two steps. First step is the formation of the dentin matrix, called predentin.
- This dentin matrix gets mineralized. Mineralization occurs in two patterns namely linear and globular.
- The spaces between calcifying globules are hypomineralized or unmineralized and are called interglobular dentin.
- It is the first formed hard tissue and is covered by enamel in the crown and cementum in the root.
- Physical and chemical properties of dentin are almost similar to that of bone but dentin is avascular and slightly harder than bone.
- Color of the dentin is light yellowish and it determines the color of the tooth; however it is modified by the nature of enamel.
- Dentin is made up of 65% inorganic and 35% of organic material and water. The mineral components of the dentin are calcium and phosphate hydroxyapatite crystals. Organic components include 91–92% of collagen (predominantly type I and small amounts of type III and V) and 8–9% of noncollagenous matrix (glycosaminoglycans and proteoglycans) or ground substances.
- The dentin is made up of closely packed microchannels called dentinal tubules.
- The course of dentinal tubules is not straight. In longitudinal sections they show a gentle "s"-shaped curvature known as primary curvature. Secondary curvatures are mild undulations present in each dentinal tubule depicting the course taken by the odontoblasts during the formation of dentin.
- Peritubular or intratubular dentin forms the inner rim of the dentinal tubule and is about 10% more mineralized than that of the intertubular dentin.
- Intertubular dentin is present between the peritubular dentin and the dentinal tubules and occupies 50% of the dentin volume.
- Odontoblastic process, also called as Tomes' fiber, is the cytoplasmic extension of the odontoblast and occupies the dentinal tubule.
- Enamel spindles are extension of odontoblastic process into the enamel before enamel is formed.
- Dentinal fluid, also called dental lymph, is present inside the dentinal tubules and is considered to be a transudate.
- Few dentinal tubules contain nerve fibers, which arrive from the Raschkow plexus of pulp through predentin.
- There are three theories put forth regarding the dentin sensitivity, namely direct neural theory, transduction theory, and hydrodynamic theory.
- Dentin formed before the root completion is known as primary dentin and the one which is formed after the root completion is known as secondary dentin.
- Mantle dentin is the first formed dentin. Circumpulpal dentin is seen adjacent to the mantle dentin and forms the bulk of the primary dentin.
- Incremental lines of the dentin are known as "imbrication lines of von Ebner" and the accentuated incremental lines are called contour lines of Owen.
- Neonatal line demarcates between the dentin developed before birth and after birth.
- Sclerotic dentin or transparent dentin occurs due to the occlusion of dentinal tubule by mineralization of involved dentinal tubules.
- Tomes' granular layer is composed of numerous closely packed minute areas of hypomineralized dentin seen in the radicular dentin adjacent to cementum.
- Reparative or tertiary dentin is formed in response to pathological stimuli.
- Dead tracts are empty dentinal tubules that occur due to the retraction or degeneration of odontoblasts and appear dark in transmitted light.
- Formation of dentin is affected in hereditary diseases like dentinogenesis imperfecta, dentin dysplasia, and regional odontodysplasia.

PRACTICE QUESTIONS

1. Write notes on physical properties and chemical composition of dentin.
2. Write notes on dentinogenesis.
3. Write notes on dentinal tubules.
4. Write notes on hypomineralized areas of the dentin.
5. What are primary and secondary dentin.
6. Theories of dentin sensitivity.
7. What is Tomes' granular layer?
8. What are dead tracts?

MULTIPLE CHOICE QUESTIONS

1. **Cells responsible for the formation of dentin are called**
   a. Osteoblasts
   b. Odontoblasts
   c. Ameloblasts
   d. Cementoblasts
2. **First formed hard tissue of the tooth is**
   a. Enamel
   b. Dentin
   c. Cementum
   d. Alveolar bone
3. **Odontoblasts are derived from**
   a. Inner enamel epithelium
   b. Outer enamel epithelium
   c. Dental papilla cells
   d. Dental sac cells
4. **Small undulations representing the course taken by the odontoblasts during dentinogenesis are called**
   a. Primary curvature
   b. Secondary curvature
   c. Contour lines of Owen
   d. Curvature of von Ebner
5. **Dentin is a vital tissue since it contains**
   a. Blood vessels
   b. Lymph vessels
   c. Odontoblasts
   d. Odontoblastic process
6. **Unmineralized dentin matrix is called**
   a. Dentinoid
   b. Predentin
   c. Prodentin
   d. Mantle dentin
7. **Dentin formed before the root completion is called**
   a. Mantle dentin
   b. Primary dentin
   c. Secondary dentin
   d. Circumpulpal dentin
8. **Incremental lines of the dentin is known as**
   a. Contour lines of Owen
   b. Incremental lines of Retzius
   c. von Ebner lines
   d. Reversal lines
9. **Contour lines of Owen are**
   a. Incremental line of dentin
   b. Accentuated incremental lines of dentin
   c. Seen in the dentinoenamel junction
   d. Also called lines of von Ebner
10. **Peritubular or intratubular dentin is**
    a. Hypomineralized
    b. More mineralized
    c. Seen in between the dentinal tubules and the intertububular dentin
    d. Forms the bulk of the dentin
11. **Sclerotic dentin is**
    a. Also called transparent dentin
    b. Formed due to the mineralization of dentinal tubules
    c. Also seen in aging tooth
    d. All of the above
12. **Tomes' granular layer is**
    a. Prominent in the crown
    b. Seen in the radicular dentin adjacent to the cementum
    c. Hypermineralized
    d. Formed due to increase in collagen
13. **von Korff fibers**
    a. Are seen during the formation of the dentin
    b. Run parallel to the odontoblasts and they fan out at the dentinoenamel junction
    c. Korff fibers are large diameter fibers made up of type III collagen
    d. All of the above
14. **Interglobular dentin is**
    a. Formed due to the failure or incomplete fusion of the calcifying globules
    b. More mineralized
    c. Carious tooth
    d. Formed due to the linear pattern of mineralization
15. **Mantle dentin is**
    a. Also called as intratubular dentin
    b. More mineralized
    c. The first formed dentin
    d. Formed after root completion
16. **Empty dentinal tubule which appear dark in reflected light under the microscope is called**
    a. Dead tract
    b. Enamel spindle
    c. Dentinal sclerosis
    d. Dentin dysplasia
17. **In dentinogenesis imperfecta**
    a. The affected teeth appear gray to yellowish-brown in color
    b. Crown is bulbous with exaggerated cervical constriction
    c. There is mutation in gene encoding dentin sialophosphoprotein
    d. All of the above

ANSWERS

1. b 2. b 3. c 4. b 5. d 6. b 7. b 8. c 9. b 10. b 11. d 12. b 13. d 14. a 15. c
16. a 17. d

BIBLIOGRAPHY

1. About I, Mitsiadis TA. Molecular aspects of tooth pathogenesis and repair: *in vivo* and *in vitro* models. Adv Dent Res. 2001;15:59.
2. Addy M, West NX, Barlow A, et al. Dentine hypersensitivity: is there both stimulus and placebo responses in clinical trials. Int J Dent Hyg. 2007;5(1):53.
3. Avery JK, Chiego DJ. Essentials of oral histology and embryology-a clinical approach, 3rd edition. US: Mosby; 2006.
4. Ballal V, Rao S, Bagheri A, Bhat V, Attin T, Zehnder M. MMP-9 in dentinal fluid correlates with caries lesion depth. Caries Res. 2017;51(5):460-465. doi: 10.1159/000479040. Epub 2017 Aug 22. PMID: 28848154.
5. Batouli S, Miura M, Brahim J, et al. Comparison of stem cell- mediated osteogenesis and dentinogenesis. J Dent Res. 2003;82(12):976.
6. Berkovitz BKB, Holland GR, Moxham BJ. Oral anatomy, histology and embryology, 4th edition. US: Elsevier; 2009.
7. Bleicher F, Couble ML, Buchaille R, et al. New genes involved in odontoblast differentiation. Adv Dent Res. 2001;15:30.
8. Bradley RM. Essentials of oral physiology, 1st edition. USA: Mosby; 1995.
9. Brizuela C, Meza G, Mercadé M, Inostroza C, Chaparro A, Bravo I, Briceño C, Hernández M, Giner L, Ramírez V. Inflammatory biomarkers in dentinal fluid as an approach to molecular diagnostics in pulpitis. Int Endod J. 2020 Sep;53(9):1181-1191. doi: 10.1111/iej.13343. Epub 2020 Jul 21. PMID: 32496605.
10. Butler WT. Dentin matrix proteins. Eur J Oral Sci. 1998;106:204.
11. Carda C, Peydro A. Ultrastructural patterns of human dentinal tubules odontoblasts processes and nerve fibers. Tissue Cell. 2006;38(2):141-50.
12. Chandra S, Chandra S, Chandra M, et al. Textbook of dental and oral histology with embryology & MCQ's, 2nd edition. NewDelhi: Jaypee Brothers Medical Publishers (P) Ltd; 2010.
13. Chatterjee K. Essentials of dental anatomy and oral histology, 2nd edition. New Delhi: Jaypee Brothers Medical Publishers (P) Ltd; 2014.
14. de Barros Pinto L, Lira MLLA, Cavalcanti YW, Dantas ELA, Vieira MLO, de Carvalho GG, de Sousa FB. Natural enamel caries, dentine reactions, dentinal fluid and biofilm. Sci Rep. 2019 Feb 26;9(1):2841. doi: 10.1038/s41598-019-38684-7. PMID: 30808878; PMCID: PMC6391475.
15. Gasga JR, Gracia G, Alvarez Fregoso, et al. Conductivity in human tooth enamel. J Mat Sci. 1999;34(9):2183.
16. Goldberg M, Kulkarni AB, Young M, et al. Dentin: structure, composition and mineralization. Front Biosci Elite Ed. 2011;3:711-35.
17. Huang GT. Dental pulp and dentin tissue engineering and regeneration: advancement and challenge. Front Biosci Elite Ed. 2011;3:788-800.
18. Khurana A, Khurana I. Human embryology, 2nd edition. India: CBS publishers and Distributor Pvt Ltd; 2012.
19. Kono RT, Suwa G, Tanijiri T. A three-dimensional analysis of enamel distribution patterns in human permanent first molars. Arch Oral Biol. 2002;147(12):867.
20. Kumat GS. Orban's Oral histology and embryology, 14th edition. India: Elsevier; 2015.
21. Li C, Jing Y, Wang K, et al. Dentinal mineralization is not limited in the mineralization front but occurs along with the entire odontoblast process. Int J Biol Sci. 2018;14(7):693-704.
22. MacDougall M, Dong J, Acevedo AC. Molecular basis of human dentin diseases. Am J Med Genet A. 2006;140:25-36.
23. Maroto M, Barberia E, Planelis P, et al. Dentin bridge formation after mineral trioxide aggregate (MTA) pulpotomies in primary teeth. Am J Dent. 2005;18(3):151.
24. Maurin JC, Delorme G, Machuca-Gavet I, et al. Odontoblast expressions of semaphorin 7A during innervation of human dentin. Matrix Biol. 2005;24(3):232.
25. Murray PE, About I, Lumley PJ, et al. Human odontoblast cell numbers after dental injury. J Dent. 2000;28(4):277.
26. Murray PE, Smith AJ, Windsor LJ, et al. Remaining dentine thickness and human pulp responses. Int Endod J. 2003;36(1):33.
27. Nanci A (Ed). Dentin, pulp complex. Ten Cate's oral histology development, structure and function, 6th edition. St Louis: Elsevier; 2005. pp. 198-239.
28. Neville BW, Damm DD, Allen CN, et al. Oral and maxillofacial pathology, 1st South Asia Edition. India: Elsevier; 2016.
29. Odell EW, Morgan PR. Biopsy pathology of the oral tissues, 1st edition. UK: Chapman & Hall; 1998.
30. Ogita Y, Iwai-Liaop Y, Higashi Y. A histological study of the organic elements in the human enamel focusing on the extent of the odontoblast process. Okajimas Falia Anat Jpn. 1998;74(6):317.
31. Provenza VD, Seibel W. Oral histology-inheritance and development, 2nd edition. USA: Lea & Febiger; 1986.
32. Qin C, Baba O, Butler WT. Post-translational modifications of sibling proteins and their roles in osteogenesis and dentinogenesis. Crit Rev Oral Biol Med. 2004;15:126.
33. Sasaki T, Garant PR. Structure and organization of odontoblasts. Anat Rec. 1996;245(2):235-49.
34. Schroeder HE. Oral structural biology, 4th edition. New York: Thieme; 1991.
35. Sivapathasundharam B. Shafer's textbook of oral pathology, 8th edition. India: Elsevier; 2016.
36. Timothy SM, Nauntofte B, Svensson P. Clinical oral physiology, 1st edition. Copenhagen: Quintessence Publishing Co. Ltd; 2004.
37. Volponi AA, Pang Y, Sharpe PT. Stem cell-based biological tooth repair and regeneration. Trends Cell Biol. 2010;20:715-22.
38. Yamakoshi Y, Hu JC-C, Fukae M, et al. Dentin glycoprotein: the protein in the middle of the dentin sialophosphoprotein chimera. J Biol Chem. 2005;280:17472.
39. Yoshiba K, Yoshiba N, Ejiri S, et al. Odontoblast processes in human dentin revealed by fluorescence labeling and transmission electron microscopy. Histochem Cell Biol. 2002;118(3):205-12.

CHAPTER 7

Pulp

B Sivapathasundharam

Chapter Outline

- Structure of Pulp   84
  - Odontoblasts and Odontoblastic Layer   85
  - Cell-free Zone of Weil   88
  - Cell-rich Zone   88
- Cells of the Pulp   88
  - Odontoblasts   88
  - Fibroblasts   88
  - Histiocytes   89
  - Dendritic Cells   89
  - Inflammatory Cells   89
- Intercellular Substance   89
  - Extracellular Matrix   89
  - Fibers of the Pulp   90
  - Blood Vessels   90
  - Lymph Vessels   90
  - Nerves   90
- Functions of Pulp   91
  - Inductive   91
  - Formative   91
  - Nutritive   91
  - Protective   91
  - Defensive and Reparative   91
- Development of Pulp   91
- Age Changes   92
  - Pulp Stones   92
  - Diffuse Calcifications   92
- Clinical Considerations   92
  - Vitality   92
  - Pulpal and Root Canal Anatomy   93
  - Pulpitis   93
  - Internal Resorption   94
  - Recession of Pulp Horns   94
  - Pulpal Changes during Exfoliation of Primary Teeth   94

Pulp is a soft connective tissue derived from ectomesenchyme and occupies the central portion of the tooth. It is enclosed all around by dentin except in the apical portion of the root, where it communicates with the apical periodontium. Pulp and dentin are developmentally, structurally, and functionally related and are often referred to as pulp-dentin complex. Pulp is responsible for the vitality of the tooth and more specifically the dentin. Anything which affects the dentin may have its effect on the pulp since the dentinal tubules start at pulp and the disturbances of the pulp may affect the quality and the quantity of the dentin produced. It is gelatinous in consistency and about 75% of its content is water. Pulp tissue is composed of cells and extracellular matrix. Similar to other connective tissues, extracellular matrix is more than the cells in volume. The shape of the pulp roughly resembles the shape of the tooth.

Pulp in the crown portion is called coronal pulp and resides in the space called pulp chamber. It is large and contains more biological elements. Pulp of the root portion is called radicular pulp and resides in the root canal or pulp canal. It acts as a conducting channel for blood vessels, lymphatics and nerves **(Figure 7-1)**. Coronal pulp has small projections known as pulp horns usually toward the cusp.

Number of pulp horns corresponds to the number of cusps. The junction between the coronal and the radicular pulp is marked by a constriction coinciding with the cervical constriction of the tooth.

The total volume of the permanent pulp organ is about 0.38 cc with a mean of 0.02 cc for the individual pulp organ. Molar pulp organ is the largest and is about four times bigger than that of the mandibular incisor pulp (the smallest pulp organ). The volume of the pulp organ gets reduced and the shape altered as age advances. The shape of the coronal pulp roughly resembles a rectangular block with six surfaces and pulp horns on the occlusal surface extend toward the cusps. The shape of the radicular pulp conforms to the shape of the root.

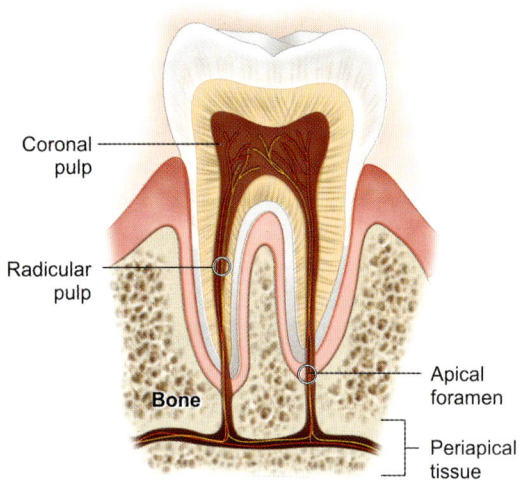

Figure 7-1: Illustration of tooth showing the components of the pulp and the periapical region.

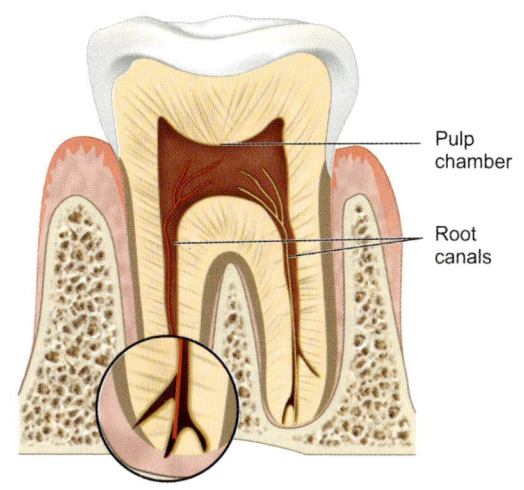

Figure 7-2: Illustration showing course of pulp canals as primary canals and accessory canals toward the apex.

Root canal and apical foramen: The root canals are also called pulp canals and they accommodate the radicular pulp. They are usually funnel-shaped, wide at cervical end and narrow down toward the apical foramen. In cross section, pulp canals appear circular, elliptical or flattened. Number of root canals usually depends on the number of roots. Some roots have more than one canal. Circular or conical roots usually have one canal, whereas elliptical or flattened roots frequently have more than one. Root canals start at the floor of the pulp chamber and end at the apical foramen and are called primary canals. The canals other than the primary (usually in branching pattern) are called accessory canals. Primary canal starts as a single canal and branches or divides anywhere during its course, sometimes to form the accessory canal **(Figure 7-2)**. Branches are more common at the apical third of the root and this may be referred as apical ramifications. Accessory canals are also called as lateral canals and they usually open at the lateral surface of the root. They are formed by the premature loss or break in the Hertwig's epithelial root sheath during root formation. Break in the root sheath causes failure of odontoblast and cementoblast differentiation from the dental papilla and dental sac respectively and results in the formation of tubular defect. Lateral canal may also be formed when the developing root encounters a blood vessel. Dentin formation around the vessels results in the development of lateral canals, which are most commonly located in the apical one-third.

Apical foramen is the opening at the root apex, through which the pulp communicates with the periodontium. Vessels and nerves enter and exit through it. The diameter of the apical foramen varies from 0.3 mm to 0.6 mm. The diameter, shape, number, and location may vary and may change as the age advances. Usually they are located at the tip of the roots; however accessory canals may open at the lateral surface of the root. The location of the apical foramen is not static, and may relocate due to secondary dentin and cementum deposition, mesial migration of the tooth or endodontic treatment. Apical foramen is usually composed of dentin, but at times may be composed of only cementum.

Root canals and the apical foramen narrow down as age advances. Sometimes root canals become obliterated due to the continued deposition of the secondary dentin.

STRUCTURE OF PULP

Pulp is a specialized loose connective tissue composed of cells and extracellular matrix (ECM) or substance **(Flowchart 7-1)**. Even mature pulp resembles the embryonic connective tissue and acts as a rich source for stem cells. Cells of the pulp include odontoblasts, fibroblasts, immunocompetent cells, and undifferentiated mesenchymal cells (mesenchymal stem cells). The intercellular matrix consists of blood vessels, nerves, fibers, and ground substance. The central zone or the pulp core contains large vessels and nerves. The peripheral zone or odontogenic zone is well-organized with histologically appreciable architecture, namely (1) odontoblastic layer, (2) cell-free zone, also known as zone of Weil, and (3) cell-rich zone **(Figures 7-3A to D)**.

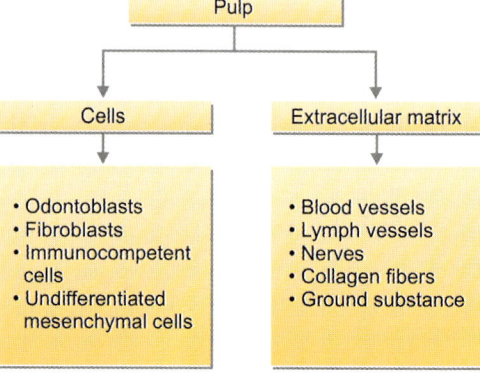

Flowchart 7-1: Structure of pulp.

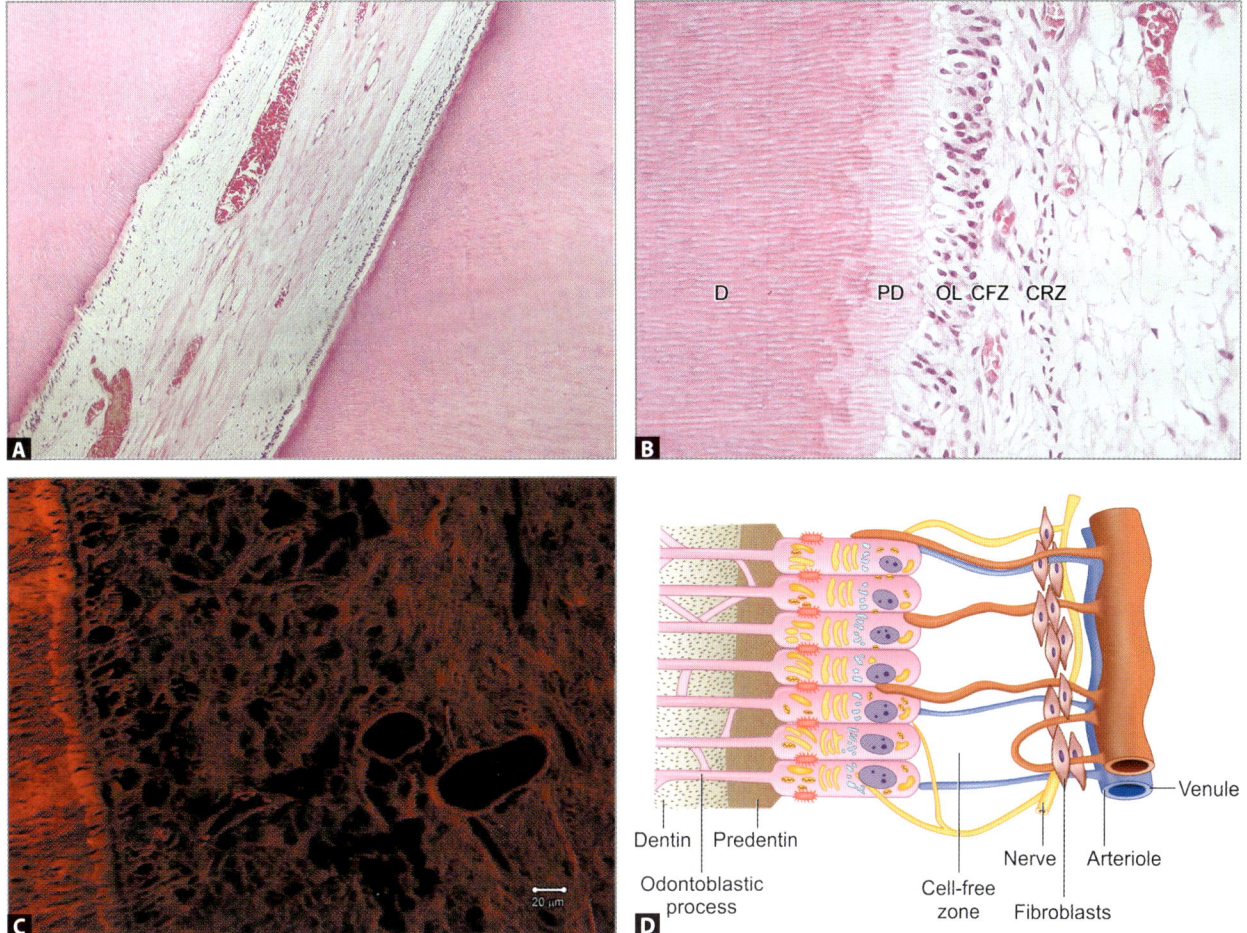

Figures 7-3A to D: (A) Pulp architecture. Hematoxylin and eosin stained section of pulp in low power; (B) High power showing dentin (D), predentin (PD), odontoblastic layer (OL), cell-free zone (CFZ) and cell-rich zone (CRZ); (C) Predentin-dentin junction in confocal microscopy; (D) Schematic representation of pulp architecture.
Source: (A and B) Pouyan Aminishakib, Postgraduate Director, Department of Oral Pathology, School of Dentistry, Tehran University of Medical Sciences; (C) Dr N Malathi, Department of Oral Pathology, Sri Ramachandra Dental College, Chennai, India, and Dr J Logeswari, Meenakshi Ammal Dental College, Chennai, India.

Odontoblasts and Odontoblastic Layer

Odontoblasts are the most characteristic, specialized, and nondividing cells with relatively long life span. Odontoblastic layer forms the peripheral portion of the pulp and lines the predentin.

The life cycle of odontoblasts starts from the peripheral cells of the dental papilla. They become preodontoblasts and then odontoblasts. Stages of odontoblasts reflect their functional activity, *i.e.* from secretory odontoblasts to transitional odontoblasts, to resting odontoblasts.

In the coronal pulp, odontoblasts are arranged in a palisaded pattern and have pseudostratified or multilayered appearance though only one layer actually exists. This is due to the different length of the cell bodies with their nuclei located at different levels **(Figures 7-4A to C)**.

Odontoblasts extend their cytoplasmic process into the dentinal tubules. Each dentinal tubule contains only one odontoblastic process. In the coronal pulp and at the cervical portion odontoblasts are tall columnar in shape. In the mid-root portion they are cuboidal or pyramidal and at the apical third they are short and flattened **(Figure 7-5)**. Number of odontoblasts per unit area in coronal pulp is more. Cell bodies of the odontoblasts are connected to each other, to the cells of the cell-rich zone, and to the cells of the pulp core by means of cell junctions and junctional complexes. This includes tight junctions, adhering junctions, and gap junctions. In gap junctions, intercellular spaces of 30–40 nm widths are present in between the adjacent odontoblasts, which provide pathway for the transport of signaling molecules. The tight junctions regulate the permeability of the dentin and help in prevention of ingress of any irritants including the microorganisms and their toxins. Gap junctions and macula adherens have also seen connecting fibroblasts and odontoblasts in cell-free zone. Due to the continuous formation of circumpulpal dentin and narrowing of pulp space, the odontoblasts in the coronal pulp become crowded, which is adjusted by programmed cell death (apoptosis).

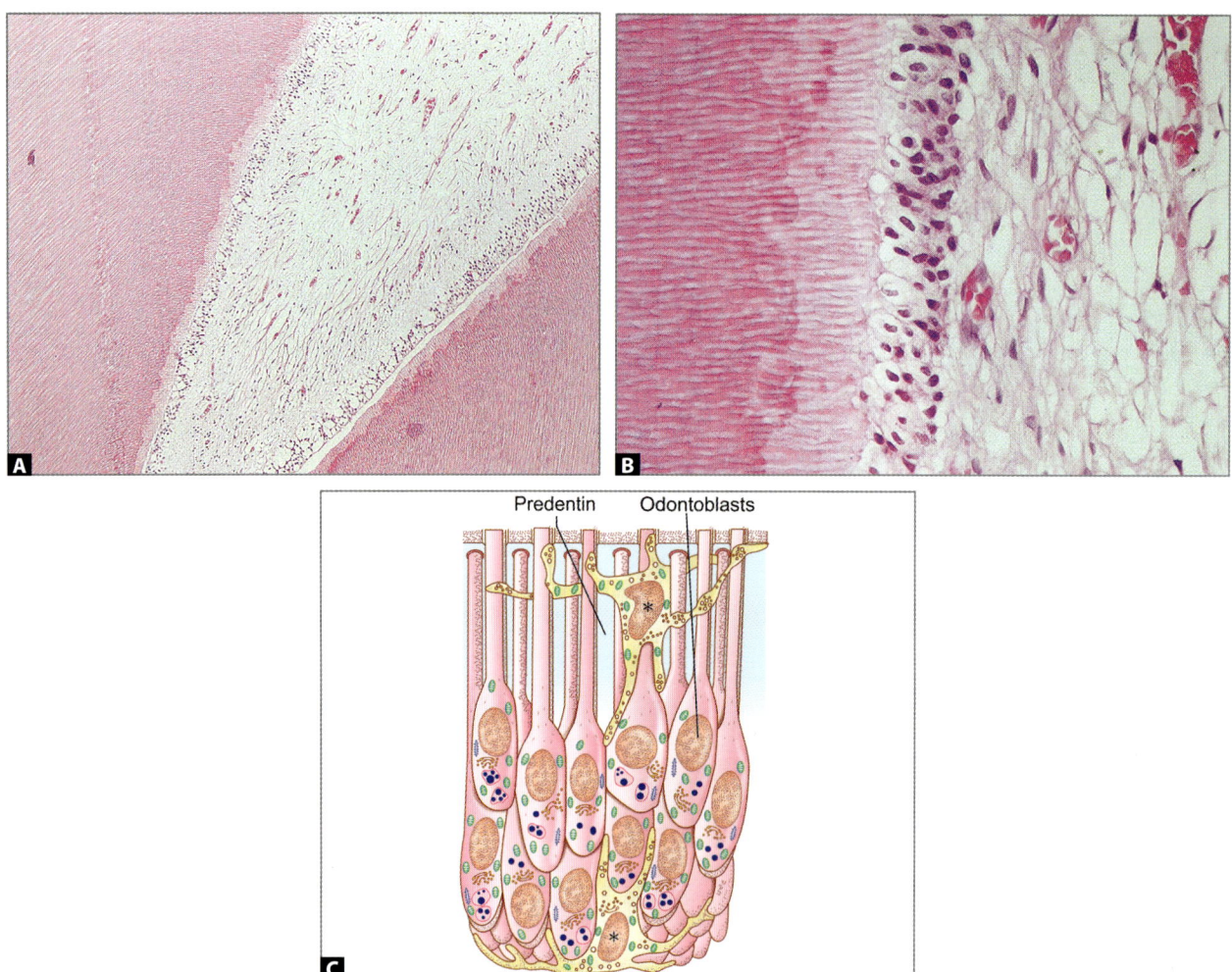

Figures 7-4A to C: (A) Hematoxylin and eosin stained section showing pseudostratified appearance of odontoblastic layer; (B) Same field in high power; (C) Schematic representation.
Source: (A and B) Pouyan Aminishakib, Postgraduate Director, Department of Oral Pathology, School of Dentistry, Tehran University of Medical Sciences.

Odontoblast has a large, oval nuclei situated basally and may contain up to four nucleoli. A well-developed Golgi apparatus is located at supranuclear position. Rough endoplasmic reticulum is more prominent. Mitochondria are evenly distributed throughout the cytoplasm. Secretory granules and filamentous material, suggestive of newly secreted proteins are also seen in the cytoplasm **(Figure 7-6)**. Morphology of the odontoblast changes according to its functional activity. Based on its functional stage, it can be typed into active or synthetic stage, transitional stage and resting stage.

Active stage: In this stage, odontoblast is ready for the synthesis of dentin. They appear elongated; cytoplasm is basophilic with basally placed nucleus. Cytoplasmic organelles are more and prominent; consist of numerous mitochondria and cytoskeletal elements scattered throughout the cell. Rough endoplasmic reticulum, well-developed Golgi apparatus, and numerous vesicles are also present. Nucleus appears basophilic with plenty of peripherally dispersed chromatin and more nucleoli.

Transitional stage: This is the intermediate stage between the active and resting stage and can be discerned only by electron microscopy. In this stage, odontoblast appears narrower and its nucleus exhibits condensed chromatin. Cytoplasmic organelles become decreased. Lysosomes and autophagic vacuoles appear in the cytoplasm.

Resting stage: In this stage, odontoblasts become smaller and crowded together. Nucleus is shifted to apical portion. Cytoplasmic organelles are fewer. Secretory vesicles are very few or absent. Supranuclear portion of the cell is devoid of organelles; though lipid-filled vacuoles may be present.

> The canalicular system of the osteocyte and odontoblast are remarkably similar, which leads to the newer perception of typing them as "odontocyte". This is supported by the demonstration of two osteocyte markers, DMP1 and E-11 in the odontoblastic process and dendrites of osteocytes.

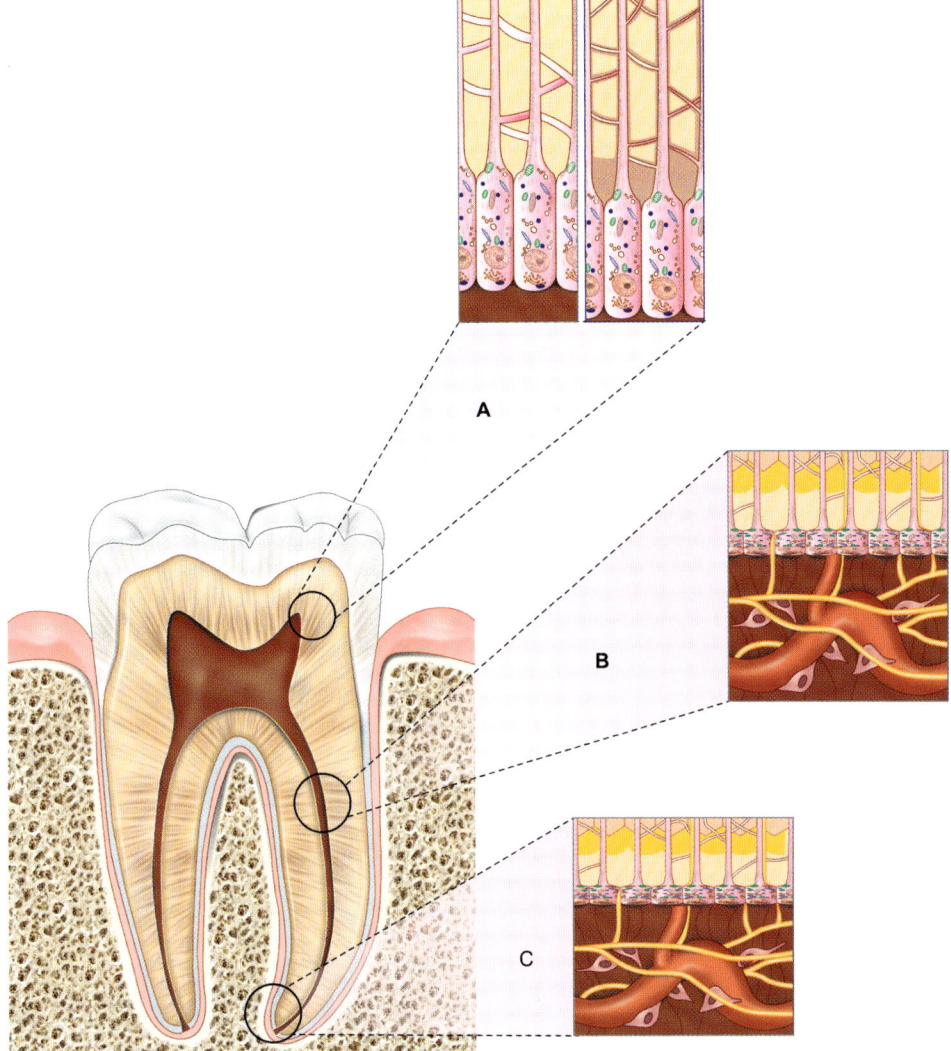

Figure 7-5: Schematic representation of odontoblasts at different locations: (A) Tall columnar in crown and cervical portion; (B) Cuboidal in midportion of the root; and (C) Flattened in apical portion of the root.

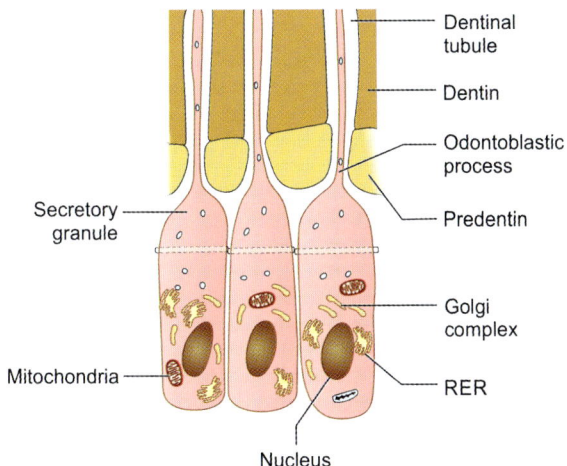

Figure 7-6: Schematic representation of odontoblasts at active stage. (RER: rough endoplasmic reticulum).

Odontoblasts secrete predentin throughout the life of the tooth although at reduced rate and in an irregular manner as age advances.

The cell body of the odontoblast is in the pulp and its cytoplasmic extension called odontoblastic process or Tomes' fiber is extended into the dentinal tubule. The diameter of the odontoblastic process is more near the cell body of the odontoblast and it becomes reduced gradually as it courses inside the dentinal tubules.

At the time of terminal differentiation, multiple processes exit from the cell body of the odontoblasts, and by the time the mantle dentin is formed, they become one single process. However, multiple lateral branches emerge from the main process and are contained within the lateral canaliculi of the dentinal tubules. The odontoblastic process contains mitochondria, secretory vesicles, microtubules, and microfilaments.

> Bone morphogenic proteins 2, 4, and 7 (BMP), epidermal growth factor (EGF), and fibroblast growth factor (FGF) have been demonstrated in the odontoblast. Other molecules such as dentin phosphoprotein, dentin sialoprotein, dentin matrix protein, decorin, and biglycan are also seen in the odontoblast and are elaborated into the ECM. While BMP, EGF, and FGF aid in wound healing, the rest of the molecules are implicated in organization and mineralization of ECM.

Cell-free Zone of Weil

This zone is of approximately 40 μm width, is seen adjacent to the odontoblastic layer, and is more prominent in the coronal pulp and inconspicuous in radicular pulp. This zone may not be present in all teeth. This is also called nuclear free or nuclear poor zone, since it contains numerous cytoplasmic processes of the fibroblasts, terminal branches of the autonomic and sensory nerves, and the major portion of the subodontoblastic capillary plexus. The fibroblastic processes present in this zone are connected to one another and to the cell bodies of the odontoblasts by means of desmosomes and to the ECM by fibronexus. This space is utilized by the inward movement of the odontoblasts during dentinogenesis. Cell-free zone thus disappears when dentin forms rapidly and reappears when dentinogenic stimuli are absent.

Cell-rich Zone

Cell-rich zone is adjacent to the cell-free zone and is seen in coronal and radicular pulp, but less distinct in the apical portion, and absent in older teeth. The inward portion of this zone is continuous with the pulp core in the crown and root. The cell types present in this zone are more or less similar to the cells of the pulp core. This zone is characterized by numerous fibroblasts, undifferentiated mesenchymal cells, macrophages, and dendritic cells. This zone is formed as a result of migration of peripheral cells from the pulp core.

■ CELLS OF THE PULP

In addition to odontoblasts, pulp contains fibroblasts, histiocytes, dendritic cells, monocytes, lymphocytes, and mast cells (**Figures 7-7A and B**).

Odontoblasts

Odontoblasts and their life cycle are already explained in detail in previous section.

Fibroblasts

They are the most abundant cell type present in the pulp and they secrete type I and III collagen fibers and ground substance. The fibroblasts are responsible for the collagen turnover by the production and destruction of the collagen fibers. They are usually associated with collagen fibers. Though fibroblasts are distributed throughout the pulp they are abundant at the cell rich zone. The young fibroblasts are polygonal in outline with large amount of cytoplasm. They have extensive cell processes and are evenly distributed. Nucleus is large, oval in outline, and stain deeply with basic dyes.

Fibroblasts are usually separated from each other by means of intercellular substance, but may have contact with the neighboring cells and ECM by cell junctions. They are motile and contractile, which helps in the formation and remodeling of connective tissue in healing process. Young pulp is more cellular than

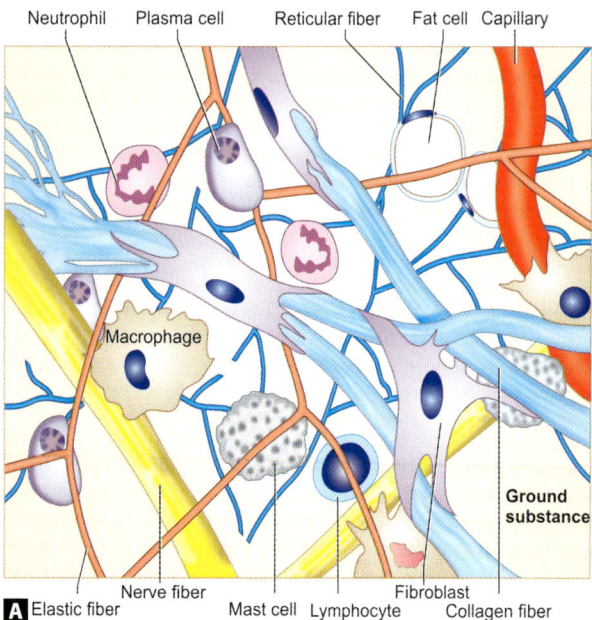
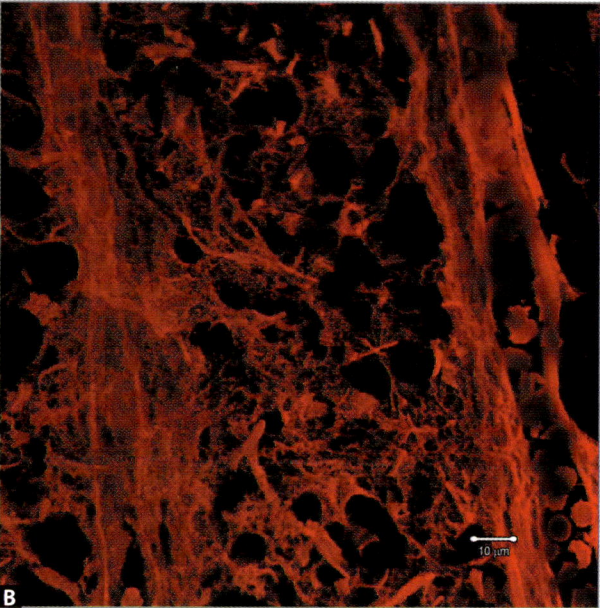

Figures 7-7A and B: (A) Schematic representation of cells and extracellular matrix of the pulp; (B) Confocal microscopic image showing pulpal capillary with RBCs inside the lumen and collagen fibers.

Source: (B) Dr N Malathi, Department of Oral Pathology, Sri Ramachandra Dental College, Chennai, India; and Dr J Logeswari, Meenakshi Ammal Dental College, Chennai, India.

mature pulp, which has a predominant fibrous component. Mature fibroblasts are stellate in shape and contain Golgi apparatus, numerous rough endoplasmic reticulum, and secretory vesicles. In older pulp, they become rounded or spindle-shaped with short processes and are known as fibrocytes. Cytoplasmic organelles become reduced in number and nuclei appear flattened with condensed chromatin.

> In pulp, fibroblasts play an active role in signaling pathway. Growth of fibroblasts and collagen synthesis is mediated by neuropeptides. They elaborate nerve growth factor (NGF) and inflammatory cytokines. NGF has a role in development and regulation of neuronal odontoblastic response. They play an important role in inflammation and repair, by secreting angiogenic factors like FGF-2 and vascular endothelial growth factor (VEGF).

Histiocytes

Tissue macrophages are called histiocytes and are present in the pulp too. Their cell outline is irregular with short blunt cytoplasmic processes. Nucleus is smaller, circular and darker than fibroblast and cytoplasm appears granular. They assume a variety of morphological forms in resting phase and may appear similar to fibroblasts. They can be demonstrated by intravital dyes like toluidine blue. They are derived from blood monocytes. They play an active role in signaling pathways in pulp similar to fibroblasts. They are closely associated with blood vessels. Their primary function is phagocytosis. In this process, the dead cells, extravasated RBCs, and foreign bodies are ingested and destroyed by the lysosomal enzymes and thereby act as a scavenger. Few subsets of macrophages participate in immune reaction by acting as antigen-presenting cells.

Activated macrophages produce interleukin 1, tumor necrosis factor (TNF), growth factors, and other cytokines.

Dendritic Cells

These are the accessory cells of the immune system and are derived from bone marrow. In the epithelium of the mucosa and epidermis of the skin, they are referred to as Langerhans cells. They are antigen-presenting cells and are about 40 µm long with multiple branched cytoplasmic process called dendrites, which extend into the dentinal tubules. They have class II MHC complexes on their cell surface. In the pulp, they usually reside at the periphery close to the predentin, but upon antigenic stimulation they migrate toward the central portion of the pulp. They take part in immunosurveillance and are responsible for the induction of T cell-mediated immunity. They bind antigens and process them for presentation to lymphocytes and macrophages. They are more in numbers in areas affected by caries, attrition, and the like. Dendritic cells also interact with the nerves and vessels in the pulp core and elicit neuroimmunologic response, which may be prime defense reaction of the pulp.

Inflammatory Cells

Lymphocytes: Lymphocytes are present in normal pulp. They increase in number during inflammation. Predominantly they are T lymphocytes but B lymphocytes may also be present in the normal pulp.

Eosinophils may be present extravascularly in normal pulp. Their cytoplasm contains eosinophilic granules and the nucleus is bilobed. Usually along with mast cells and basophils, they regulate the mechanism associated with allergy and asthma. They also produce cytokines and growth factors and are increased in number during inflammation.

Mast cells and plasma cells are present in the pulp during inflammation. Mast cells contain granules in their cytoplasm and they stain metachromatically. Plasma cells are derivatives of B lymphocytes and their number is increased during chronic inflammation. They are oval in shape with eccentrically-placed nucleus. Chromatin is pushed towards the nuclear membrane and gives the appearance of a "cartwheel" or "clock face". Cytoplasm appears basophilic. The function of the plasma cell is to produce antibody. A good marker for human plasma cell is CD 27.

Dental pulp stem cells (DPSC): Stem cells are multipotent cells, have the potential to differentiate into a variety of cell types, and exhibit self-renewal ability. Stem cells can be broadly classified into three types, namely embryonic stem cells, adult stem cells, and induced pluripotent stem cells. Embryonic stem cells are derived from the undifferentiated inner cell mass of a human embryo. They are easier to manipulate *in vitro* and have greater differentiation potential. Adult stem cells occur in a number of tissues including skin, adipose tissue, peripheral blood, bone marrow, pancreas, brain, hair follicles, and oral tissues such as dental papilla, dental pulp, periodontal ligament, etc. Their capacity for self-renewal and differentiation is limited. Induced stem cells are produced by conversion of adult stem cells into embryonic stem cells through genetic reprogramming.

Existence of stem cells within the dental pulp has been reported in permanent and deciduous teeth and is referred to as DPSC. These cells offer a promising source of autologous cells, and their similarities with bone marrow stromal cells suggest applications in regenerative medicine.

In addition to the above mentioned cells, there are other blood vascular elements that migrate from the blood vessels of the pulp in response to inflammation.

INTERCELLULAR SUBSTANCE

Intercellular substance is secreted by fibroblasts and consists of fibers and ground substance. Ground substance is also referred to as ECM. Fiber component is primarily made up of collagen.

Extracellular Matrix

Extracellular matrix or ground substance also known as extrafibrillar matrix is chiefly made up of glycosaminoglycans and proteoglycans. Glycosaminoglycans are hydrophilic and contribute to the tissue fluid pressure of the pulp. This acts as a scaffold and stabilizes the structure and provides biochemical and structural support to cells. It plays a major role in controlling the activity of cells, in terms of their development, migration, division, and function. Further it acts as a medium for the transport of nutrients from the blood vessels to the cells and metabolites and waste from the cells to the blood vessels. The major component of the ECM is collagen, which forms around 25–32% of the dry weight. The nonfibrous content of the ECM is gel-like in nature with high water content. The appearance may vary from finely granular to fibrillar. It may exhibit clear spaces in between.

Fibers of the Pulp

The principal fiber component of the pulp is collagen, secreted by the fibroblast. Type I collagen is the major component of the pulp. Type III collagen may also be present. The ratio between the type I and type III collagen is 60:40. Pulpal collagen exhibits the typical 64 nm periodicity with the length ranging from 10 nm to 100 nm. In young pulp, they are very thin with the diameter ranging from 10 nm to 12 nm. They are scattered irregularly throughout the pulp, however in the periphery they are more organized and aligned parallel to the predentin. As pulp matures, smaller fibrils are transformed into fiber bundles with greater dimension and organization. Further the cellularity decreases with aging. Apart from type I and III, pulp also contains type V and type VI in smaller amounts as a mesh work.

Tropocollagen, the collagen macromolecule, is the building block of collagen, which is formed intracellularly within the fibroblasts but assembled into collagen fibers extracellularly. Tropocollagen aggregates with the other collagen macromolecules to form the collagen fibers. The mechanism involved in the macromolecular aggregation is suggested to be the electrostatic forces of the charged group of adjacent macromolecules. Collagen turnover is also enabled by the fibroblasts. Collagen breakdown involves the enzyme collagenase. Fibrocytes are implicated in collagen removal and remodeling.

Fibronectin is a cell adhesion molecule, serves to anchor the cells to the collagen or proteoglycan unit, and organizes cellular interaction with ECM. It is found in the pulp similar to other connective tissues. Noncollagenous microfibrils of 10–14 nm diameter are also present in the pulp.

Blood Vessels

Pulp is richly supplied with blood by afferent arterioles and drained by venules. Its average capillary density is higher than most of the other tissues. Similar to the other tissues, blood vessels of the pulp provide oxygen and nutrients and remove waste and other toxic materials from the dental pulp. Arterioles are about 50–100 μm in diameter and the venules are around 100–150 μm in diameter. Blood vessels enter and exit through apical foramen and other accessory canals and foramen if present. The communication between the vessels of the pulp and the periodontium is not only at the periapical region, but also in other portions where accessory canals are present. The afferent and efferent vascular channels of the pulp and the periodontal ligament have common parent vessels at the periapical region, which in turn are from the inferior and superior alveolar arteries and veins. Small and relatively narrow arteries and thin-walled arterioles enter the pulp canals; form a stalk-like bundle, which travels through the central portion and laterally along the walls of the root canals. They run straight to reach the coronal pulp. Arteriole consists of three layers. The inner layer is called tunica intima, which is made up of endothelial cells. The outer layer is called tunica adventitia formed by connective tissue coat. The middle layer formed by smooth muscles is known as tunica media.

Blood vessels during their course, give off branches and these branching are extensive in coronal pulp.

These branches form plexus along the periphery at the subodontoblastic zone in coronal and radicular pulp and consist of arteriovenous anastomoses. Arteriovenous anastomoses are direct connection between the arteriole and a venule to bypass the capillary circulation. Loops from these plexus penetrate between the odontoblasts.

Capillaries are the terminal portion of the circulatory system. The diameter of a capillary may vary from 7 μm to 10 μm and consists of single layer of endothelial cells supported by basement membrane. Capillaries are wrapped by pericytes which are contractile cells. They act like smooth muscle cells and help in capillary constriction and dilatation.

Capillaries near the odontoblastic region are usually fenestrated. The fenestrations are minute pores containing a thin membrane covering, composed of cytoplasm of the endothelial cells and the basement membrane. Cells and other substances exit into the extracellular space through these fenestrations. Arteriovenous anastomoses and fenestrations help to reduce the intrapulpal pressure during inflammation.

The velocity and the pressure of the blood is higher in pulp when compared to other tissues. The diameter of the lumen of the arterioles increases and the thickness of the vessel wall decreases, once they enter the pulp. Usually the arterioles occupy the center portion of the pulp core. The velocity of blood flow in the pulp is estimated to be around 20–60 mL/minute per 100 g of tissue.

Lymph Vessels

These are thin-walled tubular structure and they usually do not contain any cells except few lymphocytes. The lymph vessels of the pulp arise at the subodontoblastic plexus and flow into thin-walled gathering vessels of varying caliber. They are more numerous in pulp core and exit the pulp via the apical foramina. Their lumen is larger and have irregular outline. Lymph capillaries are lined by a layer of endothelial cells, whose continuity is interrupted by minute spaces. These discontinuities allow entry and exit of lymph and other materials into the interstices of the pulp, thereby help to maintain the pulpal pressure.

Nerves

Pulp is a richly innervated organ. Nerve fibers enter the pulp along with blood vessels through the apical foramen. Approximately 350–700 myelinated and 1,000–2,000 nonmyelinated axons enter the apical foramen in a young molar tooth. They form neurovascular bundles with the blood vessels. Both myelinated and unmyelinated nerves are present in the pulp. Unmyelinated nerve fibers that run in proximity with the blood vessels are mostly sympathetic in nature and belong to autonomic nervous system. They regulate vasoconstriction by supplying to the smooth muscles of the vessels. Myelinated nerve fibers are somatosensory afferent fibers and arise from the trigeminal nerve. They register only pain sensation.

The nerves that enter the apical foramen are in the form of thick bundles. They pass from the radicular pulp to the coronal pulp, where they branch extensively in the cell-free zone of Weil just adjacent to the odontoblastic layer to form the parietal plexus otherwise known as plexus of Raschkow. This layer is more obvious in the coronal pulp than the radicular pulp. It is made up of both myelinated (diameter ranges from 2 μm to 5 μm) and unmyelinated axons. From this layer the nerves pass into the odontogenic zone and terminate in between the odontoblasts and few even extend into the dentinal tubule along with the odontoblastic process. The parietal plexus forms gradually and becomes prominent after root completion. As the nerves ascend coronally, there is discontinuity present in the investing perineurium. Further, myelinated axons lose their myelin sheath resulting in increase in the number of unmyelinated nerves in coronal pulp.

The nerve terminals are very close to the cell membrane of the odontoblasts and many indent the surface of the odontoblasts. No synaptic relationship between the nerve endings and the odontoblasts has been demonstrated so far. Predentin is also shown to contain some nerve fibers. Nerve terminals are made up of round or oval enlargements containing microvesicles, granules, and mitochondria of the terminal filaments. These nerve endings are supposed to function as pain receptors.

The primary afferent neurons of the peripheral nervous system involving the trigeminal nerve are broadly divided into—A-beta fibers, concerned with light touch and proprioception, and A-delta, and C fibers. A-delta and C fibers encode pain. Pulp responds to any kind of stimuli in the form of pain.

A-delta fibers have faster conduction and are responsible for the sharp or pricking pain. They primarily respond to mechanical stimuli rather than thermal or chemical stimuli. C fibers are relatively slower conductors and are implicated in dull ache. Unlike A-delta fibers, C fibers respond to mechanical, chemical, and thermal stimuli and conduct pain associated with tissue damage. Pulpal pain mediated by C fibers is dull, aching, and throbbing in nature in contrast to the sharp and pricking type of dentinal pain produced by the A-delta fibers. Usually pulpal pain is not localized since it does not have proprioceptive neurons and has high degree of convergence in the central nervous system (CNS).

FUNCTIONS OF PULP

Inductive

Ectomesenchymal cells adjacent to the oral ectoderm condense and exert primary inductive influence in tooth formation. Later this portion of the ectomesenchyme becomes dental papilla, which in turn is called pulp, once the tooth is formed. Dental papilla, the precursor of the pulp, interacts with the developing enamel organ to form a specific tooth type.

Formative

Odontoblasts, the cells of the pulp, are responsible for the formation of dentin. Though their cytoplasmic extension called odontoblastic processes are placed in dentinal tubules, their cell bodies are located in the pulp.

Nutritive

The avascular dentin is nourished by the vascular pulp. The dental lymph otherwise known as the dentinal fluid, which fills the dentinal tubule is the ultrafiltrate of capillary blood of the pulp.

Protective

The sensory nerves supply the pulp and respond to all kinds of stimuli in the form of pain. This forms an important protective mechanism of the tooth from any injury. Sympathetic nerves of the pulp control the pulpal circulation.

Defensive and Reparative

Pulp has good reparative capacity. Retraction of odontoblastic process or calcification of the affected tubules occurs to prevent the entry of bacteria or their toxins in case of dental caries or other physical or chemical assault. Tertiary dentin (formed by the damaged odontoblasts) or reparative dentin (formed by the newly differentiated odontoblasts) protects the pulp from further injury. If the irritant reaches the pulp, an inflammatory response is elicited. It is already stated that pulp has defense and inflammatory cells. If the inflammation is not so severe, pulpal injury will heal; if not, it will result in the death of the pulp.

DEVELOPMENT OF PULP

Pulp develops from the dental papilla. Though it is logical to assume that dental papilla transforms into pulp immediately after the differentiation of odontoblasts and dentin formation, development of pulpal architecture is not an overnight event. Once the enamel organ transforms from bud to cap stage, the cells and the intercellular substance in the center portion of the dental organ are recognized as dental papilla.

During the proliferation of dental papilla, they exert inductive influence on the epithelial enamel organ. In bell stage the peripheral layer of the dental papilla cells differentiates into odontoblasts and central cells into fibroblasts. Odontoblasts secrete dentin and during dentinogenesis the dental organ attains the shape and size of the future tooth crown. The dental papilla continues to proliferate. As the dentin wall thickens, the space taken up by the dental papilla is reduced. In the vicinity of the odontoblastic layer, dendritic cells (antigen presenting cells) appear. Along with the Hertwig's epithelial sheath and root formation, the dental papilla also proliferates, but is limited by the progressive narrowing of the space resulted due to the radicular dentin formation.

Close to the epithelial diaphragm, papilla cells proliferate more and form "pulp proliferation zone", which provides new cells needed for root lengthening. As long as the root formation continues the apical opening is wide. This wide open apex is narrowed down to an apical foramen some time after eruption. The conversion of dental papilla into pulp occurs with decrease in the cellular concentration and increase in the fibrous component. Fibroblasts of the young pulp are very active in collagen synthesis.

Development of blood vessels in the pulp starts at the early bell stage. Prior to root formation, blood vessels entering the dental papilla gather together in groups. The number and location of these vessel groups correspond to the number of roots of the particular tooth. They enter the dental papilla cells from the vascular trunks of the jaw. Few vessels enlarge and run through the pulp core toward the cuspal portion. During the course they leave numerous minute branches, which form vascular plexus in the subodontoblastic area. During primary dentinogenesis, this vasculature develops in the odontogenic zone and shows increased vessel fenestrations for odontoblast nutrition. With the completion of primary dentin formation, there is decrease in fenestrations and withdrawal of vessels from the odontoblastic layer. But the odontoblasts move inward as it lays down dentin, which results in the increased vascularity of the odontoblasts layer from the subodontoblastic zone.

The ingrowth of nerve fibers of the trigeminal ganglion to the dental papilla occurs at a comparatively late developmental stage. Nevertheless the tooth germ is innervated as early as in cap stage. The first nerve fibers to appear in the pulp are related to the blood vessels. Though these fibers are sensory they are associated with the control of blood flow. Large number of nerve fibers enters the pulp before root formation. Subodontoblastic plexus or plexus of Raschkow is established after the root completion.

AGE CHANGES

As the age of the individual advances, the volume of the pulp is reduced due to the continued formation of secondary dentin, fitting into the phrase, "grow to become small". Progressive secondary dentin formation and deposition of tertiary or reparative dentin result in partial or complete obliteration of pulp chamber and/or the pulp canals **(Figures 7-8)**.

Number of odontoblasts and fibroblasts is reduced. The reduction in cellular density is pronounced in the root. Changes in the cellular elements include decrease in size and organelle content.

Older pulp is less vascular and more fibrous. There is gradual increase in the fiber content and is generalized throughout the pulp. Localized fibrosis and scarring are not uncommon. Vascularity of the pulp decreases with age, due to decrease in the number of vessels and the formation of atherosclerotic plaques. Calcification of the vessel is also common near the apical region.

The sensitivity will be reduced due to the degeneration of myelinated and unmyelinated axons. This is complemented by the formation of dead tracts, dentinal sclerosis, and reparative dentin formation.

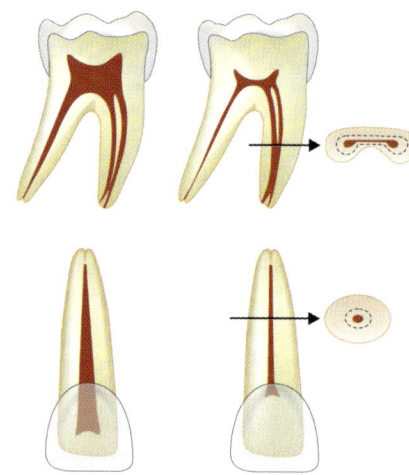

Figure 7-8: Reduction in the volume of pulp canal and chamber.

Pulp Stones

Pulp stones or denticles are calcified masses seen in the pulp chamber or pulp canals. They are classified into true pulp stones and false pulp stones. True pulp stones contain dentinal tubules surrounded by a layer of odontoblasts and false pulp stones are concentric nodules of calcification **(Figures 7-9A and B)**.

Pulp stones may be single or multiple and are seen usually at the orifice of the pulp chamber or within the root canal. False pulp stones may be formed by the calcification of a thrombi or dead cells and true pulp stone is formed by the displaced odontoblasts or inclusion of remnants of the Hertwig's epithelial root sheath.

Pulp stones that lie freely within the pulp surrounded by soft tissue are called free pulp stones **(Figure 7-10)**. Attached pulp stone is the one which is attached to the wall of the pulp chamber or canal and the embedded pulp stone is completely embedded within the dentin. Secondary dentin deposition converts the free pulp stone into attached or embedded pulp stone. Incidence of pulp stones increases with age and are regarded as age-related change rather than pathology.

Diffuse Calcifications

There may be irregular areas of dystrophic calcification in the pulp core, which appear as many tiny spicules of calcifications. This is due to the calcification of collagen fiber bundle or may originate in relation to the blood vessels or nerve trunks. Diffuse calcifications are usually found in pulp canals.

CLINICAL CONSIDERATIONS

Vitality

In clinical practice, every effort is made to preserve the vitality of the tooth. The vital tooth alone can respond to any pathological stimuli to provoke response or reparative dentin formation and can seal off the dentinal tubules to prevent the entry of any microbial or chemical irritants that can damage the pulp. A nonvital tooth is brittle and is liable for fractures.

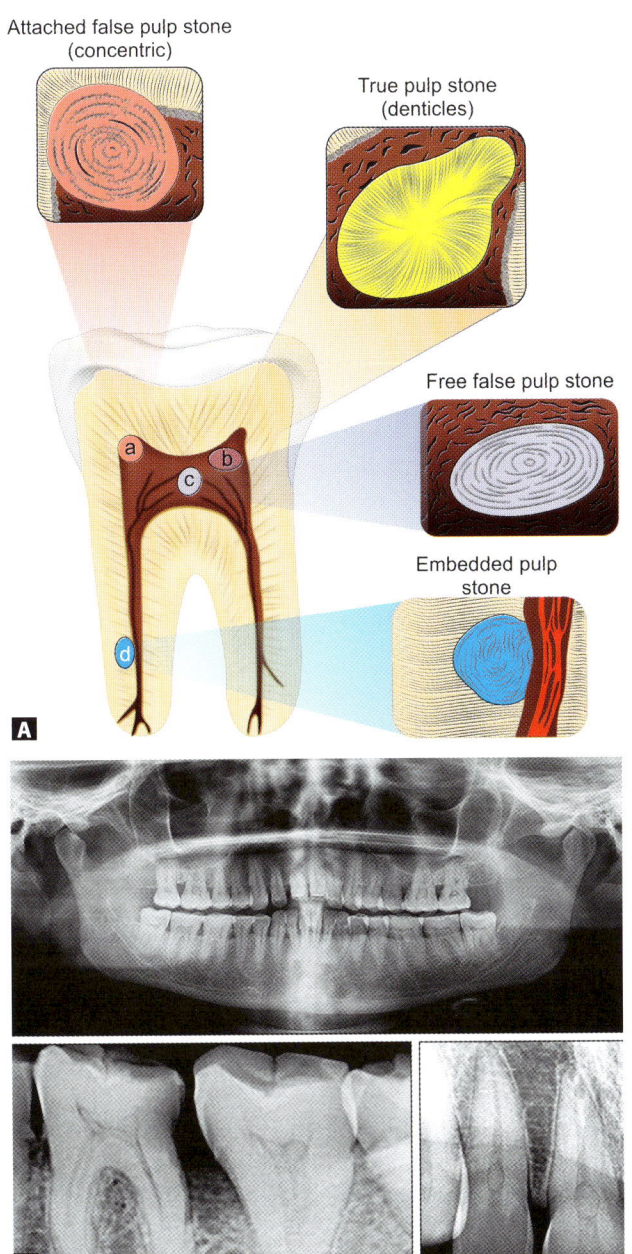

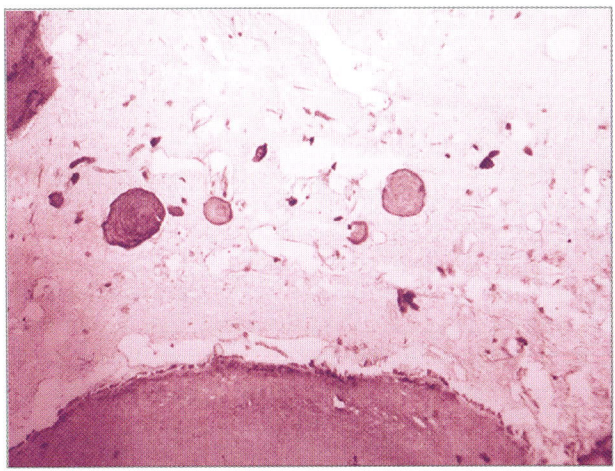

Figure 7-10: Hematoxylin and eosin stained section shows multiple free pulp stones within the pulp chamber.

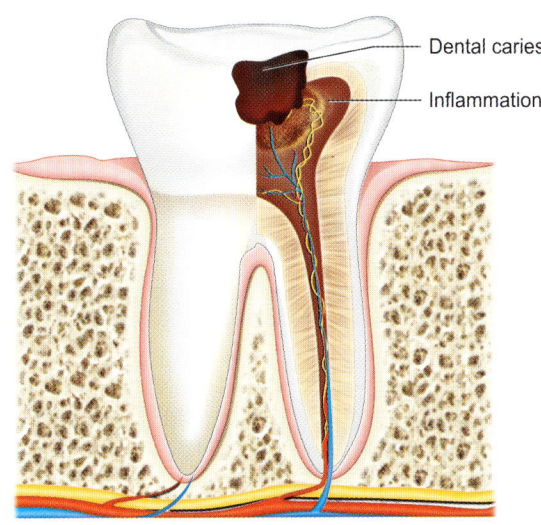

Figure 7-11: Pulpitis.

Figures 7-9A and B: Pulp stones: (A) Schematic representation of true and false pulp stone; (B) Radiographic appearance of pulp stones.

The assessment of vitality is an essential diagnostic procedure in endodontic practice. Vitality of the tooth depends on the vascular status of the pulp, but the vitality tests performed in dental practice can only check the neural status of the pulp rather than the vascular circulation. Pulse oximeter and laser Doppler flowmeter which can check the circulation are still at the experimental stage.

Pulpal and Root Canal Anatomy

Anatomy of the root canal system varies from tooth to tooth and person to person. A thorough knowledge of root canal anatomy is a must for a good endodontic practice. However, presence of lateral and accessory canals, obliteration of canals, and curved canals pose a challenge to the endodontists.

Pulpitis

The most common cause for odontalgia (toothache) is pulpitis. It is nothing but the inflammation of the pulp **(Figure 7-11)**. Since pulp resides in a rigid chamber, the accumulating inflammatory edema causes increase in the pulpal pressure, which affects the nerves. This results in intolerable pain, which can mimic neuralgia at times. This is very common in case of closed pulpitis. In open pulpitis, the pain is relatively less due to the escape of inflammatory edema and less pressure built up. Since pulpal nerve fibers are not represented individually in the sensory cortex, localization of pulpal pain is also difficult.

Many a time pulpal inflammation ends in self-strangulation of the pulp and majority of the endodontic procedures involve removal of the pulp and filling the root canal with inert materials.

Internal Resorption

It is an unusual condition where the pulpal walls begin to resorb centrally within the tooth. This may be due to the inflammatory hyperplasia of the pulp. Tooth may be asymptomatic except for a pink-hued area on the crown.

Recession of Pulp Horns

There is reduction in the size of the pulp chamber and diameter of the pulp canal with aging. This is due to the continued deposition of secondary dentin. This may also result in recession of the pulp horns. Response of the pulp to any stimuli in older teeth is much less when compared to young teeth due to the increase in thickness of the dentin and degeneration of the pulpal nerve endings.

Pulpal Changes during Exfoliation of Primary Teeth

Primary dentition sheds to enable the permanent teeth to erupt. Resorption of deciduous tooth root occurs during shedding, which involves a resorptive cell called odontoclast. Odontoclasts are analogous to osteoclasts of the bone. During resorption, number of cells in the pulp decreases with increase in the fiber content. Nerve fibers degenerate but the vascularity remains intact till the tooth exfoliates.

> **Points to Remember**
> - Pulp is the only soft tissue present inside the tooth.
> - It resides in the pulp chamber in the crown and pulp canals in the root.
> - Pulp is richly vascular and innervated, gives vitality to the tooth and reacts to any external stimuli by pain.
> - Pulp is developed from dental papilla, which in turn is from ectomesenchyme.
> - Pulp organ organized into odontoblastic zone, cell-free zone, cell-rich zone and pulp core.
> - Volume of the pulp reduces as the age advances due to secondary dentin formation.
> - During aging, number of cells in the pulp decreases and fiber content increases.
> - Pulp stones are also called denticles. They are nodular calcified masses seen in the pulp chamber or root canal.
> - Pulp stones may lie freely in the pulp, attached to the dentin wall or embedded in the dentin.
> - Inflammation of the pulp is called pulpitis.
> - Vital pulp alone reacts to any external stimuli.
> - Vitality of the pulp depends on the vascular status of the pulp.

PRACTICE QUESTIONS

1. What is odontogenic zone?
2. Write about odontoblastic layer
3. What are all the contents of pulp core?
4. Cells of the pulp.
5. Write about development of pulp.
6. Write notes on blood vessels of the pulp.
7. Write notes on nerves of the pulp.
8. What are all the functions of pulp?
9. Write about age changes seen in pulp.
10. What are pulp stones?
11. What is pulpitis?

MULTIPLE CHOICE QUESTIONS

1. **Pulp is derived from**
   a. Ectoderm
   b. Mesoderm
   c. Ectomesenchyme
   d. Endoderm
2. **Which one of the following is not true?**
   a. Pulp horns are small extensions seen towards the cuspal portion of the tooth
   b. Number of pulp horns corresponds to the number of cusps
   c. Pulp horns are seen in the radicular pulp also
   d. Recession of pulp horns occurs as a result of aging
3. **Volume of the pulp is more in**
   a. Incisors
   b. Canines
   c. Premolars
   d. Molars
4. **The most abundant cells seen in the pulp are**
   a. Odontoblasts
   b. Defense cells
   c. Fibroblasts
   d. Endothelial cells

5. **Subodontoblastic plexus is also known as**
   a. Venous plexus
   b. Plexus of Raschkow.
   c. Pulp core
   d. Lymphatic plexus
6. **Cell free zone is**
   a. Not seen in the pulp chamber
   b. Seen in the radicular pulp
   c. Used by the odontoblasts to move while forming dentin
   d. Richly vascular
7. **Pulp dentin complex is so named because**
   a. Pulp is adjacent to the dentin
   b. Pulp and dentin are developmentally, structurally, and functionally related
   c. Pulp forms primary dentin
   d. Blood vessels of the pulp enter the dentin
8. **Extracellular matrix**
   a. Is not related the activity of cells, in terms of their development, migration, division, and function.
   b. is chiefly made up of fibroblasts and odontoblasts
   c. act as a scaffold and stabilizes the structure and provides biochemical and structural support to cells.
   d. Help in the development of pulp
9. **The major fiber component of the pulp is**
   a. Elastic fibers
   b. Type I collegen
   c. Type III collagen
   d. Unmyelinated nerve fibers
10. **Which one of the following is not a function of pulp**
    a. Formative
    b. Sensory
    c. Resorptive
    d. Nutritive
11. **Pulp stones are**
    a. Also called denticles
    b. Seen in aging pulp
    c. Of two types, true denticles and false denticles
    d. All of the above
12. **Age changes of the pulp involves the following except**
    a. Reduced vascularity of the pulp
    b. Recession of pulp horn
    c. Pulpal inflammation
    d. Fibrosis
13. **True pulp stone**
    a. Are concentric calcified masses
    b. Contains dentinal tubules
    c. Calcified thrombi
    d. Seen in younger pulp
14. **Vitality of the pulp depends on**
    a. Nerve status
    b. Lymphatic status
    c. Vascular status
    d. Odontoblasts

ANSWERS

1. c   2. c   3. d   4. c   5. b   6. c   7. b   8. c   9. b   10. c   11. d   12. c   13. b   14. c

BIBLIOGRAPHY

1. About I, Mitsiadis TA. Molecular aspects of tooth pathogenesis and repair: in vivo and in vitro models. Adv Dent Res. 2001;15:59.
2. Aeinechi M, Eslami B, Ghanbariha M, et al. Mineral trioxide aggregate (MTA) and calcium hydroxide and pulp-capping agents in human teeth: a preliminary report. Int Endod J. 2003;36(3):225-31.
3. Angelova A, Takagi Y, Kaneko T, et al. Immunocompetent cells in the pulp of human deciduous teeth. Arch Oral Biol. 2004;49(1):29-36.
4. Khurana A, Khurana I. Human Embryology, 2nd edition. India: CBS Publishers and Distributor Pvt Ltd; 2012.
5. Avery JK, Chiego DJ. Essentials of Oral Histology and Embryology—A Clinical Approach, 3rd edition. US: Mosby; 2006.
6. Avery JK. Structural elements of the young normal human pulp. In: Siskin M (Ed). The Biology of the Human Dental Pulp. St. Louis: Mosby; 1973.
7. Bender IB. Pulpal pain diagnosis—a review. J Endod. 2000;26(3):175-9.
8. Berkovitz BKB, Holland GR, Moxham BJ. Oral Anatomy, Histology and Embryology, 4th edition. US: Elsevier; 2009.
9. Carda C, Peydró A. Ultrastructural patterns of human dentinal tubules odontoblasts processes and nerve fibers. Tissue Cell. 2006;38(2):141-50.
10. Casagrande L, Mattuella LG, De Arauio FB, et al. Stem cells in dental practice: perspectives in conservative pulp therapies. J Clin Pediatr Dent. 2006;31(1):25-7.
11. Edds AC, Walden JE, Scheetz JP, et al. Pilot study of correlation of pulp stones with cardiovascular disease. J Endod. 2005;31(7):504-6.
12. Espina AT, Castellanos AV, Fererira JL. Age related changes in blood capillary endothelium of human dental pulp: an ultrastructural study. Int Endod J. 2003;36(6):395.
13. Fried K, Nosrat C, Lillesaar C, et al. Molecular signaling and pulpal nerve development. Crit Rev Oral Biol Med. 2000;11(3):318.
14. Gasga JR, Gracia G, Fregoso A, et al. Conductivity in human tooth enamel. J Mat Sci. 1999;34(9):2183-8.
15. Gronthos S, Brahim J, Li W, et al. Stem cell properties of human dental pulp stem cells. J Dent Res. 2002;81(8):531-5.
16. Huang GT, Gronthos S, Shi S. Mesenchymal stem cells derived from dental tissues vs. those from other sources: their biology and role in regenerative medicine. J Dent Res. 2009;88(9):792-806.
17. Huang GT. Dental pulp and dentin tissue engineering and regeneration: advancement and challenge. Front Biosci Elite Ed. 2011;3:788-800.

18. Schroeder HE. Oral Structural Biology, 4th edition. New York: Thieme; 1991.
19. Ikawa M, Komatsu H, Ikawa K, et al. Age-related change in the human pulpal blood flow measured by laser Doppler flowmetry. Dent Traumatol. 2003;19(1):36-40.
20. Chatterjee K. Essentials of Dental Anatomy and Oral Histology, 2nd edition. India: Jaypee Brothers Medical Publishers (P) Ltd; 2014.
21. Kono RT, Suwa G, Tanijiri T. A three-dimensional analysis of enamel distribution patterns in human permanent first molars. Arch Oral Biol. 2002;147(12):867.
22. Kumat GS. Orban's Oral Histology and Embryology, 14th edition. India: Elsevier; 2015.
23. MacDougall M, Dong J, Acevedo AC. Molecular basis of human dentin diseases. Am J Med Genet A. 2006;140:25-36.
24. Martinez EF, Machado de Souza SO, Correa L, et al. Immunohistochemical localization of tenascin, fibronectin, and type III collagen in human dental pulp. J Endod. 2000;26(12):708.
25. Mathieu S, EL-Battari A, Dejou J, et al. Role of injured endothelial cells in the recruitment of human pulp cells. Arch Oral Biol. 2005;50(2):109.
26. Matsumoto Y, Zhano B, Kato S. Lymphatic networks in the periodontal tissues and dental pulp as revealed by histochemical study. Microsc Res Tech. 2002;56(1):50.
27. Mitsiadis TA, Rahiotis C. Parallels between tooth development and repair: conserved molecular mechanisms following carious and dental injury. J Dent Res. 2004;83(12):896.
28. Miura M, Gronthos S, Zhao M, et al. SHED: stem cells from human exfoliated deciduous teeth. Proc Natl Acad Sci USA. 2003;100:5807-12.
29. Miwa Z, Ikawa M, Iijima H, et al. Pulpal blood flow in vital and nonvital young permanent teeth measured by transmitted- light photo plethysmography: a pilot study. Pediatr Dent. 2002;24(6):594.
30. Murray PE, Smith AJ, Windsor LJ, et al. Remaining dentine thickness and human pulp responses. Int Endod J. 2003;36(1):33.
31. Murray PE, Windsor LJ, Smyth TW, et al. Analysis of pulpal reactions to restorative procedures, materials, pulp capping and future therapies. Crit Rev Oral Biol Med. 2002;13(6):509.
32. Nakamura Y, Hammarstrom L, Lundberg E, et al. Enamel matrix derivative promotes reparative processes in the dental pulp. Adv Dent Res. 2001;15:105.
33. Nanci A (Ed). Dentin, pulp complex. Ten Cate's Oral Histology Development, Structure and Function, 6th edition. St. Louis: Elsevier; 2005. pp. 198-239.
34. Neville BW, Douglas DD, Allen CM, et al. Oral and Maxillofacial Pathology, 1st South Asia edition. India: Elsevier; 2016.
35. Nosrat IV, Widenfalk J, Oison L, et al. Dental pulp cells produce neurotrophic factors, interact with trigeminal neurons in vitro, and rescue motor neurons after spinal cord injury. Dev Biol. 2001;238(1):120.
36. Odell EW, Morgan PR. Biopsy Pathology of the Oral Tissues, 1st edition. UK: Chapman & Hall; 1998.
37. Oyama M, Myokai F, Ohira T, et al. Isolation and expression of FIP-2 in wounded pulp of the rat. J Dent Res. 2005;84(9):842.
38. Piattelli A, Rubini C, Floroni M, et al. bcl-2, p53, and MIB-1 in human adult dental pulp. J Endod. 2000;26(4):225-7.
39. Bradley RM. Essentials of Oral Physiology, 1st edition. USA: Mosby; 1995.
40. Chandra S, Chandra S, Chandra M, et al. Textbook of Dental and Oral Histology with Embryology & MCQ's, 2nd edition. India: Jaypee Brothers Medical Publishers (P) Ltd; 2010.
41. Schroeder HE. Oral Structural Biology, 4th edition. New York: Thieme; 1991.
42. Schwendicke F, Lamont T, Innes N. Removing or controlling? How caries management impacts on the lifetime of teeth. Monogr Oral Sci. 2018;27:32-41.
43. Sivapathasundharam B. Shafer's Textbook of Oral Pathology, 9th edition. India: Elsevier; 2020.
44. Soares DG, Anovazzi G, Bordini EAF, et al. Biological analysis of simvastatin-releasing chitosan scaffold as a cell-free system for pulp-dentin regeneration. J Endod. 2018;44(6):971-6.
45. Tecles O, Laurent P, Zvgouritsas S, et al. Activation of human dental pulp progenitor/stem cells in response to odontoblast injury. Arch Oral Biol. 2005;50(2):103.
46. Miles TS, Nauntofte B, Svensson P. Clinical Oral Physiology, 1st edition. Copenhagen: Quintessence Publishing Co. Ltd; 2004.
47. Provenza VD, Seibel W. Oral Histology–Inheritance and Development, 2nd edition. USA: Lea & Febiger; 1986.
48. Volponi AA, Pang Y, Sharpe PT. Stem cell-based biological tooth repair and regeneration. Trends Cell Biol. 2010;20: 715-22.
49. Yamakoshi Y, Hu JC-C, Fukae M, et al. Dentin glycoprotein: the protein in the middle of the dentin sialophosphoprotein chimera. J Biol Chem. 2005;280:17472-9.
50. Zmijiewska C, Surkyk-Zasada J, Zabel M, et al. Development of innervation in primary incisors in the foetal period. Arch Oral Biol. 2003;48(11):745-52.

CHAPTER

Cementum

Punnya V Angadi, B Sivapathasundharam

CHAPTER OUTLINE

- Physical Properties 98
- Chemical Composition 98
  - » Inorganic Content 98
  - » Organic Content 99
- Cells of Cementum 99
  - » Cementoblasts 99
  - » Cementocytes 99
  - » Differences between Cementocytes and Osteocytes 100
  - » Cementoclasts 100
- Fibers of the Cementum 101
- Structure 102
- Classification of Cementum 103
- Cementogenesis 103
- Cementoid 106
- Incremental Lines of Cementum 106
- Hyaline Layer of Hopewell–Smith 107
  - » Attachment of Periodontal Ligament Fibers to Cementum 107
- Cementodentinal Junction 107
- Cementoenamel Junction 107
- Functions of Cementum 108
- Age Changes 108
- Clinical Considerations 109

INTRODUCTION

Cementum is a hard, avascular connective tissue that covers the roots of the teeth. It was first demonstrated in 1835 by two pupils of the classical physiologist Jan Evangelista Purkinje. Cementum originates at the cervical portion of the tooth, where the enamel ends at knife edge. It continues till the apex of the root and surrounds the apical foramen **(Figure 8-1)**. It may extend to line the dentinal wall in the apical portion of the root canal at times. Though cementum is considered to be a part of the tooth, it may also be considered as a component of the attachment apparatus, the periodontium, due to life-long incorporation of periodontal ligament fibers. It has resemblance in architecture to bone.

Cementum forms an integral part of the periodontium, which includes alveolar bone, periodontal ligament and gingiva. Cementoblasts are the cells responsible for cementum formation and are derived from dental sac or follicle.

Cementum gives attachment to the fibers of the periodontal ligament and firmly adheres to the dentin on its inner aspect. It is deposited throughout the life like dentin and there is always a thin layer of unmineralized cemental matrix on the surface. In healthy individuals, cementum is not visible clinically, since it usually covers the entire root which is embedded in the alveolar bone.

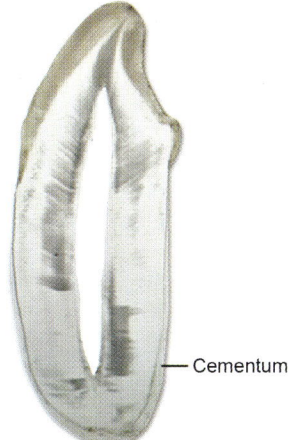

Figure 8-1: Ground section showing the cementum surrounding root dentin.

Cementum is an ectomesenchymal derivative and resembles bone in some physical, chemical, and structural characteristics. But bone is vascular while cementum is avascular and has no nerves in the matrix. Further, unlike bone, cementum lacks the Haversian system and has no

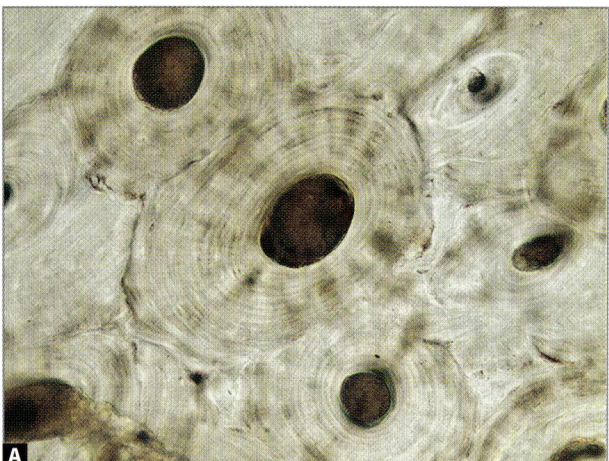
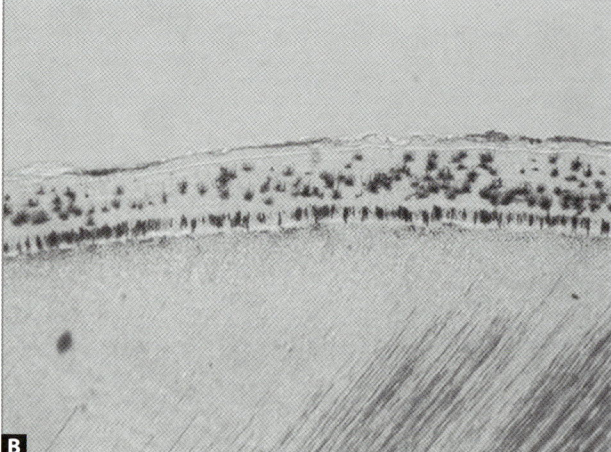

Figures 8-2A and B: (A) Haversian system in bone and (B) the avascular cementum.

marrow spaces **(Figures 8-2A and B)**. Growth of cementum is by apposition similar to bone and involves remodeling, which is slower than bone. It can resist resorption better than bone, a feature that is important, and enables orthodontic tooth movement. The reasons attributed for this phenomenon include differences in the physicochemical or biological properties between bone and cementum, the properties of precementum, increased density of Sharpey's fibers in cementum, and the close proximity of the cell rests to the cementum layer.

> Osteoblasts have a role in the differentiation and stimulation of osteoclasts, which cause bone resorption. They respond to parathyroid stimulation in the resorption process. In contrast, cementoblasts do not respond to parathyroid hormone and other cytokines, which is suggested to be a reason for its resistance to resorption.

In addition to serving as a medium for the attachment of collagen fibers from periodontal ligament and in securing the tooth to the alveolus, it also helps in adaptive and reparative processes. Cementum seals the radicular dentin surface by covering the open end of the dentinal tubules. Some regard cementum as the calcified component of the periodontal ligament. Cementum is restricted to the root in humans, however, in some mammals, cementum may be present on the crowns as an adaptation to their herbivorous diet.

PHYSICAL PROPERTIES

The color of the cementum varies from pale yellow to dark yellow. Unlike the shiny enamel surface, the cemental surface appears dull **(Figures 8-3A and B)**. The color of the cementum is lighter than that of the dentin. On the radiograph, it appears less radiopaque than enamel or dentin. It appears less yellow and less translucent, when compared to bone, and it is difficult to differentiate cementum from bone based on the color alone.

Permeability of the cementum is more than the dentin but decreases with age. Permeability varies depending on the type of cementum.

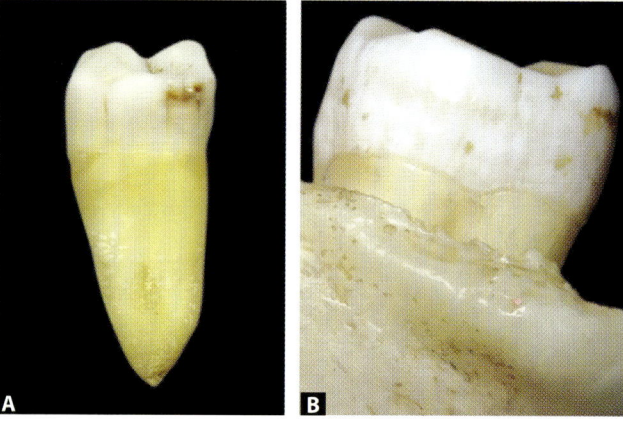

Figures 8-3A and B: (A) Mandibular premolar showing the difference in the appearance of enamel and cementum; (B) Mandibular molar showing the similarity in color of the cementum and bone.

Hardness of the cementum is less than that of the dentin but similar to bone. The hardness of the dental hard tissues in descending order is enamel, dentin, and cementum.

The thickness of the cementum varies between teeth and different regions of the same tooth. At the cementoenamel junction (CEJ), it is thinnest (about 20–50 μm) and thickest at the apical region of all the teeth and the interradicular areas of the multirooted teeth (150–200 μm). The relative softness of cementum along with its thinness in the cervical area predisposes it to be removed easily by abrasion especially in the context of gingival recession.

CHEMICAL COMPOSITION

Inorganic Content

Cementum is the relatively less mineralized tissue of the tooth. It has 45–50% of inorganic content and 50–55% of organic content, which includes 33% of organic and 22% of

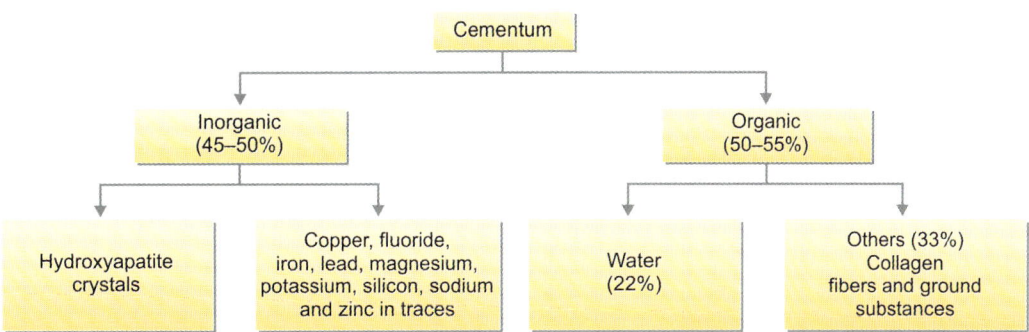

Flowchart 8-1: Chemical composition of cementum.

water by volume **(Flowchart 8-1)**. The inorganic content is composed predominantly of calcium and phosphate in the form of hydroxyapatite crystals, which are thin, plate-shaped, and similar to those of the bone (55 nm wide, 8 nm thick). Other forms of calcium are also present in cementum at higher levels than that of dentin and enamel. Trace elements such as copper, fluoride, iron, lead, magnesium, potassium, silicon, sodium, and zinc are also present in minute quantities. The trace element concentration is more on the external surface. Cementum has the highest fluoride content of all mineralized tissues, which attributes to its permeability. It is more in acellular cementum than cellular cementum.

Organic Content

The principal organic component of cemental matrix is collagen. Type I collagen (comprises 90% of the organic content) is the predominant form of collagen present in the cementum. Other types of collagen associated with cementum include type III and XII. Type V, VI, and XIV have also been found in cementum in trace amounts. Additionally, it also has proteoglycans and glycoproteins.

The noncollagenous proteins of the cementum are similar to that of bone and they include bone sialoprotein, dentin matrix protein 1, dentin sialoprotein, fibronectin, osteocalcin, osteopontin, proteoglycans, proteolipids, tenascin, alkaline phosphatase, and many growth factors. Amino acid analysis of collagen shows that it is similar to that found in bone and dentin. Osteopontin is located in the incremental lines and sialoprotein in cemental matrix. Cementum-derived attachment protein (CAP) is located in the matrix of mature cementum and in cementoblasts. It is a 56 kDa or 65 kDa collagenous protein that promotes the attachment of the mesenchymal cells to the extracellular matrix (ECM). Bone sialoprotein and osteopontin plays an important role in mineralization process by binding collagen fibrils and hydroxyapatite. After mineralization, they serve to maintain the structural integrity of cementum. Cementum is rich in glycosaminoglycans, particularly chondroitin sulfate.

> Cementum-derived attachment protein is seen only in cementum and not in bone. So this may be used as a marker to differentiate cementum and bone.

> Similar to bone, cementum also contains transforming growth factor beta (TGFβ), platelet-derived growth factor, fibroblast growth factor, insulin-like growth factor, epidermal growth factor, and various bone morphogenetic proteins (BMPs).

CELLS OF CEMENTUM

Cementoblasts

Cementoblasts are the cells responsible for the formation of cementum. During root formation, Hertwig's epithelial root sheath breaks up and the dental sac cells come in contact with the root dentin to differentiate into cementoblasts. They secrete the organic matrix consisting of collagen and protein polysaccharides. Later, they also take part in mineralization.

Cementoblasts usually line the cementoid (cemental matrix) between the attached portion of the periodontal ligament fibers **(Figures 8-4A and B)**. They resemble osteoblasts and the size ranges between 8 μm and 12 μm. They are usually cuboidal to squamous in shape with a centrally placed large vesicular nucleus and prominent nucleoli. The cytoplasm of cementoblasts is strongly basophilic and similar to other secretory cells, it contains numerous mitochondria, Golgi apparatus, and rough endoplasmic reticulum.

The secretory end of the cementoblast exhibits irregular borders. Many cytoplasmic extensions arise from the cell body of the cementoblast, which are called as cementoblastic processes. These processes are directed toward periodontal ligament as they derive their nutrition from it. Cementoblastic processes interdigitate with those of the neighboring cementoblasts. Cytoplasmic processes are short for the cementoblasts residing at the cervical third than those on the apical third. The active cementoblasts are round, plump cells with large number of organelles, and during the resting period they become flattened with less organelles and referred to as resting cementoblasts.

Cementocytes

During the formation of cellular cementum, some cementoblasts become embedded in the unmineralized cemental matrix to become cementocytes. They are structurally and functionally similar to the osteocytes of the bone. They are present between layers of cementum and lie in spaces called lacunae. Cementocytes are cuboidal in shape

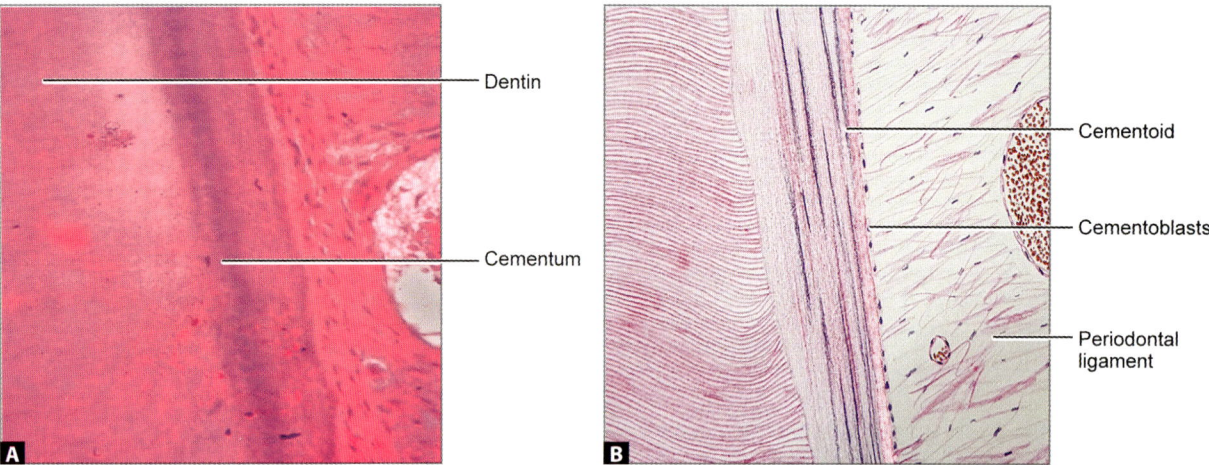

Figures 8-4A and B: (A) Hematoxylin and eosin stained section of cementum; (B) Schematic representation showing cementoid and cementoblasts.

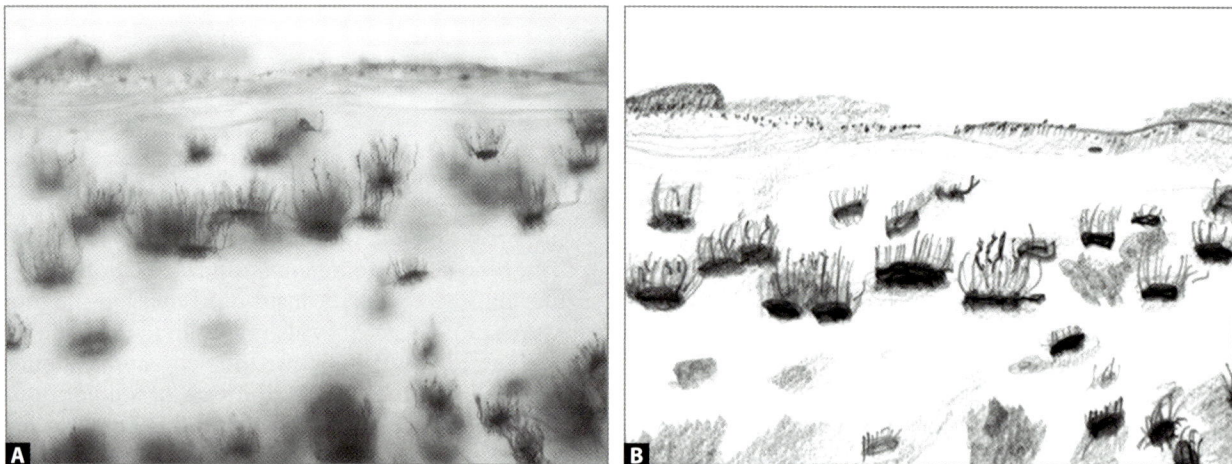

Figures 8-5A and B: (A) Ground section; and (B) Schematic representation showing cementocytes with their processes facing toward the periodontal ligament.

with long cytoplasmic processes about 10–30 in number and residing in a tubular space known as canaliculi. The cell process may have contact with those of the neighboring cells and exhibit gap junctions. Most of them are directed toward the periodontal ligament as they derive their nutrition from blood vessels in periodontal ligament **(Figures 8-5A and B)**. It has sparse organelles compared to cementoblast and are therefore considered to be resting or inactive cementoblasts. In contrast to the osteocytes of the bone, cementocytes are more widely dispersed and more randomly arranged. The diameter of the cell is around 8–12 µm, while the length of cytoplasmic processes is many times longer than that of the diameter of the cell body.

Many of the lacunae do not contain vital cementocytes. With aging, the thickness of the cementum increases, so the cells which are in deeper portions get deprived of nutrition. In such lacunae, the cells undergo degeneration and the lacunae become empty. In ground sections, the cells are lost and replaced by air and debris in those voids, which give a dark appearance. In decalcified sections, the cementocytes in the lacunae are retained but appear shrunken.

The cementocytes in the deeper layer have fewer cytoplasmic organelles, dilated endoplasmic reticulum, and sparse mitochondria indicating that these cells are degenerating or marginally active. Still deeper, there are definite signs of degeneration, characterized by cytoplasmic clumping and vesiculation.

Cementocytes are relatively inactive cells. They lay down some amount of matrix, which is present in perilacunar space or around the lacunae. They do not have any role to play in tissue homeostasis.

Differences between Cementocytes and Osteocytes (Figures 8-6A and B)

Table 8-1 describes the differences between cementocytes and osteocytes.

Cementoclasts

Cells responsible for the resorption of cementum are known as cementoclasts. They are also termed as odontoclasts and resemble osteoclasts of the bone. Cementoclasts are not seen normally, since cementum is less susceptible to resorption. However, cemental resorption is evident during shedding of deciduous teeth and in case of excessive orthodontic pressure.

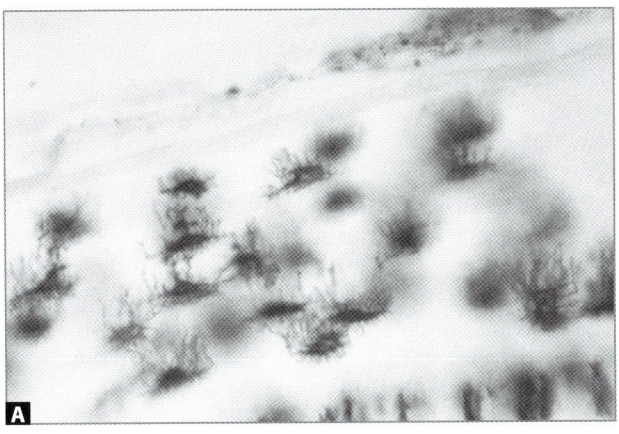
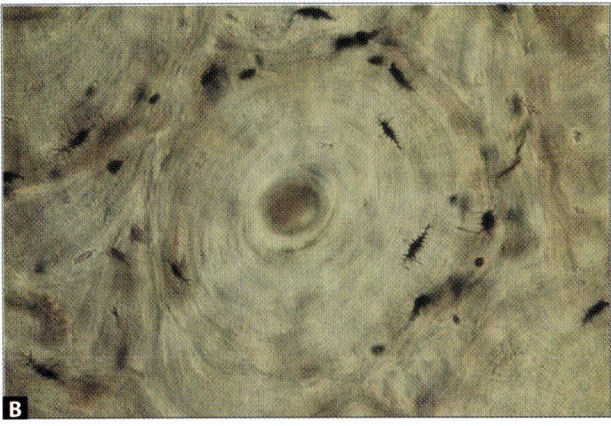

Figures 8-6A and B: Ground sections showing: (A) Cementocytes in cementum; (B) Osteocytes in Haversian system.

TABLE 8-1: Differences between cementocytes and osteocytes.

Cementocyte	Osteocyte
Entrapped cells of cementum	Entrapped cells of bone
Present in apical one-third and intraradicular areas (cellular cementum)	Present throughout bone
Widely and randomly distributed. They are not found around the blood vessels to form osteon, since cementum is avascular	Regularly distributed, usually found around the blood vessels to form osteon and are relatively close to each other
Cell processes are directed toward periodontal ligament	Run in all directions
Less in number per unit area	More in number

Cementoclasts appear as vacuolated and multinuclear or mononuclear cells with large amount of ribosomes and mitochondria. Cytoplasm exhibits projections toward the resorbing cemental surface called as brush border or ruffled border (similar to osteoclasts). They are observed in the resorbing cemental surface in Howship's lacunae, similar to bone.

FIBERS OF THE CEMENTUM

There are two types of fibers present in the cementum namely—intrinsic and extrinsic fibers.

Intrinsic fibers are collagen fibers laid down by cementoblasts. They are thin and short fibers with a diameter of about 1–2 μm and fully mineralized but cannot be identified distinctly in histological sections. They are present parallel to root surface and perpendicular to the extrinsic fibers.

Extrinsic fibers are collagen fibers of the inserted portion of the periodontal ligament secreted by fibroblasts of the periodontal ligament. They are directed either oblique or perpendicular to the root surface. The inserted portion of the extrinsic fibers is called Sharpey's fibers **(Figures 8-7A and B)**. These fibers are thick, coarse, and present in bundles with a diameter of around 5–7 μm. The extrinsic fibers are more in acellular cementum. They are thick and fully mineralized. In cellular cementum, the outer portion of the extrinsic fibers is mineralized and the innermost cores are not mineralized.

Intrinsic fibers are usually not seen in ground sections. The extrinsic fibers are not seen in cellular cementum.

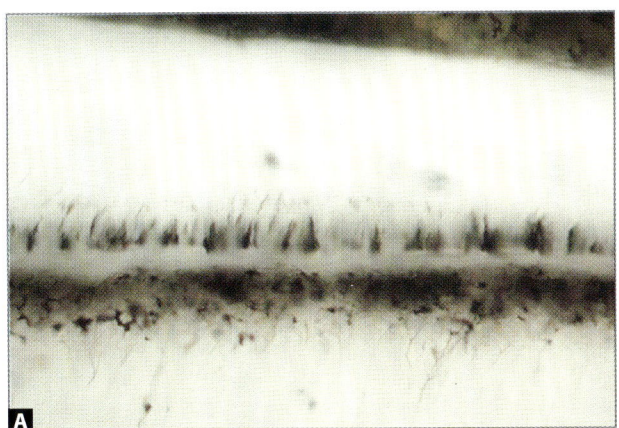
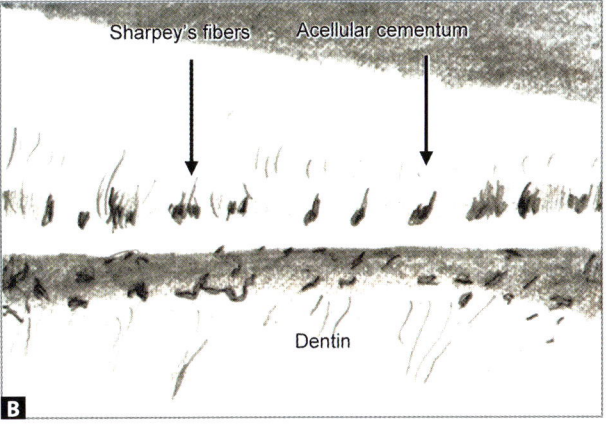

Figures 8-7A and B: (A) Ground section; and (B) Schematic representation of Sharpey's fibers in acellular cementum arranged in bundles perpendicular to cementum.

In contrast, they are seen as black spaces or thin black lines in ground sections, referred to as Sharpey's fiber spaces in cellular cementum. This is due to the air entrapment into the unmineralized cores, where the organic content is lost during the preparation of ground sections.

STRUCTURE

Cementum can be viewed as a unit containing cementoblasts, cementoid, and fully mineralized tissue. Cementum is basically categorized into two types namely—cellular and acellular based on the presence or absence of cementocytes. However, in humans it is further categorized into the following types, based on the presence or absence of fibers and their types; (1) acellular, afibrillar cementum; (2) acellular extrinsic fiber cementum; (3) cellular intrinsic fiber cementum; (4) cellular mixed fiber cementum; and (5) mixed stratified cementum.

Acellular afibrillar cementum does not contain cementocytes and detectable collagen fibers. This cementum is sparsely distributed and is composed of mineralized matrix. It is usually seen in the cervical enamel or in between fibrillar cementum and dentin. It is formed after the pre-eruptive enamel maturation and shortly before or during tooth eruption. It is also formed after eruption. This is also called coronal cementum, since it is normally seen over enamel and dentin adjacent to the CEJ. It is formed due to the premature loss of reduced enamel epithelium, which leads to the differentiation of cementoblasts from the dental sac cells. These cementoblasts form fibril-free matrix comprised of afibrillar collagen onto the enamel surface, which subsequently mineralize. It may be deposited in the form of cemental spurs or cemental islands.

> Cementum islands occur when a portion of reduced enamel epithelium is lost. The dental sac cells come in contact with the mature enamel to deposit cementum that does not contain fibers in its collagen matrix. It usually occurs coronal to the CEJ and is rarely seen in occlusal surface of posterior teeth.

Acellular extrinsic fiber cementum consists of inserted portion of periodontal ligament fibers (Sharpey's fibers) and cementum devoid of cementocytes **(Figures 8-8A and B)**. It is seen in single rooted teeth, where it extends from the cervical margin to the apical third. The extrinsic fibers are attached perpendicular to the surface of the cementum. The inserted fiber bundle is mineralized except for the inner core. The Sharpey's fibers run through the entire thickness of the cementum if it is thin. Upon further deposition of cementum, more amounts of fibers are incorporated into it. But the attachment of tooth to alveolar bone *per se* is limited to the most superficial portion of the cementum. Incremental lines are seen in a regular fashion and are closer together, since it forms at a slower rate. It is considered to be formed by the cells of the periodontal ligament fibroblasts. The ground substance is elaborated by cementoblasts.

Cellular intrinsic fiber cementum is comprised of cementoblasts and the collagen fibers secreted by them. It is more rapidly formed and less mineralized. This type of cementum is not formed during normal root formation; instead it is formed as a part of reparative process or on the unerupted or impacted teeth. In this type of cementum, collagen fibers intermingle with that of dentin. As cementum formation progresses, some of the cementoblasts get entrapped in the cemental matrix and become cementocytes. Collagen fibrils are haphazardly placed in the initial rapid phase, but subsequently they get oriented parallel to the surface.

Cellular mixed fiber cementum: As the name indicates, it contains cells (cementocytes), intrinsic fibers, (collagen fibers secreted by the cementoblasts), and extrinsic fibers, the inserted portion of the periodontal ligament fibers (secreted by the fibroblasts of the periodontal ligament).

It is predominantly a product of cementoblasts and formed at a faster rate and is relatively less mineralized. The intrinsic fibers secreted by the cementoblasts and the extrinsic fibers formed by the periodontal ligament intermingle with each other in a complex manner.

Mixed stratified cementum contains a mix of cellular intrinsic fiber cementum with acellular extrinsic fiber cementum in the apical third of the root and in furcation areas. This cementum is typed as mixed stratified cementum, the thickness of which ranges from 100 to 1000 µm.

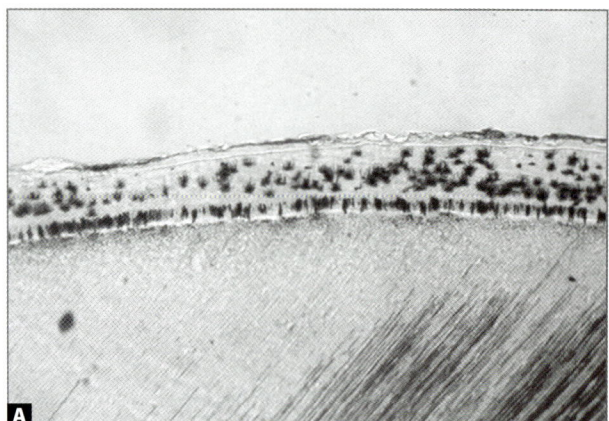 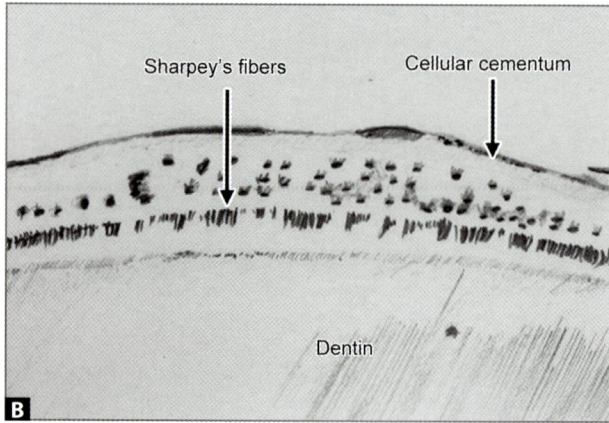

Figures 8-8A and B: (A) Ground section; and (B) Schematic representation of Sharpey's fibers in cellular cementum.

CLASSIFICATION OF CEMENTUM

The classification of cementum according to three factors has been discussed in **Box 8-1**.

The location of cellular and acellular cementum is not definite. The acellular cementum usually extends from the CEJ till the apex and is present more in coronal half of the root, while the cellular cementum is located in the apical third. Occasionally, layers of cellular and acellular cementum may alternate in any pattern. Rarely, acellular cementum can be found on cellular cementum and cellular cementum is frequently found on acellular cementum **(Figures 8-9A and B)**.

Cellular cementum comprises the entire thickness of apical cementum, being thickest at the apex, and contributes to the length of the root by its growth. The growth is in an appositional manner **(Figures 8-10A and B)**.

The collagen fibers of cellular and acellular cementum are arranged in a very complex manner with barely discernible pattern. The acellular cementum has mainly extrinsic fibers that are perpendicular to the root surface while the cellular cementum has both extrinsic and intrinsic fibers. The differing orientation gives different colors under polarized light **(Table 8-2)**.

> **BOX 8-1:** Classification of cementum according to three factors.
>
> - Time of formation:
>   - Primary
>   - Secondary
> - Presence or absence of cells within its matrix:
>   - Cellular
>   - Acellular
> - Origin of collagenous fibers of the matrix:
>   - Intrinsic fibers by cementoblast activity
>   - Extrinsic fibers by incorporation of periodontal ligament fibers
>
> Accordingly the cementum is categorized into the following types:
> - Acellular afibrillar cementum
> - Acellular extrinsic fiber cementum
> - Cellular intrinsic fiber cementum
> - Cellular mixed fiber cementum
> - Mixed stratified cementum

CEMENTOGENESIS

Formation of cementum is known as cementogenesis. It starts pre-eruptively during the development of the root and it continues after root development and eruption. As long as the functioning periodontal ligament is present, cemental deposition continues throughout the life. Primary cementum thus appears to be the main tissue that attaches the periodontal ligament to the tooth, while the secondary cementum probably forms in response to the functional demands of the attachment apparatus.

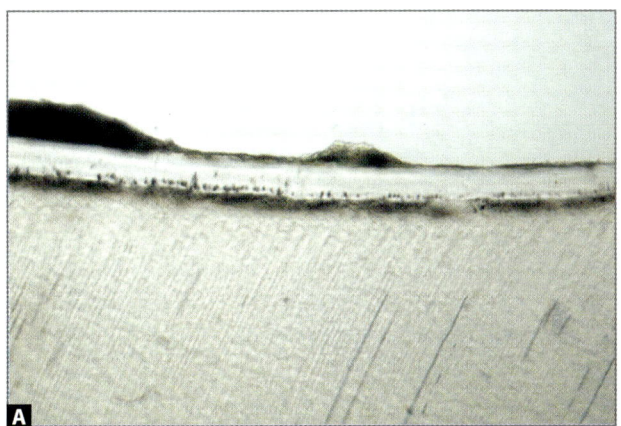 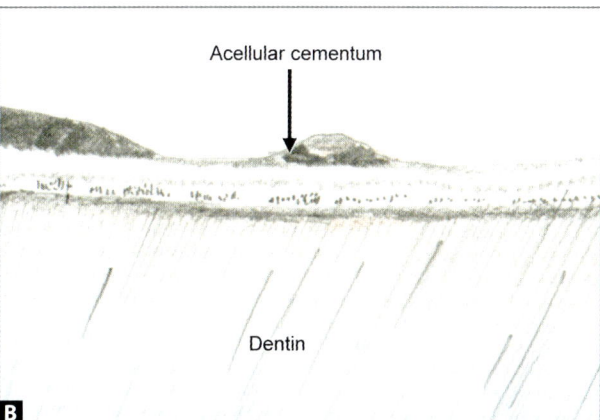

Figures 8-9A and B: (A) Ground section; and (B) Schematic representation of acellular cementum.

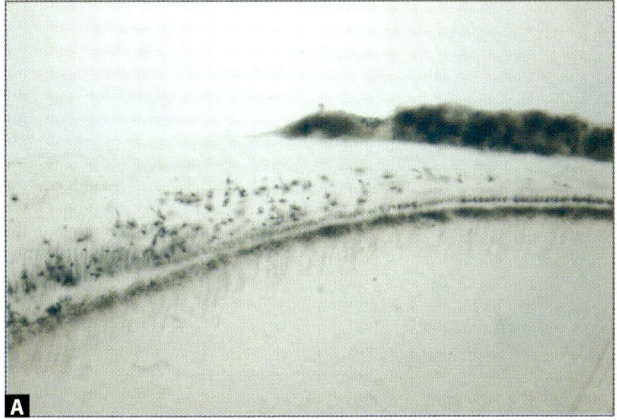 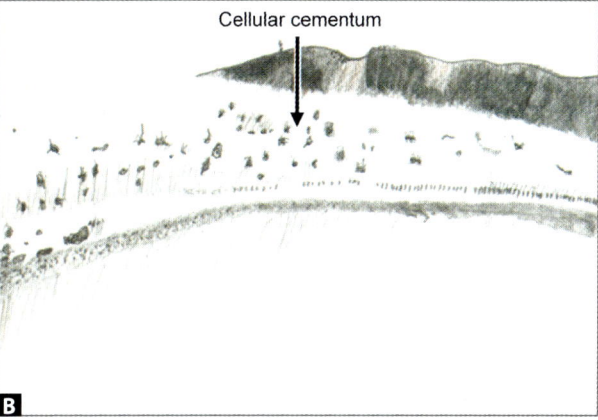

Figures 8-10A and B: (A) Ground section and (B) Schematic representation of cellular cementum.

CHAPTER 8: Cementum

TABLE 8-2: Differences between acellular cementum and cellular cementum.

Acellular cementum	Cellular cementum
Cementocytes are absent	Cementocytes are present
First laid down	Laid down later
Also known as primary cementum	Secondary cementum
Seen in coronal half	Apical one-third and interradicular areas
Laid down slowly	Laid down rapidly
Incremental lines are thin and close	Incremental lines are thick and wide apart
Width 50 µm	Width 200–300 µm
Less permeable	More permeable
More mineral content	Less mineral content
Less intrinsic fibers	More intrinsic fibers
Cementoid layer is thin	Cementoid layer is thicker
Border between acellular cementum and dentin less distinct	Border between cellular cementum and dentin more distinct
Provides attachment for the tooth	Has an adaptive role in response to tooth wear and movement. Associated with repair of the periodontal tissues

Wnt signaling is important in regulating root formation, especially may play a role in the regulation of radicular dentinogenesis. Wnt signaling also interacts with other signaling pathways to control root formation.

During root development, BMP signaling is actively involved in regulating cell fate decisions, during Hertwig's epithelial root sheath formation, and the differentiation of odontoblasts. BMP 2, 3, 4, and 7 are expressed during the initiation of tooth root development. BMP signaling also controls the patterning of root development.

After the crown formation completes, more specifically after the cessation of amelogenesis, the inner and outer enamel epithelium of the dental organ proliferates toward the future root, as a two-layered sheet of somewhat flattened epithelial cells. This is called Hertwig's epithelial root sheath. This is devoid of stellate reticulum and stratum intermedium **(Figure 8-11)**. Hertwig's epithelial root sheath is separated from the dental papilla and dental sac by basal lamina.

Root formation, which consists of the formation of radicular dentin and cementum, also involves epithelial–mesenchymal interactions, similar to crown formation. The cells of the root sheath induce the peripheral dental papilla cells to differentiate into odontoblasts. These odontoblasts secrete the organic matrix of the first formed predentin, which comprises of some collagen fibrils and ground substance. As the odontoblasts secrete the dentin matrix, they retreat toward the pulp. But at the initial few microns, they do not leave behind the typical odontoblastic process. This portion contains predominantly obliquely arranged collagen fibers and some perpendicularly oriented fibers with no clearly discerned dentinal tubules. This structureless layer of about 10 µm thickness is known as hyaline layer. This layer is in contact with the root sheath for a while.

The epithelial root sheath cells are functionally active and secrete bioactive molecules, which play a major role in root formation. This is accomplished by the epithelial–mesenchymal interactions concerned with the induction of odontoblasts and cementoblasts and/or the mineralization process. These bioactive molecules of the root sheath cells consist of enamel-related proteins, which together with the hyaline layer form cementum–dentin boundary. Thus, this layer is contributed by both the epithelial root sheath cells and the odontoblasts.

Collagen I, bone sialoprotein, and alkaline phosphatase are cementoblast markers expressed by Hertwig's epithelial root sheath, which suggests that the Hertwig's epithelial root sheath directly contributes to the cementoblasts pool of the periodontal ligament through epithelial–mesenchymal transition (EMT).

Soon the Hertwig's epithelial root sheath is broken down or becomes perforated (probably by the programmed cell death), which results in contact between the newly formed radicular

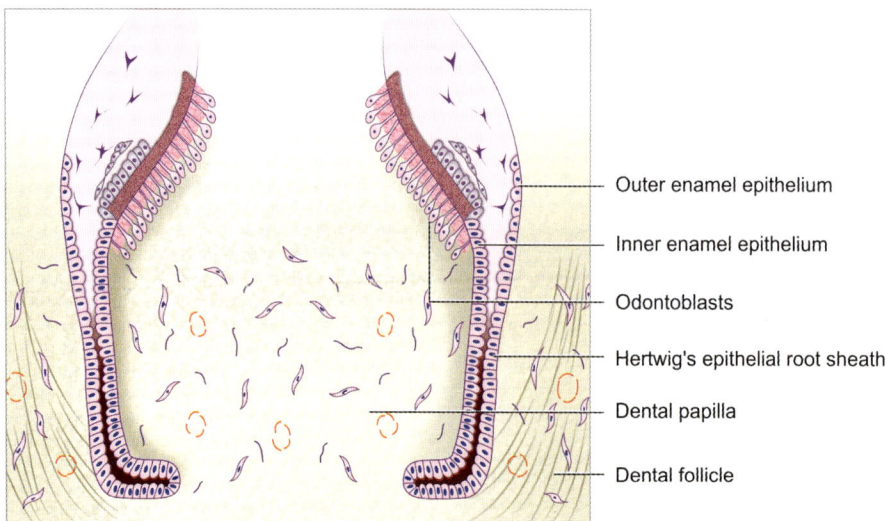

Figure 8-11: Formation of Hertwig's epithelial root sheath.

dentin with the cells of the dental sac. This interaction enables the dental sac cells to differentiate into cementoblasts. These cementoblasts lay down a layer of cemental matrix (cementoid), which consists of collagen fibrils and ground substances **(Figure 8-12)**. It is to be noted here that the fibrous component of the initial cemental matrix is not only derived from the cementoblasts but also from the cells of the dental sac. These initially formed fibrils intermingle with the fibrils of the hyaline layer. The subsequent mineralization produces a firm bond between the dentin and the cementum.

Hertwig's epithelial root sheath does not completely degenerate during or after root formation but become the epithelial cell rests of Malassez and reside in the periodontal ligament **(Figure 8-13)**. This may contribute to cementum regeneration and repair.

In the cervical third to one half of the root, the cementoblasts border the formed cementum as a cementogenic layer, since cementogenesis occurs in a sequential layered pattern. Beyond that, the cementoblasts get entrapped in the matrix they formed and become cellular cementum. This is because in the apical half or third of the root the specific areas of the matrix mature and mineralize without following a sequential pattern. Cementum formation continues in this fashion throughout the life.

> Cementoblasts apart from secreting collagen fibers, also secrete other noncollagenous proteins, which include osteopontin, bone sialoprotein, cementum attachment protein, and growth hormones. These are implicated in cell differentiation, cell growth, cell migration, cell attachment, and mineralization.

After the formation of hyaline layer, the odontoblasts migrate toward the inner portion of the pulp leaving behind the cytoplasmic process called odontoblastic process. The mineralization of the hyaline layer starts in the mid portion and proceeds both outward and inward. So the mineralization of the outermost portion (on the cemental side) is slightly delayed and progresses to cementum. Mineralization always lags several microns behind matrix formation. The mineralization of cementum is an ordered event and this

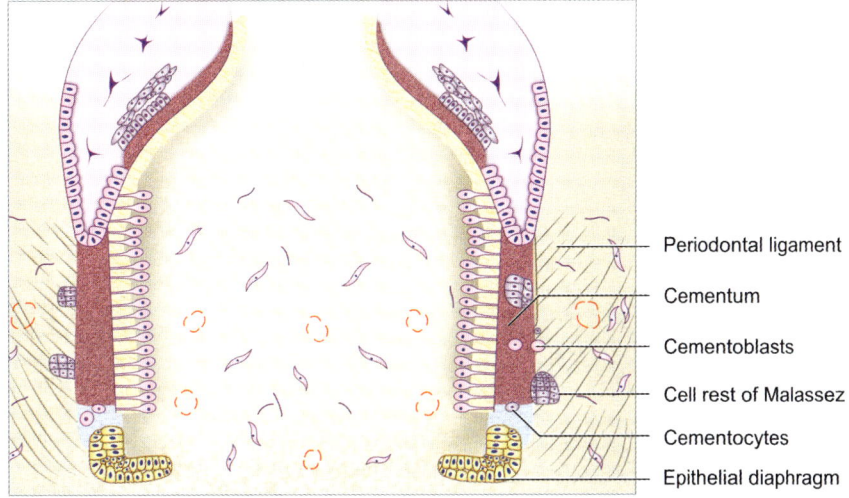

Figure 8-12: Hertwig's epithelial root sheath break down and cementum formation.

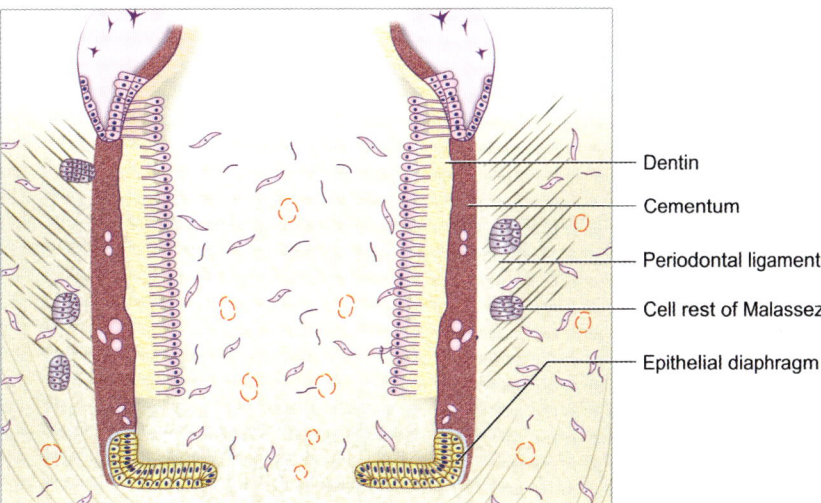

Figure 8-13: Cell rests of Malassez in the periodontal ligament.

involves deposition of mineral apatites on, in, and between the collagen fibers. These apatite crystals are needle and plate-shaped and morphologically similar to those of dentin and bone.

CEMENTOID

The unmineralized cemental matrix known as cementoid, also called as precementum, covers the cemental surface. This cementoid tissue is lined by cementoblasts. The thickness of cementoid varies from 3 to 5 µm and contains collagen fibers, ground substance, etc., and appears eosinophilic and amorphous under light microscope. During active cemental deposition, the thickness of cementoid increases.

Growth of cementum is a rhythmic process and comprises of matrix (cementoid) formation and mineralization. As new layer of cementoid is formed, the old one mineralizes. Collagen fibers from the periodontal ligament pass between the cementoblasts and enter precementum to get embedded. These embedded fibers known as Sharpey's fibers in cementum serve to attach the tooth to alveolar bone. Each Sharpey's fiber has a number of collagen fibers that pass into the cementum and are referred to as extrinsic fibers. The fiber insertion sites appear as 3–6 µm hemispherical domes on the cemental surface.

INCREMENTAL LINES OF CEMENTUM

The rhythmic deposition of cementum (phases of activity and rest) is reflected by incremental lines. This rhythmicity is not regular as in enamel or dentin. Thus the incremental lines are unevenly separated and the precise periodicity between them is not known. These incremental lines are called as *lines of Salter* (**Figures 8-14 and 8-15**).

The incremental lines in acellular cementum are thin and close because it is laid down slowly, while the incremental lines in cellular cementum are thick and far apart as it is laid down rapidly. These incremental lines are formed due to disturbance in both matrix formation and mineralization. Histochemical studies have shown that the incremental lines in cementum are highly mineralized areas with less collagen and more ground substance than other portions of cementum. They are best visualized in decalcified sections. Recent evidences suggest that the incremental lines are rich in osteopontin and that this might aid the cohesion of the matrix molecules at this site.

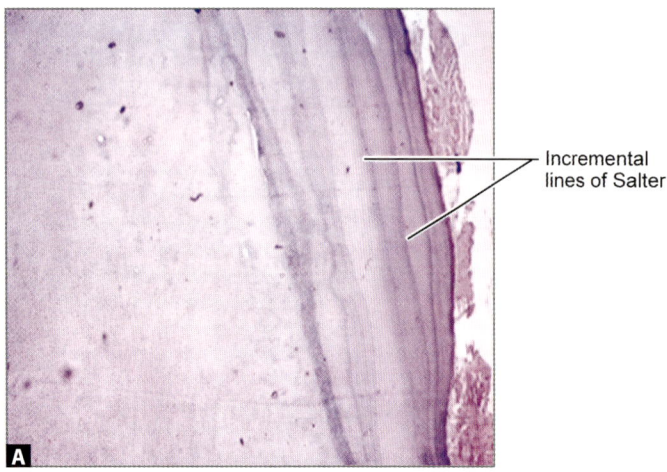
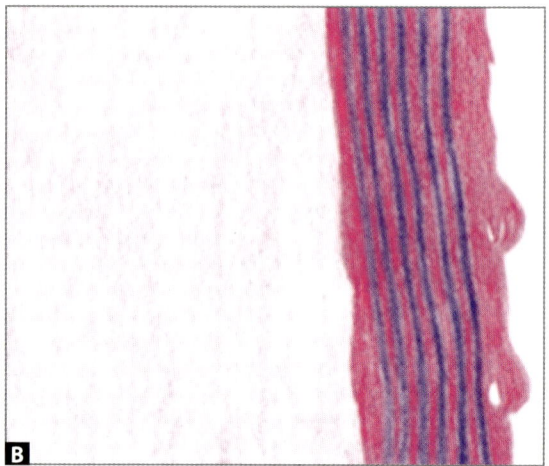

Figures 8-14A and B: (A) Hematoxylin and eosin-stained section; and (B) Schematic representation showing the incremental lines of Salter in acellular cementum.

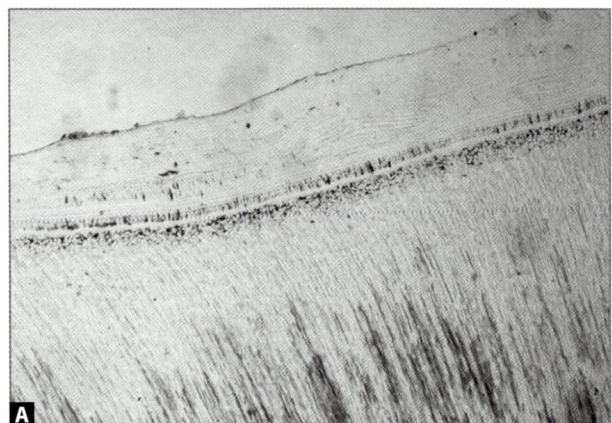
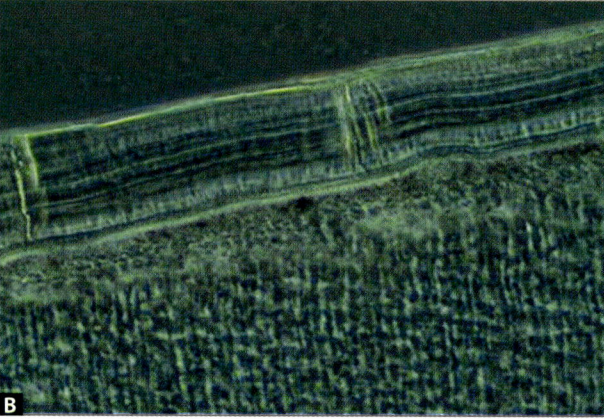

Figures 8-15A and B: (A) Incremental lines of cementum in ground section; and (B) under phase contrast microscopy.
Source: (B) Dr Bala Subramanya Goutham and Dr Sujatha Ramachandra, KIIT University, Bhubaneswar, Odisha, India.

HYALINE LAYER OF HOPEWELL-SMITH

At the cementodentinal junction (CDJ) or in between the CDJ, a narrow band of clear hyaline layer is present. This is known as hyaline layer of Hopewell-Smith and is implicated in the attachment of dentin to the cementum.

This layer contains enamel matrix like protein and dentin proteins. After the break down of Hertwig's epithelial root sheath, the inner enamel epithelial cells form the hyaline layer. This occurs subsequent to the formation of radicular dentin. Periodontal ligament fibers are attached initially into this layer.

It is not known whether it has to be included in periodontium, since it appears to have a role in attaching cementum to dentin. The initial collagenous fibers of primary cementum are embedded within it and therefore could be considered in functional terms as a tissue of tooth support. It differs, however, for the fact that it has different developmental origin, which does not involve the dental follicle.

Attachment of Periodontal Ligament Fibers to Cementum

The fibers of periodontal ligament run into the organic matrix of cementoid that is secreted by the cementoblasts. Subsequent mineralization of the cementoid will incorporate the extrinsic fibers as Sharpey's fibers into the cementum. It has been estimated that for acellular extrinsic fiber cementum, there are approximately 30,000 principal fibers of periodontal ligament attached to the cemental tissue per square millimeter.

CEMENTODENTINAL JUNCTION

The interface between the cementum and dentin is of special importance, since it is formed by two different mineralized tissues. The CDJ junction is regular and smooth in permanent teeth, while some amount of scalloping may be seen in deciduous teeth. The attachment of cementum to dentin in either case is quite firm although the nature of the attachment is not fully understood. It is seen in decalcified and stained light microscopic sections but further details are not distinctly evident in electron microscope.

> Sometimes, dentin is separated from cementum by a zone known as *intermediate cementum layer*, the thickness of which can be around 10–50 µ, and does not resemble either dentin or cementum. Usually, found in apical two-thirds of roots or molar and premolars and is rarely observed in incisors or deciduous teeth. It may be a continuous layer or present in patches.

Intermediate cementum is a form of secondary cellular intrinsic fiber cementum restricted to the apex of the tooth. It contains entrapped debris derived from either Hertwig's epithelial root sheath or odontoblastic layer. It is not involved in tooth attachment and has no functional significance. The term intermediate cementum has been incorrectly used to describe the hyaline layer. It is seen close to the dentin surface so it is suggested that it has got dentinal origin as this layer is said to contain dilated terminal endings of dentinal tubules. Branching spaces are sometimes seen in continuity with dentin.

CEMENTOENAMEL JUNCTION

Cementum and enamel usually meet at the cervical region of the tooth and form the CEJ. In 10% of the teeth, they do not meet and the root dentin is exposed resulting in hypersensitivity and increased risk of dental caries **(Figures 8-16A and B)**. This is attributed to the failure of degeneration of the Hertwig's epithelial root sheath in the cervical portion. As a result, the dental sac cells do not come in contact with root dentin to differentiate into cementoblasts to form cementum.

In 60% of teeth, cementum overlaps cervical enamel to a short distance **(Figures 8-17A and B)**. This is attributed to the premature degeneration of reduced enamel epithelium covering the enamel at the cervical region. In such situations, the dental sac cells differentiate into cementoblasts and lay down a layer of cementum directly over enamel. This type of cementum is acellular and afibrillar. As described previously, it does not contain fibrillar collagen. If such afibrillar cementum remains in contact with connective tissue cells for a long time, fibrillar cementum with typical collagen fibrils (with 64 nm periodicity) may be deposited on it, thus the thickness of cementum over the cervical enamel increases.

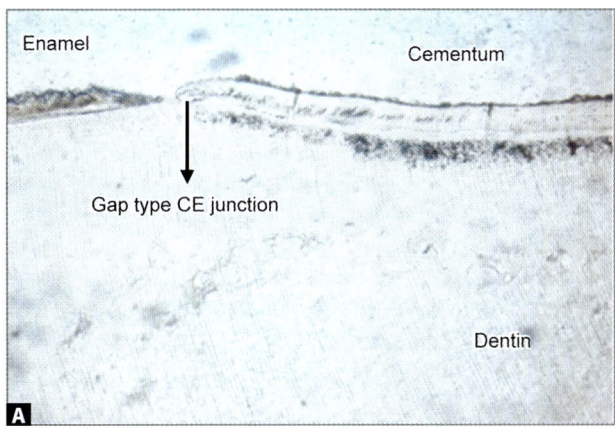 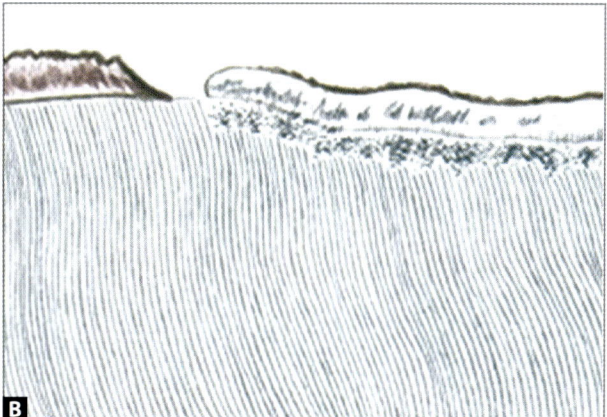

Figures 8-16A and B: (A) Ground section; and (B) schematic representation of gap type of cementoenamel (CE) junction.
Source: (B) Dr Carmen Chuah Ming Ke.

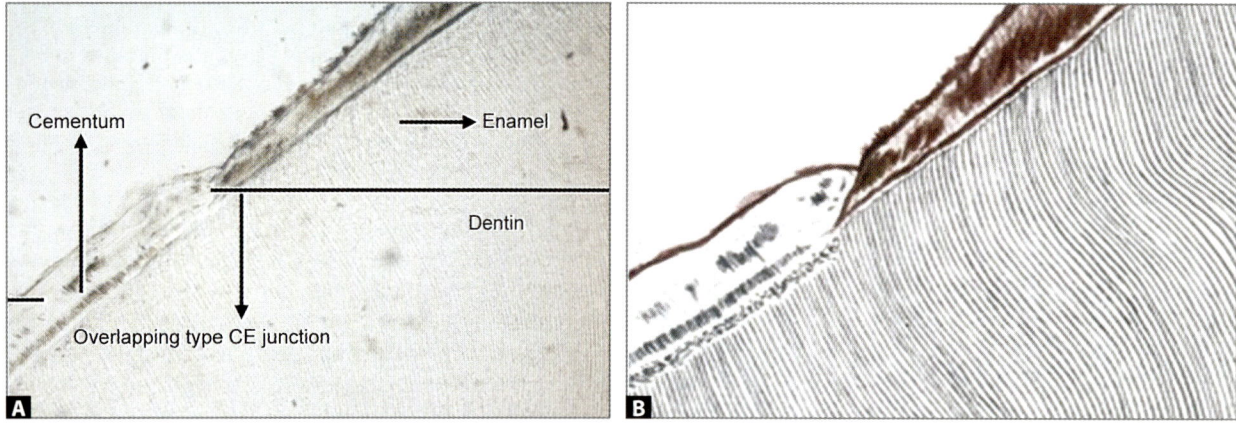

Figures 8-17A and B: (A) Ground section; and (B) Schematic representation of overlapping type of cementoenamel (CE) junction.
Source: (B) Dr Carmen Chuah Ming Ke.

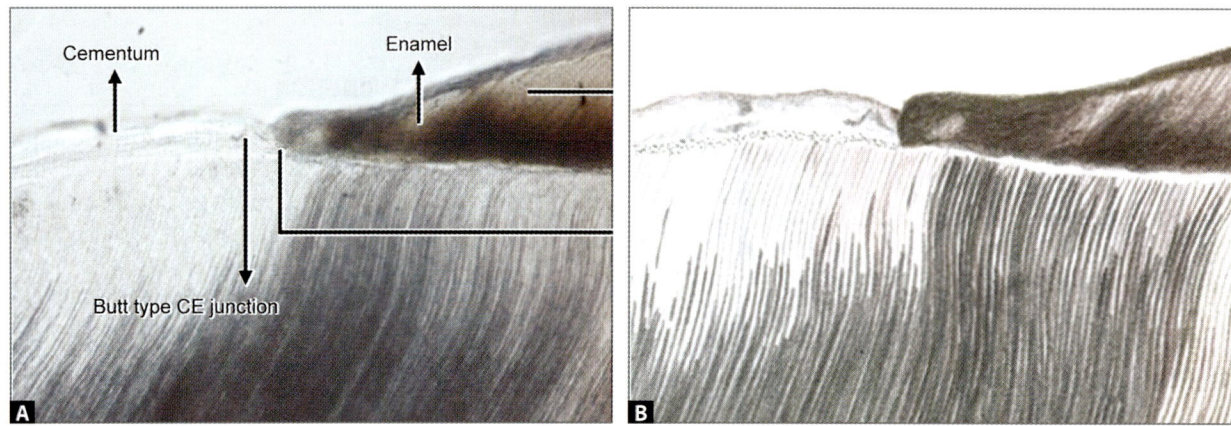

Figures 8-18A and B: (A) Ground section; and (B) Schematic representation of butt type cementoenamel (CE) junction.
Source: (B) Dr Carmen Chuah Ming Ke.

Cementum and enamel meet end to end as a butt joint with no overlapping in 30% of teeth **(Figures 8-18A and B)**. The type of CEJ varies along the circumference of each tooth and above mentioned three types of junction may be present even in a single tooth.

FUNCTIONS OF CEMENTUM

Supportive: Cementum serves as a medium for attachment of periodontal ligament to tooth and thus aids in attaching the tooth to the alveolus. Since dentin is made up of tubules, the periodontal ligament fibers cannot be incorporated into it directly. Cementum seals off the opening of the dentinal tubule on the outer aspect and provides attachment to the fibers of the periodontal ligament.

In cementum, continuous deposition and minimal resorption occurs in contrast to the bone, where deposition and resorption occurs alternatively in a rhythmic manner. Continuous cemental deposition has functional importance. Repeated apposition of cementum represents aging of tooth and functionally the tooth is as old as the last cementum layer laid down on the root surface.

Cementum enables reattachment of periodontal ligament and maintains the periodontal ligament width by continuous deposition of cementum throughout the life. The periodontal ligament fibers shift in position due to forces, functional stresses, and get re-embedded by the cementum. Proximal wear or tooth loss causes tooth to be drifted or shifted in position and the periodontal ligament has to be realigned, for which cementum helps.

Maintaining the occlusal relationship: Shortening of the tooth occurs due to physiologic occlusal wear as in attrition and in pathologic conditions (*e.g.* bruxism). This is compensated by the cementum deposition at the apex thus allowing for functional adaptation.

Reparative: Damage to roots, like fracture and resorption, can be repaired by the deposition of new cementum. This repaired cementum is usually demarcated from normal cementum by repair lines.

As cementum is the slowest growing tissue compared to other periodontal tissues, it will be the last tissue to be added to root surface after occlusal loss.

AGE CHANGES

Continuous formation of cellular cementum as age advances results in increase in the thickness. Increased thickness occurs particularly in apical third and furcation areas of the root. Constriction of apical foramen and obstruction of the apical canal occurs because of the cemental deposition in the apical zone.

With aging, cemental surface becomes irregular due to calcification of some of the fibers of the periodontal ligament. Cementum resorption is also one of the characteristic features of aging. Cementocytes are viable in the lacunae near the surface. In the deeper portion, cementocytic lacunae appear empty.

CLINICAL CONSIDERATIONS

Abnormal thickening of cementum is known as hypercementosis. It may involve single tooth or affect all teeth. Hypercementosis may be localized or generalized to involve the entire tooth surface **(Figures 8-19A and B)**.

If the over growth improves the functional qualities of cementum, it is called cementum hypertrophy, while the term cemental hyperplasia is used when the growth occurs in nonfunctional teeth or if it is not correlated with the function.

Localized cemental hypertrophy is manifested by occurrence of a spur or prong-like over growth of cementum, usually seen in teeth, which are subjected to heavy masticatory stress. This is to provide increased surface area for the attachment of periodontal ligament fibers, thus complimenting its function.

Hypercementosis is associated with many neoplastic and nonneoplastic conditions. Generalized hypercementosis occurs in Paget's disease of the bone.

Hypercementosis occurs in nonfunctioning teeth, which may extend around the entire root or may be localized to small areas. They are characterized by reduced number of Sharpey's fibers embedded in the root.

Chronic periapical inflammation sometimes results in extensive hyperplasia, which may be circumscribed and surround the root like a cuff. Calcified knoblike or spherical projections found on the hyperplastic cementum are termed as excementoses, which are developed around degenerated or calcified epithelial rests.

Since cementum is avascular, it is resistant to resorption than bone and thus facilitates orthodontic tooth movement. The degenerative processes are affected by interference in circulation. When tooth is moved by orthodontic appliance; the pressure side (direction to which the tooth moves) there will be bone resorption, while in the tension side, bone deposition.

Cementum may resorb due to severe trauma or excessive occlusal stress. Resorption may extend to involve root dentin in severe cases. The damage is repaired by deposition of cellular/acellular cementum or alternate layers of both. Repair lines demarcate the repaired tissue and the normal cementum. If the cementum deposited re-establishes the former outline of root, then it is referred to as anatomic repair. Functional repair is characterized by deposition of a thin layer of cementum on the surface of deep resorption, which does not reconstruct the former root outline and a bay-like recess remains. In such areas, the periodontal space is restored to its normal width by formation of a bony projection, so that proper functional relationship will result. The outline of alveolar bone in these cases follows that of the root surface.

Root fracture may occasionally be repaired by the formation of cemental callus, but unlike fracture in the bone, this callus does not remodel to the original dimensions of the tooth. Teeth subjected to severe blow may result in tear of cementum usually at CEJ or in cementum or in dentin.

Hypercementosis can occur in tooth affected by chronic infection or subjected to excessive occlusal stress. The excess cementum formed, anchors the tooth tightly to the socket and may lead to fracture while extraction, thus emphasizing the need for preoperative radiographs.

Cementum is exposed through gingival recession. As only few layers of cementum cover the root, the exposed cementum is quickly worn off with mechanical friction, exposing the deeper dentin, and leading to extrinsic staining and dentinal hypersensitivity.

The incidence of cemental caries increases in older adults as gingival recession is a common feature in them. It is a chronic condition that forms a large, shallow lesion that slowly invades into dentin, and then into the pulp tissue.

Cementum, though resembles bone, does not contain nerves. Thus, cementum is nonsensitive. Scaling does not produce pain, however, if cementum is removed, exposure of the underlying dentin results in sensitivity.

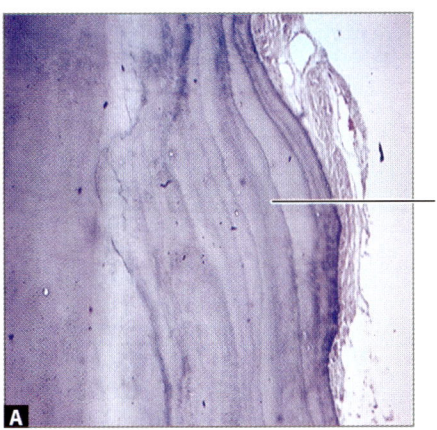
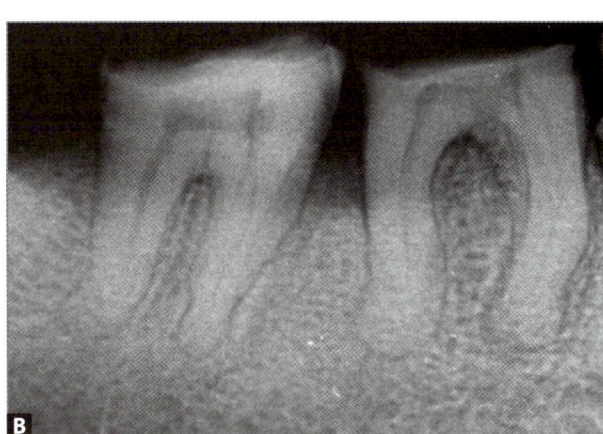

Figures 8-19A and B: Hypercementosis: (A) Photomicrograph; (B) Radiograph.

Plaque and its byproducts can cause physical, chemical, and structural alterations in cementum in teeth with deep periodontal pockets. Cementum becomes hypermineralized due to calcium, phosphorus, and fluoride deposition from the oral environment in cases of pathologically exposed cemental surface.

Alteration in cementum surface is important in practice of periodontics, as it may interfere with healing during periodontal therapy. Various procedures (mechanical— root planning and chemical) are available to remove pathologically altered cementum, so that new cementum can be deposited.

The aim of regenerative periodontal therapy is to induce new cementum formation and restoration of soft tissue attachment to the cementum. Cementum regeneration requires cementoblasts and molecular factors regulating their recruitment and differentiation are not completely understood.

A variety of chemotactic factors, adhesion molecules, growth factors, and ECM constituents participate together in the recruitment of cementoblast progenitors, their expansion, and differentiation. The mechanism by which selection of cementoblast progenitors is achieved is unclear, and it most likely involves specific integrins and signaling events.

Cementicles are spherical calcified masses made up of acellular extrinsic fiber cementum seen in the periodontal ligament.

Points to Remember

- Cementum is a hard, avascular connective tissue that covers the roots of the teeth and forms an integral part of the periodontium.
- Cementum gives attachment to the fibers of the periodontal ligament and firmly adheres to the dentin on its inner aspect thus holds the tooth in the socket.
- Cementum is derived from dental sac or follicle and cells responsible for cementum formation are called cementoblasts.
- Cells of cementum include cementoblasts, cementocytes and cementoclasts.
- Cementocytes are the entrapped cementoblasts in the cemental matrix. They have cytoplasmic processes directed towards the periodontal ligament.
- Cementoclasts are the cells responsible for the resorption of the cementum. They are multinucleated cells and resemble osteoclasts of the bone.
- The fibers of cementum include; intrinsic fibers, the collagen fibers laid down by cementoblasts and extrinsic fibers, the inserted portion of the periodontal ligament.
- Cementum can be classified into two types, *i.e,* cellular and acellular cementum based on the presence and absence of cementocytes.
- The acellular cementum usually extends from the CEJ till the apex and is present more in coronal half of the root, while the cellular cementum is located in the apical third.
- Cementoid, also called as precementum is the unmineralized cemental matrix that covers the cemental surface.
- The incremental lines of cementum called as lines of Salter represent the rhythmic deposition of cementum (phases of activity and rest).
- A narrow band of clear hyaline layer called hyaline layer of Hopewell–Smith is present at the cementodentinal junction (CDJ) or in between the CDJ. This is implicated in the attachment of dentin to the cementum.
- Cementum and enamel usually meet at the cervical region of the tooth and form the cementoenamel junction (CEJ). Overlap CEJ (60%), Butt CEJ (30%) and Gap CEJ (10%) are three types of CEJ.
- Functions of cementum include supportive, reparative and maintenance of occlusal relationship.
- Hypercementosis is abnormal thickening of cementum. It may involve single tooth or affect all teeth; may be localized or generalized to involve the entire tooth surface.

PRACTICE QUESTIONS

1. Describe physical and chemical properties of cementum. Identify the types of cemento-enamel junction with well labelled diagrams.
2. Classify cementum. Describe in detail the histology of cementum and its clinical significance.
3. Describe the gross microscopic anatomy of cementum. Add a note on cementogenesis.
4. Discuss hypercementosis.
5. Discuss in brief types of cementum.
6. Describe the chemical composition of cementum.
7. Discuss Sharpey's fibers.

MULTIPLE CHOICE QUESTIONS

1. **Avascular component of periodontium is:**
   a. Alveolar bone
   b. Periodontal ligament
   c. Cementum
   d. Gingiva
2. **Which calcified component of the tooth contains highest concentration of fluoride?**
   a. Enamel
   b. Dentin
   c. Cementum
   d. Pulp
3. **Primarily organic portion of cementum consists which of the following collagen fibrrs?**
   a. Type-I
   b. Type-II
   c. Type-IV
   d. Type-VII

4. Cementum is thinnest at which of the following site?
   a. Cementoenamel junction
   b. Middle 3rd of root
   c. Towards apex
   d. DEJ
5. Cementum is thickest at which of the following site?
   a. CEJ
   b. Middle 3rd of root
   c. Towards apex
   d. DEJ
6. Acellular cementum is found in which of the following area?
   a. Cervical and middle 3rd of root
   b. Apical 3rd of root
   c. Only in furcation areas
   d. Only in cervical areas
7. Cellular cementum is found in which of the following area?
   a. Cervical and middle 3rd of root
   b. Middle 3rd of the root
   c. Apical 3rd and furcation area of root
   d. C-E Junction
8. Intermediate cementum layer is predominately seen in which of the following areas?
   a. Cervical 3rd of molar and premolar roots
   b. Apical 2/3rd of molar and premolar roots
   c. Apical 2/3rd of canine root
   d. Cervical 1/3rd of canine root
9. In most instances, at C-E Junction:
   a. Enamel overlaps cementum
   b. Cementum overlaps enamel
   c. Cementum and enamel form butt joint
   d. Cementum and enamel never meet each other
10. Cementodentinal junction in deciduous teeth is:
    a. Straight
    b. Irregular
    c. Sometimes scalloped
    d. Smooth
11. The main difference between cellular cementum and acellular cementum is:
    a. Presence of cementocytes
    b. Presence of Sharpey's fibers
    c. Presence of lamellae
    d. Presence of incremental lines
12. Which of the following surrounds an apical foramen?
    a. Cementum always
    b. Dentin always
    c. Cementum and dentin
    d. Cementum and enamel
13. The embedded collagen fibers in cementum that radiate from periodontal ligament are called as:
    a. Circular fibers
    b. Oblique fibers
    c. Sharpey's fibers
    d. Horizontal fibers
14. Intrinsic fibers of the cementum is formed by:
    a. Fibroblasts of the periodontal ligament
    b. Cementoblasts
    c. Osteoblasts
    d. Odontoblasts
15. What is the primary function of cementum?
    a. Contributes to the size and strength of root portion of the tooth
    b. Protects the root dentin
    c. Furnish a medium for attachment of collagen fibers that bind the tooth to alveolar bone
    d. It serves as major reparative tissue for root surface
16. Which one of the following is not a function of cementum?
    a. Nutritive
    b. Reparative
    c. Supportive
    d. Maintaining the occlusal relationship
17. The condition where the overgrowth of cementum increase functional efficiency is called as:
    a. Cementum hyperplasia
    b. Cementum hypertrophy
    c. Cementoma
    d. Cementoblastoma
18. Calcifies masses seen in the periodontal ligament are called:
    a. Denticles
    b. Precementum
    c. Cementoid
    d. Cementicles

ANSWERS

1. c   2. c   3. a   4. a   5. c   6. a   7. c   8. b   9. b   10. c   11. a   12. a   13. c   14. b   15. c
16. a   17. b   18. d

BIBLIOGRAPHY

1. Ao M, Chavez MB, Chu EY, et al. Overlapping functions of bone sialoprotein and pyrophosphate regulators in directing cementogenesis. Bone. 2017;105:134-47.
2. Avery JK, Chiego DJ. Essentials of oral histology and embryology: a clinical approach, 3rd edition. St. Louis: Mosby; 2006.
3. Avery JK. Oral development and histology, 3rd edition. New York: Thieme; 2002.
4. Bartold PM, Miki Y, McAllister B, et al. Glycosaminoglycans of human cementum. J Periodontol. 1988;23:13-7.
5. Beck F, Tucci J, Russell A, et al. The expression of the gene coding for parathyroid hormone-related protein (PTHrP) during tooth development in the rat. Cell Tissue Res. 1995;280(2):283-90.
6. Berkovitz BKB, Holland GR, Moxham BJ. Oral anatomy, histology and embryology, 4th edition. US: Elsevier; 2009.
7. Bosshardt DD, Schroeder HE. Cementogenesis reviewed: a comparison between human premolars and rodent molars. The Anatomical Record. 1998;245(2):267-92.

8. Bosshardt DD, Schroeder HE. Initial formation of cellular intrinsic fiber cementum in developing human teeth. A light- and electron- microscopic study. Cell Tissue Res. 1992;267: 321-35.
9. Bosshardt DD, Schroeder HE. Initiation of acellular extrinsic fiber cementum on human teeth: A light- and electron- microscopic study. Cell Tissue Res. 1991;263:311-24.
10. Bosshardt DD, Selvig KA. Dental cementum: the dynamic tissue covering of the root. Periodontol 2000. 2007;13(1):41-75.
11. Carlson BM. Human embryology and developmental biology, 5th edition. Philadelphia: W.B. Saunders; 2014.
12. Catón J, Tucker AS. Current knowledge of tooth development: patterning and mineralization of the murine dentition. J Anat. 2009;214(4):502-15.
13. Chatterjee K. Essentials of dental anatomy and oral histology, 2nd edition. India: Jaypee Brothers Medical Publishers (P) Ltd; 2014.
14. Davidovich Z (Ed). The biological mechanisms of tooth eruption and root resorption. Birmingham: EBSCO Information Services; 1988.
15. Denton GB. The discovery of cementum. J Dent Res. 1939;18:239.
16. Fiorellini JP, Kao DWK, Kim DM, et al. Anatomy of the Periodontium. Carranza's Clinical Periodontology. US: Saunders; 2012. pp. 12-27.
17. Foster BL, Ao M, Willoughby C, et al. Mineralization defects in cementum and craniofacial bone from loss of bone sialoprotein. Bone. 2015;78:150-64.
18. Foster BL, Nagatomo KJ, Bamashmous SO, et al. The progressive ankylosis protein regulates cementum apposition and extracellular matrix composition. Cells Tissues Organs. 2011;194(5):382-405.
19. Foster BL. Methods for studying tooth root cementum by light microscopy. Int J Oral Sci. 2012;4(3):119-28.
20. Gaunt WA, Osborn JW, Ten Cate AR. Advanced dental histology, 2nd edition. Bristol: John Wright & Sons Ltd; 1971.
21. Harris EF. Odontogenesis: a companion to dental anthropology. US: John Wiley & Sons, Inc; 2016.
22. Hillson S. Development, function, and evolution of teeth (review). Human Biol. 2001;73:903-4.
23. Ho SP, Balooch M, Goodism ME, et al. Ultrastructure and nanomechanical properties of cementum dentin junction. J Biomed Mater Res. 2006;68a:343-51.
24. Ho SP, Sulyanto RM, Marshall SJ, et al. The cementum–dentin junction also contains glycosaminoglycans and collagen fibrils. J Struct Biol. 2005;151(1):69-78.
25. Hurng JP, Kurylo MP, Marshall GW, et al. Discontinuities in the human bone–PDL–cementum complex. Biomaterials. 2011;32(29):7106-17.
26. Jang AT, Lin JD, Choi RM, et al. Adaptive properties of human cementum and cementum dentin junction with age. J Mech Behav Biomed Mater. 2014;39:184-96.
27. Kallenbach E, Piesco NP. The changing morphology of the epithelium-mesenchyme interface in the differentiation of growing teeth of selected vertebrates and its relationship to possible mechanisms of differentiation. J Biol Buccale. 1978;6:229-40.
28. Khurana A, Khurana I. Human embryology, 2nd edition. India: CBS Publishers and Distributor Pvt Ltd; 2012.
29. Kumar GS. Orban's oral histology and embryology, 14th edition. India: Elsevier; 2015.
30. Lisi S, Peterková R, Peterka M, et al. Tooth morphogenesis and pattern of odontoblast differentiation. Connect Tissue Res. 2003;44(1):167-70.
31. Mckee MD, Zalzal S, Nanci A. Extracellular matrix in tooth cementum and mantle dentin: localization of osteopontin and other noncollagenous proteins, plasma proteins, and glycoconjugates by electron microscopy. Anat Rec. 1996;245(2):293-312.
32. Mitsiadis TA, Graf D. Cell fate determination during tooth development and regeneration. Birth Defects Res C Embryo Today. 2009;87:199.
33. Mitsiadis TA, Smith MM. How do genes make teeth to order through development? J Exp Zool B Mol Dev Evol. 2006;306(3):177-82.
34. Mjör IA, Fejerskov O. Histology of the human tooth, 2nd edition. Copenhagen: Munksgaard; 1979.
35. Monnouchi S, Maeda H, Yuda A, et al. Mechanical induction of interleukin-11 regulates osteoblastic/cementoblastic differentiation of human periodontal ligament stem/progenitor cells. J Periodontal Res. 2014;50(2):231-9.
36. Nanci A. Ten Cate's oral histology, development, structure, and functions, 8th edition. India: Elsevier; 2012.
37. Olson SH, Arzate H, Narayanan AS, et al. Cell attachment activity of cementum proteins and mechanism of endotoxin inhibition. J Dent Res. 1991;70:1272-7.
38. Rajkumar K, Ramya R. Textbook of oral anatomy, histology, physiology and tooth morphology, 2nd edition. India: Wolters Kluwer Health; 2017.
39. Ren LM, Wang WX, Takao Y, et al. Effects of cementum–dentine junction and cementum on the mechanical response of tooth supporting structure. J Dent. 2010;38(11):882-91.
40. Schoenwolf GC, Bleyl S, Brauer P. Larsen's human embryology, 5th edition. US: Elsevier; 2015.
41. Schroeder HE. Biological problems of regenerative cementogenesis: synthesis and attachment of collagenous matrices on growing and established root surfaces. Int Rev Cytol. 1992;142:1-59.
42. Trainor PA. Neural crest cells. US: Academic Press; 2014.
43. Villegas-mercado CE, Agredano-moreno IT, Bermúdez M, et al. Cementum protein 1 transfection does not lead to ultrastructural changes in nucleolar organization of human gingival fibroblasts. J Periodontal Res. 2018.
44. Yamamoto T, Domon T, Takahashi S, et al. The regulation of fiber arrangement in advanced cellular cementogenesis of human teeth. J Periodontal Res. 2010;33(2):83-90.
45. Yamamoto T, Hasegawa T, Yamamoto T, et al. Histology of human cementum: its structure, function, and development. Jpn Dent Sci Rev. 2019;52(3):63-74.
46. Yamamoto T, Wakita M. The development and structure of principal fibers and cellular cementum in rat molars. J Periodontal Res. 1991;26(3):129-37.
47. Yang B, Sun H, Song F, et al. Yes-associated protein 1 promotes the differentiation and mineralization of cementoblast. J Cell Physiol. 2017;233(3):2213-24.
48. Yoo YJ, Yang JY. Understanding of cementum formation by the Wnt/β-Catenin signaling. J Dent Hyg Sci. 2016;16(6):401-8.

CHAPTER

Periodontal Ligament

Anil Sukumaran, B Sivapathasundharam

CHAPTER OUTLINE

- Development of Periodontium   114
  - » Development of the Cells of the Periodontal Ligament   114
  - » Collagen Fiber Formation within the Periodontal Ligament   114
- Structure of Periodontium   116
  - » Cellular Composition   116
  - » Formative Cells   116
  - » Resorptive Cells   117
  - » Progenitor Cells   118
  - » Defense Cells   118
- Periodontal Fibers   118
  - » Principal Fibers   119
  - » Secondary Fiber System   120
  - » Sharpey's Fibers   121
- Interstitial Tissue   121
  - » Blood Vessels   121
  - » Innervation   121
- Ground Substance   122
- Functions of the Periodontal Ligament   122
  - » Physical Function—Supportive   122
  - » Formative and Remodeling Function   122
  - » Nutritive and Sensory Function   122
  - » Regenerative   122
  - » Eruptive   122
- Age Changes   122
- Clinical Considerations   123

INTRODUCTION

The periodontium consists of tissues that surround and anchor the tooth in the maxillary and mandibular alveolar process. These tissues include the gingiva and gingival attachment to the tooth, cementum, periodontal ligament (PDL), and alveolar bone **(Figure 9-1)**. It is derived from the dental follicle, which originates from the mesenchyme influenced by the migrated neural crest cells.

Fibers of the PDL are inserted into the cementum on the tooth side and alveolar bone on the other side. At the alveolar crest, its fibers are continuous with the connective tissue of the gingiva. The PDL thus provides the principal anchoring mechanism of the tooth to the alveolar bone. Along with the two hard tissue components, *i.e.*, cementum of the tooth and the alveolar process, it forms a functional unit and acts like a joint referred to as *syndesmosis*. The width of PDL ranges from 0.1 to 0.4 mm and is generally narrowest at the midpoint of the root. The PDL also has a blood supply to provide nutrients to the surface and the alveolar bone; cells for repair and remodeling the cementum, periodontal ligament, and alveolar bone, and a sensory nerve network to provide tactile information on the position of the tooth (proprioception). Thus, the PDL and associated structures have supportive, nutritive, regenerative, and sensory functions.

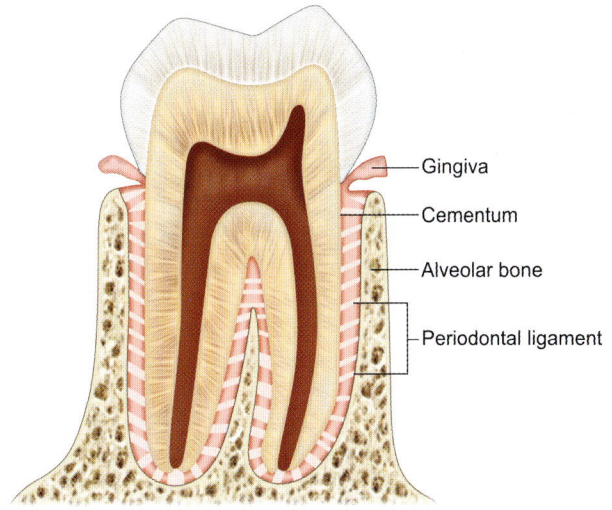

Figure 9-1: Tissues of periodontium.

DEVELOPMENT OF PERIODONTIUM

Development of PDL is a highly organized event. During tooth development, the dental papilla differentiates into odontoblasts, which form dentin and the pulp, while the dental sac or follicle gives rise to cementum, PDL, and alveolar bone. The dental sac is formed by the condensation of the ectomesenchymal tissue—its cells differentiate into cementoblasts, fibroblasts, and osteoblasts. The dental sac comprises of cells and fibers. Anatomically, the dental sac or follicle consists of the dental follicle proper and the perifollicular mesenchyme, which partly surround the tooth bud. A poorly populated zone of loose connective tissue separates these layers. The dental follicle proper remains attached to the tooth bud, while the perifollicular mesenchyme remains associated to the bony trabeculae.

The development of the PDL begins prior to tooth eruption and develops together with the root formation. At the bell stage of tooth development, the proliferation of the inner and outer enamel epithelium forms the cervical loop of the tooth bud. This sheath of epithelial cells, known as Hertwig's epithelial root sheath, grows apically between the dental papilla and the dental sac and is separated from them by basement membrane. The sheath encircles the dental papilla and separates it externally from dental sac cells.

During the development of PDL, the timing and the order of events occurring varies between deciduous and permanent teeth and also between tooth families. At the beginning of the PDL formation, the space between the alveolar bone and the cementum consists of haphazardly arranged short fiber bundle extending from the cemental surface to the surrounding bone. This is followed by the synthesis of collagen fibers, predominantly type I collagen fibers, which arrange themselves as collagen bundles from the cemental surface to the bone and secure the anchoring of the tooth to the bone. This initial attachment is modified later by the eruptive tooth movement. When the teeth are completely erupted and make the occlusal contact, the ligament fibers take on their final arrangement.

Development of the Cells of the Periodontal Ligament (Figures 9-2A and B)

The dental follicle cells, located between the alveolar bone and the epithelial root sheath, are composed of two subpopulations with distinct morphological characteristics and locations; mesenchymal cells of the dental follicle proper and the perifollicular mesenchyme. The perifollicular mesenchymal cells, probably the undifferentiated fibroblasts, contain little cytoplasm, minimal amount of rough endoplasmic reticulum, mitochondria, free ribosomes, and inactive Golgi bodies. Intercellular spaces between these cells are wide; nevertheless they are connected to one another by means of long thin cytoplasmic processes.

With the onset of root formation, these cells gain the cytoplasmic organelles essential for the protein synthesis. The intercellular space is filled with the secretion consisting of collagen fibers and ground substance. During root and PDL formation, there is remarkable increase in the cells, which

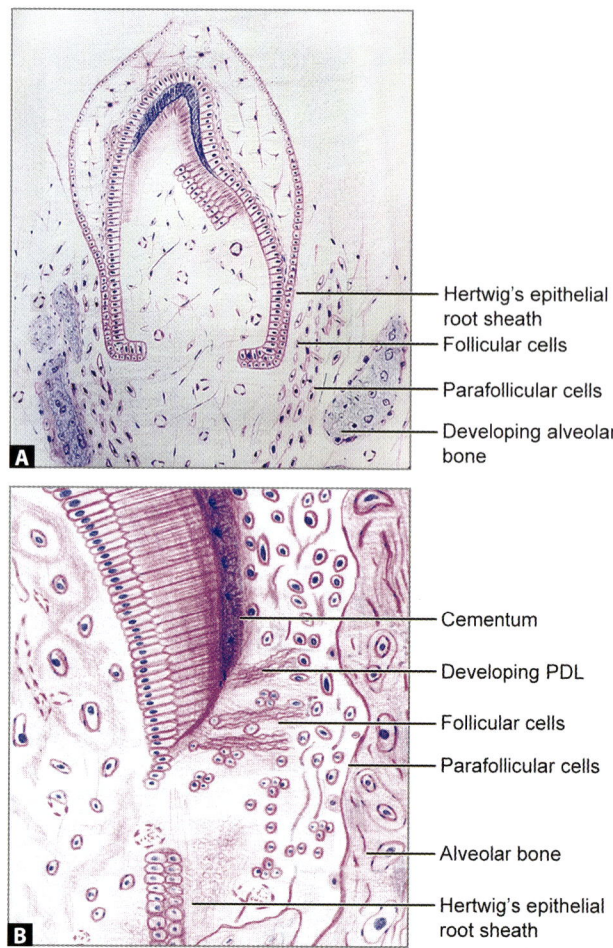

Figures 9-2A and B: Development of cells of the periodontal ligament: (A) Hertwig's epithelial root sheath; (B) Follicular and perifollicular cells.

form the connective tissue. The probable source could be the stem cells, which are lying perivascularly in this region. Osteoclasts also appear at the surface of the alveolar bone, as bone remodeling should occur during the eruption.

The developing periodontal ligament, as well as the mature periodontal ligament, contains undifferentiated stem cells that retain the potential to differentiate into osteoblasts, cementoblasts, and fibroblasts. There are structural differences between the fibroblasts of the developing periodontal ligament of the erupting tooth and the periodontal ligament of the erupted tooth.

Collagen Fiber Formation within the Periodontal Ligament

Initially, the collagen fibers become embedded in the cementum and are laid down coronally within the PDL region. The initial orientation is nearly parallel to the root surface. The fibers that are deposited apical to the cementoenamel junction form the ligament. Fibers insert themselves within the cementum matrix from the cementoenamel junction and proceed coronally after one-third of root is formed. This process closely follows the outline of the newly forming root. At this stage, none of the collagen fibers are inserted into the alveolar bone.

Collagen fiber formation differs for the deciduous teeth and permanent molars (without predecessors) and the permanent incisors, canine, and premolars. In teeth without predecessors, the alveolar bone appears before the beginning of the tooth eruption. The borders of the alveolar bone are located far occlusally than the developing tooth root, since the tooth germ lies deep within the bony compartment. The forming collagen fibers are attached to the wall of the alveolar bone on one end and on the other end, they are embedded in the newly formed cementum. As a result, initially the fiber bundles are obliquely or almost parallelly oriented to the forming tooth. This obliquity changes during tooth eruption.

The first group of fibers to be formed is the dentogingival and the transseptal fibers of the gingival fiber group. As far as the principal fibers of the periodontal ligament are concerned, the first formed fiber group is the alveolar crest group, followed by horizontal group and oblique group and finally the apical fibers.

Preeruptively all the periodontal fiber groups run in an occlusoapical direction, from the alveolar bone to the cementum. As the tooth erupts they get reoriented gradually, as a result of coronal displacement of the fiber, which end at the cementum. Thus, the orientation of the fiber bundles of the PDL depends on the stage of tooth eruption **(Figure 9-3)**.

The development of PDL occurs later for the teeth with deciduous predecessors. Majority of the fibers that run from the alveolar bone to the cementum are not formed until during or after completion of tooth eruption. After the crown has entered into the oral cavity, the transseptal fibers of the gingiva and the cementoalveolar fibers of the PDL are formed. As the tooth is nearing the occlusal plane, the coronal half of the cementoalveolar fibers are formed. The apical fibers are formed once the tooth reaches the functional occlusion.

Maturation begins from the cementoenamel junction and proceeds apically. This involves reorientation of fiber bundles perpendicularly to the tooth and alveolar bone surface and forming Sharpey's fibers in bone and cementum. Remodeling of periodontal ligament fibers proceeds from mineralized surfaces toward the central part of the ligament, which is the last to be remodeled **(Figure 9-4)**.

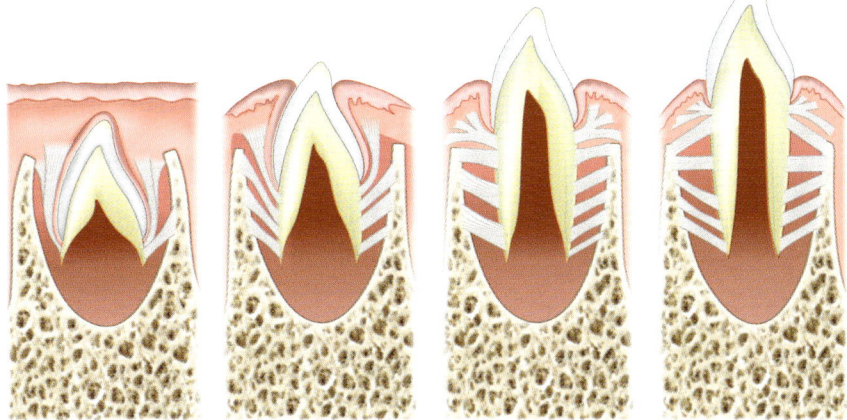

Figure 9-3: Formation of principal fiber groups of the periodontal ligament.

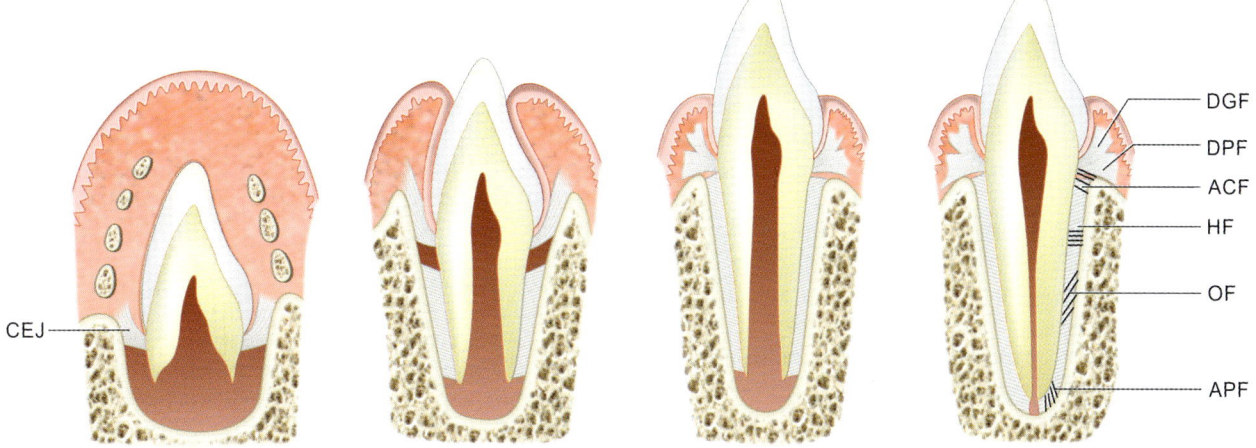

Figure 9-4: Remodeling of periodontal ligament fibers.
(CEJ: Cementoenamel junction; DGF: Dentogingival fibers; DPF: Dentoperiosteal fibers; ACF: Alveolar-crest fibers; HF: Horizontal fibers; OF: Oblique fibers; APF: Apical fibers)

STRUCTURE OF PERIODONTIUM

The PDL is a soft connective tissue that covers the root of the tooth and attaches it to the bone of the tooth socket. Similar to the other connective tissues, PDL is also composed of cells and extracellular substance. The major portion of the extracellular component is formed by the dense fibrous connective tissue in the background of the ground substance. These fibers are predominantly collagen fibers with minor volume of oxytalan fibers and reticulin fibers. The fibers of the PDL are attached on one side to the root cementum and on the other side to the alveolar bone of the tooth socket. The PDL not only connects the tooth to the alveolar process but also supports the tooth in the socket and absorbs mechanical loads placed on the tooth, thus protecting the tooth in its socket.

Cellular Composition

The healthy PDL contains several cell populations comprising of fibroblasts, bone-associated cells (osteoblasts and osteoclasts), cementoblasts, endothelial cells, epithelial cell rests of Malassez, defense cells, and cells associated with the sensory system. These cells help to maintain the integrity of periodontal ligament, cementum and alveolar bone.

Cells of periodontal ligament are categorized as:
- *Synthetic or formative cells*:
  - Fibroblasts
  - Osteoblasts
  - Cementoblasts
- *Resorptive cells*:
  - Osteoclasts
  - Cementoclasts
  - Fibroblasts
- *Progenitor cells*
- *Other cells*:
  - Epithelial cell rests of Malassez
  - Defense cells:
    - Mast cells
    - Macrophages
    - Eosinophils

Formative Cells

These cells are actively involved in the formation or renewal of periodontal tissue components namely—PDL, cementum, and alveolar bone. Any actively synthesizing cell will have the following features:
- *Large amount of cytoplasm*—to accommodate more synthetic organelle.
- *Large vesicular nucleus*—to produce more ribosome for RNA transcription.
- *More number of mitochondria*—to supply adequate energy for the synthetic activity.
- *Increased rough endoplasmic reticulum*—to synthesize the specific protein actively.
- *Golgi apparatus*—to modify the protein secreted.
- *Membrane bound vesicles*—actually contain the packed secretory product.

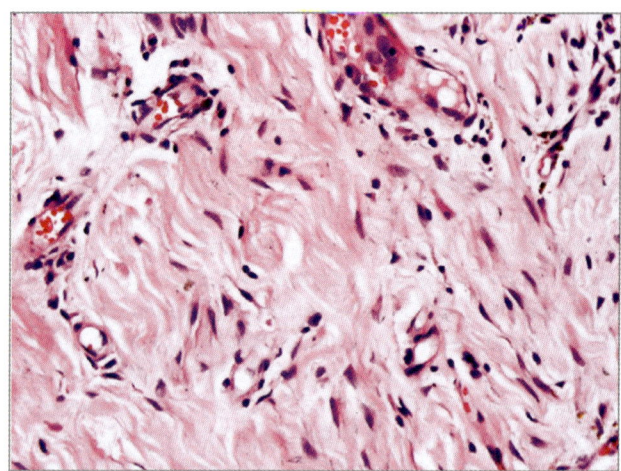

Figure 9-5: Fibroblasts.

All these features are present in the formative cells of the PDL, which include fibroblasts, cementoblasts, and osteoblasts.

Fibroblasts

They are the predominant cell type present in the PDL and form about 25–30% of the cells present in the PDL **(Figure 9-5)**. Fibroblasts of the periodontal ligament are not very similar to the fibroblasts of other connective tissue. Developmentally fibroblasts near the cemental surface are derived from the ectomesenchymal cells of the investing layer of the dental papilla, whereas those near the alveolar bone are from the perivascular mesenchyme. PDL fibroblasts are responsible for the formation and remodeling of the PDL fibers and metabolism of extracellular matrix component. The collagen turnover rate in the PDL is much more than any other connective tissue due to the fibroblast phagocytosis and collagenase secretion.

They presumably have a signaling system to maintain PDL width and thickness. PDL contains a variety of fibroblast subpopulations with different functional characteristics. A subpopulation of osteoblast-like fibroblasts, rich in alkaline phosphatase, has been identified in the PDL. These cells have the capacity to give rise to bone cells and cementoblasts. They are also responsible for the production of acellular extrinsic fiber cementum in the mature PDL.

Fibroblasts of the PDL are evenly distributed with their long axis parallel to the course of the collagen fibers. They are attached to the neighboring fibroblasts by means of adhering junction and gap junction, and to the fibers by means of *fibronexus*.

> Fibronexus is a cell surface specialization made up of intracellular actin filaments and extracellular fibronectin filaments. Fibronectins are an important class of matrix glycoproteins, whose primary role is to attach the cells to a variety of extracellular matrices. They are cell adhesive proteins and possess specific high-affinity binding sites for cell-surface receptors, collagen, fibrin, and sulfated proteoglycans.

They are stellate or spindle-shaped cells containing a prominent nucleus, which has single distinct nucleolus, and clearly defined nuclear pores. They also have cilia oriented in front of the nucleus. Fibroblasts play a major role in the development, maintenance, and repair of PDL and gingival connective tissue. Cilia coordinate a series of signaling pathways critical to fibroblast migration during development and in repair. Further, PDL fibroblasts are contractile and motile and generate forces for eruption of the tooth. Fibroblasts synthesize collagen, reticulin, oxytalan, and elastic fibers as well as the glycoproteins and glycosaminoglycans of the amorphous extracellular matrix. They also produce growth factors and cytokines such as platelet-derived growth factor (PDGF), bone morphogenetic protein (BMP), insulin-like growth factor 1 (IGF-1), and interleukin-1 (IL-1).

Periodontal ligament fibroblasts are phenotypically different from gingival fibroblasts. They consist of subtypes with distinct phenotypes and synthesize higher quantities of chondroitin sulfate and lesser quantities of heparan sulfate and hyaluronan sulfate. Cyclic adenosine monophosphate (cAMP) and alkaline phosphatase expression is more in PDL fibroblasts than in the gingival fibroblasts. Developmentally gingival fibroblasts are from the mesoderm and periodontal fibroblasts are from ectomesenchyme.

Osteoblasts

These cells within the PDL are found on the surface of the alveolar bone. The osteoblasts in active state form a layer of cuboidal cells, which exhibit strong basophilic cytoplasm **(Figure 9-6)**. A prominent nucleus lies towards the basal end of the cell and a pale juxtanuclear area indicates the site of Golgi complex. Similar to fibroblasts, they are seen to contain a prominent rough endoplasmic reticulum and numerous mitochondria and vesicles. The Golgi complex however appears more localized and extensive than in the fibroblast. They maintain contact with the adjacent osteoblasts by means of desmosomes and tight junctions.

Periodontal ligament was earlier referred to as *pericementum* or dental periosteum since the osteoblastic layer was akin to the cellular layer or the cambium layer of the periosteum and the periodontal ligament was considered as the fibrous layer of the periosteum.

Cementoblasts

These cells are responsible for secreting the organic matrix of cementum. They appear as a distinct layer of cells, similar to osteoblastic layer of the bone, but as an interrupted layer on the root surface **(Figure 9-7)**. They exhibit desmosomes and gap junctions. Cementoblasts secreting cellular cementum have cytoplasmic processes and those depositing acellular cementum do not have prominent cementocytic processes. Synthetically active cementoblasts appear basophilic due to the presence of abundant rough endoplasmic reticulum.

Resorptive Cells

Osteoclasts

These are large multinucleated cells that resorb the bone. The precursor cells of the osteoclasts are circulating monocytes. The osteoclasts have a ruffled border and are located adjacent to the resorbing surface **(Figure 9-8)**. Osteoclasts are characterized by expression of tartrate resistant acid phosphatase (TRAP), specified osteoprotegerin (OPG), cathepsin K, and chloride channel 7 (ClCN7). Along with the osteoblasts and cementoblasts, they maintain the homeostasis of the PDL.

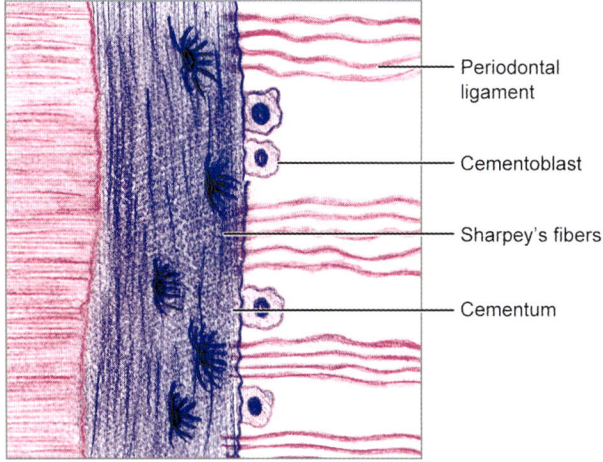

Figure 9-7: Cementoblasts.

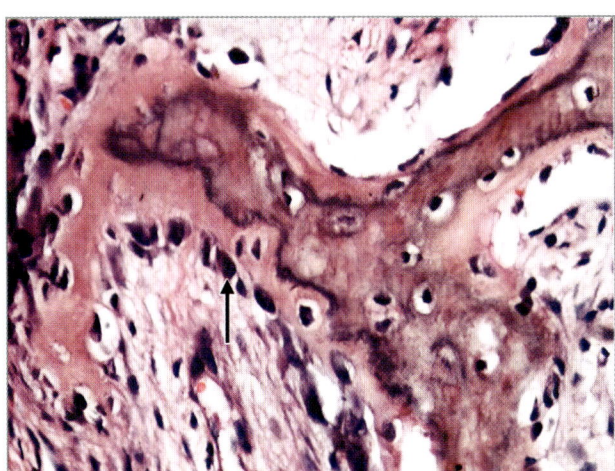

Figure 9-6: Osteoblasts.

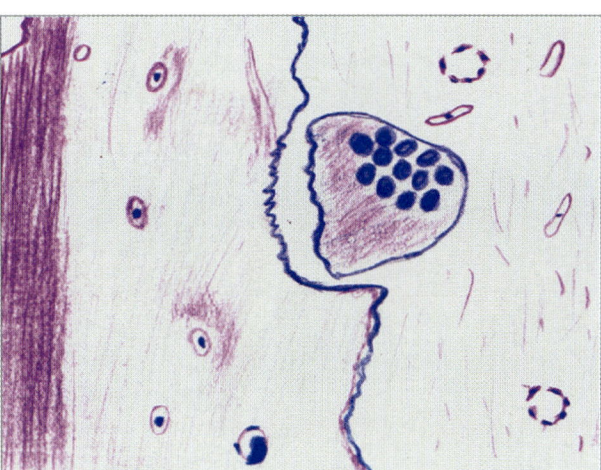

Figure 9-8: Multinucleated osteoclast in resorption bay.

Osteoblasts synthesize receptor activator of nuclear factor kappa-B ligand (RANKL), which regulates the formation of multinucleated osteoclasts from their precursors as well as their activation and survival in normal bone. This suggests that osteoblasts control osteoclast differentiation, but not function. OPG prevents excessive bone resorption by binding to RANKL and preventing it from binding to its receptor RANK on the osteoclast.

Progenitor Cells

Stem Cells in the Periodontal Ligament

Experimental studies have shown that a population of progenitor cells with the potential to differentiate into several distinct mesenchymal cell types can be isolated from the PDL. Periodontal ligament stem cells can differentiate into cells that form bone, cementum, cartilage, fat, muscle, neuron and glial-like cells. Periodontal ligament stem cells on hydroxyapatite or tricalcium phosphate scaffolds implanted into periodontal defects in experimental animals or the alveolus after tooth extraction form cementum and PDL. Thus, there is considerable interest in the therapeutic potential of these stem cells for treatment of periodontal defects.

Epithelial Cell Rests of Malassez

These cells originate from the degeneration of Hertwig's epithelial root sheath to form quiescent cell rests that persist as the sole epithelial cells in the periodontium. As soon as the radicular dentin is formed the continuity of the Hertwig's epithelial sheath breaks down. The remnants of the root sheath persist as epithelial cell rests. They are seen as a network, strands, islands or tubule-like structures in the PDL, near and parallel to the surface of the root. Some of them may be incorporated into the cementum. These cells are responsible for maintaining the constant width of the PDL and their additional role is in the regeneration of periodontal tissues **(Figure 9-9)**. They become reduced in volume as age advances. Their clinical significance is origin of odontogenic cysts or tumors from them.

Defense Cells

Mast cells are derived from the myeloid stem cell that is a part of the immune system. They are round or oval in outline with a diameter of about 12–15 μm. The cells contain numerous basophilic granules in their cytoplasm, which usually obscure the small and round nucleus. Apart from their role in allergy and anaphylaxis, mast cells play an important role in healing, angiogenesis, immune tolerance, and defense against pathogens. The basophilic cytoplasmic granules have been shown to contain heparin and histamine. The physiologic role of heparin in mast cells does not appear to be clear, whereas mast cell histamine plays a role in the inflammatory reaction and they degranulate in response to antigen–antibody reaction on their surface **(Figure 9-10A)**.

Macrophages present in the PDL are located adjacent to the blood vessels and are responsible for phagocytosis. They also secrete growth factors that regulate fibroblasts.

Eosinophils **(Figure 9-10B)** and *adipose cells*, although scarce, are also present in the lamina propria of the gingiva. Normal gingiva contains small foci of plasma cells. Lymphocytes are found in the connective tissue near the base of the sulcus. Neutrophils can be seen in relatively high numbers in both the gingival connective tissue and the sulcus. These inflammatory cells are usually present in small amounts in clinically normal gingiva.

PERIODONTAL FIBERS

The collagen fibers of the periodontium collect to form bundles with a diameter of about 5 μm. The collagen fibril diameters of the human PDL are relatively small when

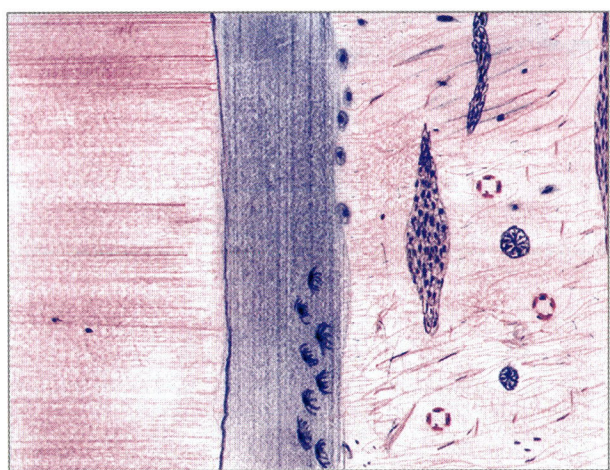

Figure 9-9: Epithelial rests of Malassez present in the form of nests in the periodontal ligament.

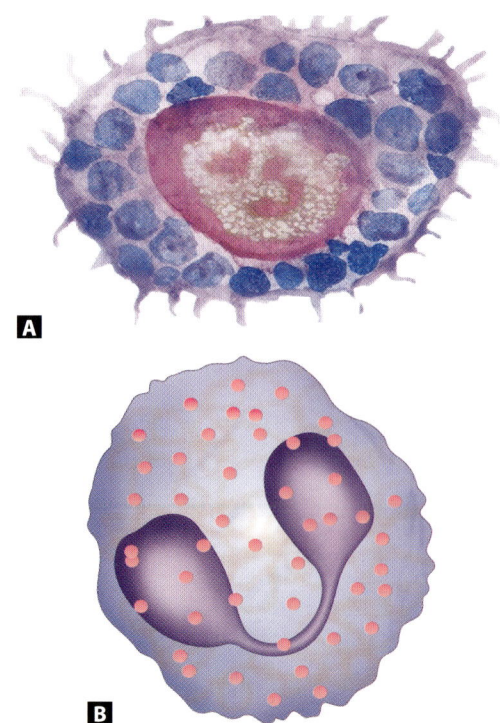

Figures 9-10A and B: (A) Mast cell with granules in the cytoplasm; (B) Eosinophils with bilobed nucleus and eosinophilic granules in the cytoplasm.

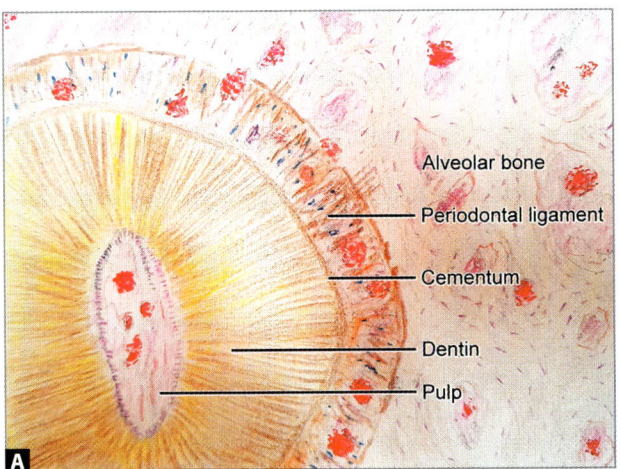 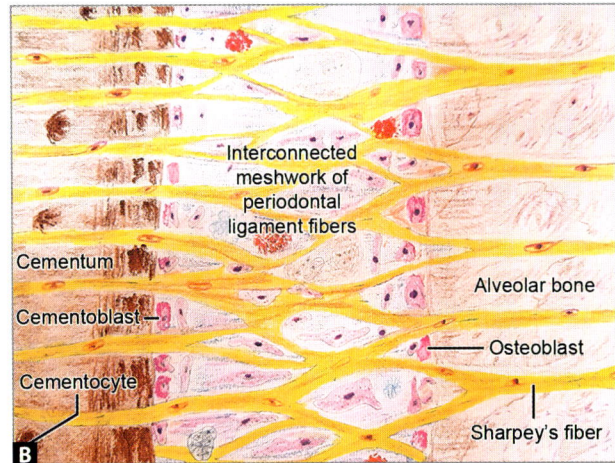

Figures 9-11A and B: (A) Cross-section of root in the alveolar bone showing periodontal ligament fibers connecting cementum and bone; (B) Periodontal ligament formed by the interconnected meshwork of collagen fibers.

compared to the collagen fibers of the other connective tissue and this may be attributed to high collagen turnover rate or the absence of mature collagen fibrils. Fibers of the periodontium are broadly divided into two, namely— gingival fibers, which are present in the lamina propria of the gingiva and surround the neck of the teeth and the PDL fibers, which surround the teeth and attach the teeth to the alveolar bone proper.

The most important fibers of the PDL are the principal fibers. These fibers are collagenous in nature and are arranged in bundles **(Figure 9-11A)**. They are usually wavy in nature to permit tooth movement. The terminal or the embedded portion of the principal fibers that insert into the cementum and bone are termed Sharpey's fibers. The principal fibers are composed primarily of type I collagen, whereas reticular fibers are made up of type III collagen. These fibers are wider on the bone end than on the cemental end. From their origin they branch into smaller fibers, which join with adjacent fibers to create an interconnected fibrous meshwork **(Figure 9-11B)**. So, the periodontal fibers may not be continuous from the cementum to the bone but form an interconnected fibrous meshwork.

Collagen V is also seen located in the interstitial spaces between the bundles or in between type I and III fibrils. Other minor collagens involved in the fibrous meshwork of the periodontal ligament are type IV, V, VI, and XII collagen, which are important to maintain the normal architecture of the PDL and play a role in regeneration of ligament during remodeling, which occurs during tooth movement.

Principal Fibers

Principal fibers of periodontal ligament have been categorized into five groups based on their anatomic location and develop sequentially in the developing root **(Figure 9-12A)**:
- Alveolar crest fibers **(Figure 9-12B)**
- Horizontal fibers **(Figure 9-12C)**
- Oblique fibers **(Figure 9-12D)**
- Periapical fibers
- Interradicular fibers

Alveolar crest fibers extend from the crest of the alveolar bone obliquely, attaching to the cementum immediately below the dentogingival junction at a position more coronal than their attachment to the bone. These fibers are attached to the fibrous layer of the periosteum of the alveolar crest. They resist forces of tilt, extrusion, intrusion, rotation, and lateral movement of the tooth.

Horizontal fibers are located just below the alveolar crest fibers and extend in a more or less horizontal direction from the alveolar bone to the cementum and resist horizontal and tipping forces. They are parallel to the occlusal plane and are normally limited to the coronal one fourth of the PDL space.

Oblique fibers extend in an oblique direction from the bone coronally and cementum apically. They are the largest group in the PDL. They bear the large part of the vertical and intrusive masticatory force and transmit it as tension to the alveolar bone.

Apical fibers are arranged radially around the apical ends of the roots. They originate from cementum of root apex, splaying apically and laterally at the fundus of the alveolar socket. They are seen only in fully formed roots and protect the vessels and nerves at the apical portion of the root. These fibers prevent tipping forces and luxation.

Interradicular fibers are seen only in multirooted teeth. They extend radially from the crest of the alveolar bone between the roots of multirooted teeth (interradicular septum) to the cementum in the furcation area of the tooth. They resist forces of tipping and torque and prevent luxation.

Although not strictly part of the PDL, there are other distinct groups of fibers that help to maintain the functional integrity of the periodontium. These groups are found in the lamina propria of the gingiva and collectively form the gingival ligament or fibers. Five groups of gingival fiber bundles exist, which include dentogingival, alveologingival, transseptal, circular, and dentoperiosteal fibers.

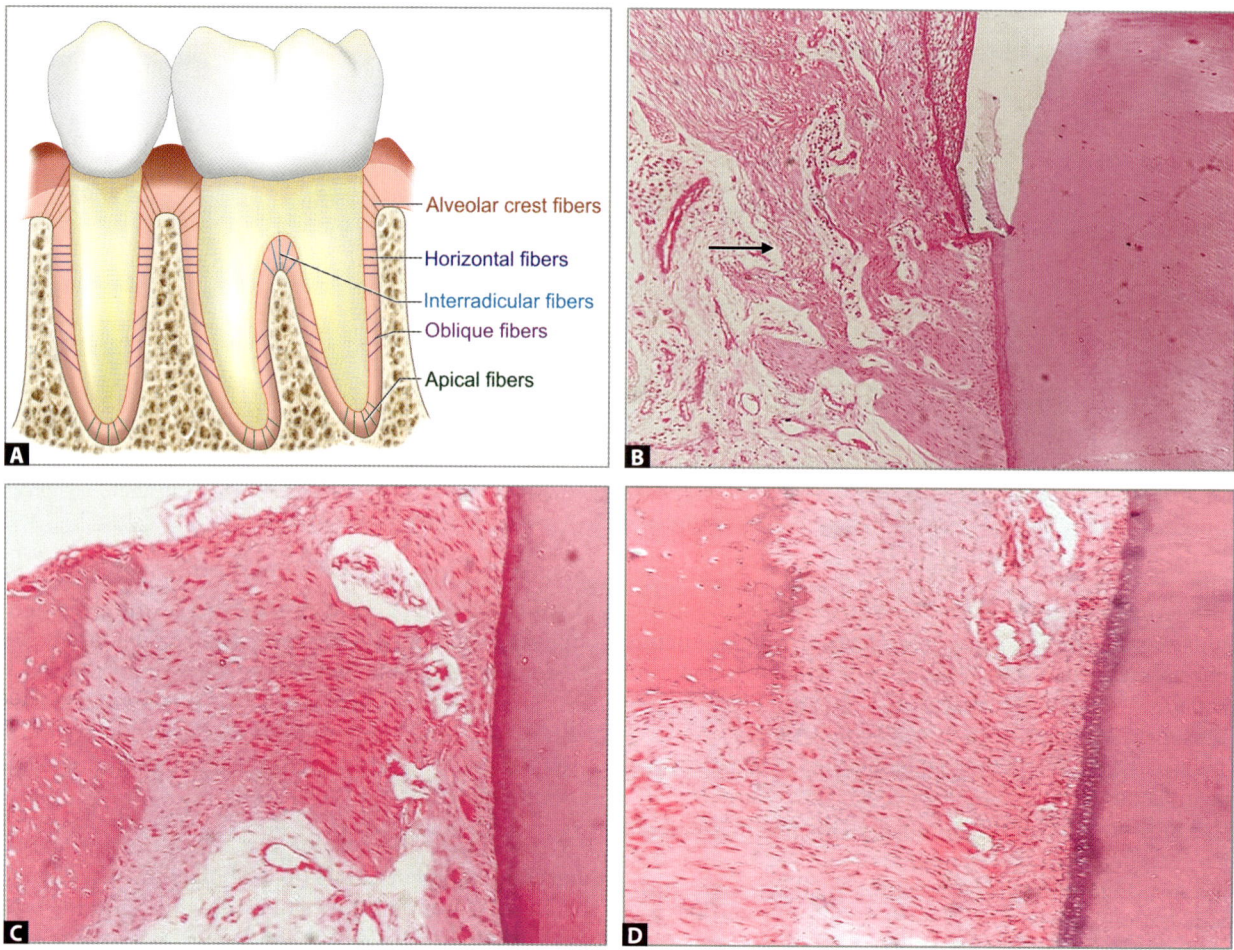

Figures 9-12A to D: (A) Principal fibers of periodontal ligament; (B) Alveolar crest group; (C) Horizontal group; (D) Oblique group.
Source: Dr N Malathi, Department of Oral Pathology, Sri Ramachandra Dental College, Chennai, Tamil Nadu, India.

Dentogingival fibers: These are the most numerous fibers, extending from cervical cementum to lamina propria of the free and attached gingiva.

Alveologingival fibers: These fibers extend from the crest of the alveolar bone into the lamina propria of the free and attached gingiva.

Transseptal fibers: They extend across the crest of the alveolar bone from the cementum of one tooth to the cementum of the adjacent tooth.

Circular fibers: Encircle the neck of the tooth, intermingling with the other fibers in this region and helping to hold the free gingiva against the tooth.

Dentoperiosteal fibers: Running apically from the cementum over the periosteum of the outer cortical plates of the alveolar process, these fibers insert into the alveolar process or the vestibular muscle and floor of the mouth.

Secondary Fiber System

In addition to the collagen fibers, the PDL also contains secondary fiber system comprised of elastic fibers. Elastic fibers serve to protect and maintain the integrity of the vascular system of the PDL during mastication. Elastic fibers are synthesized by fibroblasts, thinner than collagen fibers, and are arranged in a branching pattern to form a three-dimensional network. They are remarkably resilient and give tissues the ability to withstand stretch and distension. These fibers are interwoven with collagen fibers to limit distensibility and to prevent tearing. Elastic fibers are composed of elastin, an important extracellular matrix protein that provides resilience and elasticity to tissues and fibrillin (glycoprotein associated with microfibrils).

Synthesis of elastic fibers occurs in three stages, namely—oxytalan fibers, which occur only as elastic microfibrils; elaunin fibers, *i.e.*, elastic microfibrils with small quantities of elastin, and fully formed elastic fibers.

Oxytalan fibers are immature elastic fibers, oriented in an apico-occlusal direction. One end of these fibers is attached to the cementum perpendicularly and the other end being attached to the wall of the blood vessels. They form a meshwork that covers the root surface. These fibers can only be demonstrated by special stains. These fibers are smaller in diameter and appear to interface with the collagen fiber bundles, supporting the collagen bundles and the blood vessel walls. They help in fibroblast migration and attachment. These fibers are similar to the microfibrils of elastic fibers and consist predominantly of the protein fibrillin.

Elaunin fibers are immature form of elastic fibers and are made up of bundles of microfibrils intermingled with small amounts of elastin. Presence of elaunin fibers is limited mainly to the apical region of the ligament in close association with blood vessels.

Mature elastic fibers are only seen associated with the walls of the large blood vessels.

Reticulin fibers are immature collagen fibers associated with the basement membrane of the blood vessels. They can be demonstrated with silver stains.

Sharpey's Fibers

> Sharpey's fibers also called as perforating fibers, were first described by William Sharpey in 1867. These are embedded portion of fibers in hard tissue. Apart from forming a part of periodontal tissue, they are also associated with muscle attachment with bones and cranial sutures.

Embedded portions of the PDL fibers on cementum and alveolar bone are called Sharpey's fibers **(Figure 9-13)**. These fibers on the cemental side are more numerous and smaller in diameter than on the bone side. The point of insertion of the PDL fibers in the alveolar bone appears as calcified projections. The inserted portion exhibits mineralization perpendicular to the long axis of the fibers. The Sharpey's fibers in the primary acellular cementum are fully mineralized, but in the cellular cementum and alveolar bone, they are only partially mineralized. The fibers are usually longer on the bone appositional side of the ligament, which is where tension is formed. Sharpey's fibers are associated with high levels of osteopontin and bone sialoprotein. The link between the Sharpey's fibers and the osteopontin and bone sialoprotein permits constant embedding of PDL into the alveolar wall.

> **Intermediate plexus**
> It was believed that the PDL fibers rather being continuous, consisted of two parts, one part arises from cementum and the other from alveolar bone. These two portions are spliced together in midway between the cementum and alveolar bone. This spliced portion was known as *intermediate plexus*. Rearrangement of the fiber ends in the plexus and enables tooth eruption without necessitating the embedding of new fibers into the tooth and the bone.

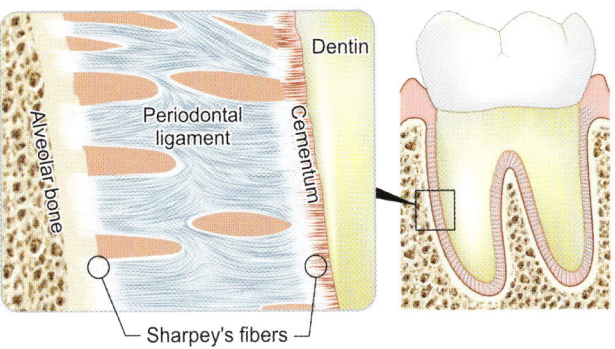

Figure 9-13: Sharpey's fibers.

The concept and existence of intermediate plexus was proposed, way back in 1923, by Sicher. According to him, this intermediate plexus consisted of dental fibers (originating from cementum) spliced to alveolar fibers (originating from alveolar bone) in the middle portion of the periodontal membrane. It was proposed that the membrane adapted to drift, attrition, and rapid growth by an unsplicing and resplicing of the fibers. But existence of such plexus was disproved as early as in 1959 and was attributed to orientation artifact.

Indifferent plexus
These were first described by Shackleford in 1971 as smallest fibers with no specific orientation and course in all directions. They anastomose extensively with the principal fibers and form a continuous fibrous matrix. Anastomoses start adjacent to bone or cementum and increase until the indifferent fiber plexus reaches maximum density a short distance from the mineralized matrix.

Intermediate and indifferent plexuses were proposed and implicated in the maintenance of tooth support while ligament remodeling occurs during tooth movement.

But the existence of these two plexus was contradicted by many workers later, based on their investigations. Accordingly, majority of the collagen fibers of the PDL were organized into well-oriented circular bundles, forming a network.

■ INTERSTITIAL TISSUE

The portion of the periodontium, lying in between these fiber group, called the interstitial tissue, composed of loose connective tissue; containing type V collagen, network of blood vessels, lymph vessels, and nerves that maintain the viability of the PDL. The function of the interstitial tissue relates to the constant stretching and contraction of the fiber bundles during the masticatory process.

Blood Vessels

The vascular supply to the PDL is mainly from inferior and superior alveolar arteries. The rich vascularity of the PDL is attributed to the vessels from the periapical region, those from the alveolar bone, which enter horizontally from the alveolar bone and from the gingival connective tissue, which enter coronally. The arterioles and the capillaries, which enter into the PDL, branch out and ramify profusely and make this tissue richly vascular. Both continuous and fenestrated capillaries are present in the PDL. The vascularity of the periodontal tissue increases from incisors to molars. Blood vessels are located closer to the alveolar bone than to the cementum.

Venous vessels accompany the arterioles and the arterial capillaries. The diameter of the venous channels is relatively bigger. Arteriovenous anastomoses, bypassing the capillary circulation is also present in PDL.

Lymphatic network follows the vascular architecture. They carry the products of metabolism from the cells and extracellular matrix and drain into the regional lymph nodes.

Innervation

Two types of nerve fibers are present in the periodontal ligament, viz autonomic and sensory. Autonomic fibers are associated with the vessels. Autonomic fibers are only sympathetic (vasomotor function) and no parasympathetic nerve fibers are present in the PDL. Sensory fibers are responsible for the perception of pain (nociception) and touch (mechanoreception). Both myelinated and unmyelinated nerve fibers are present in the PDL. Smaller diameter fibers are responsible for pain and large fibers respond to forces applied to the tooth and the supporting structures. They are also responsible for proprioception (ability to perceive the position and movements). Mechanoreceptors responsible for proprioception detect tooth-to-tooth contact during mastication and reflexly control the mandibular movements. They are activated by tooth movements as little as 1–3 microns. Thus, the receptors in the PDL together with the proprioceptors in muscles, tendons, and temporomandibular joint, play a major role in the regulation of masticatory movements and forces.

Nerve fibers enter the PDL from the periapical region and through the alveolar bone along the blood vessels. Both groups together form nerve plexus. Most of them enter as myelinated fibers and gradually lose their myelin sheath to end as free nerve endings, Ruffini-like mechanoreceptors, tactile (Meissner's) corpuscles or spindle-like pressure, and vibration endings. The nerve fibers of the PDL are generally present closer to the alveolar bone.

It is believed that the periodontal sensory innervation may interact with immunocompetent cells to assist their migration to the area of inflammation, *e.g.*, to take part in the remodeling during orthodontic tooth movement.

The nerve fibers of the PDL are from superior and inferior alveolar branches of trigeminal nerve.

GROUND SUBSTANCE

The extracellular part of the PDL consists of fibers and ground substance secreted by the fibroblasts. Ground substance is an amorphous background material that binds tissue and fluids, the latter serving for the diffusion of gases and metabolic substances. The PDL ground substance has been estimated to be 70% water and is thought to have a significant effect on the tooth's ability to withstand loads. There is an increase in tissue fluids within the amorphous matrix of the ground substance in areas of injury and inflammation.

FUNCTIONS OF THE PERIODONTAL LIGAMENT

The functions of the periodontal ligament are categorized as physical, formative and remodeling, nutritive, and sensory.

Functions of periodontal ligament:
- Supportive
- Formative
- Nutritive
- Sensory
- Regenerative

Physical Function—Supportive

The physical functions of the PDL include attachment of tooth to the alveolar bone, absorb the occlusal loads applied to the teeth during function and dissipate them to the bone. It protects the vessels and nerves from injury due to mechanical forces by providing a viscoelastic cushion by virtue of its fibers and hydraulic fluid systems.

The PDL serves supportive function by attaching the tooth to the surrounding alveolar bone proper. By its inherent resilience, PDL serves as a shock-absorber by mechanisms that provide resistance to light as well as heavy forces.

Formative and Remodeling Function

Cells of the PDL participate in the formation and resorption of cementum and bone. Variations in cellular enzyme activity are correlated with the remodeling process. The PDL is constantly undergoing remodeling. Old cells and fibers are broken down and replaced by new ones, and mitotic activity can be observed in the fibroblasts and the endothelial cells.

Nutritive and Sensory Function

The PDL supplies nutrients to the cementum, bone, and gingiva by way of the blood vessels and it also provides lymphatic drainage.

Periodontal ligament is supplied by nerve fibers that can transmit sensation of touch, pressure, and pain to higher centers. The nerve fibers enter the PDL from periapical area through channels from the alveolar bone. By its proprioceptors, it plays an important role in the regulation of occlusal contact and masticatory movements.

Regenerative

The PDL serves the major remodeling function by providing cells that are able to form as well as resorb all the tissues that make up the attachment apparatus, *i.e.*, bone, cementum, and the PDL. Undifferentiated ectomesenchymal cells, located around blood vessels, can differentiate into the specialized cells that form bone (osteoblasts), cementum (cementoblasts), and connective tissue fibers (fibroblasts). Bone and tooth resorbing cells (osteoclasts and odontoclasts) are generally multinucleated cells derived from blood-borne macrophages.

Eruptive

Periodontal ligament also plays an important part in the eruption of teeth and healing. According to one of the theories of tooth eruption, PDL fibroblasts move actively and pull the tooth from its site of development to the occlusal plane.

AGE CHANGES

As age advances, there is reduction in the number and functional activity of periodontal ligament fibroblasts, which include the mitotic activity and synthesis ability. Reduction in the organic matrix production and vascularity and an increase in the number of elastic fibers are noted during aging. Increased arteriosclerotic changes have also been reported in PDL as a result of aging. The width of the PDL is generally reduced due to continuous deposition of cementum and bone.

CLINICAL CONSIDERATIONS

The thickness of the periodontal ligament varies from 0.1 to 0.4 mm with a mean of around 0.2 mm. In the middle portion of the root, the width of the PDL is relatively thin and this portion acts as a fulcrum for the physiologic tooth movement. The ligament is thicker in functioning than in nonfunctioning teeth. Also, it is wider in areas of tension than in areas of compression.

The primary role of PDL is to support the tooth in the bony socket. Its thickness varies in individuals and in different teeth in the same person. The cells of the PDL are capable of remodelling the ligament and adjacent bone when functional forces are altered or the ligament is damaged. The PDL plays a key role in protecting the tooth from being resorbed by the normal remodelling process that occurs in the alveolar bone.

Orthodontic tooth movement depends on the resorption and formation of both bone and PDL. These activities can be stimulated by properly regulated pressure and tension. If the movement of the tooth is within physiological limits, the compression of the periodontal ligament on pressure side results in bone resorption, whereas on the tension side there is bone apposition. Application of the large forces results in the necrosis of PDL and alveolar bone and damage to the cementum. Blood vessels are occluded and the blood supply is cut off when excessive forces are applied, which can cause localized necrosis of the ligament. However, this may be repaired by migration of cells from adjoining vital periodontal ligament. When ligament continuity is not re-established, localized resorption and ankylosis may occur.

Chronic periodontitis is a multifactorial inflammatory disease associated with plaque biofilms and characterized by progressive destruction of the periodontium. Its primary features include the loss of periodontal tissue support, manifested through clinical attachment loss and radiographically assessed alveolar bone loss, presence of periodontal pocketing and gingival bleeding **(Figures 9-14 and 9-15)**. Chronic periodontitis accounts for a substantial proportion of edentulism and masticatory dysfunction and has a plausible negative impact on general health and quality of life.

Stage 4 periodontitis (aggressive periodontitis) is a highly destructive form of periodontitis affecting primarily young individuals, including conditions formerly classified as early-onset periodontitis and rapidly progressing periodontitis.

Periodontal abscess is a localized accumulation of pus located within the gingival wall of the periodontal pocket, resulting in a significant tissue breakdown. The primary detectable signs/symptoms associated with a periodontal abscess may involve ovoid elevation in the gingiva along the lateral part of the root and bleeding on probing **(Figure 9-16)**. Other signs/symptoms that may also be observed include pain, suppuration on probing, deep periodontal pocket, and increased tooth mobility.

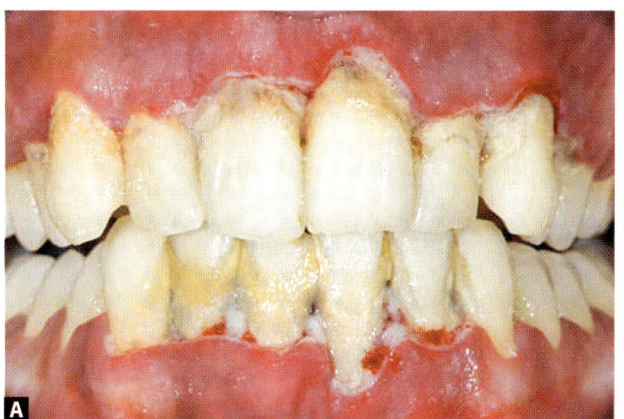
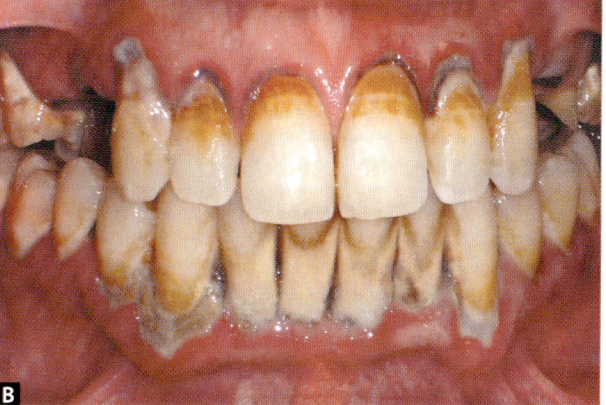

Figures 9-14A and B: Clinical appearance of chronic periodontitis.

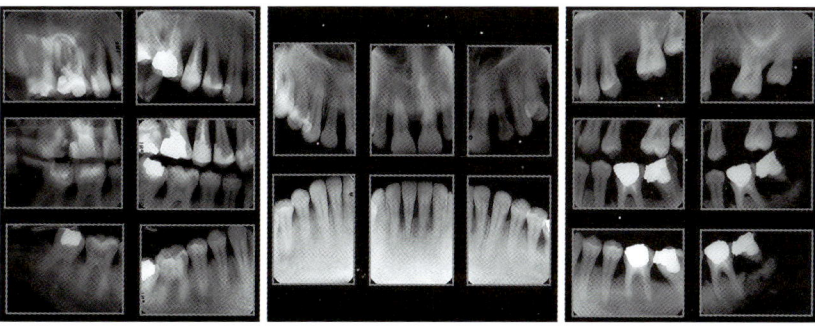

Figure 9-15: Intraoral radiographs showing alveolar bone loss in chronic periodontitis.

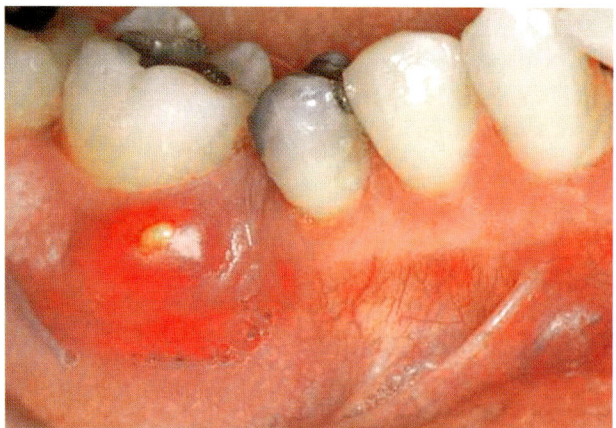

Figure 9-16: Periodontal abscess.

Points to Remember

- The periodontal ligament is a unique connective tissue that attaches tooth to the alveolar bone.
- It supports the tooth in its socket, provides nutrients and sensory perception to the tooth, and maintains cementum and the alveolar bone of the tooth socket.
- It holds a pivotal role in maintenance of mechanical resistance and support of mechanical load exerted by the forces of mastication.
- The PDL cellular constituents include fibroblasts, as well as osteoblasts, osteoclasts and cementoblasts, cementocytes.
- Other cell types present within PDL include epithelial cell rests of Malassez, macrophages, nerve cells, endothelial cells, epithelial cells and mesenchymal progenitor populations.
- The extracellular component is mainly formed of fibrous element, predominantly populated by defined bundles of collagen type I, II and XII fibers.
- The ability of periodontal ligament to remodel and allow for tooth movement is particularly important in maintenance of the periodontium.
- The cementum anchors the periodontal ligament to the tooth and seals the ends of the open dentinal tubules.
- The periodontal ligament, cementum, and alveolar bone act as a functional unit to support and maintain the teeth in the oral cavity.
- The functions of the periodontal ligament include supportive, formative, nutritive, sensory and regenerative.
- Age changes of periodontal ligament include reduction in the number and functional activity of fibroblasts, which include the mitotic activity and synthesis ability, reduction in the organic matrix production and vascularity and an increase in the number of elastic fibers.
- Increased arteriosclerotic changes have also been reported in PDL as a result of aging. The width of the PDL is generally reduced due to continuous deposition of cementum and bone.
- Chronic periodontitis is the common cause for tooth loss.

PRACTICE QUESTIONS

1. Write short notes on periodontal ligament fibers.
2. Write notes on development of periodontal ligament.
3. Enumerate the functions of the periodontal ligament.
4. Write notes on cells of the periodontal ligament.
5. Write notes on principal fibers of periodontal ligament.
6. Write notes on gingival fibers.

MULTIPLE CHOICE QUESTIONS

1. Periodontal fibers which are consistent and reconstructed even after the destruction of the alveolar bone:
   a. Apical fibers
   b. Alveolar crest fibers
   c. Oblique fibers
   d. Transseptal fibers
2. Type III collagen is mainly found in:
   a. Principal fibers
   b. Sharpey's fibers
   c. Reticular fibers
   d. None of the above
3. The following group of fibers is absent in an incompletely formed root:
   a. Oblique group
   b. Horizontal group
   c. Apical group
   d. Alveolar crest group
4. Which of the following is not correct about periodontal ligament?
   a. It is shaped like hourglass
   b. It is narrow at axis of rotation
   c. It is thicker on mesial side of root.
   d. None of the above
5. The function of fibroblast in periodontal ligament include:
   a. Synthesis of collagen
   b. Degradation of collagen
   c. Both (a) and (b)
   d. None of the above

6. **Largest fiber group in periodontal ligament is:**
   a. Transseptal fibers
   b. Oblique fibers
   c. Horizontal fibers
   d. Apical fibers
7. **The width of periodontal ligament is around:**
   a. 0.2 mm
   b. 0.5 mm
   c. 0.75 mm
   d. 6 mm
8. **The thickness of periodontal ligament is maximum in:**
   a. Teeth with light function
   b. Teeth with heavy function
   c. Teeth which are functionless
   d. The third molar teeth
9. **Embedded portion of the fibers of the PDL in both the cementum and alveolar bone are referred to as:**
   a. Oblique fibers
   b. Principal fibers
   c. Transseptal fibers
   d. Sharpey's fibers
10. **Periodontal ligament derives its blood supply from:**
    a. Gingiva
    b. Bone marrow
    c. Both of the above
    d. None of the above
11. **The vascular supply of periodontal ligament is:**
    a. In the form of net-like plexus that runs closer to alveolar bone than to cementum
    b. Greatest in the middle third of the single rooted teeth
    c. In the form of net-like plexus that runs closer to cementum than to alveolar bone
    d. Greatest in the middle third of the multirooted teeth
12. **Which of the following fibers regulate the blood flow of periodontal ligament?**
    a. Mature elastin fibers
    b. Oxytalan fibers
    c. Elaunin fibers
    d. Collagen-type III
13. **Radiograph of a periodontal ligament of a tooth which has lost its antagonist shows:**
    a. Widening of the periodontal ligament space
    b. Increased density
    c. Narrowing of the periodontal ligament space
    d. Sclerotic changes
14. **Predominant connective tissue cells of periodontal ligament are:**
    a. Fibroblasts
    b. Epithelial rests of Malassez
    c. Osteoclasts
    d. Osteoblasts
15. **Which of the following are the pressure receptors of periodontal ligament?**
    a. Free nerve endings
    b. Meissner's corpuscles
    c. Spindle like nerve endings
    d. Ruffini-like receptors
16. **Age changes in the periodontal ligament include which of the following?**
    a. Increased fibroplasia
    b. Increased vascularity
    c. Increased thickness
    d. decreased cellularity
17. **The periodontal ligament fibers that mainly prevent the extrusion of teeth are:**
    a. Horizontal fibers
    b. Interradicular fibers
    c. Alveolar crest fibers
    d. Transseptal fibers
18. **The periodontal ligament develops from:**
    a. Pulpal tissue
    b. Dental papilla
    c. Inner dental epithelium
    d. Dental sac
19. **An actively synthesizing periodontal cell have the following features, *except*:**
    a. Large amount of cytoplasm
    b. Large vesicular nucleus
    c. Less number of mitochondria
    d. Increased rough endoplasmic reticulum
20. **What kind of fibers form the majority of the periodontal ligament?**
    a. Elastic fibers
    b. Argyrophil fibers
    c. Collagen fibers
    d. Oxytalan fibers
21. **The cells originating from the degeneration of Hertwig's epithelial root sheath to form quiescent cell rests are called:**
    a. Resorptive cells
    b. Epithelial cell rests of Malassez
    c. Progenitor cells
    d. Synthetic or formative cells
22. **Which of the following statement is not correct about osteoblasts?**
    a. These cells are found on the surface of the alveolar bone
    b. The osteoblasts in active state form a layer of cuboidal cells
    c. These are large multinucleated cells that resorb the bone
    d. They maintain contact with the adjacent cells by means of desmosomes and tight junctions.
23. **The synthetic or formative cells of periodontal ligament includes all of the following cells, *except*:**
    a. Fibroblasts
    b. Osteoblasts
    c. Cementoblasts
    d. Cementoclasts

ANSWERS

| 1. d | 2. c | 3. c | 4. c | 5. c | 6. b | 7. a | 8. b | 9. d | 10. c | 11. a | 12. b | 13. c | 14. a | 15. c |
| 16. d | 17. c | 18. d | 19. c | 20. c | 21. b | 22. c | 23. d | | | | | | | |

BIBLIOGRAPHY

1. Aaron JE. Periosteal Sharpey's fibers: a novel bone matrix regulatory system. Front Endocrinol (Lausanne). 2012;3:98.
2. Avery JK, Chiego DJ. Essentials of Oral Histology and Embryology: A Clinical Approach, 3rd edition. US: Mosby; 2006.
3. Bartold PM, Mcculloch CA, Narayanan AS, et al. Tissue engineering: a new paradigm for periodontal regeneration based on molecular and cell biology. Periodontol 2000. 2000;24:253-69.
4. Bartold PM, Narayanam AS. Molecular and cell biology of healthy and diseased periodontal tissue. Periodontol 2000. 2006;40:29-49.
5. Bartold PM, Shi S, Gronthos S. Stem cells and periodontal regeneration. Periodontol 2000. 2006;40:164-72.
6. Berkoritz BK. Periodental ligament: structural and clinical correlates. Dent Update. 2004;31:46-50.
7. Berkovitz BKB, Holland GR, Moxham BJ. Enamel. In: Oral Anatomy, Histology and Embryology, 3rd edition. St Louis: Mosby; 2002. pp. 101-18.
8. Berkovitz BKB, Holland GR, Moxham BJ. Oral Anatomy, Histology and Embryology, 4th edition. US: Elsevier; 2009.
9. Bernick S. The organization of the periodontal membrane fibres of the developing molars of rats. Arch Oral Biol. 1960;2:57-63.
10. Bosshardt DD. Biological mediators and periodontal regeneration: a review of enamel matrix proteins at the cellular and molecular levels. J Clin Periodontol. 2008;35(Suppl 8):87-105.
11. Bradley RM. Essentials of Oral Physiology, 1st edition. USA: Mosby; 1995.
12. Bradley RM. Essentials of Oral Physiology, 1st edition. USA: Mosby; 1995.
13. Carmichael GG, Fullmer HM. The fine structure of the oxytalan fiber. J Cell Biol. 1966;28:33-6.
14. Cho MI, Garant PR. Development and general structure of the periodontium. Periodontol 2000. 2000;24:9-27.
15. Cohen B, Kramer IRH. Scientific Foundations of Dentistry, 1st edition. Great Britain Letterpress; 1976.
16. Dori F, Nikolidakis D, Huszar T, et al. Effect of platelet rich plasma on the healing of intrabony defects treated with an enamel matrix protein derivative and a natural bone mineral. J Clin Periodontol. 2000;35:44.
17. Eccles JD. Studies on the development of the periodontal membrane: the principal fibres of the molar teeth. Dent Pract Dent Rec. 1959;10:31-5.
18. Everts V, Niehof A, Jansen D, et al. Type VI collagen is associated with microfibrils and oxytalan fibers in the extracellular matrix of periodontium, mesenterium and periosteum. J Periodontal Res. 1998;33:118-25.
19. Frans Van den Berg. Extracellular matrix. In: Schleip R, Findley TW, Chaitow L, Huijing PA (Eds). Fascia: the tensional network of the human body: the science and clinical applications in manual and movement therapy. New York: Churchill Livingstone; 2012. pp. 165-70.
20. Fullmer HM. Connective tissue components of the periodontium. In: Miles AEW (Ed). Structural and Chemical Organization of Teeth, Volume II. New York: Academic Press; 1967. pp. 349-414.
21. Grant D, Bernick S. Formation of the periodontal ligament. J Periodontol. 1972;43:17-25.
22. Grant DA, Bernick S, Levy BM, et al. A comparative study of periodontal ligament development in teeth with and without predecessors in marmoset. J Periodontol. 1972;43:162-9.
23. Gronthos S, Mrozik K, Shi S, et al. Ovine periodontal ligament stem cells: isolation, characterization, and differentiation, potential. Calcif Tissue Int. 2006;79:310-7.
24. Higashi S. The elastic fibers in the periodontal membrane and cementum of human teeth (in Japanese). Shikwa Gakuho. 1964;64:453-77.
25. Johnson RB, Pylypas SP. A re-evaluation of the distribution of the elastic mesh work within the periodontal ligament of the mouse. J Periodontal Res. 1922;27:239-49.
26. Khoshhal M, Amiri I, Gholami L. Comparison of in vitro properties of periodontal ligament stem cells derived from permanent and deciduous teeth. J Dent Res Dent Clin Dent Prospects. 2017;11:140-8.
27. Khurana A, Khurana I. Human Embryology, 2nd edition. New Delhi: CBS Publishers and Distributor Pvt. Ltd; 2012.
28. Kielty CM, Sherratt MJ, Marson A, et al. Fibrillin microfibrils. Adv Protein Chem. 2005;70:405-36.
29. Kielty CM, Sherratt MJ, Shuttleworth CA. Elastic fibres. J Cell Sci. 2002;115:2817-28.
30. Kumar GS. Orban's Oral histology and Embryology, 14th edition. India: Elsevier India (P) Ltd; 2015.
31. Kuroiwa M, Chihara K, Higashi S. Electron microscopic studies on Sharpey's fibres in the alveolar bone of rat molars. Kaibogaku Zasshi. 1994;69(6):776-82.
32. Lekic P, Rojas J, Birek C, et al. Phenotypic comparison of periodontal ligament cells in vivo and in vitro. J Periodontal Res. 2001;36:71-9.
33. Lindhe J, Lang NP, Karring T. Clinical Periodontology and Implant Dentistry, 2nd Volume, 5th edition. US: Willey- Blackwell; 2008.
34. Mcculloch CA, Lekic P, Mckee MD. Role of physical forces in regulating the form and function of the periodontal ligament. Periodontol 2000. 2000;24:56-72.
35. Miles TS, Nauntofte B, Svensson P. Clinical Oral Physiology, 1st edition. Copenhagen: Quintessence Publishing Co. Ltd; 2004.
36. Moss-Salentijn L, Hendricks-Klyvert M. Dental and Oral Tissues, 3rd edition. Philadelphia: Lea and Febiger; 1990.
37. Nakahara T, Nakamura T, Kobayashi E, et al. In situ tissue engineering of periodontal tissues by seeding with periodontal ligament-derived cells. Tissue Eng. 2004;10:537-44.
38. Nanci A, Bosshardt DD. Structure of periodontal tissues in health and disease. Periodontol 2000. 2000;40:11-28.
39. Nanci A. Ten Cate's Oral Histology: Development, Structure, and Function, 7th edition. US: Elsevier; 2008.
40. Neville BW, Damm DD, Allen CM, et al. Oral and Maxillofacial Pathology, 1st South Asia edition. India: Elsevier; 2016.
41. Newman MG, Takei H, Klokkevold PR, et al. Carranza's Clinical Periodontology, 10th edition. Philadelphia: WB Saunders; 2006.
42. Park JC, Kim JM, Jung IH, et al. Isolation and characterization of human periodontal ligament (PDL) stem cells (PDLSCs) from the inflamed PDL tissue: in vitro and in vivo evaluations. J Clin Periodontol. 2011;38:721-31.
43. Polimeni G, Xiropaidis AV, Wikesjö UM. Biology and principles of periodontal wound healing/regeneration. Periodontol 2000. 2006;41:2006.
44. Provenza DV, Seibel W. Oral Histology: Inheritance and Development, 2nd edition. USA: Lea and Febiger; 1986.

45. Rimoin DL, Tiller GE. Skeletal dysplasias and connective tissue disorders. In: Gleason CA, Devaskar SU (Eds). Avery's Diseases of the Newborn, 9th edition. US: Elsevier; 2012. pp. 258-76.
46. Rincon JC, Xiao Y, Young WG, et al. Production of osteopontin by cultured porcine epithelial cell rests of Malassez. J Periodontal Res. 2005;40:417-26.
47. Saffar JL, Lasfargues JJ, Cherruah M. Alveolar bone and the alveolar process: the socket that is never stable. Periodontol 2000. 1997;13:76.
48. Sawada T, Sugawara Y, Asai T, et al. Immunohistochemical characterization of elastic system fibers in rat molar periodontal ligament. J Histochem Cytochem. 2006;54(10):1095-1103.
49. Schroeder HE. Oral Structural Biology, 4th edition. New York: Thieme; 1991.
50. Sims MR. Oxytalan-vascular relationships observed in histologic examination of the periodontal ligaments of man and mouse. Arch Oral Biology. 1975;20:713-6.
51. Sivapathasundharam B. Shafer's Textbook of Oral Pathology, 8th edition. India: Elsevier; 2016.
52. Sonoyama W, Seo BM, Yamaza T, et al. Hertwig's epithelial root sheath cells play crucial roles in cementum formation. J Dent Res. 2007;86(7):594.
53. Ten Cate AR. The development of the periodontium: a largely ectomesenchymally derived unit, periodontol 2000. 1997;13:9.
54. Wise GE, King GJ. Mechanisms of tooth eruption and orthodontic tooth movement. J Dental Res. 2008;87:414-34.

CHAPTER

Alveolar Bone

B Sivapathasundharam

CHAPTER OUTLINE

- Physical Properties 129
- Chemical Composition 129
- Classification of Bones 129
  - According to the Shape 129
  - According to the Development 130
  - According to the Macrostructure 130
  - According to the Microstructure 132
- Formation of Bone 133
  - Intramembranous Ossification 134
  - Endochondral Ossification 135
  - Mineralization of Bone Matrix 136
- Cells of the Bone 136
  - Osteoprogenitor Cells 136
  - Osteoblasts 136
  - Osteoid 137
- Osteocytes 138
- Osteoclasts 138
- Bone Remodeling 140
  - Incremental Lines (Resting Lines) 141
  - Reversal Lines 141
- Alveolar Bone 141
- Development of Maxilla and Mandible 141
  - Maxilla 141
  - Mandible 142
- Development of Alveolar Process 145
- Structure of Alveolar Bone 145
  - Alveolar Bone Proper 145
  - Supporting Alveolar Bone 146
- Remodeling of Alveolar Bone 146
- Age Changes 147
- Clinical Considerations 147

INTRODUCTION

Alveolar bone is that part of maxilla or mandible, which accommodates the teeth through periodontal ligament attachment **(Figure 10-1)**. Attachment of tooth to the alveolar bone is a peg-in-socket type of fibrous joint known as "Gomphosis". It is considered to be a joint, since a limited movement of the teeth is possible due to masticatory force. The fibers of the periodontal ligament are attached on one end to the cementum and on the other end to the alveolar bone. The embedded portions of the periodontal ligament fibers are here also called "Sharpey's fibers" **(Figure 10-2)**. The existence of the alveolar bone depends on the presence or absence of teeth. When a tooth or teeth are lost the alveolar bone resorbs. If teeth are developmentally missing as in anodontia, the alveolar bone is poorly developed. Apart from accommodating teeth, it transmits the forces of mastication to the jaw bone.

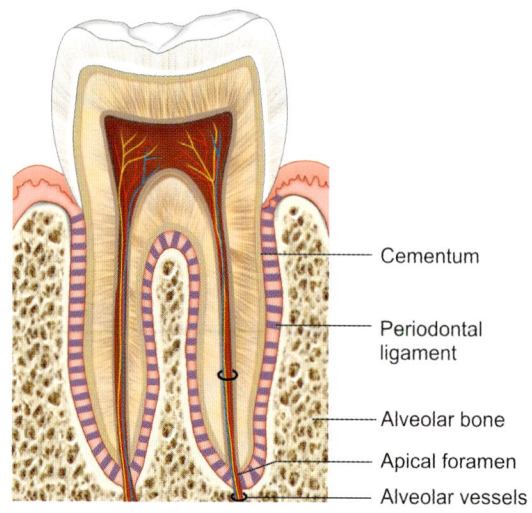

Figure 10-1: Tooth in alveolar socket.

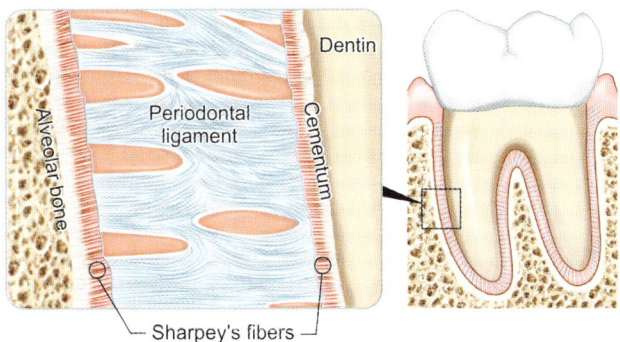

Figure 10-2: Sharpey's fibers (embedded portion of the periodontal ligament fiber).

Bone is a vascular and mineralized connective tissue, which gives the skeletal framework and acts as a reservoir of calcium. With the muscle attachment it helps in locomotion. Further it protects the visceral organs. It also has synthetic role by way of producing blood cells. Bone marrow, the soft tissue present within the bone, contains *hematopoietic* stem cells, capable of producing blood cells. The yellow bone marrow of the long bones acts as a storage of fats. By absorbing or releasing alkaline salts, bone buffers the blood against excessive pH changes. Bone remodels actively according to the functional needs. Knowledge of bone in general is essential for better understanding of the anatomy and physiology of the alveolar bone.

PHYSICAL PROPERTIES

Although apparently hard and rigid, bones exhibit a considerable degree of elasticity, which is important for the skeleton's ability to withstand any impact. Compact bones have been found to have tensile strength in the range of 700–1,400 kg/cm^2 and compressive strength in the range of 1,400–2,100 kg/cm^2. These values are of the same general order as for aluminum or mild steel, but bone has an advantage of being considerably lighter when compared to these minerals. The physical properties of the bone depend on the variation in mineral–collagen ratio; less mineral tends to provide greater flexibility and more mineral, increases the brittleness.

> Bone resists compressive forces best and the tensile forces least. It also resists forces applied along the axis of its fibrous component. Thus, fracture of the bone occurs usually as a result of tensile and slicing stresses.

CHEMICAL COMPOSITION

Similar to the dental hard tissues, bone too is made up of inorganic and organic components and water. Living bone contains 10–20% water. Of its dry mass, approximately 60–70% is inorganic. Most of the rest is collagen, but bone also contains a small amount of other substances such as proteins and inorganic salts.

The inorganic component is in the form of calcium phosphate hydroxyapatite [$Ca_{10}(PO_4)_6(OH)_2$] crystals. The organic component consists mainly of type I collagen fibers and small quantity of type V and type III collagen within the ground substance. Hydroxyapatite crystals are arranged parallel to the long axes of collagen bundles and many actually lie in voids within the bundles themselves. Around 5% are composed of noncollagenous proteins including—osteonectin, osteocalcin, bone morphogenetic protein (BMP), bone proteoglycan, bone sialoproteins, etc.

Osteonectin anchors the collagen to the bone mineral, while osteocalcin is a calcium-binding protein and is involved in bone mineralization. The ground substance is made up of glycoproteins, proteoglycans, lipids, etc. The composition of bone mineral is much more complex and contains additional ions such as silicon, carbonate, and zinc.

CLASSIFICATION OF BONES

Bones can be classified in many ways. They may be classified according to the shape, development, structure, and microstructure.

According to the Shape

They are classified as long bones, short bones, flat bones, irregular bones, and sesamoid bones.

Long bones typically have an elongated shaft and two expanded ends one on either side. The shaft is known as diaphysis and the ends are called epiphyses. Normally the epiphyses are smooth and articular (forming part of the joint). The shaft is tubular and has a central medullary cavity, where it accommodates the bone marrow. The epiphyses are covered by compact bone at the periphery and cancellous bone at the center. Hyaline cartilage covers the articulating surface of the epiphysis. Examples of long bone include humerus, femur, radius, ulna, tibia, and fibula **(Figure 10-3)**.

Short bones are short in posture and can be of varied shapes and are named according to their shape. Examples of this type of bones include—cuboid, cuneiform, scaphoid, trapezoid, etc. All the carpal and tarsal bones are included in this category.

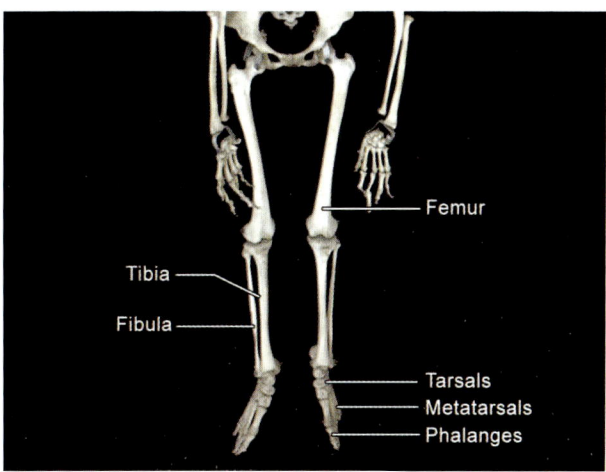

Figure 10-3: Long bones and short bones.

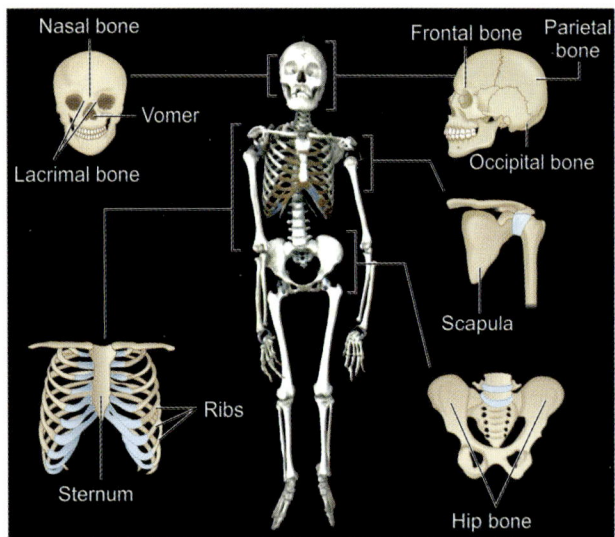

Figure 10-4: Flat bones.

Flat bones appear flat, thin, and curved with two prominent surfaces. Predominantly they resemble shallow plates and form boundaries of certain body cavities. Spongy bone is present in between the two surfaces and no distinct marrow cavity is seen. Examples include scapula, ribs, sternum, etc. **(Figure 10-4)**.

Irregular bones do not have any specific shape and appear completely irregular. They are mainly made up of cancellous bone covered by a layer of compact bone. Vertebrae, pelvic bone, and bones in the base of skull are made up of irregular bone **(Figure 10-5)**.

Sesamoid bones: The word sesamoid is derived from the Latin word "sesamum" (sesame seed) to denote its small size. They are in the form of nodules, embedded in tendons and joint capsules. They do not possess any periosteum and their ossification takes place after birth. Examples of this type of bones are patella, pisiform, and fabella. They develop in locations where there is considerable pressure, tension, friction or stress **(Figure 10-6)**.

Sutural bones: These are named after their location and not the shape and are usually seen in sutural lines. They are also called wormian bones. Since the number of sutural bones is more, they are not named **(Figure 10-7)**.

According to the Development

Depending on the development, the bones are classified into membranous bones and cartilaginous bones.

Membranous bones are also known as dermal or mesenchymal bones. They develop directly from the sheet-like membrane of the embryonic connective tissue, the mesenchyme. Flat bones of the skull, mandible, and clavicle are examples of membranous bones.

Cartilaginous bones are formed from the preformed cartilage models. Examples of this type of bones include bones of limbs, vertebral column, and thoracic cage.

Some bones are formed partly from cartilage model and partly from mesenchymal condensation and are known as membrocartilaginous bones. Mandible, clavicle, occipital, and sphenoid bones are membrocartilaginous bones.

According to the Macrostructure

According to the macrostructure, they are typed as compact and cancellous bone.

Compact bone is the strongest and densest form of bone in the body and forms the cortex (outer covering) and appears

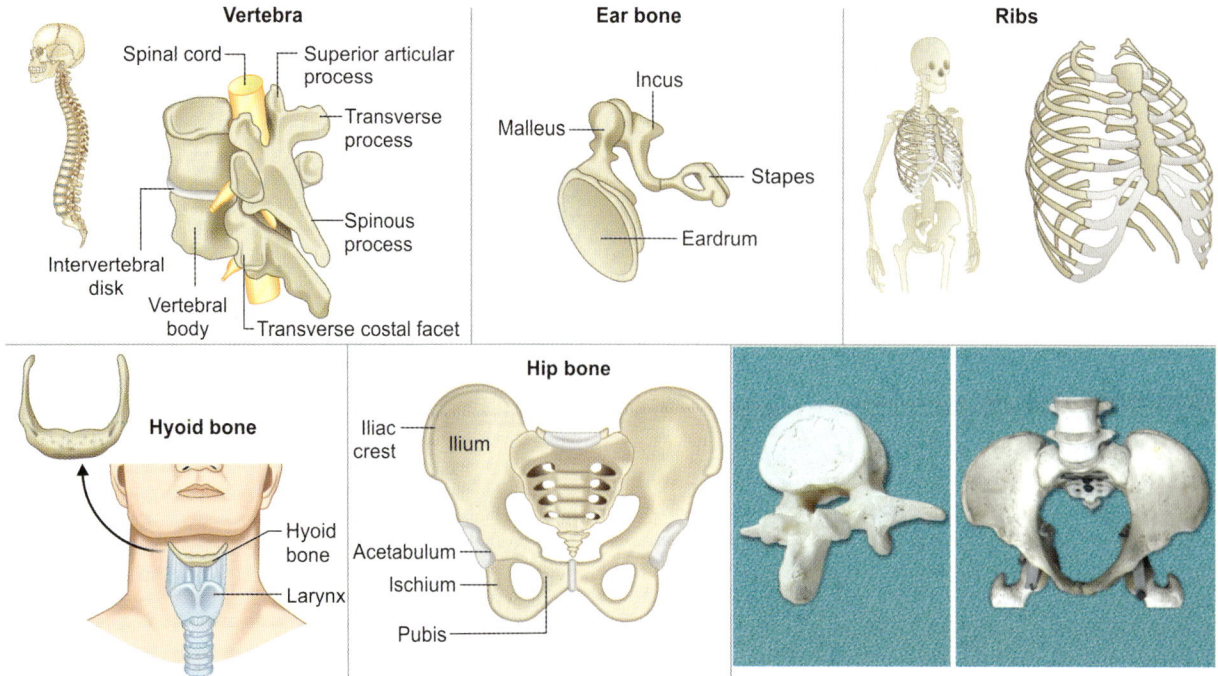

Figure 10-5: Irregular bones.

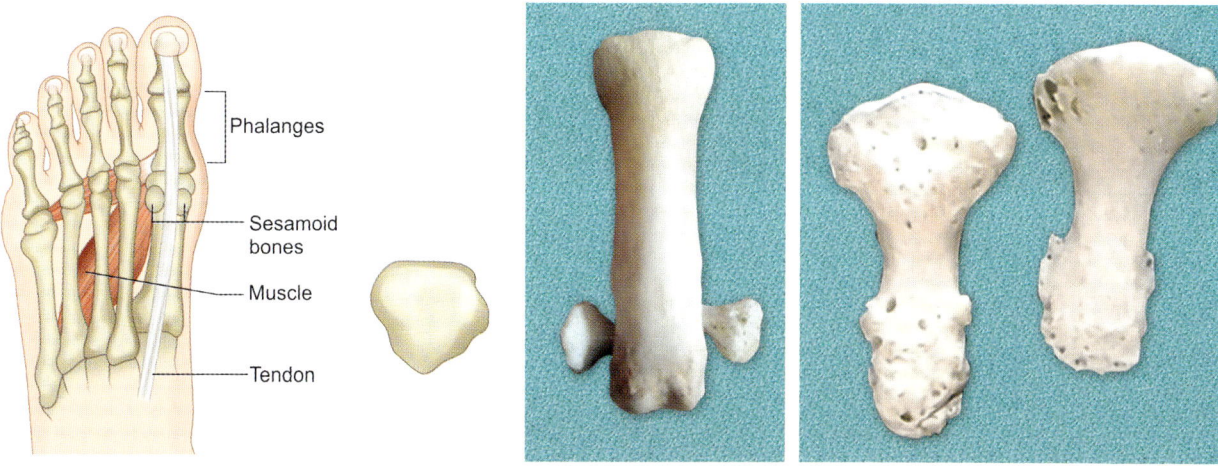

Figure 10-6: Sesamoid bone.

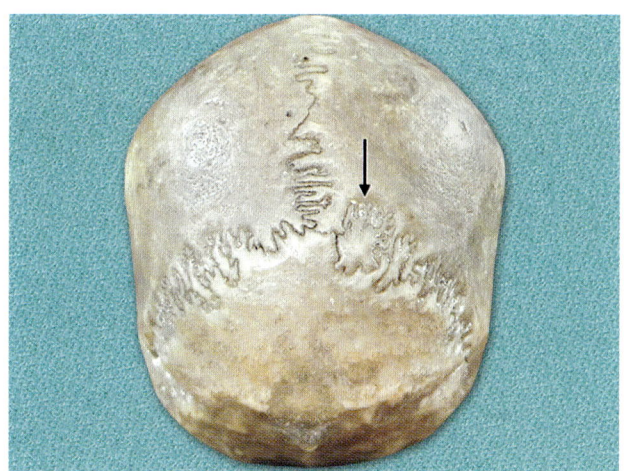

Figure 10-7: Sutural bones.

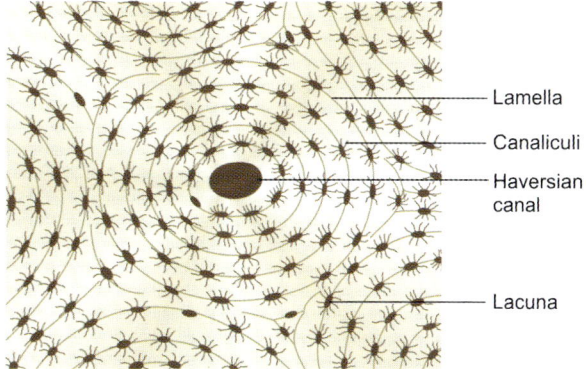

Figure 10-8: Schematic representation of Haversian system consists of concentric lamellae surrounding the Haversian canal.

smooth, white, and solid. Compact bone forms 80% of the human skeleton. Bony matrix is solidly filled with organic ground substance and inorganic salts, leaving only tiny spaces called the lacunae, which contain the osteocytes. Compact bone is covered by periosteum on the outer surface and endosteum on the inner surface.

The structural and functional unit of the compact bone is known as *osteon*, or Haversian system **(Figures 10-9A and B)**. Osteon is a cylindrical structure made up of concentric sheets or layers of calcified matrix called lamellae **(Figure 10-8)**. Center of each osteon contains a canal called *Haversian canal*, which contains blood vessels, nerves, and lymphatic vessels **(Figures 10-9A and B)**. The blood vessels supply blood to the interior spongy bone as well as the living cells, the osteocytes, housed within the lamellae. These vessels and nerves branch off at right angles through a perforating canal known as *Volkmann's canal*, to extend to the periosteum and endosteum **(Figure 10-10)**.

> Bone which contains lamellae is also known as lamellar bone. Based on the location, these lamellae are classified into concentric lamellae (surround the Haversian canal in a circular pattern), interstitial lamellae (located in between the concentric lamellae), and circumferential lamellae (run parallel to the entire circumference of the bone and encircle the concentric and interstitial lamellae).

Immature compact bone does not contain osteons and has a woven structure.

Periosteum is the thin yet tough outermost layer of the compact or cortical bones. It has two layers, namely outer fibrous layer and inner cellular (cambium layer) or osteogenic layer **(Figure 10-11)**. The fibrous layer is made up of collagen fibers that support the bone and firmly connect it to the surrounding structures. Osteogenic cells in the periosteum play a vital role in the growth and repair of bone. The periosteum is very active during development and repair.

Endosteum is made up of thin cellular layer, which contains quiescent osteoblasts and osteoprogenitor cells **(Figure 10-12)**. Osteoprogenitor cells act as reservoir for the new bone-forming cells, the osteoblasts.

Cancellous bone: It is also known as spongy bone or trabecular bone and is made up of trabeculae and marrow (the soft tissue) **(Figures 10-13A and B)**. It is less dense compared to compact bone and accounts for 20% of the skeleton. Cancellous bone is

132 CHAPTER 10: Alveolar Bone

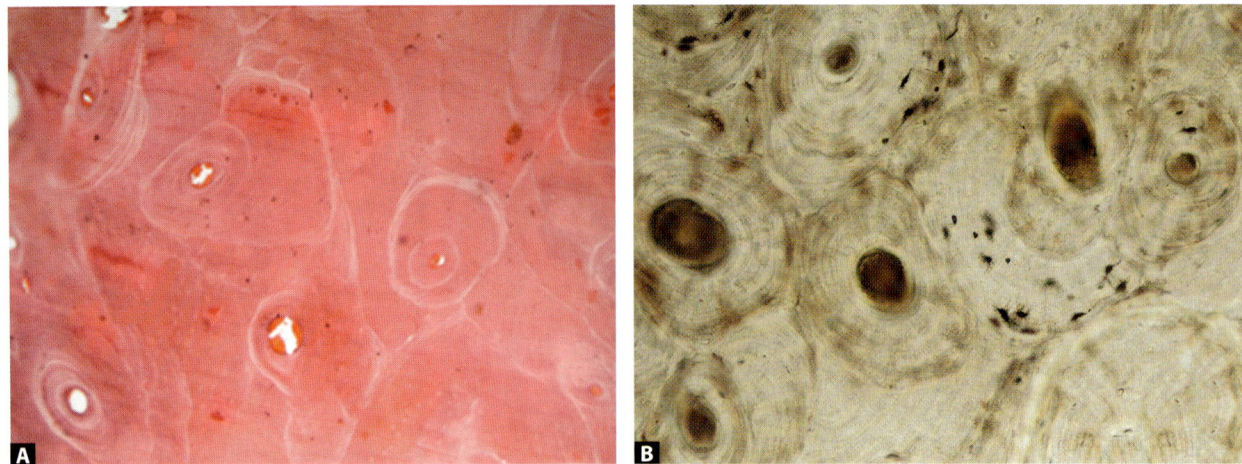

Figures 10-9A and B: Haversian system: (A) Hematoxylin and eosin stained section; and (B) ground section.

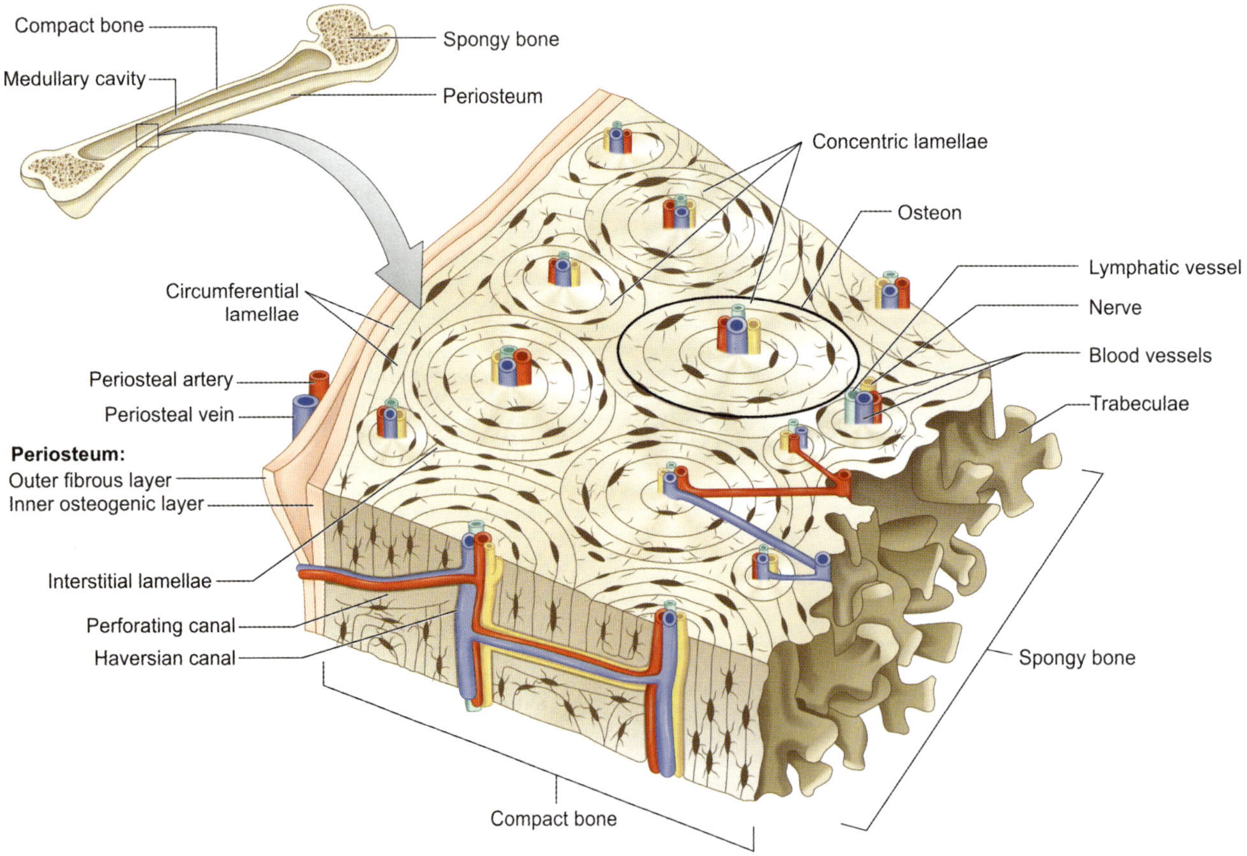

Figure 10-10: Structure of compact bone.

richly vascular and usually contains red bone marrow, where the production of blood cells (hematopoiesis) occurs. The volume of the cancellous bone is ten times higher than that of the compact bone.

According to the Microstructure

Based on the microstructure, bone can be classified as fine fiber bundle bone and coarse woven bone.

Fine fiber bundle bone: It is the matured, lamellated bone in which there is regular and parallel alignment of collagen fibers into sheets or lamellae and is mechanically strong.

Coarse woven bone: It is characterized by a haphazard organization of collagen fibers and is mechanically weak. This usually occurs when the bone is rapidly laid down (in repair and during the development of embryo). Here the new bone is laid over the pre-existing connective tissue. The new collagen

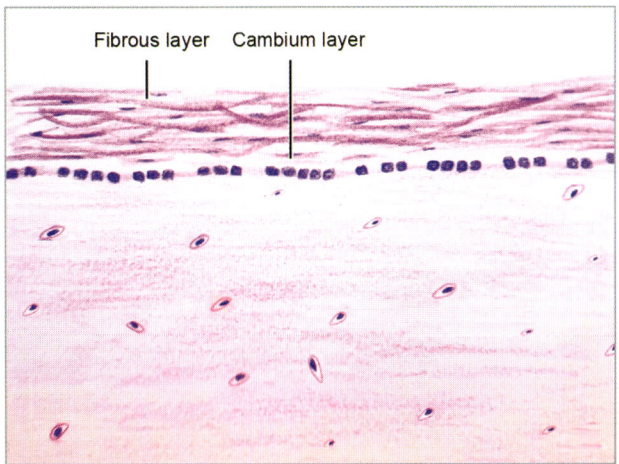

Figure 10-11: Layers of periosteum.

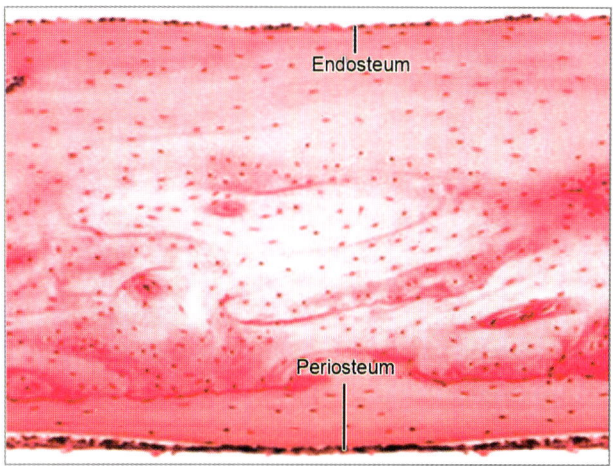

Figure 10-12: Endosteal layer.

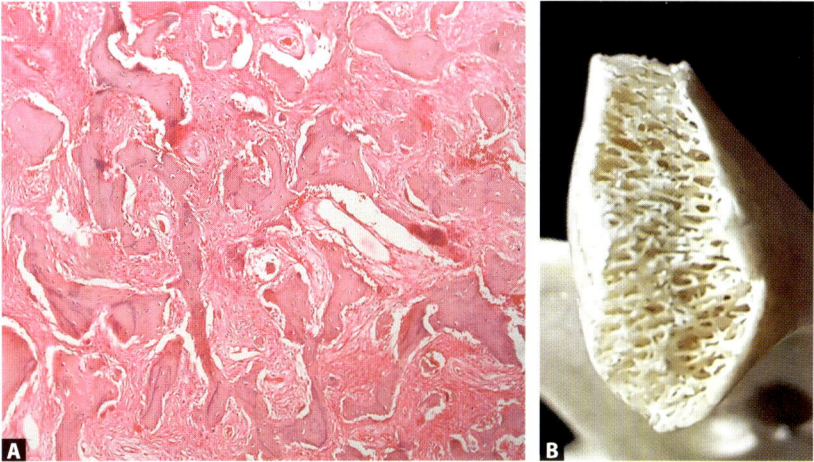

Figures 10-13A and B: Structure of cancellous bone: (A) Microscopic; (B) Macroscopic.

formed by the osteoblasts and the pre-existing collagen of the connective tissue together constitutes the fibrous matrix of the new bone. This fibrous matrix comprises of collagen fibers of varying thickness and orientation and many are in continuation with the adjacent soft connective tissue. This type of bone is called coarse woven bone or embryonic bone **(Figure 10-14)**.

The differences between the fine fiber bundle bone and the coarse woven bone are given in **Table 10-1**.

FORMATION OF BONE

It is also known as osteogenesis or ossification and involves the laying down of new bone by the bone-forming cells called osteoblasts. During the early stages of embryogenesis, the embryo's skeleton is made up of fibrous membranes and hyaline cartilage. During 6th or 7th week of intrauterine life, the actual process of bone formation begins. There are two osteogenic pathways—intramembranous ossification and endochondral ossification—but bone is the same regardless of the pathway that produces it. Both involve the transformation of a pre-existing mesenchymal tissue into bone. Intramembranous ossification involves direct conversion of mesenchyme into bone. This process occurs primarily in the bones of the skull. In endochondral ossification, the mesenchymal cells differentiate into cartilage, which is later replaced by bone.

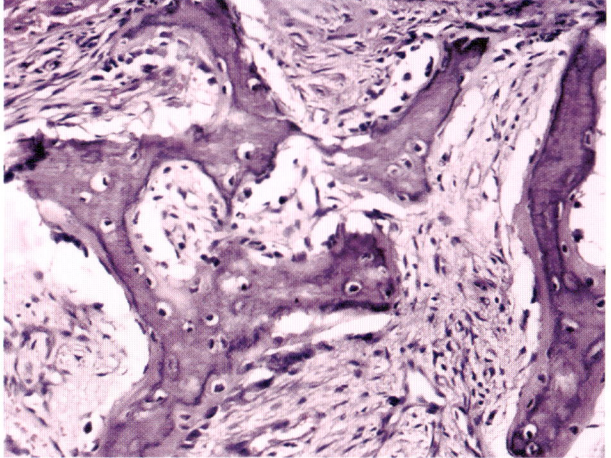

Figure 10-14: Woven bone in fibrous matrix.

TABLE 10-1: Difference between fine fiber bundle bone and coarse woven bone.

Fine fiber bundle bone	Coarse woven bone
Also known as mature bone or lamellar bone	Known as immature bone
Collagen fibers arranged distinctly and orderly	Intertwined coarse and fine collagen fiber bundles arranged irregularly
Interfibrillar space is less and consists of tightly packed osteons forming a solid mass	Interfibrillar space is more, which is occupied by mineral crystals and acidic proteins
Slowly deposited	Rapidly formed and have high turnover rate
Mineralizes slower	Mineralizes faster
In H and E staining appears more eosinophilic	In H and E staining appears more basophilic due to its higher proteoglycan content
Enriched with osteocalcin	Enriched with Bone sialoprotein (BSP) and bone acidic glycoprotein (BSP-75)
Portion of lamellar matrix of a given bone is resorbed at one time	Can be entirely removed by osteoclasts
Collagen mediated mineralization occurs	Matrix vesicles initiate mineralization
Fewer osteocytes are present	Numerous large osteocytes are present
Osteocytes are flattened	Osteocytes are isodiametric
Seen postnatally	Usually seen prenatally, or during healing of a fracture
Lamellated	Nonlamellated
Lamellae are arranged in concentric circles around blood vessels or parallel to periosteum	Lamellae are arranged irregularly
Closely packed/fused or large trabeculae are evident with small marrow spaces	Distantly placed small trabeculae are evident with large marrow spaces

Intramembranous Ossification

The flat bones of the face, most of the cranial bones, and the clavicles are formed through this process. During intramembranous ossification in the skull, the ectomesenchymal cells proliferate and condense into compact nodules. Some of these cells differentiate into capillaries, while others will become osteogenic cells and then osteoblasts **(Figure 10-15)**. The osteoblasts secrete the bone matrix called osteoid, which consists of collagen precursors and other organic proteins that are able to bind calcium. The osteoid mineralizes within a few days and hardens, thereby entrapping the osteoblasts within. The entrapped osteoblasts are called osteocytes **(Figure 10-16)**. As osteoblasts transform into osteocytes, osteogenic cells in the surrounding connective tissue differentiate into new osteoblasts at the edges of the growing bone. The mechanism of intramembranous ossification involves BMPs and the activation of a transcription factor called core binding factor alpha 1 (*Cbfa1*). Cbfa1 is an important transcription factor for osteoblastic differentiation and osteogenesis. BMP is also a potent inducer of differentiation of pluripotent mesenchymal cells into osteoblast lineage and bone formation.

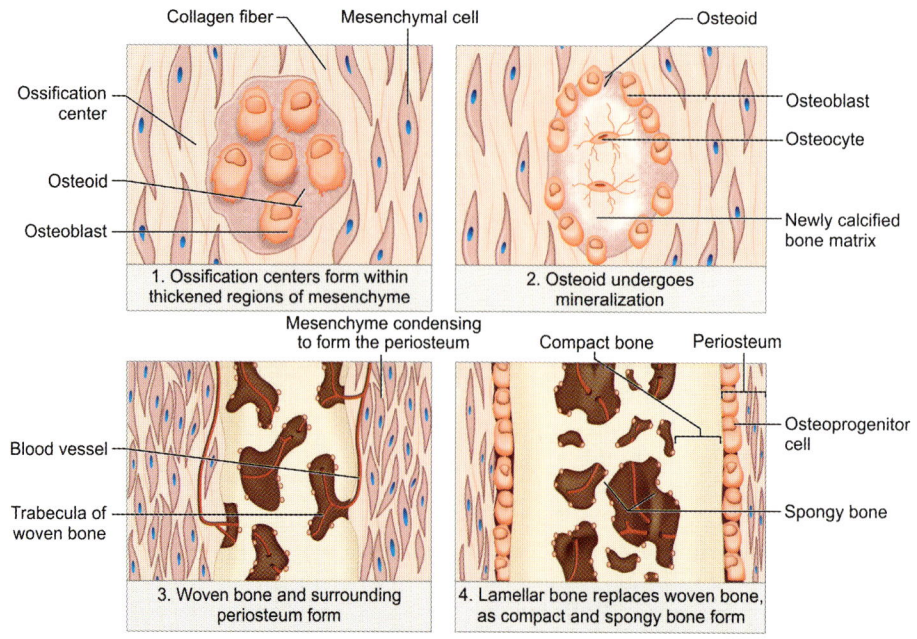

Figure 10-15: Steps in intramembranous ossification.

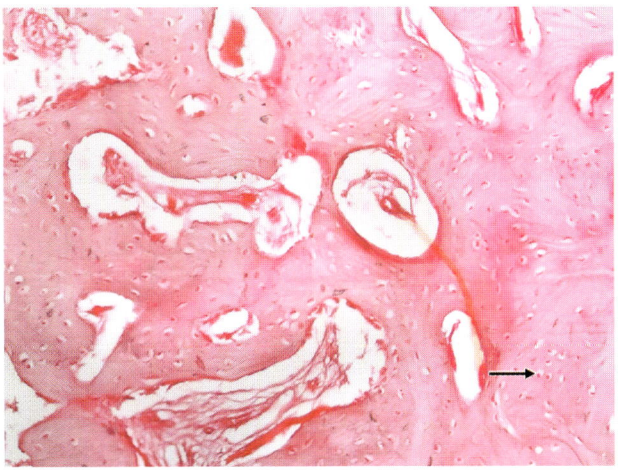

Figure 10-16: Osteocytes.

Several groups of osteoid come together around the capillaries to form a trabecular matrix, while osteoblasts on the surface of the newly formed cancellous bone become the cellular layer of the periosteum. The periosteum then secretes compact bone over the surface of the cancellous bone. The bone trabeculae crowd nearby blood vessels, which eventually condense into red bone marrow. The new bone continuously remodels under the action of osteoclasts.

Endochondral Ossification

In this process, bone develops by replacing the hyaline cartilage. Cartilage does not become bone. Instead, cartilage formed from the aggregated mesenchymal cells, serves as a template to be completely replaced by new bone. The process of endochondral ossification takes much longer time than intramembranous ossification. Bones at the base of the skull and long bones form by endochondral ossification.

There are five stages in the process of endochondral ossification. In the first stage, the mesenchymal cells are committed to differentiate into cartilage-forming cells (chondroblasts). In second stage, the committed mesenchyme cells condense into compact nodules and differentiate into chondroblasts. During third stage, the chondroblasts proliferate rapidly to form the model for the bone. In the fourth stage, the chondroblasts stop dividing and increase their volume dramatically, becoming hypertrophic chondrocytes. Chondrocytes are mature cartilage cells entrapped within the cartilaginous matrix. These large chondrocytes alter the matrix they produce to enable it to become mineralized.

> Chondroblasts are actively dividing immature **cartilage forming** cells, which first form extracellular matrix. Chondroblasts entrapped within the cartilaginous matrix are called chondrocytes. They are differentiated cells, involved in the diffusion of the nutrients, maintenance, and repair of the extracellular matrix of the cartilage.

The final stage involves the invasion of the cartilage model by blood vessels. The hypertrophic chondrocytes die by apoptosis and this space will become bone marrow. As the cartilage cells die, a group of cells that surround the cartilage model differentiate into osteoblasts. These osteoblasts begin forming bone matrix on the partially degraded cartilage. Eventually, the entire cartilage is replaced by bone. Thus, the cartilage tissue serves as a model for the bone to be formed **(Figure 10-17)**.

As already described, the coarse woven bone is formed by the deposition of new bone over the pre-existing connective tissue. The collagen of the pre-existing connective tissue and the newly laid down collagen are in varying thickness and orientation, giving the woven appearance.

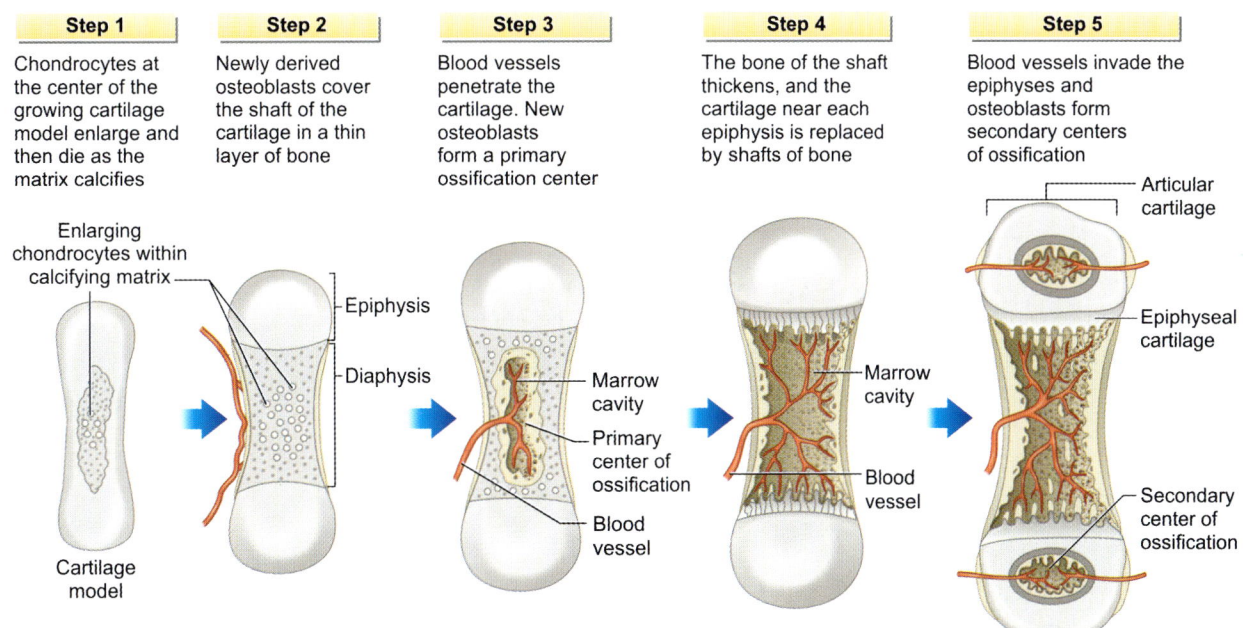

Figure 10-17: Endochondral ossification.

The lamellar bone is laid down in two ways. They can be laid down concentrically around the blood vessels to form osteons. Alternatively, it may be formed as sheets on the surface of the bone as circumferential lamellae.

Mineralization of Bone Matrix

The term mineralization refers to the process by which an inorganic substance precipitates in an organic matrix. Normal bone contains about 60–70% of inorganic material and the rest is organic substance and water. The major mineral content of bone is calcium phosphate hydroxyapatite [$Ca_{10}(PO_4)_6(OH)_2$] crystals.

Mineralization of bone is a well-organized process in which crystals of calcium phosphate are produced by the osteoblasts and are laid down within the bone matrix, the osteoid. Osteoid is composed of collagen fibers and ground substance. When matrix matures, there is expression of alkaline phosphatase and several other proteins, including osteocalcin, osteopontin, and bone sialoproteins. These are calcium and phosphate-binding proteins, thought to regulate ordered deposition, amount, and size of the hydroxyapatite crystals.

Bone alkaline phosphatase increases the phosphorus concentrations in the local environment and removes the phosphate-containing inhibitors of hydroxyapatite crystal growth, or modify phosphoproteins to control their ability to act as nucleators. Mineral crystals are deposited first in between the ends of collagen fibrils of the matrix, then on the surface of the collagen fibril and inside the collagen fibril. This progresses gradually in the intercollagen fibril area and noncollagen fibril area, where small rod-like crystals are deposited densely. As bone matures, hydroxyapatite crystals enlarge by crystal growth and aggregation **(Figure 10-18)**.

Mineralization of bone is regulated by hormones like Vitamin D, parathyroid, etc., osteoblasts, osteocytes, osteoclasts, and cell products. Calcium ions, inorganic phosphate, and pyrophosphate play a significant role in controlling bone mineralization process. Vitamin D plays an indirect role in enhancing the mineralization of the osteoid. It stimulates the intestinal absorption of calcium and phosphorus so as to achieve enough calcium concentration. It also promotes differentiation of osteoblasts and stimulates osteoblast expression of bone-specific alkaline phosphatase, osteocalcin, osteonectin, etc. Promoters of bone mineralization include dentin matrix protein 1 and bone sialoprotein.

CELLS OF THE BONE

Osteoprogenitor Cells

They are mesenchymal stem cells that can undergo cell division and differentiate into osteoblasts. Osteoprogenitor cells are seen in bone marrow, inner layer of periosteum, and endosteum. These cells are most active during bone growth, but large numbers are reactivated in adult life in bone repair. First they differentiate into preosteoblasts and then mature to become osteoblasts whose function is to form bone matrix. Osteoblasts progress through a series of maturational stages and ultimately become mature osteocyte **(Figure 10-19)**.

> There is a large reservoir of cells in the body capable of forming bone throughout life. However, lot of studies support the view that there may be different types of precursor pools, any or all of which may be important in situations requiring new bone formation and replacement or expansion of the osteoblast population.

Osteoblasts

They are the cells of mesenchymal origin and responsible for the formation of bone. Active osteoblasts appear cuboidal, may be rounded to polygonal occasionally, and exhibit a basophilic cytoplasm. Osteoblasts may be uninucleated or occasionally multinucleated and are placed eccentrically, away from the bone forming front **(Figure 10-20)**. There is increased amount of rough endoplasmic reticulum and Golgi apparatus. Nucleus is spherical and lies toward the basal end. Osteoblasts contact one another by means of cell junctions of different kind (adherens, gap, and tight junction). They are seen lining the osteoid (unmineralized bone matrix) over the forming bone surface.

The procollagen molecules secreted in the rough endoplasmic reticulum are transferred to the Golgi apparatus from where they are discharged as secretory vesicles through exocytosis. Extracellularly these molecules are arranged as fibrils to form a part of the osteoid. Apart from secreting the formative components of the bone, osteoblasts also secrete growth factors, cytokines, and prostaglandins. These molecules control osteoblasts' own activity.

Osteoblasts are derived from the osteoprogenitor of the mesenchyme. Periosteum also serves as a reservoir of osteoblasts particularly during fracture healing.

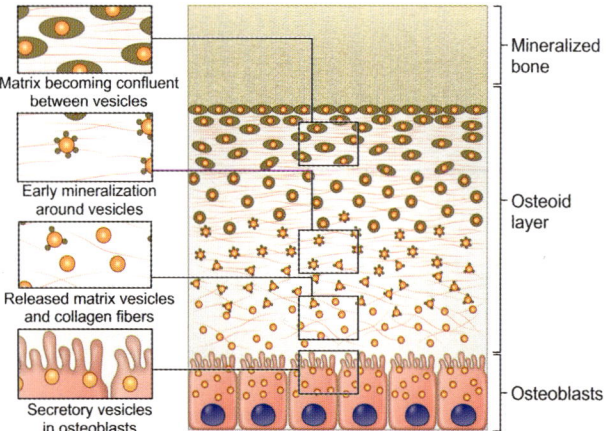

Figure 10-18: Mineralization of bone matrix.

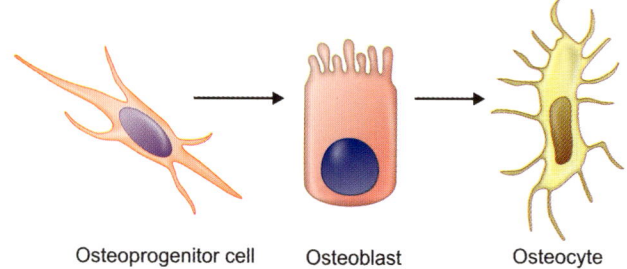

Figure 10-19: Derivatives of osteoprogenitor cell.

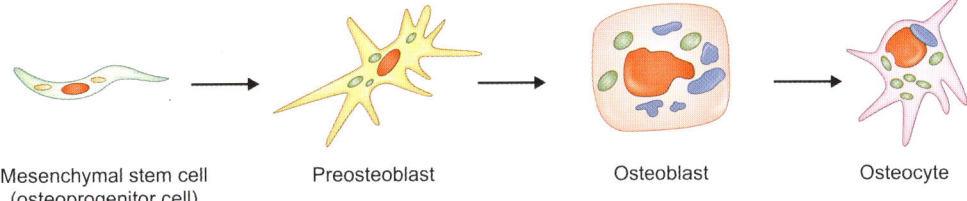

Figure 10-20: Differentiation of osteoblast.

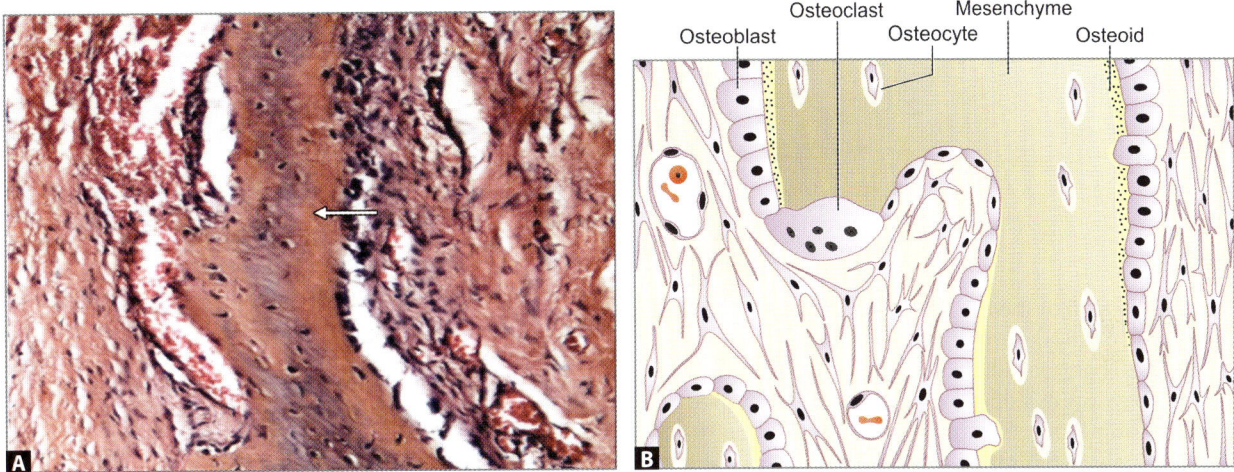

Figures 10-21A and B: Bone cells and osteoid formation. (A) Hematoxylin and eosin stained section and (B) schematic representation.

Osteoid is elaborated by the osteoblast all around its cell body. Osteoblasts get in the matrix with the cytoplasmic processes resulting in the formation of lacunae and canaliculi, respectively. The entrapped osteoblasts are called osteocytes (Figures 10-21A and B).

Functions of osteoblasts include production of type I collagen and noncollagenous protein matrix, and modification of the organic matrix by withdrawal or modification of proteoglycans and glycoproteins. Further they initiate mineralization by secreting several promotor or regulators of mineralization particularly phosphoproteins and providing additional inorganic phosphate by action of membrane-bound alkaline phosphatase, which act as the seed. Osteoblastic cells also play a role in bone resorption through osteoclasts by the secretion of receptor activator of nuclear factor kappa B ligand (RANKL).

Bone morphogenetic proteins
They are a group of growth factors that belong to the transforming growth factor beta (TGF-β) superfamily. Initially they are believed to be involved in the formation of bone and cartilage, but are now considered to constitute a group of essential morphogenetic signals and orchestrating the tissue architecture throughout the body. They have an important role during development in the embryonic patterning and early skeletal formation. BMPs also play an important role in postnatal bone formation. They induce the mesenchymal stem cells to differentiate into osteoblasts. Till now there are more than 20 types of BMPs that have been identified, but only BMP-2, 4, 6, 7, and 9 have been shown to possess significant osteogenic properties. RUNX gene on chromosome 6p21 encoding a transcription factor Cbfa-1 is involved in osteoblast differentiation and skeletal morphogenesis.

Osteoid

Unmineralized bone matrix secreted by the osteoblasts is called osteoid and is analogous to the predentin or cementoid (Figure 10-22). It is seen over the surface of actively forming bone with the thickness of about 5–10 μm. As detailed earlier the osteoid is composed of type I collagen, arranged more or less parallel to the bone surface, and embedded in the ground substance. The staining property of the osteoid differs from that of the matrix associated with the mineralized bone. Other than type I collagen, the osteoid contains some components which are specific to the osteoblast lineage and used as markers for osteoblasts. These include osteocalcin, osteoblast transcription factor, and Cbfa-1.

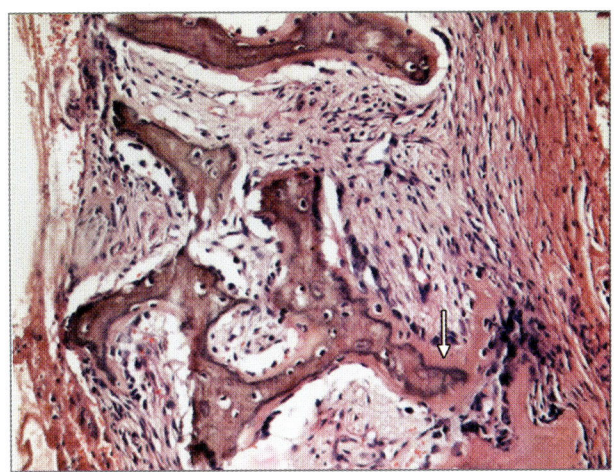

Figure 10-22: Osteoid.

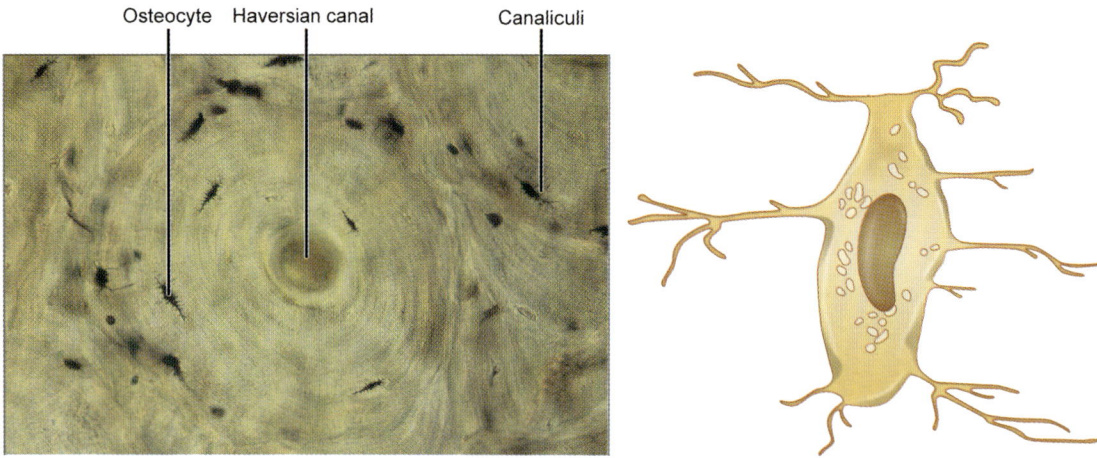

Figure 10-23: Structure of osteocytes.

Osteocytes

They are entrapped or incorporated osteoblasts in the bone, which are terminally differentiated. During the formation of bone matrix, osteoblasts get embedded within the bone matrix (osteoid) to become osteocytes. They are stellate-shaped and are the most numerous cell types of the bone **(Figure 10-23)**. During the transition from osteoblasts to mature osteocyte, the cells lose a large part of their cellular organelles. Their cell processes are packed with microfilaments. The number of osteoblasts that get entrapped to become osteocytes depends on the rate at which the bone is forming. In woven bone formation and bone repair osteocytes are more. The space where the osteocytes reside is known as lacunae **(Figure 10-24)**. The osteocytes have cytoplasmic processes and are accommodated in a tubular space called canaliculi. Canaliculi connect the lacunae containing osteocytic cell body, with each other through gap junctions and with the exterior, *i.e.*, with the periosteal and endocortical surfaces of cortical bone, the lumen of blood vessels and Haversian canals, as well as the surfaces adjacent to the bone marrow on endocortical and cancellous bone surfaces. The lacunar-canalicular system also distributes osteocyte- secreted molecules within the bone or bone marrow microenvironment.

Osteocytes are considered a major source of molecules that regulate the activity of osteoclasts and osteoblasts. The integrity of the bone is maintained by the viable osteocytes. Further they are sensitive to mechanical strain, and in response to such stresses, communicate with surface osteoblasts and osteoclasts through canaliculi, and are actively involved in bone turnover.

Osteoclasts

Osteoclasts are specialized cells responsible for the resorption of bone. This function is critical in the maintenance, repair, and remodeling of bones. Bone is a dynamic tissue that is continuously being broken down and restructured. Resorption process also helps to regulate the blood calcium level.

Osteoclasts release hydrogen ions through the ruffled border into the resorption bays through the action of carbonic anhydrase ($H_2O + CO_2 \rightarrow 3^- + H^+$). This acidifies and aids in the dissolution of the mineralized bone matrix into Ca^{2+}, H_3PO_4, $H_2CO_3^-$, water, and other substances.

> Experiments suggest that osteoclasts play a role in the modulation of activity of the osteoblasts. Osteoclasts, tumor osteoclast-like cells, and chicken and human multinucleated giant cells produce a soluble factor that controls the collagen synthesizing activity of the osteoblasts.

Morphology

Osteoclasts are large multinucleated cells. The diameter of the osteoclasts is about 150–200 μm. The shape of the osteoclasts is variable since it is motile. The cell membrane of the osteoclast adjacent to resorbing bone forms a "ruffled border" or "brush border" consisting of multiple infoldings of the cell membrane **(Figure 10-25)**. This extensively folded ruffled border facilitates bone removal by considerably increasing the surface area of the cell, for secretion and uptake of the resorption contents and is a morphologic characteristic of an osteoclast that is actively resorbing the bone. It secretes acid and proteases across the ruffled border and these dissolve the minerals of bone and destroy the organic matrix. The cytoplasm is abundant, pale-staining, and has many acid phosphatase and lysosome containing vesicles and vacuoles. Mitochondria are

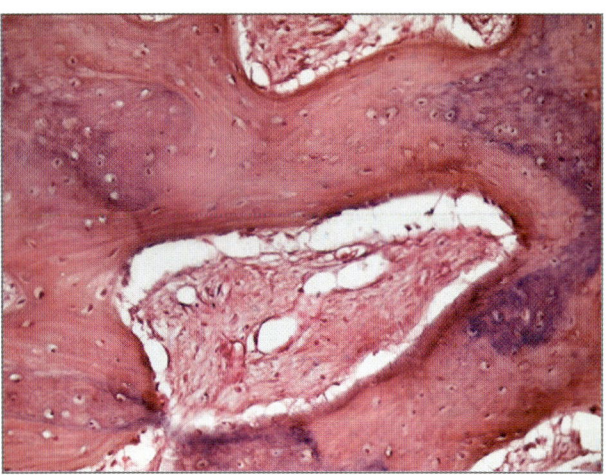

Figure 10-24: Osteocytes in lacunae.

CHAPTER 10: Alveolar Bone

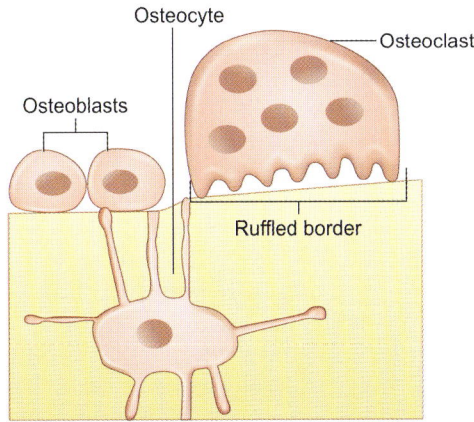

Figure 10-25: Structure of osteoclast.

more numerous adjacent to the ruffled border. Golgi bodies are extensive and are arranged in stacks. Microtubules in the cytoplasm help to transport vesicles between Golgi bodies and the ruffled border. The number of nuclei varies from 10 to 20. Individual nuclei within a single cell are small, round or oval, are uniform in size, and have a single prominent nucleolus.

Osteoclasts are usually seen in a bay-like depression in the bone surface usually not covered by osteoid. These depressions are called resorption bays, or Howship's lacunae **(Figures 10-26A and B)**. There are only 2–3 cells seen per 1 mm^3 of bone.

Formation

There has been considerable debate regarding the origin of osteoclasts. Previously it was believed that the osteoblasts and osteoclasts are of the same lineage, and osteoblasts fuse together to form osteoclasts. Currently it is accepted that the osteoclast is a hematopoietic cell derived from granulocyte macrophage colony forming unit (CFU-GM) and branches from the monocyte–macrophage lineage early during the differentiation process **(Figure 10-27)**. Osteoclast formation requires the presence of RANKL and macrophage colony-stimulating factor (M-CSF).

> Receptor activator of nuclear factor kappa B ligand is a member of the tumor necrosis factor family (TNF), and is essential in osteoclastogenesis. Osteoclast differentiation is inhibited by osteoprotegerin (OPG), which is produced by osteoblasts and binds to RANKL thereby preventing interaction with RANK. OPG is a member of TNF superfamily and represents a mature protein of 380 amino acids.

TNF-alpha stimulates osteoclast differentiation in the presence of M-CSF through a mechanism independent of the RANKL system.

Resorption and Regulation

In the resorption process, osteoclasts break down the tissue in bones and release the minerals, resulting in a transfer of calcium from bone to the blood. Osteoclasts produce a number of enzymes; chief among them is acid phosphatase. This enzyme dissolves collagen of the organic matrix and the calcium and phosphorus of the inorganic portion of bone. Bone is first broken into fragments; the osteoclast then engulfs the fragments and digests them within cytoplasmic vacuoles. Calcium and phosphorus liberated by the breakdown of the mineralized bone are released into the bloodstream.

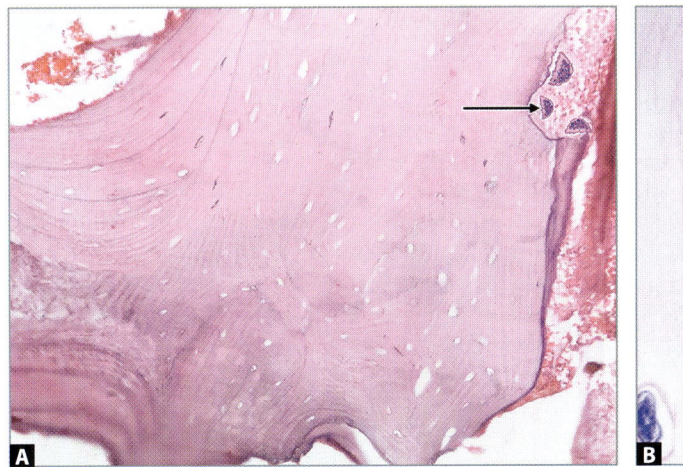
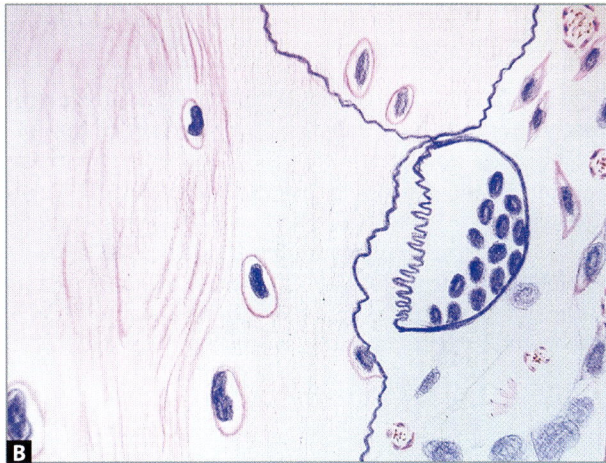

Figures 10-26A and B: (A) Osteoclasts in Howship's lacunae; (B) Schematic representation.

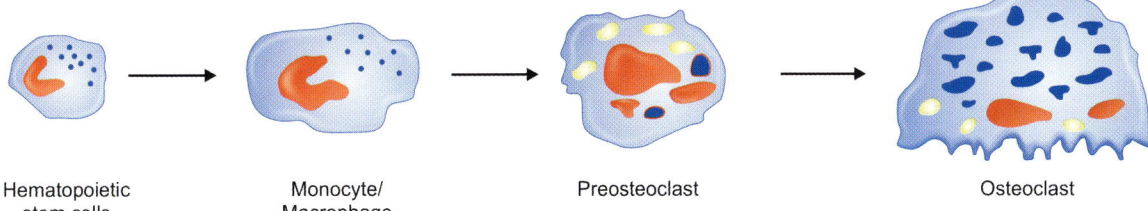

Figure 10-27: Formation of osteoclast.

Osteoclastic bone resorption is a two-phase process, which involves the solubilization of the mineral salts and the degradation of noncollagen bone matrix and collagen fibrils. It is assumed that the collagen fibrils are digested extracellularly in the resorption zone since recognizable collagen fibrils have been reported within cytoplasmic vacuoles of the osteoclasts. So the suggested hypothesis is, the osteoclastic resorption of bone involves the participation of two different cell types. Accordingly, osteoclastic bone resorption is initiated by osteoclasts that demineralize areas of bone and degrade noncollagen bone matrix. After the osteoclasts have moved away or become partially detached from the demineralized site, the exposed collagen fibrils are phagocytosed by mononuclear, fibroblast-like or monocyte-derived cells. This is supported by the fact that mononuclear cells are often found in close association with osteoclasts in Howship's lacunae and the resorbing bone produces a substance that is chemotactic for human monocytes. Also fibroblasts in the vicinity of osteoclasts in periodontal ligament contain many intracellular collagen fibrils associated with lysosome-like structures, whereas osteoclasts lack such profiles. There are indications that osteoclasts in different bony sites preferentially use different enzymes. Osteoclast–osteoblast communication occurs during bone remodeling.

It is generally accepted that bone resorption can be stimulated by parathyroid hormone (PTH) and inhibited by calcitonin. Estrogen suppresses the production of cytokines (IL-1 and IL-2) involved in bone resorption. Vitamin D3 promotes differentiation of osteoclast from monocyte–macrophage precursors *in vitro*. Bisphosphonates restrain bone resorption through injury and apoptosis to the osteoclasts.

■ BONE REMODELING

Bone is a metabolically active organ that undergoes continuous remodeling throughout the life. The process of removal of old bone and formation of new bone is called remodeling. Bones undergo a lifelong process of remodeling–formed bone tissue is removed and new bone tissue is formed. It is a highly regulated process that maintains a balance between bone resorption and formation, thus maintaining the skeletal integrity. Bone remodeling serves to adjust bone architecture to meet changing mechanical needs and it helps to repair microdamages in bone matrix preventing the accumulation of old bone. Further it plays an important role in maintaining plasma calcium homeostasis.

In general, when stress is applied to the bone, the body responds by activating osteoblasts to produce mineral matrix and form additional layers of cortical bone. When stress on the bone decreases, osteoclasts break down the mineral matrix to release mineral ions into the blood and reduce the bone mass. Thus, these processes help to control, sustain, preserve and provide the strength and mass to bones depending on what the body's activity level dictates. They also regulate mineral homeostasis either by storing extra minerals in cortical bone or releasing minerals into the blood when the body is mineral-deficient.

The remodeling process consists of three successive phases namely, resorption, during which osteoclasts remove the old bone; reversal, mononuclear cells appear on the bone surface; and formation, osteoblasts lay down new bone until the resorbed bone is completely replaced. During remodeling or maturation, the immature or woven bone is converted into mature bone **(Figure 10-28)**.

The woven bone consists of bone trabeculae and the soft tissue, comprising the marrow and its associated blood vessels. New bone is laid down in layers or lamellae over the surface of the trabeculae facing the marrow. This results in diminution of the volume of the soft tissue and ultimately only the blood vessels remain. This is called primary osteon. Osteocytes in this osteon appear large and irregular **(Figure 10-29)**.

Secondary osteon is formed by the resorption of the primary osteon and the woven bone and replacement with the soft tissue. New bone is laid down in the concave resorbed area. The secondary osteon is demarcated from the remaining unresorbed bone by a line called reversal line.

The regulation of bone remodeling is both systemically and locally mediated. The major systemic regulators include parathyroid hormone, calcitriol, and other hormones such as growth hormone, glucocorticoids, thyroid hormones, and sex hormones. Factors such as insulin-like growth factors (IGFs), prostaglandins, tumor growth factor-beta (TGF-beta), bone morphogenetic proteins (BMP), and cytokines are involved as well. Local mediators include a number of cytokines and growth factors.

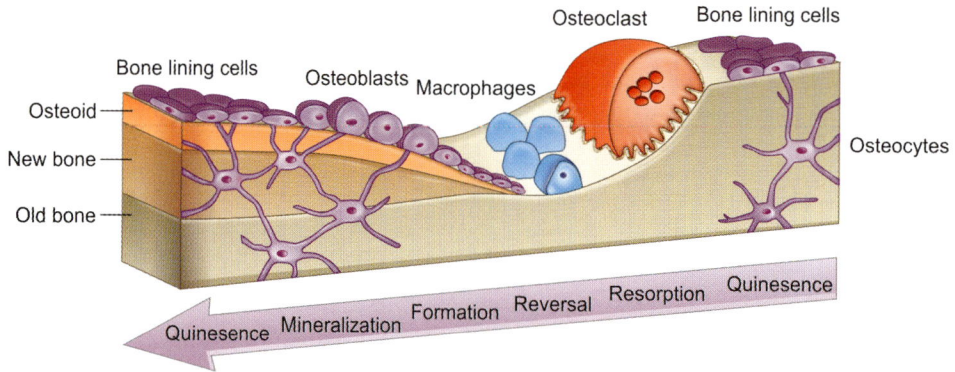

Figure 10-28: Steps in bone remodeling.

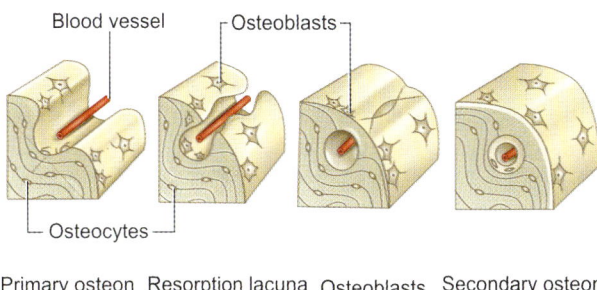

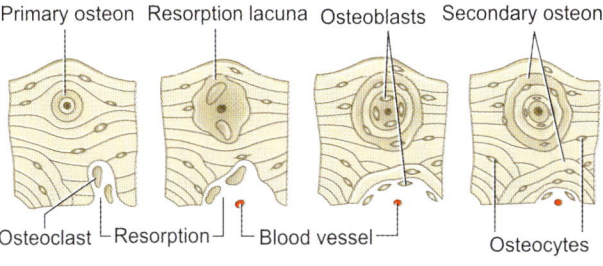

Figure 10-29: Bone remodeling.

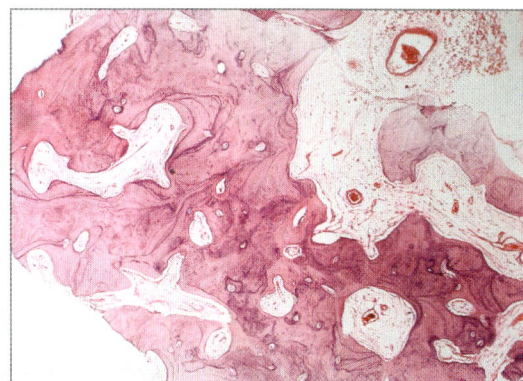

Figure 10-31: Reversal lines.

ALVEOLAR BONE

As defined earlier it is that part of maxilla or mandible that forms the socket to accommodate the teeth. The boundary between the body of the maxilla or the mandible and their respective alveolar bone is indistinct. It is a tooth-dependent structure. The shape of the alveolar processes depends on the size, shape, and position of the teeth **(Figure 10-32)**. Apart from accommodating the roots of the teeth, alveolar bone absorbs and distributes the masticatory forces generated during chewing; it also supplies nutrition to the periodontal ligament via the blood vessels. Further while supporting the deciduous teeth, it houses and protects the developing permanent teeth and helps in the eruption of deciduous and permanent teeth. The alveolar process consists of an outer bony plate (cortical plate) of varying thickness, covered by periosteum on the facial and lingual sides, an inner perforated bony plate (cribriform plate) called alveolar bone proper, and the spongy bone between the cortical plate and the alveolar bone proper **(Figure 10-33)**.

The cortical plate and the alveolar bone proper meet at the alveolar crest.

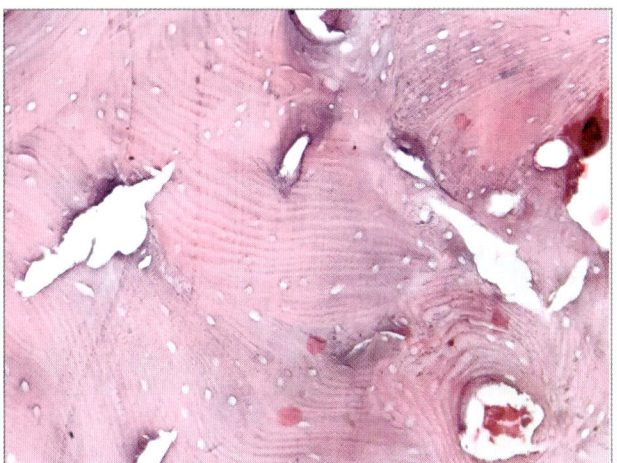

Figure 10-30: Resting lines.

Further there is an association between muscle activity and bone formation or resorption. Bone resorption is accelerated when there is absence of muscular activity. When there is muscle activity, tension is transmitted to the bone. Osteocytes produce prostaglandins and IGF-1, which stimulate the osteoblasts to form bone.

Incremental Lines (Resting Lines)

Similar to hard tissues of the tooth, bone is also formed in a rhythmic pattern. There exists a period of activity and period of rest. This is reflected by the incremental lines. These lines are hypomineralized and parallel to each other **(Figure 10-30)**.

Reversal Lines

These lines demarcate the region of resorbed bone and the newly forming bone, *i.e.*, the remodeling site. They appear hematoxylin, scalloped and irregular **(Figure 10-31)**.

DEVELOPMENT OF MAXILLA AND MANDIBLE

Maxilla and mandible develop from the first branchial arch and both develop by intramembranous ossification.

Maxilla

Maxilla, which is a hollow pyramidal structure, develops in the mesenchyme of the maxillary process from the mandibular arch (the first branchial arch). It contributes to the formation of middle third of the face, lateral wall and floor of the nasal cavity, floor of the orbit, and roof of the oral cavity. Maxilla develops from the center of ossification of the maxillary process and there is no separate premaxillary ossification center in human. In the 8th week of intrauterine life, the center of ossification begins immediately lateral to and slightly below the infraorbital region, where it gives off its anterior superior dental branch, close to the site of developing deciduous canine tooth. This ossification center

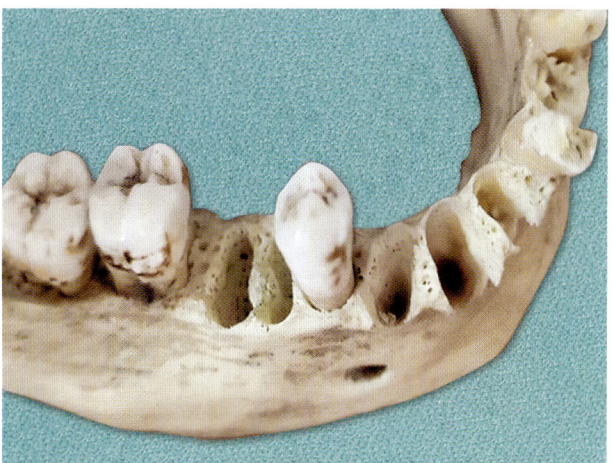

Figure 10-32: Mandibular bone showing different shapes of alveolar socket.

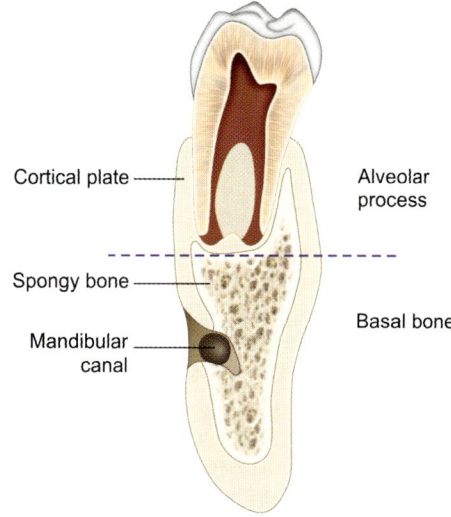

Figure 10-33: Parts of the alveolar process.

is associated with the cartilage of the nasal capsule. This serves as the primary cartilage, as there is no primary cartilage present in the maxillary arch. A secondary cartilage, from the zygomatic process also contributes to the development of maxilla. Growth of the maxilla is initiated from the center of ossification and spreads posteriorly below the orbit toward the developing zygoma; anteriorly toward the developing incisor region; upward to form the frontal process of maxilla; downward to form the alveolar plate of maxilla and medially into the palatine process to form the hard palate **(Figures 10-34A and B)**. The medial and lateral alveolar plates, which extend as a downward growth, form a trough of bone around the maxillary tooth germs. Premaxilla, which is the incisor bearing part of the maxilla, was thought to have a separate center for ossification. But it has been found that ossification in the incisor-bearing region develops from the body of maxilla itself. Medial alveolar plate is formed at the junction between the body of the maxilla and palatal process. Also the development and growth of maxilla is little influenced by secondary cartilages, which appear in the region of zygomatic or malar process, margins of the alveolar plate, and in the midline of developing hard palate.

In the initial stages, the body of the maxilla is relatively small due to the nondevelopment of sinus. In the 4th month of intrauterine life, maxillary sinus appears as an outgrowth from the lateral wall of the nasal cavity. At this stage, the sinus is in the size of a small pea. It enlarges with the growing maxilla after birth and attains a fully developed stage following the eruption of the permanent dentition. Development of sinus forms a hollow in the maxilla separating its upper or orbital surface from its lower or dental surface.

Sutural growth, development of alveolar process, subperiosteal bone formation, enlargement of maxillary sinus, and bone remodeling (resorption and deposition) contribute to the growth of maxilla. Surrounding structures like orbital, nasal, and oral cavities are also associated with maxillary growth and thereby is not an isolated developmental process. Sutural growth continues until 10 years of age and the maxilla articulates with the other bones of skull by frontomaxillary, zygomaticomaxillary, zygomaticotemporal, and pterygopalatine sutures. All the sutures contribute to the forward and downward growth of the maxilla. The height of the maxilla is determined by the development of

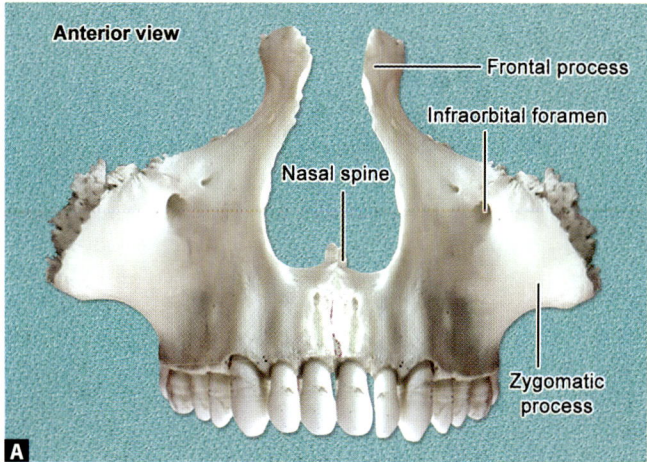
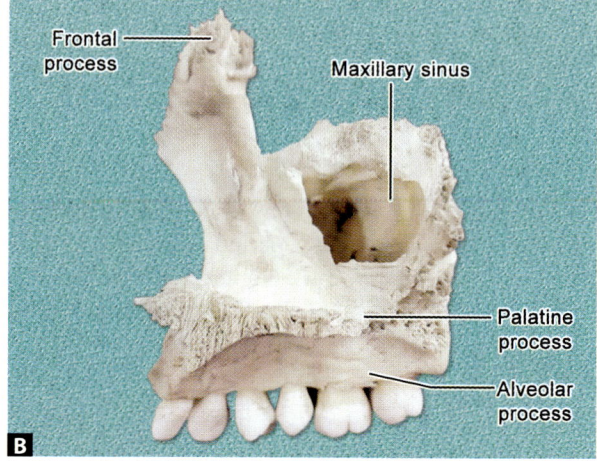

Figures 10-34A and B: Parts of the maxilla.

alveolar process especially during the eruption of permanent dentition. Maxillary sinus, which occupies most of the body of the maxilla, contributes to its growth by a process called pneumatization, which involves bone resorption on the sinus side (inner portion) and bone deposition on the facial surface of the maxillary process. Bone remodeling at the floor of the nasal cavity also increases the height of the maxilla **(Figure 10-35)**.

At birth, the maxilla is greater in its transverse and anteroposterior dimension when compared to its height. The body of the maxilla is little more than the alveolar process and the frontonasal process is prominent. The tooth-bearing areas reach almost to the floor of the orbit. Maxillary sinus will be like a furrow on the lateral wall of the nose. As age advances, the bone reverts to its infantile condition in its size by reduction in the height of the body and alveolar process following tooth loss.

Mandible

Mandible the strongest, largest, and the only movable bone of the skull, develops within the mandibular process of mandibular arch **(Figure 10-36)**. Meckel's cartilage, the cartilage of first arch is closely associated anatomically to the developing mandible but does not contribute much to its development. In the 6th week of intrauterine life, this cartilage extends as a rod of cartilaginous tissue, from the developing ear region to the symphysis, providing a framework for the formation of bone. Mandibular nerve, which is a branch of trigeminal nerve is closely associated with this Meckel's cartilage and divides itself into lingual nerve on the medial aspect and inferior alveolar nerve on the lateral aspect. Further, the inferior alveolar nerve in turn divides into incisor and mental branches.

Condensation of mesenchyme occurs during 7th week of intrauterine life, at the site close to future mental foramen,

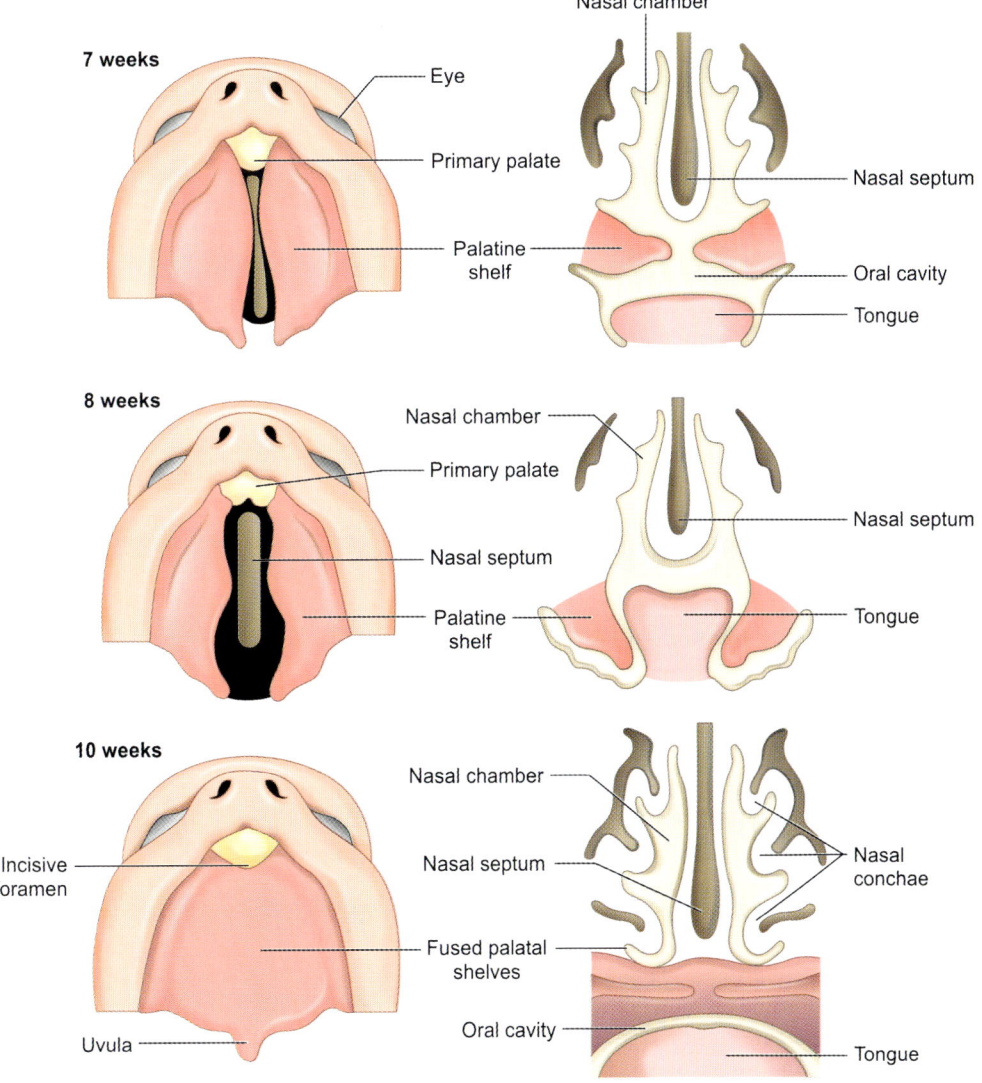

Figure 10-35: Development of the maxilla.

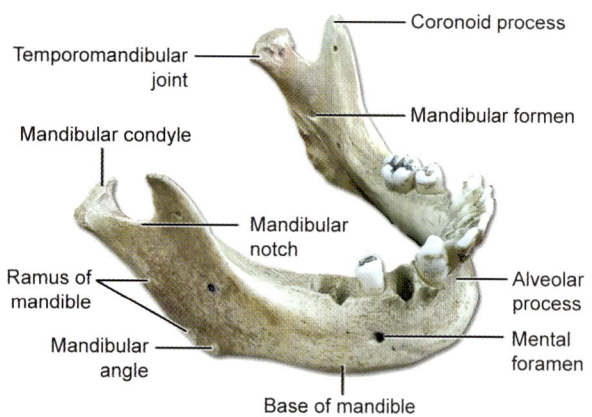

Figure 10-36: Structure of the mandible.

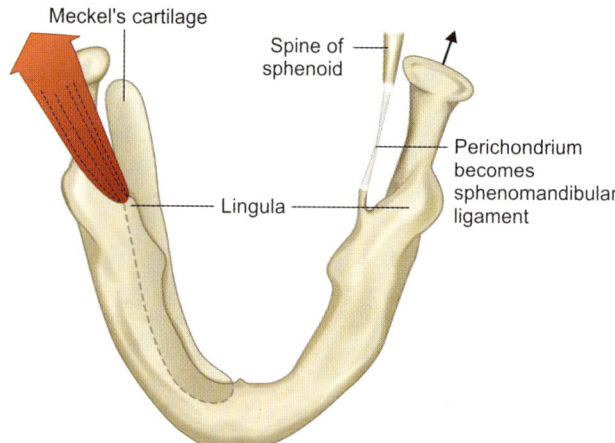

Figure 10-38: Divergent spread of ossification.

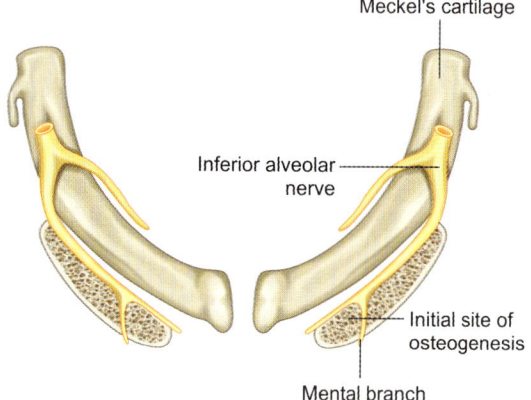

Figure 10-37: Development of mandible.

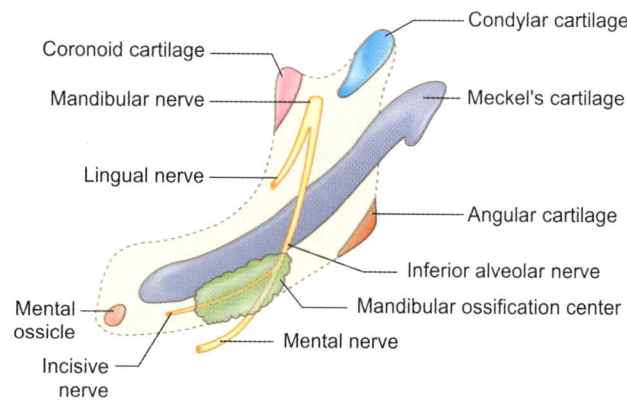

Figure 10-39: Secondary cartilages.

which is marked as a center for ossification **(Figure 10-37)**. Continuous deposition of bone on the lateral aspect of Meckel's cartilage in a forward, backward, and upward direction corresponding to the future body of the mandible. The two cartilaginous processes on either side with bone deposition on its lateral aspect approximate with each other at the midline but remain separated for a short period after birth. The trough-shaped cavity is then transformed into a canal by the joining of lateral and medial plates with the nerve at its center. Extension of ossification in a backward direction until a point where the mandibular nerve divides contributes to the increase in the size of mandible. Subdivision of the bony trough takes place by the formation of medial and lateral alveolar plates to accommodate the developing tooth germs. Thus the entire body of the mandible is formed with the teeth occupying individual compartments along with the neurovascular bundles within its own body canal.

A divergent spread of ossification occurs posteriorly in the mesenchyme of first arch, turning away from the Meckel's cartilage, which is marked by lingula in the adult mandible (point of entry for inferior alveolar nerve) **(Figure 10-38)**. Rapid spread of ossification from this region contributes to the development of ramus and the rudimentary mandible is thus formed mostly by intramembranous ossification by 10 weeks of development. Although not much significant tissue is contributed by Meckel's cartilage, it terminates itself in its posterior extremity to form incus and malleus of the inner ear, sphenomalleolar and sphenomandibular ligament behind the body of mandible and nodular remnants in the symphysis region until birth.

Secondary cartilages, which contribute to the further growth of mandible, develop between 10th and 14th week *in utero*. These cartilages include condylar, coronoid, and symphyseal **(Figure 10-39)**. Condylar cartilage is the largest and most important of all the three as it serves as an important center of growth of the mandible up to 16th year of life. It occupies most of the developing ramus at 12 weeks of development by attaining a cone-shaped or carrot-shaped mass, which is converted sooner into bone by endochondral ossification. A thin layer of cartilage remains at the end of 20 weeks and this remnant persists until the end of second decade of life. The developing condyle articulates with the temporal bone above by the condensation of mesenchyme between these two structures to form temporomandibular joint. Coronoid cartilage, which surmounts the anterior and upper border of coronoid process, is a transient growth cartilage that disappears before birth. Symphyseal cartilage, which are two in number on each side, appear in between the opposing end of Meckel's cartilage and disappear soon after birth.

At birth, the body of the mandible is greater than the ramus in size and the mandible on either side are separated at the

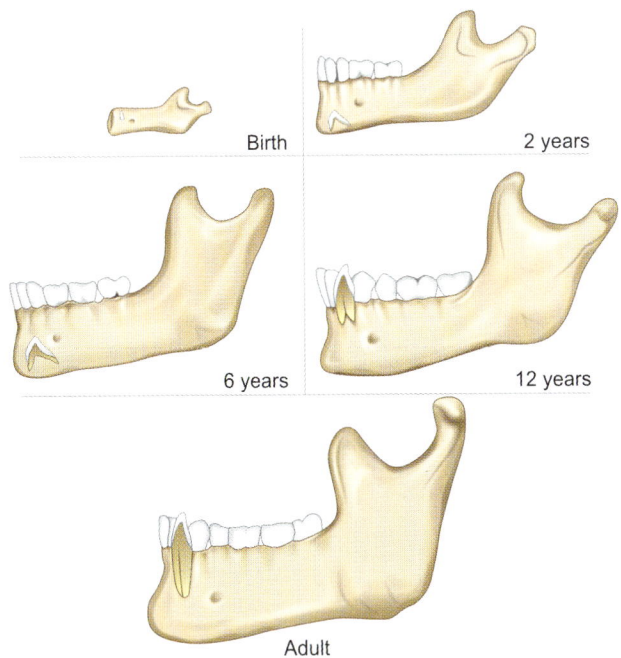

Figure 10-40: Growth of the mandible.

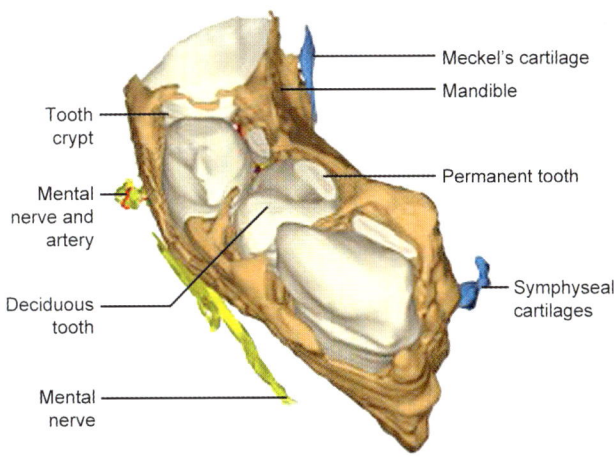

Figure 10-41: Tooth crypt.

symphysis. During the second year, ossification of the symphysis takes place resulting in the formation of single bone. As age advances, growth of the mandible in terms of height, width, and length occurs by remodeling of bone in the body, ramus, condylar, and coronoid processes **(Figure 10-40)**.

DEVELOPMENT OF ALVEOLAR PROCESS

Root development and the development of the supporting tissues of the tooth occur simultaneously. The supporting tissues of the tooth, namely-cementum, periodontal ligament, and alveolar bone have a common origin, *i.e.*, from the cells of the dental sac.

Alveolar process develops only during the eruption of the teeth. In early stage this bone forms a thin eggshell of support known as tooth crypt **(Figure 10-41)**. At the end of the 2nd month of intrauterine life, the developing maxilla and mandible form a groove which is open toward the oral cavity. Tooth germs at late bell stage develop within this bony crypt along with their associated vessels and nerves. Individual tooth germs are separated from one another by the formation of septum in between the adjacent tooth germs. Dental sac is present between the vertical bony septum and the developing tooth.

According to the growth of the jaws, the tooth germs exhibit bodily movements by bone remodeling. Alveolar process begins to be distinct when there is formation of the root. As the roots develop, the alveolar processes increase in height. The cells of the dental sac differentiate to become osteoblasts and form the alveolar bone proper. During this time the dental sac cells also differentiate into fibroblasts and cementoblasts to form periodontal ligament and cementum.

> At birth, maxilla and mandible contains ten primitive tooth crypts separated from one another by interdental septa. Deciduous teeth are contained in these crypts. These primitive tooth crypts occupy the larger part of the body of the maxilla and mandible.

The developing deciduous teeth and the permanent first molar are covered occlusally by the oral mucosa. The permanent molars at first are completely surrounded by bone. The mandibular permanent tooth germs lie first at the corresponding deciduous tooth germs bony compartment and acquire their own bony crypt, after the deciduous teeth begin to erupt. Later a horizontal plate of bone develops, which separates the dental crypt from mandibular canal.

When the alveolar processes are forming, their free border grows more rapidly and the crest of the alveolar process is composed of chondroid bone (has the characteristics of both the bone and cartilage). During intrauterine life, the developing alveolus, similar to the rest of the skeleton is formed from an embryonic type of bone. This is gradually replaced by mature lamellar bone of compact or spongy type.

STRUCTURE OF ALVEOLAR BONE

Alveolar bone has two parts, namely alveolar bone proper and supporting alveolar bone, which consists of the cortical plate and the spongy bone in between the two bony plates. The thickness of the alveolar bones varies between teeth and different regions of the same tooth. It is usually thinner at the crest and thicker at the apical portion of the socket.

Alveolar Bone Proper

It is a thin lamellae of bone that forms the inner wall of the tooth sockets. It is of 0.1–0.4 mm thick, surrounds the root of the teeth, and gives attachment to the periodontal ligament fibers. It is called cribriform plate (lamina cribrosa) since it is perforated by the many openings that transmit the interalveolar nerves and vessels **(Figure 10-42)**. Though it has perforations, on radiograph it appears as radiopaque, known as lamina dura, due to the presence of compacted lamellae **(Figure 10-43)**. The bony partition between two adjacent teeth is called interdental septum, which is made up entirely of cribriform plate. Interradicular septum again made up of cribriform plate lies in between the roots of multirooted teeth. Interdental and interradicular arteries, veins, lymph vessels, and nerves lie in canals called perforation canals of Zuckerkandl and Hirschfeld **(Figure 10-44)**.

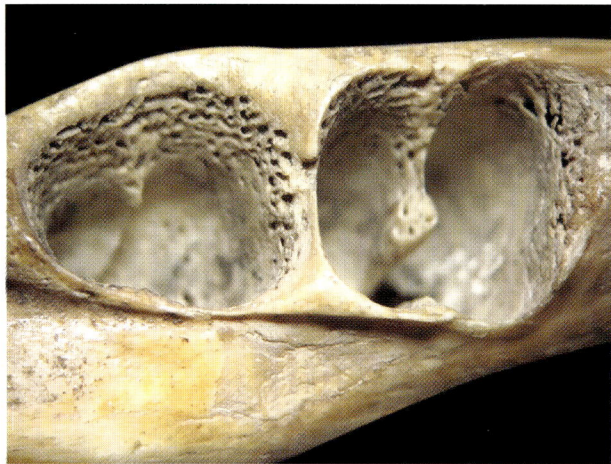

Figure 10-42: Cribriform plate.

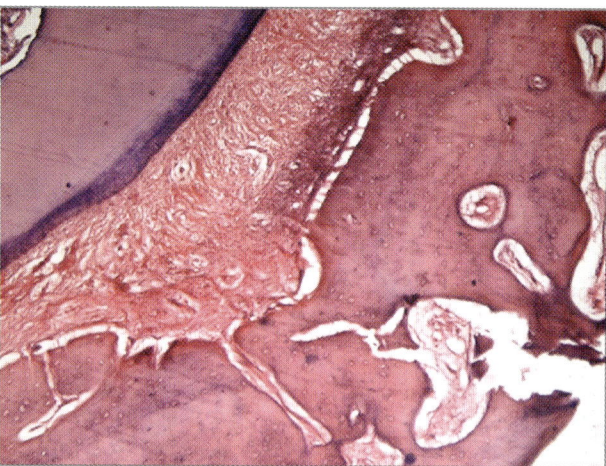

Figure 10-45: Sharpey's fibers.

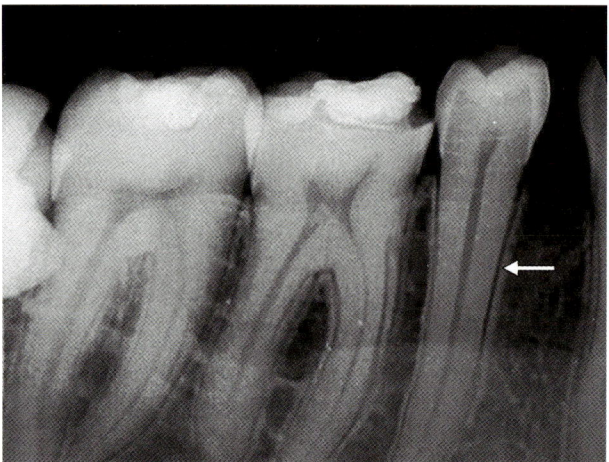

Figure 10-43: Lamina dura (arrows).
Source: Dr Ragu Ganesh, Department of Oral Medicine, Meenakshi Ammal Dental College, Chennai, Tamil Nadu, India

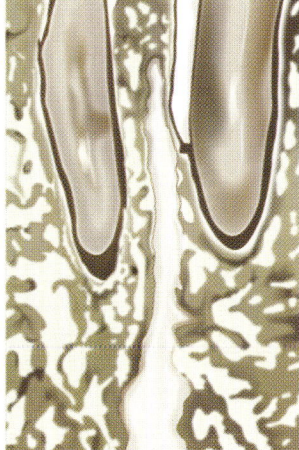

Figure 10-44: Canal of Zuckerkandl and Hirschfeld.

Alveolar bone consists mainly of bundle bone, since bundles of periodontal ligament fibers are inserted into it. The surface of the alveolar bone proper adjacent to the periodontal ligament consists of multiple layers of bone parallel to the alveolar socket wall. This bony plate is penetrated by bundles of Sharpey's fibers, which are embedded perpendicular to the surface **(Figure 10-45)**.

Supporting Alveolar Bone

It consists of cortical plate or the alveolar cortex and the cancellous bone in the center portion. The structure of the cortical plate is similar to other compact bone of the body, made up of lamellar bone, and consists of Haversian system and interstitial lamellae **(Figure 10-46)**. The thickness of the alveolar cortex is variable. It is more pronounced in the mandible and thicker in some places, than that of the maxilla. It is generally thicker in lingual side than the facial side. The cancellous bone or the spongiosa is comprised of network of delicate trabeculae interspersed in the marrow space **(Figure 10-47)**. The marrow is usually of fatty type. Red marrow or hematopoietic marrow is found in angle of the mandible and maxillary tuberosity. Maxillary alveolar process contains more cancellous bone than the mandible. The bony trabeculae within the cancellous bone vary in thickness and are typed as fine, medium, and coarse. Further based on the arrangement of the trabeculae, they are categorized into type I and type II. Type I the trabeculae are laid parallel to the body of the bone in layers compared to the ladder, more pronounced in mandible compared to the maxilla. The distinct trajectory pattern in mandible is well accommodated in this pattern. In type II, the trabeculae are randomly arranged and comparatively more in number and are noticed in delicate interdental and interradicular bone along with few areas of maxilla.

▮ REMODELING OF ALVEOLAR BONE

During the jaw growth and tooth eruption, remodeling takes place extensively in the alveolar processes. Periosteal and endosteal new bone formation occurs during this period with the remodeling of the entire Haversian system and interstitial bone. Alveolar bone turnover rate is higher than that of other bones. Though bone is actively being remodeled as in alveolar process, complete replacements by secondary osteon never occurs.

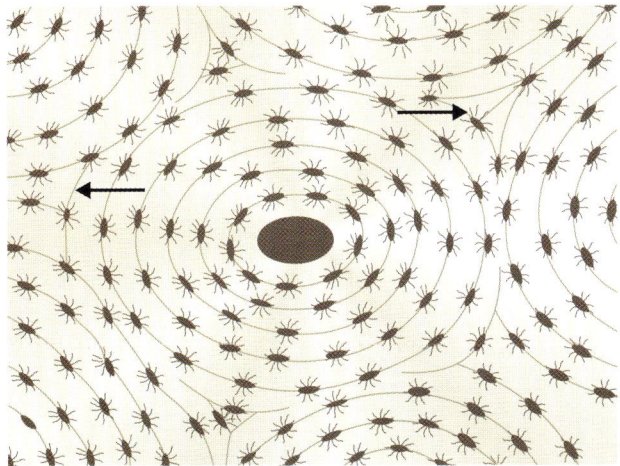

Figure 10-46: Interstitial lamella.

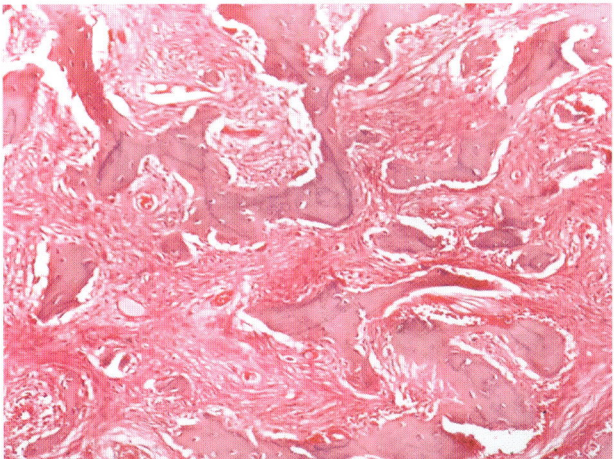

Figure 10-47: Cancellous bone.

Osteoprotegerin, also known as osteoclastogenesis inhibitory factor (OCIF), protects bone from excessive resorption by binding to RANKL and preventing it from binding to RANK. Osteoclast differentiation is regulated by RANKL/RANK signaling. This signaling also helps in activation and survival of osteoclasts in normal bone remodeling. Osteoprotegerin acts as a decoy receptor for RANKL. By binding to RANKL, OPG prevents RANK-mediated nuclear factor kappa B (NF-κB) activation, which is a central and rapid acting transcription factor for immune-related genes, and a key regulator of inflammation, innate immunity, and cell survival and differentiation.

AGE CHANGES

Bone changes occur during normal aging in both sexes. The equilibrium between the bone formation and resorption changes with increasing age, resulting in loss of bone tissue. In aging bone, the mineral content is reduced, and is prone for osteoporosis—a condition in which bones are less dense, more fragile, and liable for fractures.

Changes are both quantitative and qualitative, which include, alterations in the dynamics of bone cell populations, resulting in uncoupling of the normal process of bone resorption and formation, changes in bone architecture (*e.g.*, rearrangement of trabeculae) and cross-sectional geometry (characterized by subperiosteal expansion and enlargement of the medullary cavity), occurrence of microfractures, localized disparity in the concentration of minerals, with hypomineralization in some areas and hypermineralization in others, changes in the properties of mineral crystals, and changes in the protein content of matrix material.

Aging results in fatty infiltration of the marrow spaces. There is reduction in the height of the alveolar bone **(Figure 10-48)**. Proliferative capacity and the formative function are reduced. The surface facing the periodontal ligament becomes irregular.

CLINICAL CONSIDERATIONS

The existence of alveolar bone is tooth-dependent. When the tooth is lost, the alveolar bone undergoes resorption. When the tooth is not formed or not erupted alveolar bone does not form completely. There is equilibrium between bone formation and resorption, which maintains the height and density. Resorption of alveolar bone occurs due to periodontitis (inflammation of the tissues of the periodontium), trauma from occlusion, and systemic diseases **(Figure 10-49)**.

Periodontitis usually starts as gingival inflammation (gingivitis). There is change in the composition of bacterial plaque, which occurs when there is transition of gingivitis to periodontitis. Inflammation spreads to involve the marrow spaces of the alveolar bone from gingiva. This is characterized by the replacement of marrow with leukocytes and fluid exudates, and proliferation of endothelial cells and fibroblasts. Further there is increase in mononuclear phagocytes and multinucleated osteoclasts, which results in resorption of the alveolar bone.

Resorption of alveolar bone is a characteristic feature in progressive periodontal diseases. Endotoxins of the gram-negative bacteria of the dental plaque cause increase in cyclic adenosine monophosphate (cAMP), which results in osteoclastic activation and resorption of the alveolar bone. Bone loss in periodontitis is of two types, namely horizontal bone loss and vertical bone loss **(Figures 10-50A and B)**.

Horizontal bone loss is characterized by reduction in the height of the alveolar crest and is more prevalent. In vertical or angular bone loss, resorption occurs adjacent to the tooth surface, resulting in a triangular defect.

Dehiscences and fenestrations represent anatomical variations concerning the shape and the morphology of the alveolar bone. A fenestration is an isolated "window" of bone loss on the facial or lingual aspect of a tooth that places the exposed root surface directly in contact with gingiva. The alveolar marginal bone is intact. When the denuded area involves the alveolar margin it is termed as dehiscence **(Figures 10-51A to C)**. Their undiagnosed or unexpected presence may affect the periodontal surgical procedures or require changes in dental implant placement protocols.

Bone resorbs on the side of pressure and apposes on the side of tension. This property is utilized in orthodontic

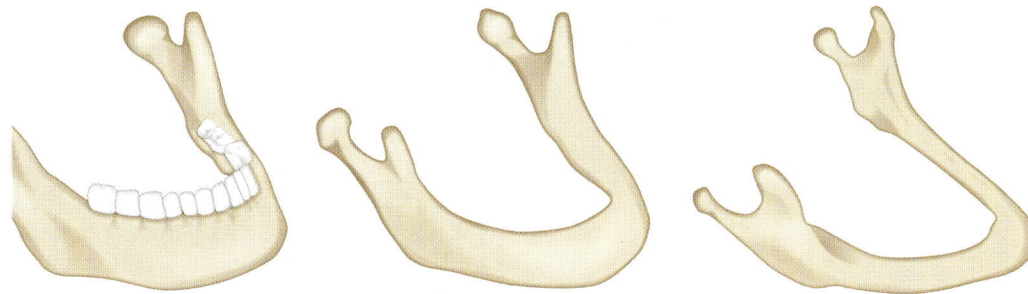

Figure 10-48: Age changes in mandible.

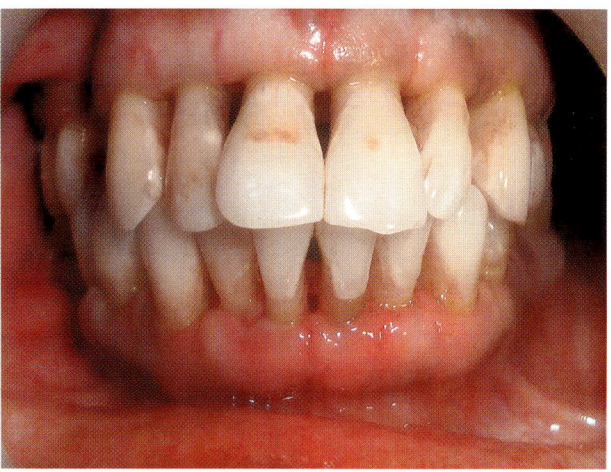

Figure 10-49: Alveolar bone resorption in periodontitis.
Source: Dr Burnice Nalinakumari, Department of Periodontics, Meenakshi Ammal Dental College, Chennai, Tamil Nadu, India.

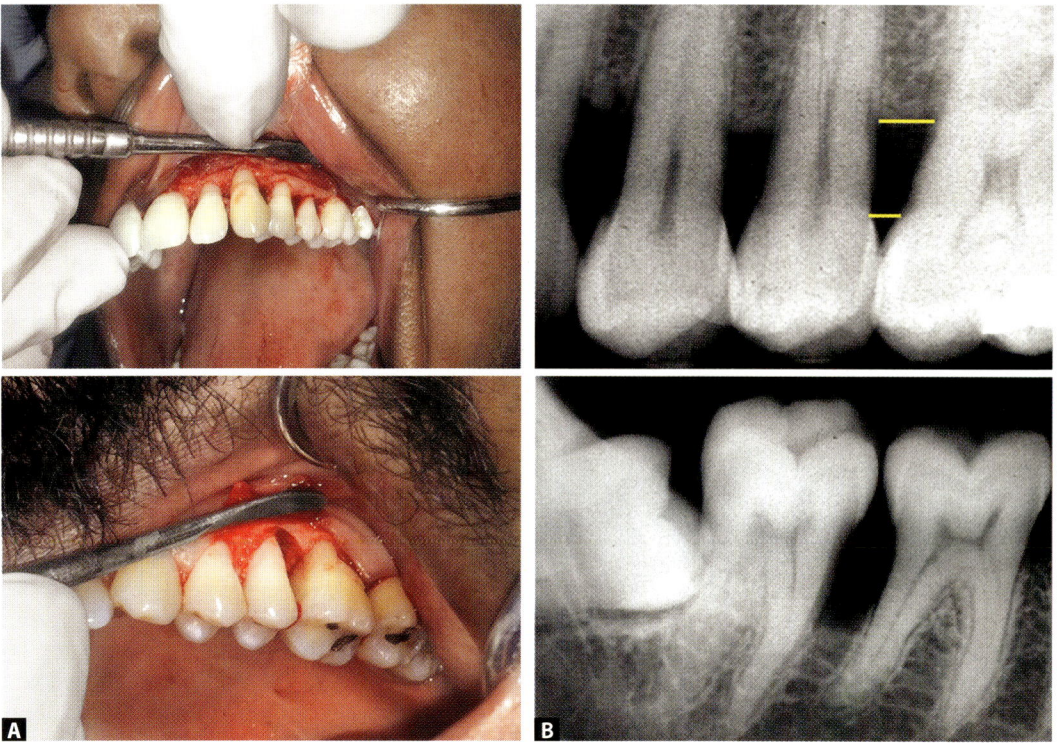

Figures 10-50A and B: (A) Horizontal bone loss; (B) Vertical bone loss.
Source: Dr Rahul Visvanathan, Department of Periodontics, Meenakshi Ammal Dental College, Chennai, Tamil Nadu, India.

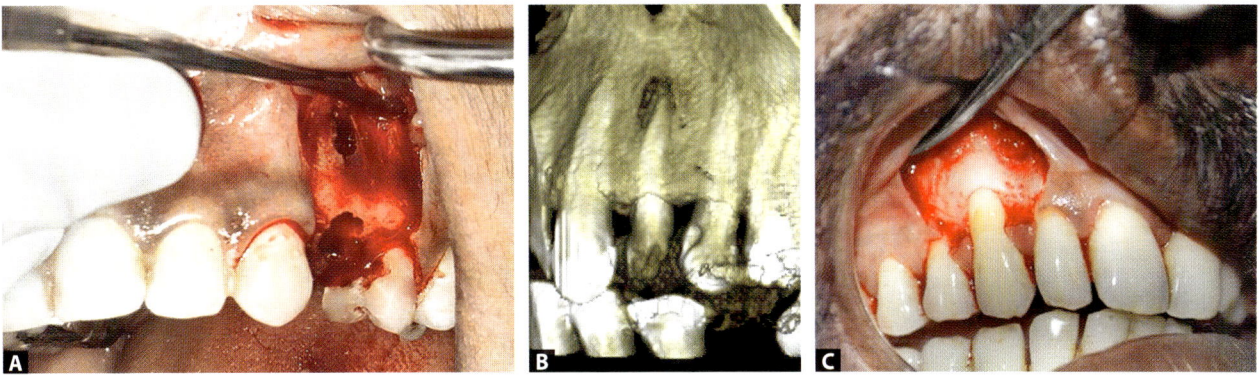

Figures 10-51A to C: (A and B) Fenestration; (C) Dehiscence.
Source: Dr Rahul Visvanathan, Department of Periodontics, Meenakshi Ammal Dental College, Chennai, Tamil Nadu, India.

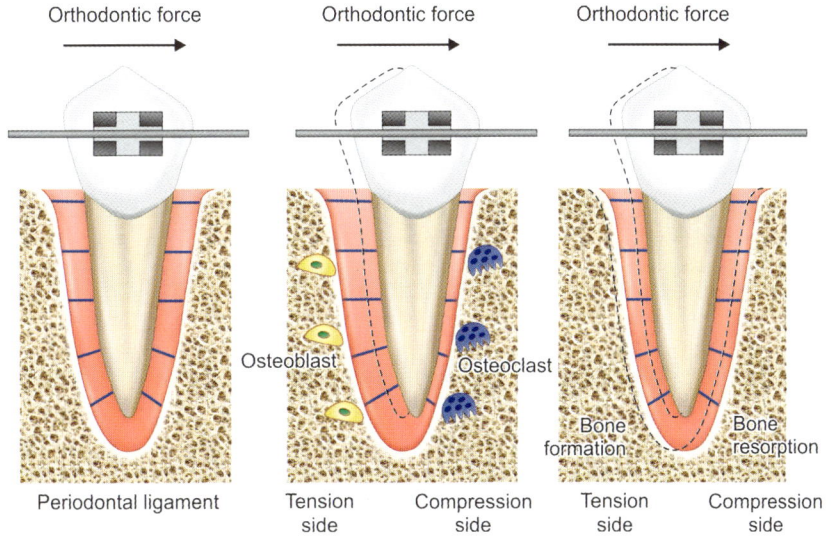

Figure 10-52: Bone remodeling during orthodontic treatment.

tooth movement **(Figure 10-52)**. In the pressure side there is compression of blood vessels and injury to the periodontium and increase in cAMP in cells, which play a role in bone resorption. The initial resorption process involves osteoblasts, which secrete collagenolytic enzymes and thereby remove the extracellular matrix to facilitate the access of osteoclasts precursors to the bone surface. Further they also elaborate cytokines and chemokines, which attract monocyte precursors and enhance osteoclasts differentiation. Osteoblasts are activated at the site of tension to produce new bone.

Occlusal forces are transmitted to the periodontal attachment apparatus and these forces can cause changes in the bone and connective tissue. Trauma from occlusion also results in destruction of alveolar bone. This may be acute or chronic. Acute trauma from occlusion can be a result of, an abrupt occlusal impact due to biting of a hard object and restorations or prosthetic appliances with high points that interfere with or alter the occlusal forces on teeth.

Chronic trauma from occlusion is more common than acute trauma. It develops from gradual changes in occlusion produced by tooth wear, drifting movement due to loss of adjacent tooth, extrusion of teeth, and parafunctional habits such as bruxism and clenching.

Apart from local causes, some of the systemic disorders also affect the alveolar bone. Primary hyperparathyroidism is a systemic disease that causes hypercalcemia and affects bone remodeling. Alveolar bone is particularly sensitive to increased levels of parathyroid hormone from either primary or secondary hyperparathyroidism. Generalized loss of lamina dura in radiographs occurs in hyperparathyroidism due to the involvement of the alveolar bone proper. Decreased cortical bone density and increased likelihood of oral tori have also been reported.

Points to Remember

- Bone is a vascular and mineralized connective tissue, gives the skeletal framework and acts as a reservoir of calcium.
- Bone is made up of 60–70% inorganic (calcium phosphate hydroxyl apatite crystals) and 30-40% of organic materials (collagen fibers and ground substance) and water.
- Bones can be classified according to the shape, development, structure, and microstructure.
- Osteoblasts are the cells responsible for bone formation. They get entrapped inside the bone matrix (osteoid) and become osteocytes. The osteoblasts secrete the bone matrix called osteoid, which consists of collagen precursors and other organic proteins. The osteoid mineralizes within a few days and hardens.
- Osteoclasts are multinucleated cells, which resorb bone. The cell membrane of the osteoclasts adjacent to resorbing bone is thrown into multiple infoldings called "ruffled border" or "brush border". Osteoclasts are usually seen in a bay-like depression called resorption bays, or Howship's lacunae.
- Formation of bone is called osteogenesis. This occurs in two steps. First there is formation of bone matrix called osteoid, which is composed of collagen fibers and ground substance. This mineralizes to form the bone. Mineralization is regulated by vitamin D, and parathyroid hormone. When matrix matures, there is expression of alkaline phosphatase and several other proteins, including osteocalcin, osteopontin, and bone sialoproteins.
- Bone is formed in two ways, *i.e,* intramembranous and endochondral ossification. In intramembranous ossification, the mesenchymal cells proliferate and condense into compact nodules. Some of these cells differentiate into capillaries, while others will become osteoblasts.
- In endochondral ossification, bone develops by replacing the hyaline cartilage. Cartilage does not become bone. Instead, cartilage formed from the aggregated mesenchymal cells, serves as a template to be completely replaced by new bone.
- Incremental lines of the bone reflect the period of activity and period of rest.
- The structural and functional unit of the compact bone is known as *osteon*, or Haversian system. Osteon is a cylindrical structure made up of concentric sheets or layers of calcified matrix called lamellae. Center of each osteon contains a canal called *Haversian canal*, which contains blood vessels, lymphatic vessels, and nerves. These vessels and nerves branch off at right angles through a perforating canal known as *Volkmann's canal*, to extend to the periosteum and endosteum.
- Fine fiber bundle bone is the matured, lamellated bone in which there is regular and parallel alignment of collagen fibers into sheets or lamellae and is mechanically strong.
- Coarse woven bone is characterized by a haphazard arrangement of collagen fibers and is mechanically weak. This usually occurs when the bone is rapidly laid down (in repair and during the development of embryo).
- The process of removal of old bone and formation of new bone is called remodeling, which is a lifelong process. Bone remodeling occurs to meet changing mechanical needs. It also plays an important role in maintaining plasma calcium homeostasis. The regulation of bone remodeling is both systemically and locally mediated.
- Reversal lines demarcate the region of resorbed bone and the newly forming bone in the remodeling site. They appear hematoxylin, scalloped and irregular.
- Alveolar bone is that part of maxilla or mandible and forms the tooth socket. It transmits the forces of mastication to the jaw bone. It also supplies nutrition to the periodontal ligament via the blood vessels. Further while supporting the deciduous teeth, it houses and protects the developing permanent teeth.
- The existence of the alveolar bone depends on the presence or absence of teeth. When teeth are lost the alveolar bone resorbs. If teeth are developmentally missing the alveolar bone is poorly developed.
- Alveolar bone develops from the dental sac cells and the alveolar process develops only during the eruption of the teeth.
- Alveolar process begins to be distinct when there is formation of the root. As the roots develop, the alveolar processes increase in height. The cells of the dental sac differentiate to become osteoblasts and form the alveolar bone proper.
- Alveolar bone has two parts, namely alveolar bone proper and supporting alveolar bone, which consists of the cortical plate and the spongy bone in between the two bony plates.
- Alveolar bone proper is made up of thin lamellae of bone that forms the inner wall of the tooth sockets. It is of 0.1–0.4 mm thick, surrounds the tooth root, and gives attachment to the periodontal ligament fibers.
- Supporting alveolar bone consists of cortical plate and the center portion is made up of cancellous bone.
- During the jaw growth and tooth eruption, remodeling takes place extensively in the alveolar processes.
- In aging the equilibrium between the bone formation and resorption is altered, resulting in loss of bone tissue. The mineral content is reduced, and is prone for osteoporosis—a condition in which bones are less dense, more fragile, and liable for fractures in aging. Aging also results in fatty infiltration of the marrow spaces. There is reduction in the height of the alveolar bone.
- Resorption of alveolar bone occurs due to periodontitis, trauma from occlusion, and systemic diseases.
- Bone resorbed on the side of pressure and deposited on the side of tension. This property is utilized in orthodontic tooth movement.
- Some of the systemic disorders also affect the alveolar bone. Primary hyperparathyroidism is a systemic disease that causes hypercalcemia and affects bone remodeling.

PRACTICE QUESTIONS

1. What is bone?
2. Write notes on development of bone.
3. Describe the development of maxilla and mandible.
4. Describe the development of alveolar process.
5. Write a notes on aging of bone.
6. Write a notes on bone remodeling.
7. Describe the structure of alveolar bone.

CHAPTER 10: Alveolar Bone

MULTIPLE CHOICE QUESTIONS

1. **Functions of bone does not include:**
   a. Gives skeletal frame work of the body
   b. Calcium reservoir
   c. Formation of cartilage
   d. Gives attachment to the muscle fibers
2. **Bone can be classified according to the following, *except*:**
   a. Shape
   b. Type of marrow
   c. Development
   d. Structure
3. **In endochondral ossification:**
   a. Mesenchymal cells condense to form bone
   b. A cartilaginous model is first formed and is replaced by bone.
   c. Cartilage is directly converted into bone
   d. Chondroblasts form the bone matrix
4. **Mandible is formed by:**
   a. Metaplastic ossification
   b. Intramembranous ossification
   c. Meckel's cartilage
   d. Second branchial arch
5. **Reversal lines:**
   a. Denote the rhythmic activity and rest
   b. Demarcate the region of resorbed bone and the newly forming bone
   c. Are seen in all hard tissues
   d. Are not seen in remodeled bone
6. **Osteoclasts are:**
   a. Multinucleated cells
   b. Responsible for bone resorption
   c. Hematopoietic cells derived from granulocyte macrophage colony forming unit
   d. All of the above
7. **Osteoclasts are seen in:**
   a. Ruffled border
   b. Osteon
   c. Volkman's canal
   d. Howship's lacunae
8. **Incremental lines:**
   a. Demarcate the region of resorbed bone and the newly forming bone
   b. Seen in all hard tissues
   c. Not seen on membranous bones
   d. Seen in aging bone
9. **Osteocytes are:**
   a. Formed from osteoprogenitor cells
   b. Responsible for bone resorption
   c. Seen in Howship's lacunae
   d. Entrapped osteoblasts
10. **Structural and functional unit of the compact bone is known as:**
    a. Lamellar system
    b. Haversian system
    c. osteoid
    d. Osteonectin
11. **Alveolar bone develops from:**
    a. Dental organ
    b. Dental papilla
    c. Dental sac
    d. Endoderm
12. **Chondroid bone:**
    a. Forms the mandible
    b. Has the characteristic of both the bone and cartilage and seen in growing free borders of the alveolar bone
    c. Is formed by endochondral ossification
    d. Is replaced by cartilage
13. **Thin lamellae of bone that forms the inner wall of the tooth sockets is called:**
    a. Supporting alveolar bone
    b. Alveolar bone proper
    c. Woven bone
    d. Cortical bone
14. **Age changes in the alveolar bone include the following, *except*:**
    a. Fatty infiltration of the marrow spaces
    b. Reduction in the height of the alveolar bone
    c. Proliferative capacity and the formative function are reduced
    d. The surface facing the periodontal ligament becomes smooth
15. **Supporting alveolar bone consists of:**
    a. Coarse woven bone.
    b. Cortical plate on the outer portion and the cancellous bone in the center portion.
    c. Sharpey's fibers.
    d. Thick compact bone in the facial surface of maxilla.
16. **Perforation canals of Zuckerkandl and Hirschfeld consists of:**
    a. Haversian vessels.
    b. Interdental and interradicular arteries, veins and lymph vessels.
    c. Inferior alveolar nerves and vessels
    d. Hematopoietic marrow
17. **In Type I, the trabeculae pattern of supporting alveolar bone:**
    a. Randomly arranged and comparatively more in number
    b. Are noticed in delicate interdental and interradicular
    c. Are laid parallel to the body of the bone in layers compared to the ladder, more pronounced in mandible
    d. Are predominantly seen in maxilla

18. **An isolated "window" of bone loss on the facial or lingual aspect of a tooth that exposes the root surface is called:**
    a. Dehiscence
    b. Horizontal bone loss
    c. Fenestration
    d. Angular bone loss
19. **Orthodontic tooth movement is based on the fact that:**
    a. Bone resorbs on the side of tension and apposes on the side of pressure
    b. Bone resorbs on the side of pressure and apposed on the side of tension
    c. Bone calcium homeostasis
    d. Osteoblasts are activated at the site of pressure to produce new bone
20. **Generalized loss of lamina dura in radiographs occurs in:**
    a. Hyperthyroidism
    b. Hyperparathyroidism
    c. Vitamin D deficiency
    d. Chronic periodontitis

ANSWERS

1. c	2. b	3. b	4. b	5. b	6. d	7. d	8. b	9. d	10. b	11. c	12. b	13. b	14. d	15. b
16. b	17. c	18. c	19. b	20. b										

BIBLIOGRAPHY

1. Agostinelli C, Agostinelli A, Berardini M, et al. Radiological evaluation of the dimensions of lower molar alveoli. Implant Dent. 2018.
2. American Society for Bone and Mineral Research President's Committee on Nomenclature. Proposed standard nomenclature for new tumor necrosis factor family members involved in the regulation of bone resorption. The American Society for Bone and Mineral Research President's Committee on Nomenclature. J Bone Miner Res. 2000;15:2293-6.
3. Berkovitz BKB, Holland GR, Moxham BJ. Oral anatomy, histology, and embryology, 4th edition. St. Louis Missouri: Mosby Elsevier; 2009.
4. Boyce BF, Xing L. Biology of RANK, RANKL, and osteoprotegerin. Arthritis Res Ther. 2007;9 (Suppl 1):S1.
5. Boyce BF, Xing L. Functions of RANKL/RANK/OPG in bone modeling and remodeling. Arch Biochem Biophys. 2008;473(2):139-46.
6. Burr DB, Allen MR. Bone cells. Basic and Applied Bone Biology. US: Academic press; 2014. pp. 27-45.
7. Chen CH, Wang L, Serdar Tulu U, et al. An osteopenic/osteoporotic phenotype delays alveolar bone repair. Bone. 2018;112:212-9.
8. Cho MI, Garant PR. Development and general structure of the periodontium. Periodontol. 2000;24:9-27.
9. Cohen B, Kramer IRH. Scientific foundations of dentistry, 1st edition. London: William Heinemann Medical Books Ltd.; 1976.
10. Furuya M, Kikuta J, Fujimori S, et al. Direct cell–cell contact between mature osteoblasts and osteoclasts dynamically controls their functions in vivo. Nat Commun. 2018;9(1):300.
11. Gulabivala K, Ng Y-L. Tooth organogenesis, morphology and physiology. Endodontics, 4th edition. US: Mosby; 2014. pp. 2-34.
12. Hattner R, Epker BN, Frost HM. Suggested sequential mode of control of changes in cell behavior in adult bone remodeling. Nature. 1965;206:489-90.
13. Johnson K. A study of the dimensional changes occurring in the maxilla following tooth extraction. Aust Dent J. 1969;14(4):241-4.
14. Karsenty G. Role of Cbfa1 in osteoblast differentiation and function. Semin Cell Dev Biol. 2000;11:343-6.
15. Katranji A, Misch K, Wang HL. Cortical bone thickness in dentate and edentulous human cadavers. J Periodontol. 2007;78(5):874-8.
16. Kumar GS. Orban's oral histology and embryology, 13th edition. India: Reed Elsevier India Pvt Ltd.; 2014.
17. Kuroki A, Sugita N, Komatsu S, et al. Association of liver enzyme levels and alveolar bone loss. A cross-sectional clinical study in Sado Island. J Clin Exp Dent. 2018;10(2):e100-6.
18. Lian JB, Stein GS. Runx2/Cbfa1: a multifunctional regulator of bone formation. Curr Pharm Des. 2003;9:2677-85.
19. Lindhe J, Cecchinato D, Bressan EA, et al. The alveolar process of the edentulous maxilla in periodontitis and non-periodontitis subjects. Clin Oral Implants Res. 2012;23(1):5-11.
20. Lindhe J, Bressan E, Cecchinato D, et al. Bone tissue in different parts of the edentulous maxilla and mandible. Clin Oral Implants Res. 2013;24(4):372-7.
21. Martin TJ, Sims NA. Osteoclast-derived activity in the coupling of bone formation to resorption. Trends Mol Med. 2005;11:76-81.
22. Matsuo K, Irie N. Osteoclast-osteoblast communication. Arch Biochem Biophys. 2008;473:201-9.
23. Nanci A. Ten Cate's oral histology: development, structure, and function, 8th edition. St. Louis Missouri: Mosby Elsevier; 2014.
24. Nakashima T, Hayashi M, Fukunaga T, et al. Evidence for osteocyte regulation of bone homeostasis through RANKL expression. Nat Med. 2011;17:1231-4.
25. Schroeder HE. Oral structural biology: embryology, structure, and function of normal hard and soft tissues of the oral cavity and temporomandibular joints, 3rd edition. New York: Thieme Medical Publishers, 1991.
26. Scott J. The development, structure, and function of alveolar bone. Dent Pract Dent Rec. 1968;1:19-22.
27. Simonet WS, Lacey DL, Dunstan CR, et al. Osteoprotegerin: a novel secreted protein involved in the regulation of bone density. Cell. 1997;89:309-19.
28. Suga S. Alveolar bone-its structure, function and reaction. Shikai Tenbo. 1983;61(5):840-56.
29. Takayanagi H. Mechanistic insight into osteoclast differentiation in osteoimmunology. J Mol Med. 2005;83:170-9.
30. Xiong J, Onal M, Jilka RL, et al. Matrix-embedded cells control osteoclast formation. Nat Med. 2011;17:1235-41.

CHAPTER 11

Tooth Eruption

B Sivapathasundharam, Logeswari Jayamani

CHAPTER OUTLINE

- Eruption   155
- Pattern of Tooth Movement   155
- Histology of Tooth Movement   157
- Theories of Tooth Eruption   159
  » Root Growth Theory   159
  » Pulp Growth Theory   159
  » Vascular Pressure Theory   159
  » Bone Growth Theory   160
  » Ligament Traction Theory   160
  » Neuromuscular Theory   161
  » Dental Follicle Theory   161
- Clinical Considerations   161
  » Premature Eruption   161
  » Delayed Eruption   161
  » Natal and Neonatal Tooth   161
  » Failure of Tooth Eruption   161
  » Supraeruption   162
  » Passive Eruption   162
  » Ectopic Eruption   162
  » Impacted and Embedded Tooth   162
  » Submerged Tooth   162

INTRODUCTION

Human is a diphyodont, *i.e.,* having two sets of teeth. The first set of teeth is called deciduous or primary teeth and the second set, the secondary or permanent teeth. Infants' jaws are small, which can accommodate few small teeth. Primary dentition serves this purpose. Tooth once formed cannot grow to increase in size. Thus, smaller deciduous teeth are replaced by more number of bigger and stronger permanent teeth, to meet the increased masticatory load of an adult jaw.

> At birth no teeth are present in the mouth. The first tooth to erupt in the oral cavity is the deciduous mandibular central incisor.

Development of dentition starts at intrauterine life and continues till adulthood. Stages in the development of dentition include predentition period, deciduous dentition period, mixed dentition period, and secondary dentition period.

Though the first evidence of tooth development appears at the 6th week of intrauterine life, eruption starts only at 6th month after birth. From birth to 6th month is called the predentition or predentate period, since no teeth are present in the mouth during this period. The alveolar arches of the infant are called gum pads that are nothing but the thickened oral mucosa, more specifically the alveolar mucosa.

Deciduous dentition period starts with the eruption of mandibular central incisors (approximately 6th month of life) and extend till the appearance of any one of the permanent tooth (usually mandibular first molars or central incisors, which erupt at about six years) **(Figures 11-1A and B)**.

In mixed dentition period, both deciduous and permanent teeth are present. This period extends from 6 to 12 years **(Figures 11-2A and B)**.

Secondary or permanent dentition period starts after all the deciduous teeth are shed. This starts at about 12 years **(Figures 11-3A and B)**.

As stated previously, first tooth to erupt in the oral cavity is deciduous mandibular central incisor and the last one to erupt is the third molar, also called as wisdom tooth. In both dentitions, mandibular teeth erupt earlier than the maxillary teeth. Teeth erupt at earlier date in girls than boys. The sequence and the chronology of eruption are depicted in **Figures 11-4 to 11-7**. However, this is not a hard and fast rule. The sequence and chronology may be altered by many systemic factors and local factors. Systemic factors include

154 CHAPTER 11: Tooth Eruption

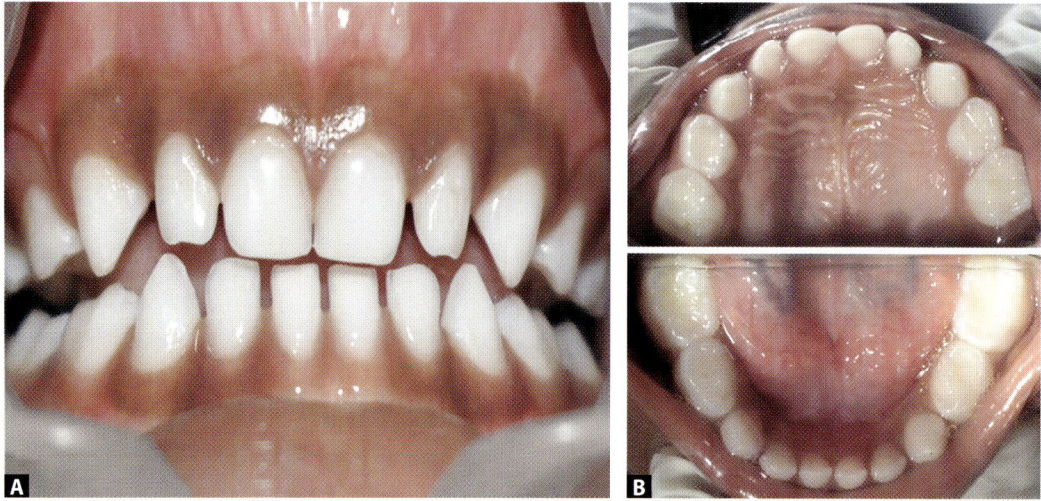

Figures 11-1A and B: Deciduous dentition.
Source: Department of Pedodontics and Preventive Dentistry, Meenakshi Ammal Dental College, Chennai, Tamil Nadu, India.

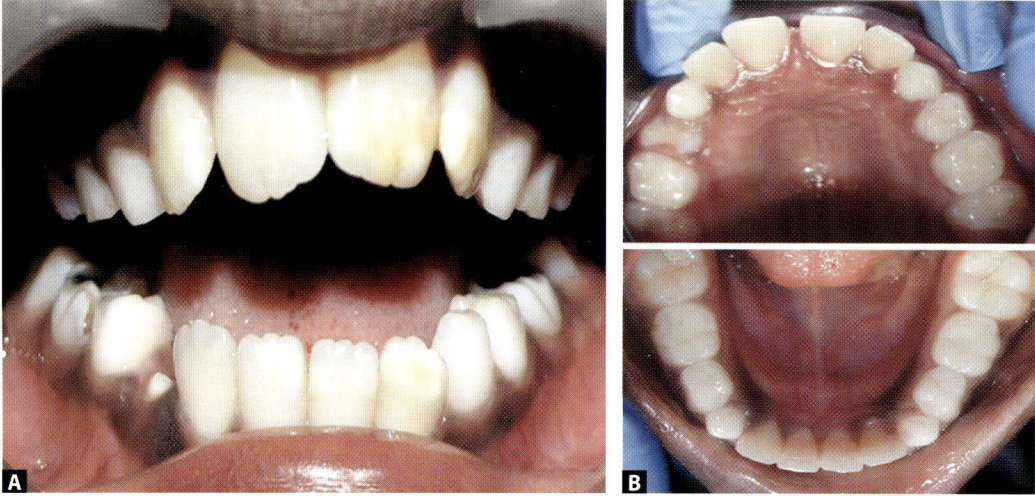

Figures 11-2A and B: Mixed dentition.
Source: Department of Pedodontics and Preventive Dentistry, Meenakshi Ammal Dental College, Chennai, Tamil Nadu, India.

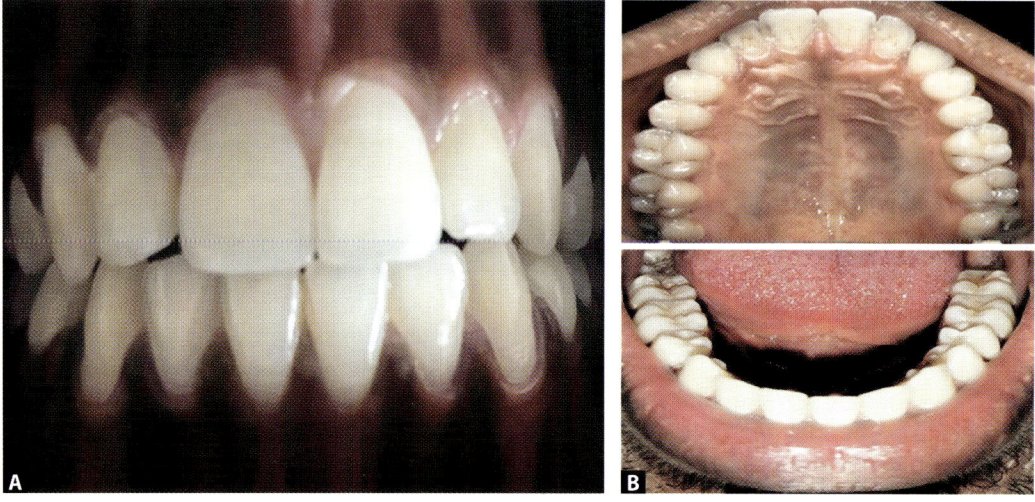

Figures 11-3A and B: Permanent dentition.

CHAPTER 11: Tooth Eruption

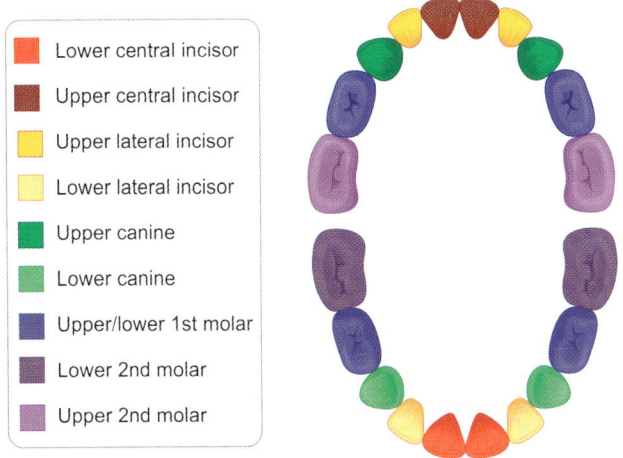

Figure 11-4: Sequence of eruption of deciduous teeth.

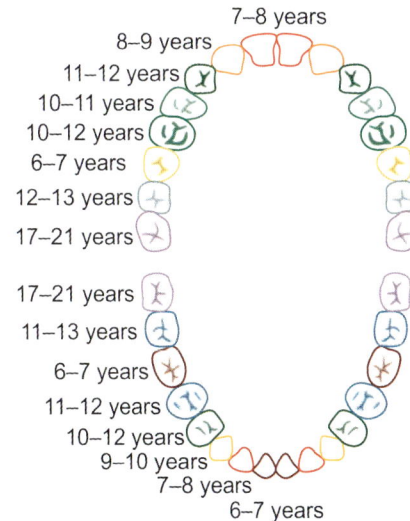

Figure 11-7: Chronology of eruption of permanent teeth.

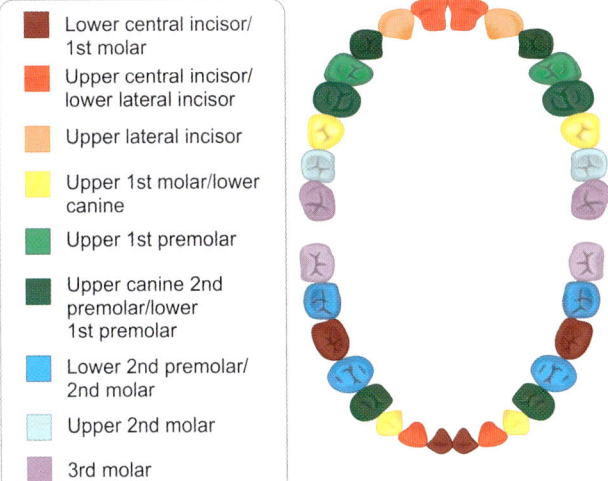

Figure 11-5: Sequence of eruption of permanent teeth.

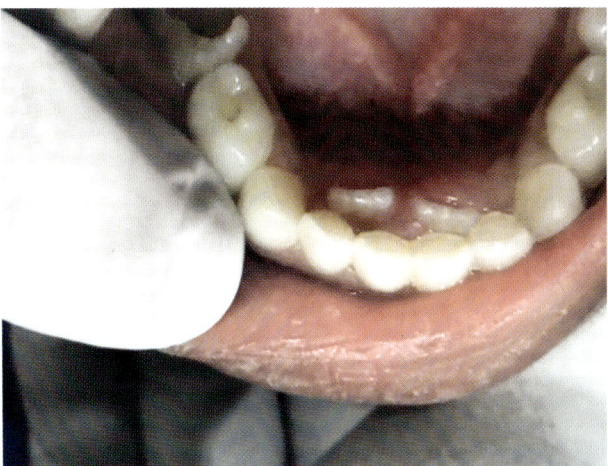

Figure 11-8: Emergence of mandibular permanent central incisors.

ERUPTION

Eruption is defined as, "axial or occlusal movement of the tooth from the site of its developmental position in the tooth crypt, to its site of functional position in the occlusal plane". The other word commonly confused with eruption is "emergence". It is the moment of appearance of any portion of the crown through the gingiva **(Figure 11-8)**. Thus, it is a stage in the dynamic process of eruption. Eruption is a continuous process, which starts after the crown formation and ends only when the tooth is lost. During eruption teeth move in three-dimensional space, not just along their long axis.

PATTERN OF TOOTH MOVEMENT

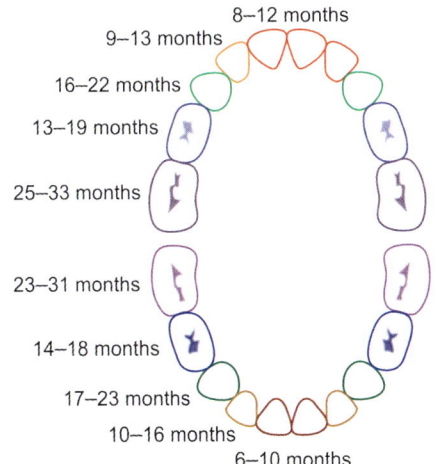

Figure 11-6: Chronology of eruption of deciduous teeth.

genetic makeup, race, nutritional, and hormonal status. Local factors include availability of space (which may depend on retention or early loss of deciduous tooth), obstruction of the eruptive path (by supernumerary tooth, odontome, cyst or tumors) and thick mucosa.

Movement of the tooth starts as early as during the development and it continues even after eruption. Tooth germ moves within its bony crypt during development in accordance with the growth of the jaws. Though its final destination is the occlusal plane, where it has to meet its antagonist and perform its function, for what it is destined to,

it keeps moving to compensate for the occlusal and proximal wear. Accordingly, the physiological tooth movements are categorized as follows:
1. Pre-eruptive tooth movement
2. Eruptive tooth movement
3. Posteruptive tooth movement

Pre-eruptive tooth movement starts from the time of initiation and formation of the tooth to the time of crown completion or till the time of the initiation of root formation. These movements occur in coordination with the positional changes of the neighboring crowns and the growth of the jaws.

Primary and secondary teeth move mesially and distally with lengthening of the jaws. Deciduous tooth germs are small during their initial development and there is good deal of space for them in the developing jaws. However, they become crowded because of their rapid growth. Anteriors move forward and molars drift posteriorly as the jaws grow in anteroposterior, mediolateral, and vertical direction.

The movement of the developing deciduous tooth germ along with the jaw growth gains enough space and relieves crowding.

Permanent teeth move within the jaws to adjust themselves, to be placed apical to or in between the resorbing roots of the deciduous teeth and also in harmony with the growing alveolar process.

At the beginning of the pre-eruptive phase, the incisal tips of the anteriors of both deciduous and the permanent teeth are at the same level and the permanent teeth are placed lingual to the deciduous teeth. As the deciduous teeth erupt, the permanent successors are positioned at the level of apical third of the roots of the deciduous anteriors **(Figures 11-9A and B)**.

Premolars and deciduous molars, occlusal planes are at the same level during the pre-eruptive period. As deciduous molars erupt, premolars move in between roots of the deciduous molars **(Figures 11-10A and B)**. Positional changes in the successional teeth are due to the eruption of the deciduous teeth and the growth of the jaws (*i.e.,* increase

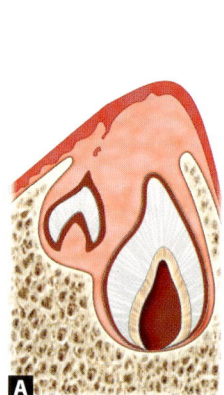
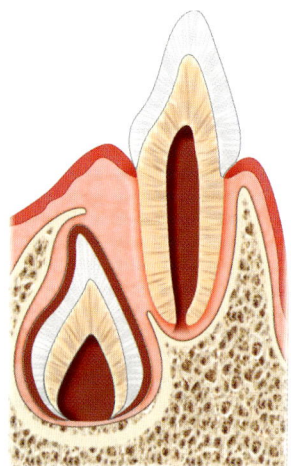
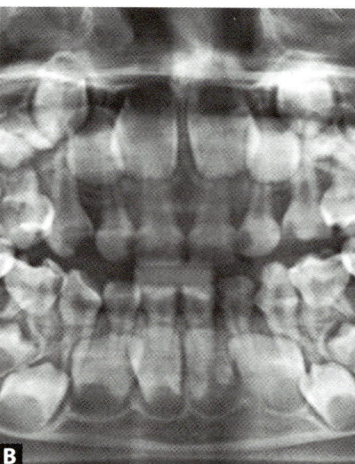

Figures 11-9A and B: At the beginning, permanent anterior teeth are placed lingual to the deciduous predecessor and occlusal plane of both are at same level. As the deciduous teeth erupt, the permanent successors are positioned at the level of apical third of the roots of the deciduous anteriors: (A) Schematic representation; and (B) Radiograph.
Source: Department of Pedodontics and Preventive Dentistry, Meenakshi Ammal Dental College, Chennai, Tamil Nadu, India.

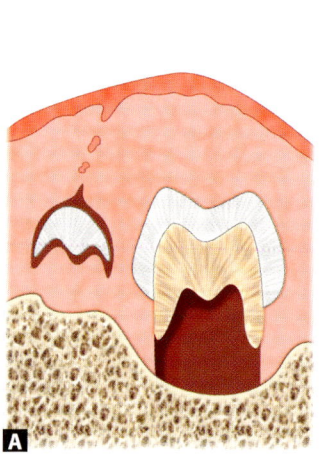
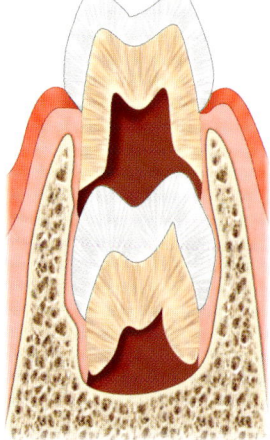
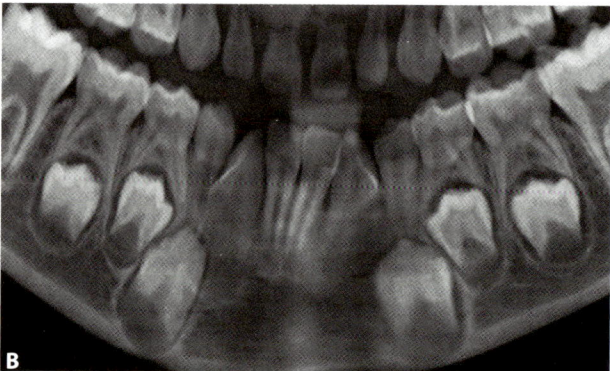

Figures 11-10A and B: Premolars and deciduous molars occlusal planes are at the same level during the pre-eruptive period. As deciduous molars erupt, premolars move in between roots of the deciduous molars: (A) Schematic representation; and (B) Radiograph.
Source: Department of Pedodontics and Preventive Dentistry, Meenakshi Ammal Dental College, Chennai, Tamil Nadu, India.

in height to accommodate the permanent teeth at a more apical position).

Permanent molars, which do not have deciduous predecessors, move in a different way. The maxillary molars develop in the maxillary tuberosity with their occlusal surface facing distally **(Figure 11-11)**. As the maxilla grows forward and downward, sufficient space is available to accommodate the permanent molars and the permanent molars swing occlusally from their distal slant. The mandibular permanent molars develop within the ramus of the mandible with their occlusal surface facing mesially **(Figure 11-12)**. They become upright as the mandible grows forward and upward.

Eruptive tooth movement starts from the root formation till the tooth reaches the occlusal plane. The direction of movement is principally axial or occlusal. During this period, four major events occur, which include—the formation of the root, movements within the bone to reach the oral mucosa, emergence of the tooth crown through the oral mucosa, and movements that occur after emergence till the tooth reaches the occlusal plane.

As the root formation continues, the jaw requires space to accommodate the lengthening roots, which is accomplished by the bone remodeling at the fundus of the future alveolar bone.

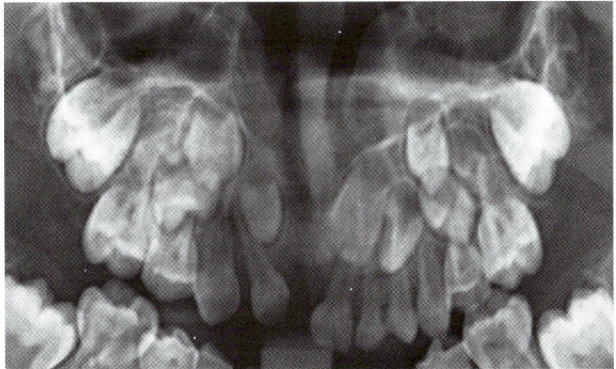

Figure 11-11: Radiograph showing permanent maxillary molars develop with their occlusal surface facing distobuccally.
Source: Department of Pedodontics and Preventive Dentistry, Meenakshi Ammal Dental College, Chennai, Tamil Nadu, India.

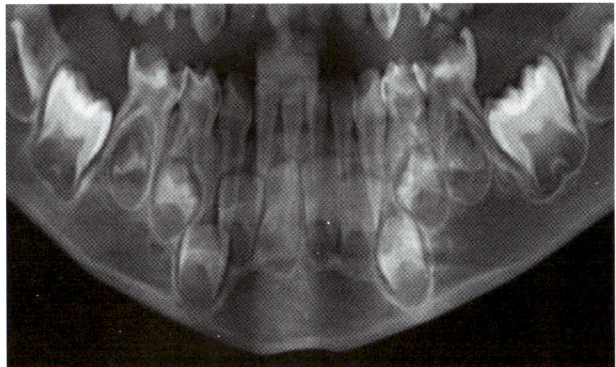

Figure 11-12: Radiograph showing permanent mandibular molars develop with their occlusal surface facing mesially.
Source: Department of Pedodontics and Preventive Dentistry, Meenakshi Ammal Dental College, Chennai, Tamil Nadu, India.

Intrabony tooth movements are mainly to accommodate the elongating roots and to enable the fusion of reduced enamel epithelium that covers the formed crown with the oral epithelium.

As the reduced enamel epithelium fuses with the oral epithelium, the crown penetrates the oral mucosa and appears into the oral cavity. Fusion of reduced enamel epithelium with the oral epithelium results in the formation of dentogingival junction.

After the emergence of the tooth crown into the oral cavity, it keeps moving occlusally till it meets its antagonist at the occlusal plane. During this phase of eruption there is gradual exposure of the tooth crown and apical shift of the dentogingival junction.

Since jaw growth continues along with the eruptive tooth movement, movements in other plane also occur in addition.

Posteruptive tooth movement: Eruption does not cease with the establishment of the occlusion. Growth of the craniofacial bones does not stop in young adulthood but is a continuous process and may proceed even into later ages. As the teeth reach their functional position in the occlusal plane and engage in masticatory function, the wear and tear starts.

The main purpose of the posteruptive tooth movement is to maintain the position of the erupted teeth while the jaws continue to grow and compensate for the occlusal (and incisal) and proximal wear. While the movement associated with the jaw growth is principally in axial direction, the one associated with the teeth wear is both axial and mesial. The latter may also result in decrease in dental arch size. The mesial drift is caused by the anterior component of occlusal force, and contraction of the transseptal fibers of the periodontal ligament.

> Pre-eruptive tooth movement, eruptive tooth movement and posteruptive tooth movement require signaling in the PTHrP (parathyroid hormone-related peptide) pathway. In the pre-eruptive phase, teeth are fully within the bony crypt. Enamel organ produces PTHrP and CSF1 (colony stimulating factor 1 [**CSF1**], also known as macrophage colony-stimulating factor [M-CSF]) which feed back to the dental follicle.
>
> In eruptive tooth movement or intraosseous phase is characterized by the spatially restricted removal of bone on the coronal side of the tooth due to signals from the dental follicle. Osteoclasts invade and resorb the bone to create an eruption pathway.

HISTOLOGY OF TOOTH MOVEMENT

Pre-eruptive tooth movement: This movement results from the combination of bodily movement of the tooth germ and its eccentric growth (one portion of the tooth germ grows while the remaining portion do not grow, resulting in change in the center of the tooth germ). Since the pre-eruptive tooth movement is predominantly intraosseous, it is mainly associated with the remodeling of the bony tooth crypt. It is brought about by the osteoblastic and osteoclastic activity. When the tooth germs make bodily movement in mesial direction, there is resorption of the mesial wall of the bony crypt and deposition of the bone at the distal wall as a fill-in process. It is not clear whether remodeling is the cause or effect of tooth movement.

Eruptive tooth movement: During this phase many significant developments occur in the developing tooth and its surrounding structures. These include root formation and development of periodontal ligament and dentogingival junction.

After the crown stage, the Hertwig's epithelial root sheath forms. This initiates radicular dentin formation by the odontoblasts, which are differentiated from the dental papilla cells. As soon as the root dentin is formed, Hertwig's root sheath breaks down and cementoblasts differentiate from the cells of the dental sac and a layer of cementum is formed over the radicular dentin. Root forms in this way.

Lengthening of the root is accommodated by the tooth movement. Formation of the periodontal ligament and alveolar bone occurs with the root development. Periodontal ligament remodels to allow the tooth movement. Fibroblasts are responsible for the remodeling of the periodontal ligament, by degrading and ingesting the collagen and synthesizing new collagen fibrils. Further the periodontal ligament fibroblasts have cytoskeleton, which make them contractile and help in tooth movement. They have contact with the neighboring fibroblasts by adhering type cell junctions and with the collagen fibers of the periodontal ligament through fibronexus. With the root elongation and tooth eruption, the alveolar bone increases in height.

For the intraosseous eruptive tooth movement two things must happen; the overlying tissues (bone, primary tooth root, and gingiva) must resorb to provide an eruptive path, and need a force for the tooth to move towards the occlusal plane.

The blood vessels decrease in number, nerve fibers and the connective tissue overlying the tooth germ degenerate. This results in the formation of an inverted triangular area of altered tissue that forms the eruption pathway. This connective tissue contains remnants of dental lamina and is known as "gubernacular cord". This strand of connective tissue extends till the lamina propria of the oral mucosa. Gubernacular cord lies in the bony canal called gubernacular canal, which can be visible in dried skull as small openings lingual to the deciduous teeth. It is believed that the gubernacular cord guides the eruption of the permanent tooth. Gubernacular canal widens by local osteoclastic activity **(Figure 11-13)**. Macrophages in the eruption pathway release hydrolytic enzymes that destroy the connective tissue including blood vessels and nerves in that area. Reduced enamel epithelium secretes proteases, which break down the connective tissue and helps in the creation of eruption path.

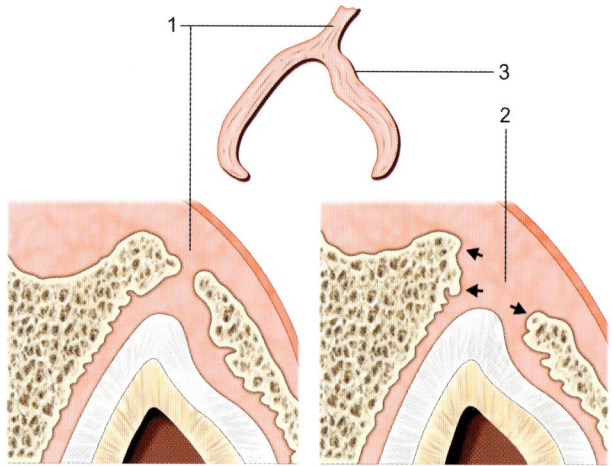

Figure 11-13: (1) Gubernacular cord; (2) canal; and (3) dental follicle.

Resorption process may be controlled by the local growth factors such as transforming growth factor-beta 1 (TGF β1) and epidermal growth factor (EGF) produced within or around the dental follicle. These factors are chemotactic to monocytes from the peripheral blood vessels around the dental sac. Osteoclasts differentiate from the monocytes and resorb the bone. Subsequent to the connective tissue changes, reduced enamel epithelium and the oral epithelium proliferates and fuses with each other. This proliferating epithelium secretes enzymes that degrade the connective tissue. These broken down products are also phagocytosed by the epithelial cells. After their fusion, the central portion of the epithelial cells degenerate and form an epithelium-lined canal, through which the tooth erupts without bleeding **(Figures 11-14A to C)**. During intraosseous phase, the rate of tooth movement is about 10 μm per day. The epithelium attached to the tooth crown subsequently forms the dentogingival junction.

> Colony stimulating factor 1 (CSF-1) and monocyte chemotactic protein plays a major role in osteoclastogenesis. Osteoprotegerin inhibits osteoclast differentiation. Its expression along with Secreted frizzled-related protein 1(SFRP-1) is down regulated in the apical region. Expression of receptor activator of nuclear factor kappa B ligand (RANKL) is more at coronal half and BMP-2 expression is more at basal half of the dental follicle. Wnt/β-catenin signaling plays a critical role in bone formation and regeneration, which occur during tooth eruption. Osteoblasts differentiation at the fundus of the alveolar crypt is accentuated during eruptive tooth movement. Also osteoblasts might influence eruption process by activating osteoclasts.

The views regarding the eruptive force still remain unclear. Periodontal ligament is considered as an unlikely source of the eruptive force, since the majority of the principal fibers of the periodontal ligament are sparsely formed and incompletely attached with the alveolar bone at this stage. Deposition of bone at the fundus of the crypt was also considered, but as stated earlier it is not clear whether the bone formed is the cause or the result of tooth movement. Local tissue fluid and vascular pressure are also suggested to produce eruptive force.

> Clusterin and TGF-β1 are two proteins that have been found to be associated with macrophage chemotaxis stimulation. Ameloblasts also secrete these proteins, which help in the breakdown of the connective tissue and participate in the process of tooth eruption. A recent study showed that miR-214 (MicroRNAs or miRNAs-a class of naturally occurring, single stranded, small noncoding RNA molecules, and their main function is to silence the mRNA and downregulate gene expression) might fine-tune clusterin and TGF-β in the secretory ameloblasts. Inactivation of miR-214 stimulates the biosynthesis of contractile proteins, but decreases the expression of proteins involved in the eruption.

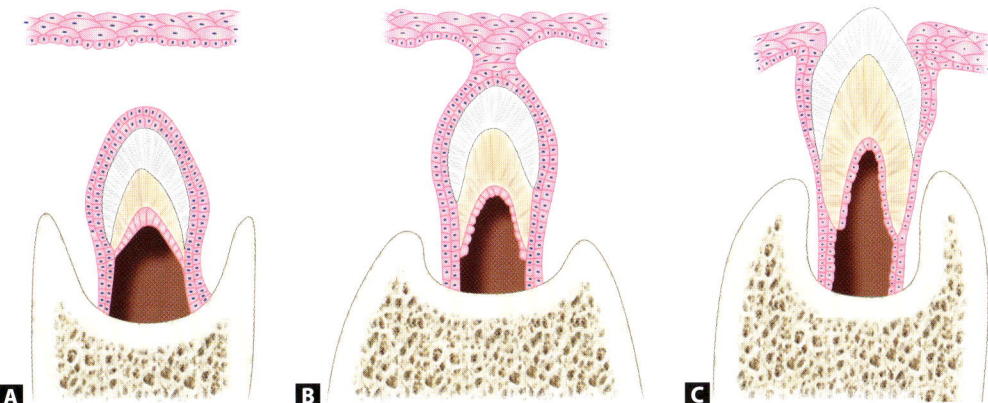

Figures 11-14A to C: Fusion of reduced enamel epithelium with the oral epithelium results in the bloodless emergence of tooth into the oral cavity: (A) Completion of crown formation; (B) Fusion with oral epithelium; (C) Eruption into oral cavity.

Posteruptive tooth movement: This occurs after the tooth reaches the occlusal plane and mainly to accommodate the growing jaws and to compensate for the occlusal and proximal wear.

Posteruptive tooth movement to accommodate the growth of the jaws and compensation for the occlusal wear consists of mainly axial or occlusal movement. Movement associated with jaw growth stops at the end of the second decade when significant jaw growth ceases. The same mechanisms responsible for pre-eruptive tooth movement operate on these occlusal movements too. The cemental deposition, which occurs at the root tip to compensate for the occlusal wear is only an infilling phenomenon.

During the root completion, the height of the alveolar process (the alveolar crest) increases and the base of the alveolar socket resorb to accommodate the formation of the root tip. The wide root canals become narrower. Later, bone deposition at the base of the alveolar socket and remodeling of periodontal ligament collagen fibers occurs.

Wearing away at the contact point results in mesial drifting of the teeth due to the anterior component of force and contraction of transseptal fibers of the periodontal ligament. In mesial drifting, there is bone resorption at the mesial wall of the alveolar socket and deposition at the distal wall. In posteruptive tooth movement, periodontal ligament plays a major role in contributing to the eruptive force. The principal fibers of the periodontal ligament are well-orientated and attached firmly to the alveolar bone after eruption. The primary eruption mechanism is believed to be either contraction of collagen as it matures or traction by the contractile fibroblasts. Vascular effects similar to pre-eruptive movement may also contribute.

THEORIES OF TOOTH ERUPTION

Eruption of tooth is a complex and well-regulated process. Many factors play a role in the eruption process. Apart from genetic factors, nutritional and hormonal status, race, ethnicity, sex, height and weight of the individual, craniofacial morphology, preterm birth, socioeconomic level, presence of systemic diseases, and local factors play a major role. Eruption process also involves signaling from a large number of genes and molecules.

Many theories have been postulated to describe the eruption process but still all are debatable. In fact, eruption occurs due to the combination of many factors.

Number of theories has been postulated to explain various aspects of tooth eruption. These include root growth theory, pulp growth theory, pulp constriction theory, vascular pressure theory, bone remodeling theory, ligament traction theory, neuromuscular theory, and dental follicle theory.

Root Growth Theory

According to this theory, lengthening of the root pushes the tooth. For this to happen it needs a fixed base. The base of the tooth crypt cannot act as fixed base, as the pressure on the bone causes resorption. Supporters of this theory proposed existence of a ligament attached to the bony wall on either side of the tooth crypt that acts as a fixed base and termed that as cushion hammock ligament. But it was proved that the so called cushion hammock ligament is pulp delineating membrane and has no bony insertion. Though root growth can produce a force, it may not be translated into an eruptive tooth movement, unless there is a fixed and rigid base to withstand the force. Apart from this, there are other factors against this theory. It is a fact that some teeth move more distance than the length of the roots (upper canine). Rootless teeth do erupt, which was proved experimentally by resecting the root and demonstrating the tooth eruption. Also if the deciduous tooth is extracted, the successor erupts rapidly even if only half root is formed. Natal and neonatal tooth erupt with incompletely formed roots. Some teeth erupt even after the root completion.

Pulp Growth Theory

This theory states that growth or constriction of the pulp generates propulsive force by growth of the dentin, growth of the pulp, and hydraulic effects within the pulp vasculature **(Figures 11-15A and B)**. But strong evidence against this theory is the eruption of tooth, in which the pulp is removed.

Vascular Pressure Theory

To certain extent, this theory overlaps with the pulp growth theory. As per this theory, the eruptive force is provided by the

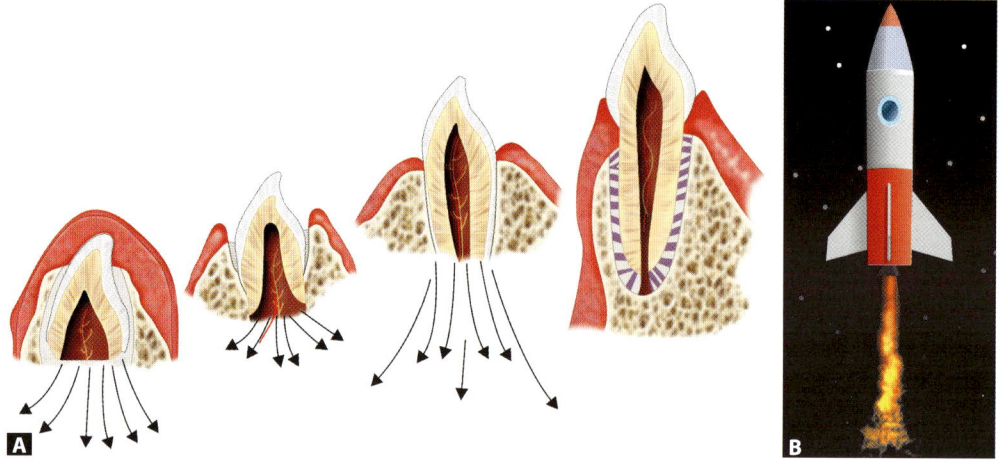

Figures 11-15A and B: Propulsive force to push the tooth toward occlusal plane by pulp growth and constriction.

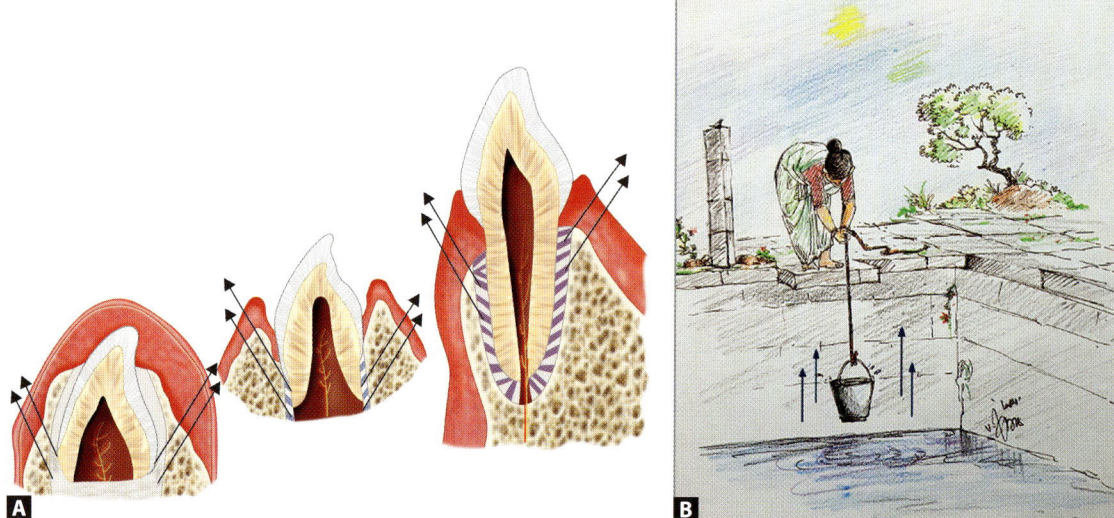

Figures 11-16A and B: Tractional force produced by periodontal ligament.

pressure in the blood vessels within the tooth and at the apical region. This is again discounted due to the fact that pulpless tooth do erupt and also the use of hypotensive drugs have no effect on the eruption rates. Further, the decrease in blood flow may cause change in the nutrients and hormones, which might affect the tissue growth that alter the rate of eruption.

Bone Growth Theory

As per this theory, bone forming at the base or the fundus of the tooth crypt pushes the tooth occlusally. But it is not clear whether the bone formed at the base is the cause or result of tooth movement.

Ligament Traction Theory

In contrast to other theories, the tooth is pulled (instead of a push) occlusally by the periodontal ligament **(Figures 11-16A and B)**. The formation of cross-linkages of the collagen fibers of the periodontal ligament results in shrinkage. This shrinking collagen exerts force that would help the tooth to erupt. Experiments preventing the collagen cross-linking did not encounter failure of eruption. The other view is that the contractile fibroblasts of the periodontal ligament exert tractional force through the fibers of the periodontal ligament or cell to cell contact. This force might lead to eruption. Studies have documented that there is no evidence that the fibroblasts exert force that is sufficient enough to move the tooth under normal physiological conditions. Further the fibroblasts *in vivo* do not exhibit the features of migratory cell or myofibroblasts (fibroblasts with contractile property).

However, the role of periodontal ligament in eruption cannot be denied since the ankylosed tooth (cementum is directly fused with the alveolar bone and no intervening periodontal ligament) and implants do not show occlusal movement or mesial drift.

If the tooth has to erupt, there should be space in the eruption path, lift or pressure from the apical region, and adaptability in the periodontal ligament. Based on these factors, Inger Kjaer (2014) proposed a hypothesis. According to which, eruption occurs due to an innervation-provoked pressure in the apical part of the tooth. However, this requires continuous adaptation from the periodontal ligament and the active movement of the crown follicle, destroying overlying bone tissue.

Neuromuscular Theory

Otherwise known as unification theory of tooth eruption; states that the synchronized forces of the orofacial musculatures, controlled by the central nervous system, are responsible for the active movements of a tooth. These forces also prepare the pathway for the molecular events, which play a role in tooth movement.

Dental Follicle Theory

According to this theory, dental follicle induces bone resorption above the developing crown and bone apposition below it. This results in the formation of an eruptive path through which the tooth moves passively.

Thus an asymmetric bone remodeling enables tooth eruption.

The importance of the dental follicle in tooth eruption was documented for a long time. Experimental removal of dental follicle resulted in failure of eruption of the tooth. When the follicle was preserved and tooth was removed and replaced with metal replica, eruption of metal replica occured normally.

Molecular studies have revealed that dental follicle, reduced enamel epithelium, stellate reticulum, and alveolar bone regulate eruption by inductive signals. It is suggested that the coronal aspect of the dental follicle regulates bone resorption and the apical aspect regulates bone formation. This is confirmed by the fact that there is a higher expression of RANKL genes (responsible for bone resorption) in the coronal half of the dental follicle and higher expression of BMP-2 genes (responsible for bone apposition) in the apical half of the follicle. BMPs regulate the expression of Cbfa1 (core binding factor alpha1), which acts as a key transcriptional regulator for osteoblast differentiation during bone formation.

> It is a proven fact that the tooth development is regulated by a cascade of mutual interactions between the epithelial enamel organ and the dental mesenchyme. Similarly the tooth eruption is regulated by the paracrine signaling of the dental follicle. Interactions between the dental follicle, the reduced enamel epithelium, and the stellate reticulum lead to the recruitment of monocytes to the dental follicle, which ultimately results in bone resorption. In addition, reduced enamel epithelium secretes proteases that aid in creating an eruption pathway through enzymatic digestion of collagens.

Most of the theories of tooth eruption discuss about the eruptive force, which push or pull the tooth toward the occlusal plane. But the origin of such force remains unclear. However, one recent hypothesis completely denies the existence of such eruptive force and suggested that follicular soft tissues detect functional bite-forces and so direct bone remodeling with the effect of enabling tooth eruption.

Thus, from the above theories, it can be construed that the eruption is not associated with a single factor instead it is multifactorial. It is a complex process and can be influenced by genetic factors, nutritional and hormonal status, race, ethnicity, sex, height and weight of the individual, craniofacial morphology, preterm birth, socioeconomic level, presence of systemic diseases, and local factors.

CLINICAL CONSIDERATIONS

Premature Eruption

As stated previously, eruption is not an overnight event; rather it is a continuous process. On occasions teeth erupt prematurely. Premature eruption may occur in systemic diseases like hyperthyroidism, hypophosphatasia, acute lymphocytic leukemia, cyclic neutropenia, histiocytosis X, cherubism, acrodynia, and Papillon–Lefèvre syndrome. Activity-dependent neuroprotective protein syndrome results in premature eruption of deciduous teeth. Rarely the exact cause for the early eruption is unknown.

Premature eruption of permanent teeth could be due to premature loss of primary teeth if the loss occurs within one year before eruption. On the contrary, if extraction is done at a very young age, the eruption of permanent teeth is delayed.

Delayed Eruption

In delayed or retarded eruption, teeth erupt well beyond the normal eruption range. This is more common than the premature eruption. This could be due to either local or systemic factors. The major local cause of delayed eruption is the presence of retained deciduous tooth, thick fibrous tissue or bone over the erupting tooth. Other causes include lack of space, traumatic injury to the periodontal ligament, and deflection of the path of eruption by trauma or cyst or tumor enlargement and presence of cyst, tumors or supernumerary tooth in the eruption path. Systemic factors associated with delayed eruption include deficiency of growth hormone, thyroid hormone, parathyroid hormone, nutritional status, genetic factors, osteopetrosis and some syndromes [hyperimmunoglobulinemia E (hyper-IgE) syndrome, Albright syndrome, Hurler's syndrome, cleidocranial dysplasia, etc.].

Natal and Neonatal Tooth

Natal teeth are those teeth that are present at the time of birth and neonatal teeth are those that erupt within 30 days of life. The most commonly involved tooth is mandibular central incisors **(Figure 11-17)**. Natal or neonatal tooth may cause problems during feeding and may cause ulceration of the tongue of the neonate. These teeth exhibit structural abnormalities such as atubular dentin, aprismatic enamel, and absence of cementum. On occasions a white hornified epithelial structure may be present on the gingiva over the ridge at birth, which can be removed easily. It was termed as predeciduous teeth.

Failure of Tooth Eruption

In this condition, one or more teeth fail to erupt completely. Failure of eruption of tooth has two broad categories,

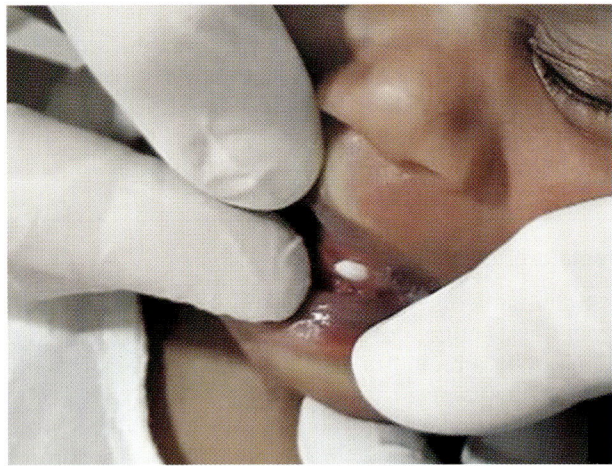

Figure 11-17: Natal tooth.
Source: Dr S Rohini, GRM Dental Clinic, Chennai, Tamil Nadu India.

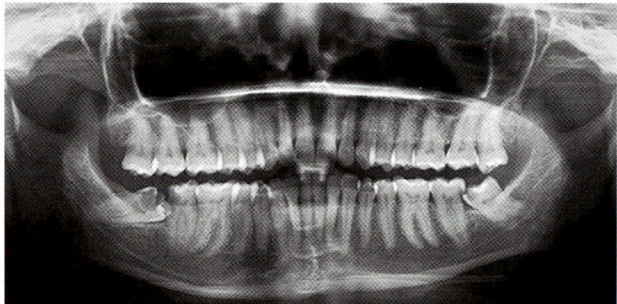

Figure 11-18: Orthopantomograph showing impacted mandibular third molars.

namely—primary failure of eruption and mechanical failure of eruption.

Primary failure of eruption may be caused by genetic factors. Here there is no obvious blockade of eruption path. The tooth may emerge into the oral cavity and fail to reach the occlusal plane. Posterior teeth are usually involved.

Mechanical failure of eruption may be caused by the physical barrier, which completely prevents the eruption. Retained deciduous tooth, supernumerary tooth, odontome, intraosseous cysts or tumors may block the eruption of the permanent successor. Ankylosed tooth and tooth that does not have inherent eruptive force also fails to erupt.

Supraeruption

This is also known as hypereruption and occurs when the opposing tooth is lost. The occlusal surface of the involved tooth crosses the occlusal plane. However, the clinical crown height is not increased, since the tooth moves in axial direction along with the alveolar bone.

Passive Eruption

This is characterized by the apical migration of dentogingival junction and exposure of more amount of crown and sometimes a portion of root (clinical crown). There is no active occlusal movement of the tooth. This gives the apparent appearance of tooth eruption.

Ectopic Eruption

This is characterized by the eruption of tooth away from its destined location. Causes would include wrong eruption path, lack of space due to smaller jaw size, premature loss of deciduous predecessors, and eruption of other permanent teeth, which occupy the space and presence of odontome or supernumerary tooth, which deflect the path of eruption.

Impacted and Embedded Tooth

Impacted teeth are unerupted or partially erupted tooth due to lack of space or by a tooth block (**Figure 11-18**). Embedded teeth are also unerupted teeth but they lack the eruptive force. These unerupted or partially erupted teeth are vulnerable for dental caries, pericoronitis, and development of odontogenic cysts or tumors. The impacted mandibular third molars weaken the angle of the mandible and make it more prone for fracture.

Submerged Tooth

These are ankylosed deciduous teeth, particularly the mandibular second molar. These teeth exhibit resorption of root to varying degree and ankylosis to the alveolar bone, thereby preventing the eruption of the succedaneous premolar. The eruption of adjacent permanent teeth and the growth of the alveolar bone make the ankylosed deciduous second molar's occlusal plane to be at a lower level giving the submerged appearance.

Points to Remember

- Eruption is axial or occlusal movement of the tooth from its developmental site to its functional position in the occlusal plane.
- Eruptive movements include pre-eruptive tooth movement, eruptive tooth movement and posteruptive tooth movement. Posteruptive tooth movement occurs to compensate for the occlusal/incisal and the mesial wear.
- During eruption the bone in the eruptive path is resorbed by osteoclasts and the connective tissue is destructed by the hydrolytic enzymes.
- Theories of eruption include root growth theory, pulp growth theory, pulp constriction theory, vascular pressure theory, bone remodeling theory, ligament traction theory, neuromuscular theory, and dental follicle theory.

PRACTICE QUESTIONS

1. Define eruption.
2. What is the purpose of having two sets of teeth in human?
3. What happens during pre-eruptive tooth movement?
4. Histology of eruptive tooth movement.
5. Lists the theories of tooth eruption.
6. What is ligament traction theory?
7. What is the difference between impacted and embedded teeth?

MULTIPLE CHOICE QUESTIONS

1. Having more than one set of teeth is known as:
   a. Diphodont
   b. Diphyodont
   c. Polyphyodont
   d. Heterodont
2. Mixed dentition period extends from:
   a. 6 months to 12 years
   b. 6 years to 12 years
   c. 6years to 18 years
   d. 6 months to 6 years
3. First tooth to erupt in the oral cavity is:
   a. Deciduous mandibular first molar
   b. Deciduous maxillary incisor
   c. Deciduous mandibular central incisor
   d. Maxillary molars
4. First permanent tooth to erupt in the oral cavity is:
   a. Mandibular central incisor
   b. Mandibular first molar
   c. Maxillary central incisor
   d. Maxillary first molar
5. Last permanent tooth to erupt in the oral cavity is:
   a. Maxillary canine
   b. Mandibular third molar
   c. Mandibular canine
   d. Maxilary third molar
6. Root growth theory is not accepted because of the following, *except*:
   a. Base of the tooth crypt cannot act as fixed base
   b. Cushion hammock ligament does not exist
   c. Rootless teeth do not erupt
   d. Some teeth move more distance than the length of the roots
7. Ligament traction theory based on the concept that:
   a. Contractile fibroblasts of the periodontal ligament exert tractional force
   b. Fibroblasts in periodontal ligament act as myofibroblasts and help in eruption
   c. Periodontal ligament fibers push the tooth toward occlusal plane
   d. Hydrostatic pressure exerted by the periodontal ligament pulls the tooth towards occlusal plane
8. The local causes of delayed eruption is due to the following, *except*:
   a. Presence of retained deciduous tooth, thick fibrous tissue or bone over the erupting tooth
   b. Deficiency of hormones
   c. Lack of space
   d. Deflection of the path of eruption by trauma or cyst or tumor enlargement
9. Natal tooth is the one which:
   a. Erupts shortly after birth
   b. Is present at birth
   c. Erupts within 30 days after birth
   d. Does not erupt at birth
10. Delayed eruption:
    a. Is more common than premature eruption
    b. May be due to presence of retained deciduous tooth, thick fibrous tissue or bone over the erupting tooth
    c. May be due to deficiency of growth hormone, thyroid hormone or parathyroid hormone
    d. All of the above
11. Embedded tooth:
    a. Has eruptive force but fails to erupt due to lack of apace
    b. Is caused by deficiency of growth hormone
    c. Does not have eruptive force
    d. Is also known as submerged tooth

ANSWERS

1. b   2. b   3. c   4. a   5. b   6. c   7. a   8. b   9. b   10. d   11. c

BIBLIOGRAPHY

1. Acquavella FJ. Delayed eruption. Why? N Y State Dent J. 1965;31:448-9.
2. Avery JK, Chiego DJ. Essentials of oral histology and embryology: a clinical approach, 3rd edition. US: Mosby; 2006.
3. Avery JK. Oral development and histology, 3rd edition. New York: Thieme; 2002.
4. Berkovitz BKB, Holland GR, Moxham BJ. Oral anatomy, histology and embryology, 4th edition. US: Elsevier; 2009.

5. Bhaskar SN. Synopsis of oral pathology, 5th edition. St. Louis: The CV Mosby Co; 1977.
6. Cahill DR, Marks SC. Tooth eruption: evidence for the central role of the dental follicle. J Oral Pathol. 1980;9:189-200.
7. Chandra S, Chandra S, Chandra M, et al. Textbook of dental and oral histology with embryology and MCQ's, 2nd edition. India: Jaypee Brothers Medical Publishers (P) Ltd; 2010.
8. Di Biase DD. Mucous membrane and delayed eruption. Trans Br Soc Study Orthod. 1969;5:149-58.
9. Frazier-Bowers SA, Koehler KE, Ackerman JL, et al. Primary failure of eruption: further characterization of a rare eruption disorder. Am J Orthod Dentofacial Orthop. 2007;131(5):578.e1-11.
10. Gerlach RF, Toledo DB, Novaes PD, et al. The effect of lead on the eruption rates of incisor teeth in rats. Arch Oral Biol. 2000;45:951-5.
11. Goho C. Delayed eruption due to overlying fibrous connective tissue. ASDC J Dent Child. 1987;54:359-60.
12. Gozes I, Van Dijck A, Hacohen-Kleiman G, et al. Premature primary tooth eruption in cognitive/motor-delayed ADNP-mutated children, Transl Psychiatry. 2017;7(2):e1043.
13. Inger Kjær. Mechanism of Human Tooth Eruption: Review Article Including a New Theory for Future Studies on the Eruption Process, Volume 2014, Article ID 341905, 13 pages, http://dx.doi.org/10.1155/2014/341905.
14. Jin Y, Wang C, Cheng S, Zhao Z, Li J. MicroRNA control of tooth formation and eruption. Arch Oral Biol. 2017;73:302-10.
15. Khan S, Brougham CL, Ryan J, Sahrudin A, O'Neill G, Wall D, et al. (2013) miR-379 Regulates Cyclin B1 Expression and is Decreased in Breast Cancer. PLoS ONE 8(7): e68753. https://doi.org/10.1371/journal.pone.0068753
16. Kumar GS. Orban's oral histology and embryology, 14th edition. India: Elsevier; 2015.
17. Marks SC, Cahill DR. Experimental study in the dog of the non- active role of the tooth in the eruptive process. Archs Oral Biol. 1984;29:311-22.
18. Marks SC, Schroeder HE. Tooth eruption: Theories and facts. Anat Rec. 1996;245:374-93.
19. Moorrees CF, Gron AM, Lebret LM, et al. Growth studies of the dentition: a review. Am J Orthod. 1969;55:600-16.
20. Nanci A. Ten Cate's oral histology, 9th edition. US: Elsevier; 2018.
21. Ondarza A, Jara L, Munoz P, et al. Sequence of eruption of deciduous dentition in a Chilean sample with Down's syndrome. Arch Oral Biol. 1997;42:401-6.
22. Provenza VD, Seibel W. Oral Histology-inheritance and development, 2nd edition. USA: Lea & Febiger; 1986.
23. Rajkumar K, Ramya R. Textbook of oral anatomy, histology, physiology & tooth morphology, 2nd edition. India: Wolters Kluwer Health; 2017.
24. Richman JM. Shedding new light on the mysteries of tooth eruption. Proc Natl Acad Sci U S A. 2019;116(2):353-55. doi:10.1073/pnas.1819412116
25. Rusmah M. Natal and neonatal teeth: a clinical and histological study. J Clin Pediatr Dent. 1991;15(4):251-3.
26. Sarrafpour B, Swain M, Li Q, et al. Tooth eruption results from bone remodeling driven by bite forces sensed by soft tissue dental follicles: a finite element analysis. PLoS One. 2013;8(3):1-18.
27. Sharma P, Arora A, Valiathan A. Age changes of jaws and soft tissue profile. Scientific World. 2014;2014:301501.
28. Sogi S, Hugar SM, Patil S, et al. Multiple natal teeth: a rare case report. Indian J Dent Res. 2011;22(1):169-71.
29. Wang XP. Tooth eruption without roots. J Dent Res. 2012;92(3):212-4.
30. Wise GE, Yao S, Henk WG. Bone formation as a potential motive force of tooth eruption in the rat molar. Clin Anat. 2007;20:632.
31. Yaseen SM, Naik S, Uloopi KS. Ectopic eruption: a review and case report. Contemp Clin Dent. 2011;2(1):3-7.
32. Zhu J, King D. Natal and neonatal teeth. ASDC J Dent Child. 1995;62(2):123-8.

CHAPTER 12

Shedding

B Sivapathasundharam

CHAPTER OUTLINE

- Order of Shedding   166
- Mechanism of Shedding   167
- Histology of Shedding   167
  » Tooth Resorption   168
  » Resorption of Pulp   169
  » Bone Resorption   169
  » Periodontal Ligament   170
- Clinical Considerations   170
  » Premature Shedding   170
  » Delayed Shedding or Retained Deciduous   170
  » Retained Root Remnants   170

"The falling leaf that tells of autumn's death is, in a subtler sense, a prophecy of spring"
—Robert Green Ingersol

INTRODUCTION

The term "shedding" or "exfoliation" refers to the physiological process of replacement of the old with the new one. The term deciduous means "falling off at maturity" and is generously used in reference to seasonally shed leaves, animal parts (like antlers of deer), and baby teeth or milk teeth in few mammals. Deciduous teeth are the first set of teeth that are developed during embryonic stage and erupt into the oral cavity after birth. They are smaller in size, less in number, and are shortly replaced by permanent or succedaneous teeth.

The term polyphyodont refers to replacement of teeth multiple times throughout the life that are seen in lower vertebrates. Diphyodont refers to having two sets of teeth, namely primary and permanent as seen in mammals. In mammals, especially in human, deciduous teeth are replaced by permanent teeth, which are stronger, larger in size, and numerically greater, to withstand the increased jaw size and masticatory load of an adult.

Shedding is most predominantly brought about by progressive resorption of alveolar bone, periodontal ligament, and roots of deciduous teeth **(Figure 12-1)**. Loss or destruction of hard tissue by cellular activity is known as resorption. It may be physiological as in shedding or pathological.

Resorption of hard tissue is regulated by systemic and local factors. Systemic factors that operate on resorption

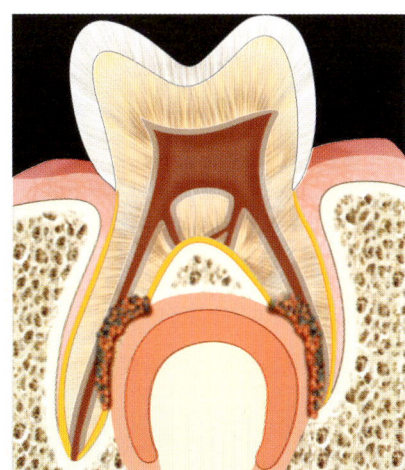

Figure 12-1: Erupting permanent tooth causing resorption.

are parathyroid hormone, 1,25-dihydroxy vitamin D3, and calcitonin. Local factors include—macrophage colony stimulating factor (M-CSF), interleukin 1(IL-1), interleukin 6 (IL-6), tumor necrosis factor-alpha (TNF-α), which include receptor activator of nuclear factor kappa-B ligand (RANKL) and osteoprotegerin (OPG) as family members and microorganisms. The process of resorption in shedding begins well in advance, precisely after the root completion of deciduous teeth. However, the time period varies for different teeth within the same jaw.

The pattern of shedding follows the pattern of eruption of the successors.

ORDER OF SHEDDING

The shedding of deciduous teeth is a well-orchestrated event. It is accompanied or followed by the eruption of successional and accessional teeth, wherein 20 deciduous teeth exfoliate and are replaced by 28 permanent teeth between the ages of 6 years and 12 years. This time period is referred to as mixed dentition period **(Figure 12-2)**. Third molars erupt between 17 and 24 years.

Deciduous mandibular incisors are the first to shed with the eruption of permanent incisors. Usually the shedding pattern is symmetrical within the same jaw. The symmetry between the left and right side of the mouth with respect to the timing of deciduous teeth shedding and eruption of permanent teeth is very interesting. Both the events are interrelated and well-programmed.

Mandibular deciduous teeth exfoliate before the maxillary teeth, but the exception is mandibular second molars. Progression of shedding starts from anterior to posterior in the lower jaw. In the upper jaw, though it is anterior to posterior, first molars shed before canines. Shedding occurs slightly earlier in girls than boys, but within the specified chronological age.

The process of shedding starts with development and positioning of permanent tooth germ in close proximity with the roots of deciduous teeth. In deciduous anterior teeth, resorption begins at the lingual aspect of the apical third of the deciduous tooth, where the developing tooth buds are located. Once the resorption reaches the labial aspect of the tooth root, the permanent tooth moves directly below the deciduous tooth root. From then on, the resorption continues in horizontal plane and proceeds axially. Ultimately the deciduous tooth exfoliates and the permanent tooth erupts and replaces it **(Figures 12-3A to D)**.

Frequently the erupting permanent mandibular incisors miss their direction and erupt lingually and leave the deciduous as retained **(Figure 12-4)**. As far as the maxillary canine is concerned, if the erupting permanent canine is misdirected, it erupts labial to the deciduous canine.

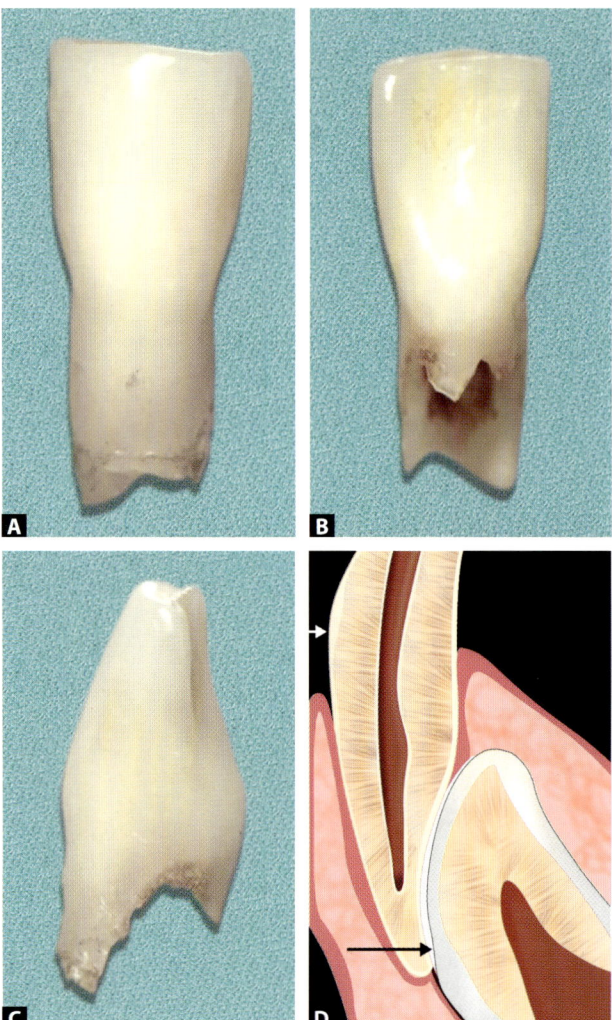

Figures 12-3A to D: (A) Labial view of deciduous mandibular central incisor with resorption; (B) Palatal view of deciduous mandibular central incisor with resorption; (C) Apicolingual resorption of deciduous mandibular central incisor; (D) Apicolingual placement of permanent incisor causing resorption of lingual aspect of the apical third of the primary tooth.

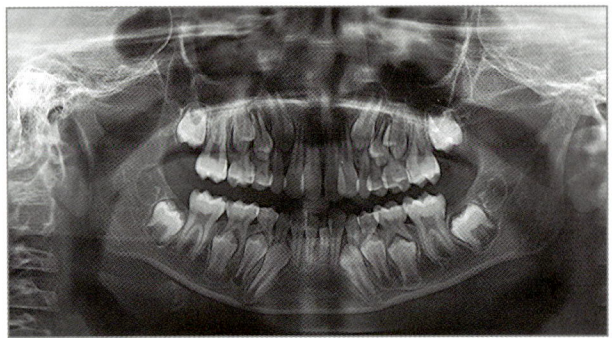

Figure 12-2: Orthopantomograph of 8 years old individual revealing mixed dentition.
Source: Dr Farzan JM and Dr Parisa Norouzi Baghaomeh, Meenakshi Ammal Dental College, Chennai, Tamil Nadu, India.

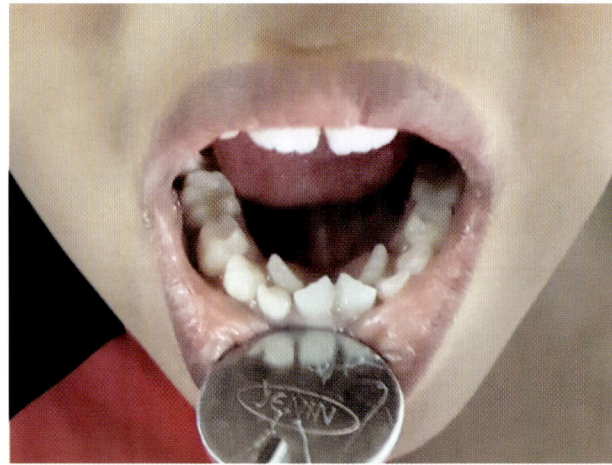

Figure 12-4: Eruption of permanent mandibular lateral incisors lingual to the deciduous teeth.

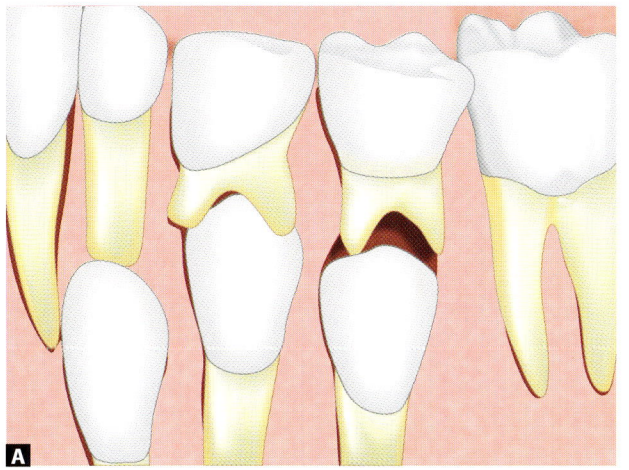
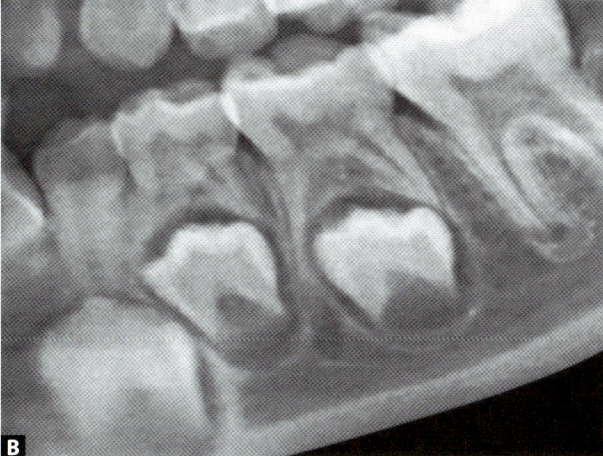
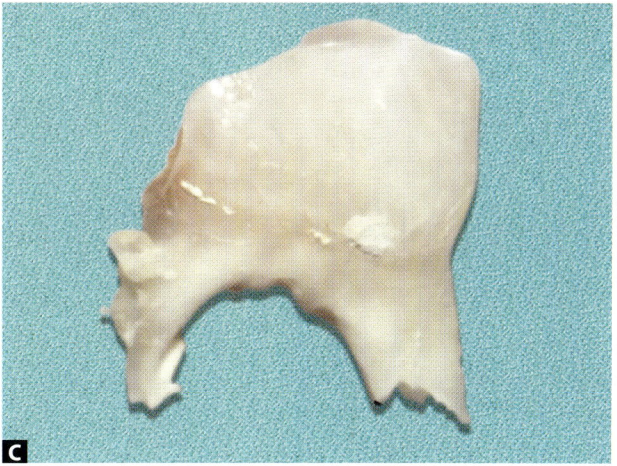

Figures 12-5A to C: (A) Placement of premolars in between the roots of the deciduous molars; (B) Radiograph showing resorption in the roots of deciduous molars and positioning of the permanent tooth bud in between the resorbed roots; and (C) Uneven resorption of deciduous molar roots.
Source: Dr Karthikeyan K, Smile Dental Clinic, Chennai, Tamil Nadu, India.

Shedding of deciduous molars begins with the development of premolars lingually **(Figures 12-5A to C)**. First resorption occurs in the interradicular bone of the deciduous molars. This is followed by the resorption of the roots of the deciduous molars on the inner aspect. The developing premolars soon move between the divergent roots of deciduous molars due to the resorption of interradicular bone and portion of deciduous tooth root, jaw growth, and the occlusal movement of the deciduous molars. This results in gaining of enough space for the premolars to grow. Resorption of deciduous molar roots is often uneven due to disparity between the interradicular distance and the successional tooth's follicle size. The resorption temporarily ceases and repair occurs by deposition of cementum like tissue.

Thus the shedding and eruption processes are not continuous; period of rest exists, which permits the repair and reattachment of deciduous tooth. However, once the eruptive forces of the successors are regained, resorption continues until the roots are completely lost and the tooth is shed.

MECHANISM OF SHEDDING

As stated previously, the process of shedding involves resorption of deciduous tooth root, periodontal ligament, and alveolar bone. Resorption of alveolar bone and periodontal ligament precedes the resorption of cementum and dentin of the tooth root. This is caused by the pressure generated from the developing and erupting permanent tooth and the degenerating periodontal ligament due to the increased masticatory load exerted by the growing jaws and muscles of mastication.

The hard tissues (bone and teeth) are resorbed by osteoclasts and odontoclasts, while periodontal ligament by fibroblasts and macrophages. Though osteoclasts and odontoclasts are the key cell types responsible for the resorption of all hard tissues, macrophages and monocytes join them in resorptive activities. These cells together exhibit a complex interplay of molecular biologic events, involving cytokines, enzymes, and hormones that influence the resorption process.

HISTOLOGY OF SHEDDING

The resorption of hard tissues, the bone and tooth and soft tissue, the periodontal ligament occur almost together, however, they begin and continue independently. As soon the permanent teeth make the eruptive movements, the roots of the deciduous teeth and interradicular septum of deciduous tooth begin to resorb from the apical region to the crown.

Tooth Resorption

The structural changes accompanying tooth resorption are first noticed at the site of erupting permanent tooth; soon the resorption continues in the vicinity of the root. In the tooth, resorption begins at the site proximal to the pressure exerted by erupting permanent successor, however, the process of resorption is proved by various experiments to be inherent and autonomous. Though the contributory role by the erupting successional tooth is undeniable, it is not a prerequisite. It is proved by the fact that if a permanent successor is missing, the shedding is delayed but never fails.

Odontoclasts are the cells responsible for the resorption of the tooth. They are structurally and functionally similar to osteoclasts. However, they differ from osteoclast by their smaller size, having fewer nuclei than osteoclasts, and having smaller or no clear zone. Since they can resorb any of the dental tissue (enamel, dentin, cementum, or pulp), they are called as odontoclasts.

The origin of odontoclasts is assumed to be similar to osteoclasts of the bone, *i.e.*, from the circulating monocyte-like cells. Further undifferentiated mesenchymal cells are also suggested to be a source for odontoclasts.

Cytokines and key transcriptional factors secreted by the dental pulp cells of deciduous teeth mediate monocyte–macrophage lineage to form osteoclasts or odontoclasts **(Figure 12-6)**.

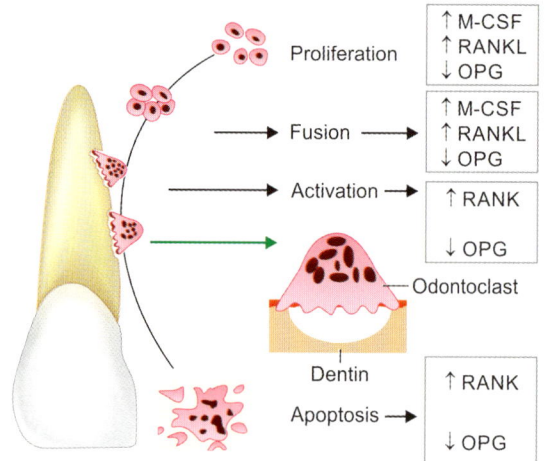

Figure 12-6: Formation of odontoclast and resorption.

Odontoclasts are found in clusters. They tend to fuse with each other to become multinucleated cells, once they attach to the resorbing surface. Mononuclear odontoclasts do exist, albeit a very smaller quantity (<4%). The cell membrane of the odontoclast is thrown into multiple villous like folds of about 2–3 μm depth to form the ruffled border or brush border (similar to osteoclasts). This increases the surface area, thereby increasing the functional area. Adjacent to the ruffled border, there is an area devoid of cytoplasmic organelles called clear zone. This region consists of actin and myosin filaments and acts as an attachment apparatus.

Cytoplasm of the odontoclasts is filled with mitochondria, ribosomes, Golgi apparatus, and plenty of vesicles presumed to be lysosomes that play an active role in resorption. Cytoplasm appears foamy due to the presence of vesicles and vacuoles. These vacuoles exhibit acid phosphatase activity. Odontoclast resides within an irregular bay similar to the Howship's lacunae of bone, indicating active resorptive process. These resorption bays are small and shallow in contrast to deep Howship's lacunae of the osteoclasts.

Odontoclasts are distributed in variable position and follow the pattern of resorption. They are found around the roots of the resorbing tooth and inside the root canals and pulp chamber against the predentin surface **(Figure 12-7)**. As far as the single rooted deciduous teeth are concerned, they exfoliate before the resorption process reaches the crown portion, so the pulpal architecture is usually intact when the teeth are shed and odontoclasts are not found in the pulp chamber. In contrast, deciduous molars exhibit complete resorption of the root and partial resorption of the crown before exfoliation. When resorption progresses to involve the

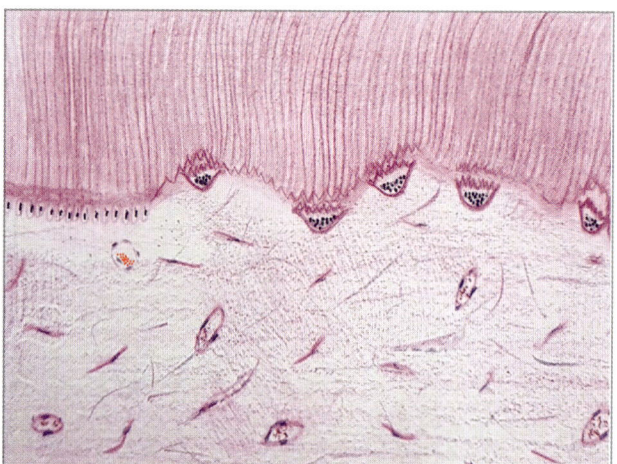

Figure 12-7: Odontoclasts resorbing dentin.

crown of the deciduous molar, the odontoblastic layer of the coronal pulp is replaced by the odontoclasts. On occasions, exfoliating deciduous molar crown appears reddish due to the thinning of the crown as a result of the resorption of the dentin and enamel.

The active resorption of tooth begins with breakdown of mineral (inorganic) content and collagen matrix (organic content) of the dentin and cementum by secretion of hydrolytic enzymes by the odontoclasts. These enzymes act as proton pumps and lower the pH, into acidic, at the confined area favoring dissolution. This is achieved by the attachment of odontoclasts to the tooth surface through the clear zone. This creates a sealed space covered by ruffled border of the odontoclast. The ruffled border acts as proton pump and elaborates hydrogen ions, which acidifies the extracellular environment **(Figures 12-8A and B)**.

The inorganic content of the tooth, made up of calcium phosphate hydroxyapatite crystals, is broken down and absorbed into the intracellular vesicles and is moved across the cell and terminally excreted into the intercellular fluid as granules. The collagenous organic matrix is denatured by collagenase enzymes, wherein the tightly packed fibrils

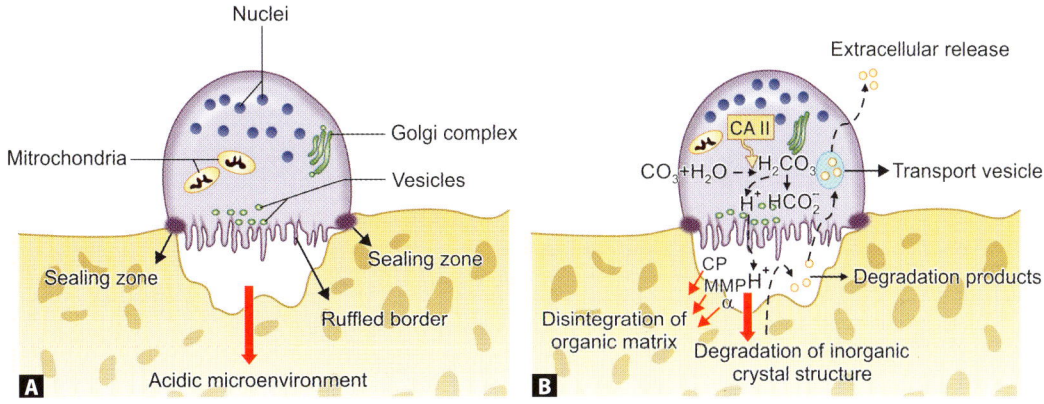

Figures 12-8A and B: Odontoclast and its components.

become loosely bound and degraded by lysosomes secreted by the odontoclasts, while the protein breaks down into amino acids by the action of protease enzyme secreted from odontoclast cells. The degradation of the organic matrix is brought about by three groups of proteinase enzymes namely- collagenases and matrix metalloproteinases (MMP), both act at neutral or just below neutral pH, and the cysteine proteinase family, which acts at an acidic pH.

As stated previously, resorption is not a continuous process. There are periods of rest and repair. Resorbed area is repaired by the deposition of cementum-like tissue secreted by the cementoblast-like cells. Alternate periods of resorption and repair result in the formation of reversal lines similar to the bone. Usually the rest period is shorter when compared to the resorption period. Loss of periodontal ligament with prolonged rest period may lead to ankylosis. However, the resorption process restarts after a rest period and ultimately causes the falling off of the deciduous teeth.

The gingival attachment of the deciduous tooth migrates apically once the deciduous tooth root is completely resorbed. This holds the deciduous tooth during the last phase of shedding.

Resorption of Pulp

Most of the time, teeth are shed with intact coronal pulp. Infrequently odontoclasts are found within the pulp chambers and the pulp canals replacing the odontoblastic layer of the pulp. The resorbing pulp is called as resorbing organ of Tomes, named after Charles S. Tomes, the first person to describe the process of tooth resorption and structural changes that occur during tooth resorption.

Histologically, resorbing pulp appears less cellular and more fibrous with reduced or no neural elements. This explains why primary teeth are relatively insensitive to tooth preparation for restorative procedures. As the resorption process nears the cementoenamel junction, the coronal pulp is infiltrated by chronic inflammatory cells and the odontoblasts begin to degenerate. The type of degeneration seen in pulp is compared to the degeneration of epithelium that covers the erupting tooth that are lost while eruption.

Similar to the RANK–RANKL of osteoblast and osteoclasts interaction, RANK receptor is expressed by odontoclasts and RANKL by odontoblasts, fibroblasts of the pulp, and periodontal ligament and cementoblasts. M-CSF and OPG is also expressed by odontoblasts, ameloblasts, and cells of the dental pulp. M-CSF upregulates RANK and downregulates the OPG, both are important for the differentiation and activation of odontoclasts. These are present both in deciduous and permanent tooth. But it is not clear why deciduous tooth root alone undergoes resorption while permanent tooth root does not normally. This might be due to the different types of RANKL and CSF-1 expressions in pulp cells of deciduous teeth. Under normal conditions, periodontal ligament cells of deciduous and permanent teeth express OPG and not RANKL, which inhibits the differentiation of odontoclasts and prevent resorption. RANKL is expressed by the periodontal ligament cells only during physiologic root resorption. Further, it is suggested that the periodontal ligament cells of the deciduous teeth produce more collagenase (MMP- 9) than the periodontal ligament cells of the permanent teeth. Also it responds to proinflammatory cytokines, such as IL1 and TNF-α enhancing the expression of matrix metalloproteinases, but not to the tissue inhibitors of metalloproteinases (TIMP).

Bone Resorption

Bone is a dynamic tissue, which undergoes physiologic turnover called remodeling throughout the life to regulate the serum calcium level and repair. Bone remodeling involves simultaneous bone resorption by osteoclasts and bone deposition by osteoblasts. Bone resorption occurring in shedding is similar to the general pattern of resorption occurring in the bone remodeling. The process of resorption includes breakdown of organic and inorganic components of the bone. The first step in the bone resorption is the acidification of the area to be resorbed. This happens beneath the ruffled border of the osteoclasts. The required H^+ ions are provided by the H^+-ATPase pump. Acidification leads to delinking of the hydroxyapatite from the collagen and dissolution of the apatite crystals. The exposed organic matrix, which consists of collagen and ground substance, is digested by the enzymes secreted by the osteoclasts. The morphology of the osteoclasts and mechanism of bone resorption are discussed in the chapter on alveolar bone.

> Bony trabeculae are covered by osteoid (the unmineralized bone matrix), surrounded by a layer of osteoblasts. Similarly dentin is lined by predentin and a continuous layer of odontoblasts, and cementum is covered by cementoid and a layer of cementoblasts.
> Osteoid protects the bony trabeculae from resorption. When resorption has to be taken place, the osteoid layer should be disrupted and the trabeculae have to be exposed to osteoclastic attachment. The osteoblasts are sensitive to bone resorptive hormones (parathormone) and cytokines and they degrade the osteoid during resorption. But the cementoblasts of the tooth are nonresponsive to hormones and cytokines. So the cementoid over the cementum and the predentin lining of the dentin is damaged by inflammatory process which enables resorption.

Periodontal Ligament

The changes in periodontal ligament are less known, since changes seen are meager. The degradation is genetically determined and occurs due to cell death without obvious inflammation. The cell death occurs either due to apoptosis (physiological programmed cell death) or functional interference happening within the cells of periodontal ligament. The periodontal ligament fibroblasts show typical signs of impaired function and series of morphological alterations such as cell shrinkage and fragmentation. Further they are rapidly phagocytosed by macrophages. The fact that programmed cell death is seen during shedding that occurs at specific ages, supports the concept that shedding is a genetically determined process. Additionally, experimental demonstration of the enzyme collagenase at the site of resorption (toward the pressure side) was suggested to facilitate the resorption of the periodontal ligament.

> Frequently, the mechanism of shedding of deciduous teeth has been always revolved around two main factors, firstly pressure from the erupting permanent tooth and secondly genetic. Various studies have been documented in favor of both.
> The experimental studies [Shapiro and Rogers (1939) and Obersztyn (1963)] reveal that deciduous tooth resorption occurs independently even in absence of permanent tooth germs, despite a delay. Further the resorption noticed in the portion of root, which is not exposed to pressure, confirms the pressure from the erupting tooth is not the only factor responsible for resorption. Further, the presence of bony partition between the permanent tooth and its deciduous predecessor present in some stage of development is against the pressure theory.
> Clinically, this is confirmed by the shedding of deciduous tooth, even in the absence of permanent tooth germ within the jaw. For example, delayed shedding of deciduous lateral incisors with congenitally missing permanent lateral incisors endorses the minimal or nil influence from developing permanent successor.
> Various studies done on eruption in monozygotic twins witnessed that shedding is determined mostly by genetic factors (in 80% of cases) while rest is by other local factors.
> Obersztyn (1963) proposed two other factors, namely trauma from increased occlusal load and local inflammation that can influence the resorption. Though clinically accelerated resorption of restored or decayed tooth (resulting from pulpal inflammation) supports this concept, these factors are not accepted by all.

Migration of dentogingival junction as well as of gingival epithelium takes place prior to shedding, and suggests that this phenomenon may play an important role in the process of exfoliation.

CLINICAL CONSIDERATIONS

Premature Shedding

Premature shedding may occur as a consequence of multiple factors namely—trauma and pulpal inflammation caused by dental caries leading to pulpal necrosis or internal resorption, which in turn initiates resorption leading to premature shedding. This may lead to improper positioning of permanent tooth due to lack of guidance or delayed eruption of permanent tooth due to formation of thick fibrous tissue over the erupting tooth.

Delayed Shedding or Retained Deciduous

The persistence of primary tooth beyond the shedding period is referred as retained deciduous. The causes for the retained deciduous tooth include missing permanent tooth, impacted tooth, ankylosis of deciduous tooth, etc. It is usually seen in relation to maxillary laterals, canines, and mandibular second molars (**Figure 12-9**).

Retained Root Remnants

On occasions, a portion of the root of the deciduous molar may be retained. When the bicuspids develop and erupt, if the space available is enough for them, a part of deciduous molar root may be left unresorbed.

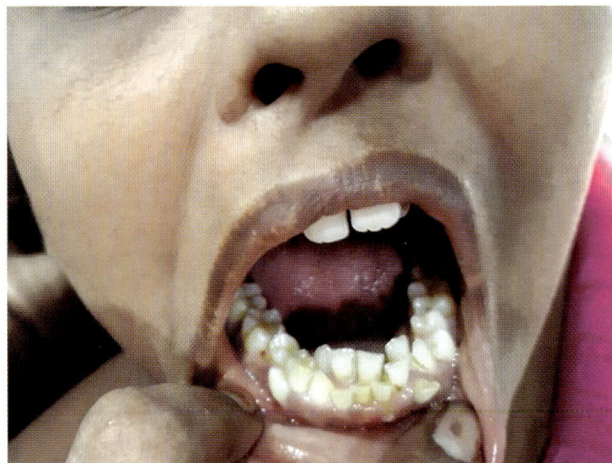

Figures 12-9: Retained deciduous teeth in mandibular anterior region.
Source: Dr S Rohini, GRM Dental Clinic, Chennai, Tamil Nadu, India.

CHAPTER 12: Shedding

Points to Remember

- Physiological process of replacement of the old with the new one is called shedding.
- Shedding is most predominantly brought about by progressive resorption of alveolar bone, periodontal ligament, and roots of deciduous teeth.
- Resorption of hard tissue is regulated by systemic and local factors.
- Deciduous incisors are the first to shed with the eruption of permanent incisors.
- Mandibular deciduous teeth exfoliate before the maxillary teeth, but the exception is mandibular second molars.
- Shedding occurs slightly earlier in girls than boys.
- Shedding and eruption processes are not continuous; period of rest exists, which permits the repair and reattachment of deciduous tooth.
- The hard tissues (bone and teeth) are resorbed by osteoclasts and odontoclasts, while periodontal ligament by fibroblasts and macrophages.
- Odontoclasts are multinucleated cells responsible for the resorption of the tooth. They are structurally and functionally similar to osteoclasts.
- Resorbing pulp appears less cellular and more fibrous with reduced or no neural elements. This is why primary teeth are relatively insensitive to tooth preparation for restorative procedures.
- Mechanism of shedding of deciduous teeth has been always revolved around two main factors, firstly pressure from the erupting permanent tooth and secondly genetic.
- Persistence of primary tooth beyond the shedding period is referred as retained deciduous.
- Submerged teeth are ankylosed deciduous molars particularly the mandibular second molar tooth, whose occlusal plane is lower than the adjacent permanent first molar and first premolar.

PRACTICE QUESTIONS

1. What is shedding?
2. Write notes on mechanism of shedding.
3. Write notes on histology of shedding.
4. Write a brief notes on odontoclasts.
5. Describe the histological changes of pulp during shedding.

MULTIPLE CHOICE QUESTIONS

1. Human dentition is:
    a. Monophyodont
    b. Diphyodont
    c. C. Polyphyodont
    d. Homodont
2. In shedding which one of the following does not occur:
    a. Resorption of alveolar bone
    b. Resorption of the periodontal ligament
    c. Resorption of the dental follicle
    d. Resorption of the roots of deciduous teeth
3. Systemic factors that operate on resorption include the following, *except:*
    a. Thyroid hormone.
    b. Parathyroid hormone
    c. 1,25-dihydroxy vitamin D3
    d. Calcitonin
4. The time period referred to as mixed dentition period is:
    a. 6 months to 6 years
    b. 6 years to 12 years
    c. 6 months to 12 years
    d. 12 years to 17 years
5. First deciduous tooth to shed is:
    a. Deciduous upper incisors
    b. Deciduous molars
    c. Deciduous mandibular incisors
    d. Deciduous mandibular second molars
6. Resorption begins at the lingual aspect of the apical third in:
    a. Deciduous mandibular molars
    b. Deciduous anterior teeth
    c. Deciduous canines
    d. Deciduous maxillary molars
7. Cells responsible for the resorption of tooth are called:
    a. Osteoblasts
    b. Fibroblasts
    c. Odontoblasts
    d. Odontoclasts
8. Resorption of hard tissues, the bone and tooth and soft tissue, the periodontal ligament:
    a. Occur almost together
    b. One after another
    c. After the resorption of pulp
    d. Follows the eruption of permanent tooth
9. Tooth resorption is a:
    a. Pathological process
    b. Continuous process
    c. Process consisting of active and rest phase
    d. A hormonally influenced process
10. Resorbing pulp is called as:
    a. Resorbing organ of Tomes
    b. Tomes' fibrosis
    c. Resorbing organ of Ranvier
    d. Pulpal odontoclastosis

11. **Resorbing pulp exhibits the following,** *except:*
    a. Increased vascularity
    b. Less cellularity
    c. More fibrous tissue content
    d. Reduced or no neural elements
12. **Which of the following tissues resorbs first:**
    a. Alveolar bone and periodontal ligament
    b. Cementum and dentin
    c. Enamel and dentin
    d. Alveolar bone and cementum
13. **Submerged or ankylosed deciduous tooth is usually the:**
    a. Maxillary deciduous lateral incisors.
    b. Mandibular deciduous second molars.
    c. Mandibular deciduous first molar.
    d. Deciduous mandibular canines.

ANSWERS

1. b   2. c   3. a   4. b   5. c   6. b   7. d   8. a   9. c   10. a   11. a   12. a   13. b

BIBLIOGRAPHY

1. Andreasen JO, Andreasen FM, Andersson L. Textbook and color atlas of traumatic injuries to the teeth, 4th edition. Oxford: Blackwell Munksgaard; 2007.
2. Ashizawa Y, Deguchi T, Okafuji N, et al. A histological study of the exfoliation of human deciduous teeth. J Dent Res. 1993;72(3):634-40.
3. Ashizawa Y, Deguchi T, Okafuji N, et al. Cementum like tissue deposition on the resorbed pulp chamber wall of human deciduous teeth prior to shedding. Acta Anat. 1993;147:24-34.
4. Ashizawa Y, Deguchi T, Okafuji N, et al. Odontoclastic resorption at the pulpal surface of coronal dentin prior to shedding of human deciduous teeth. Arch Histol Cytol. 1992;55:273-285.
5. Ashizawa Y, Deguchi T, Okafuji N, et al. Odontoclastic resorption of the superficial nonmineralized layer of predentine in the shedding of human deciduous teeth. Cell Tissue Res. 1994;277:19-26.
6. Avery JK, Chiego DJ. Essentials of oral histology and embryology: a clinical approach, 3rd edition. US: Mosby; 2006.
7. Avery JK. Oral development and histology, 3rd edition. New York: Thieme; 2002.
8. Berkovitz BKB, Holland GR, Moxham BJ. Oral anatomy, histology and embryology, 4th edition. US: Elsevier; 2009.
9. Burgess TL, Qian Y, Kaufman S, et al. The ligand for osteoprotegerin (OPGL) directly activates mature osteoclasts. J Cell Biol. 1999;145:527-38.
10. Chandra S, Chandra S, Chandra M, et al. Textbook of dental and oral histology with embryology and MCQ's, 2nd edition. India: Jaypee Brothers Medical Publishers (P) Ltd; 2010.
11. Chatterjee K. Essentials of dental anatomy and oral histology, 2nd edition. India: Jaypee Brothers Medical Publishers (P) Ltd; 2014.
12. Cutler CW, Jotwani R. Dendritic cells at the oral mucosal interface. J Dent Res. 2006;85(8):678-89.
13. Davidovitch Z, Lynch P, Shanfeld JL. Immunohistochemical localization of interleukins in dental and paradental cells during tooth eruption and root resorption in kittens. In: Davidovich Z (Ed). The Biological Mechanisms of Tooth Eruption and Root Resorption. Birmingham: EBSCO Media; 1988. pp. 355-64.
14. Domon T, Osanai M, Yasuda M, et al. Mononuclear odontoclast participation in tooth resorption: the distribution of nuclei in human odontoclasts. Anat Rec. 1997;249(4):449-57.
15. Gaunt WA, Osborn JW, Ten Cate AR. Advanced dental histology, 2nd edition. Bristol: John Wright & Sons Ltd; 1971.
16. Haralabakis NB, Yiagtzis SC, Toutountzakis NM. Premature or delayed exfoliation of deciduous teeth and root resorption and formation. Angle Orthod. 1994;64(2):151-7.
17. Harokopakis-Hajishengallis E. Physiologic root resorption in primary teeth: molecular and histological events. J Oral Sci. 2007;49(1):1-12.
18. Haschek W, Bolon B, Rousseaux C, Wallig M (Eds). Fundamentals of toxicologic pathology, 3rd edition. US: Academic Press; 2017.
19. Herzberg AJ, Raso DS, Silverman JF. Color Atlas of normal cytology, 1st edition. USA: Churchill Livingstone; 1999.
20. Jenkins GN. The physiology and biochemistry of mouth, 4th edition. US: Blackwell Publications; 1978. pp. 197-214.
21. Kang MK, Mehrazarin S, No-Hee P. Oral mucosal stem cells-identification, characterization, and clinical and disease implications. In: Vishwakarma A, Sharpe P, Shi S, Ramalingam M (Eds). Stem Cell Biology and Tissue Engineering in Dental Sciences. US: Elsevier Inc.; 2015.
22. Kumar GS. Orban's oral histology and embryology, 14th edition. India: Elsevier; 2015.
23. LaGrow Asa J. Record keeping of shedding of deciduous teeth and eruption of permanent teeth. AJO-DO. 1937;23(1):44.
24. Nanci A. Ten Cate's oral histology, 9th edition, US: Elsevier; 2018.
25. Obersztyn A. Experimental investigation of factors causing resorption of deciduous teeth. J Dent Res. 1963;42:600.
26. Odell EW, Morgan PR. Biopsy pathology of the oral tissues, 1st edition. UK: Chapman & Hall; 1998.
27. Ozaki S, Kaneko S, Podyma-Inoue KA, et al. Modulation of extracellular matrix synthesis and alkaline phosphatase activity of periodontal ligament cells by mechanical stress. J Periodontal Res. 2005;40:110-7.
28. Park JY, Chung H, Choi Y, et al. Phenotype and tissue residency of lymphocytes in the murine oral mucosa. Front Immunol. 2017;8:250.
29. Provenza VD, Seibel W. Oral histology—Inheritance and Development, 2nd edition. USA: Lea & Febiger; 1986.
30. Rathbone JM, Hadgraft J. Absorption of drugs from the human oral cavity. Int J Pharm. 1991;74:9-24.
31. Renshaw AA. Aspiration cytology—a pattern recognition approach, 1st edition. China: Elsevier; 2005.

32. Robson F, Ramos-Jorge ML, Bendo CB, et al. Prevalence and determining factors of traumatic injuries to primary teeth in preschool children. Dent Traumatol. 2009;25(1):118-22.
33. Rogers WM, Shapiro HH. Experiments dealing with factors influencing the shedding of deciduous teeth. J Dent Res. 1939;18:73.
34. Russo FB, Pignatari GC, Fernandes IR, et al. Epithelial cells from oral mucosa: How to cultivate them? Cytotechnology. 2016;68(5):2105-14.
35. Sahara N, Okafuji N, Toyoki A, Ashizawa Y, Yagasaki H, Deguchi T, et al. A histological study of the exfoliation of human deciduous teeth. J Dent Res. 1993;72(3):634-40.
36. Schroeder HE. Differentiation of human oral stratified epithelia. Basel, Switzerland: S Karger; 1981.
37. Shannon DB, McKeown ST, Lundy FT, et al. Phenotypic differences between oral and skin fibroblasts in wound contraction and growth factor expression. Wound Repair Regen. 2006;14:172-8.
38. Shapiro HH, Rogers WM. Experiments dealing with factors influencing the shedding of deciduous teeth. J Dent Res. 1939;18:73.
39. Squier C, Brogden K. Human oral mucosa, development, structure and function. Oxford: Wiley-Blackwell; 2011.
40. Squier CA, Kremer MJ. Biology of oral mucosa and oesophagus. J Natl Cancer Inst Monogr. 2011;29:7-15.
41. Szpaderska AM, Zuckerman JD, DiPietro LA. Differential injury responses in oral mucosal and cutaneous wounds. J Dent Res. 2003;82:621.
42. Tsai MT, Chen Y, Lee CY, et al. Noninvasive structural and microvascular anatomy of oral mucosae using handheld optical coherence tomography. Biomed Opt Express. 2017;8(11):5001-12.
43. Tyrovola JB, Spyropoulos MN, Makou M, et al. Root resorption and the OPG/RANKL/RANK system: a mini review. J Oral Sci. 2008;50(4):367-76.
44. Wu YM, Richards DW, Rowe DJ. Production of matrix-degrading enzymes and inhibition of osteoclast-like cell differentiation by fibroblast-like cells from the periodontal ligament of human primary teeth. J Dent Res. 1999;78:681-9.
45. Yildirim S, Yapar M, Srmet U, et al. The role of dental pulp cells in resorption of deciduous teeth. Oral Surg Oral Med Oral Pathol Oral Radiol Endod. 2008;105:113-20.

CHAPTER 13

Oral Mucous Membrane

B Sivapathasundharam, Preethi S

Chapter Outline

- Functions of Oral Mucous Membrane   174
- Boundaries of the Oral Cavity   175
- Clinical Appearance and Regional Variations   175
  » Oral Frenum   176
- Classification of Oral Mucosa   177
- Components of the Oral Mucosa   177
  » Oral Epithelium   179
  » Basement Membrane and Basal Lamina   188
  » Connective Tissue   188
- Masticatory Mucosa   193
  » Hard Palate   193
  » Gingiva   194
- Lining Mucosa   201
  » Lips   201
  » Buccal Mucosa   202
  » Alveolar Mucosa   202
  » Vestibular Fornix   203
  » Floor of the Mouth   203
  » Soft Palate   203
- Specialized Mucosa   204
  » Ventral Surface of Tongue   204
  » Dorsal Surface of Tongue   204
- Development of the Oral Mucosa   208
- Age Changes   208
- Clinical Considerations   209

INTRODUCTION

Surface of the body is covered by the skin and the body cavities are lined by the mucous membrane. Mucous membrane is a moist pliable sheet, lining the body cavities and covers the internal organs. It merges with the skin surface externally at the openings. Its moistness is due to serous and mucous secretions. Oral mucous membrane or the oral mucosa lines the oral cavity proper and the vestibular cavity.

The oral cavity is an interesting part of the human body, anatomically located between the skin on the exterior and the gastrointestinal tract on the interior. Oral mucosa extends from the skin adjacent to the vermillion border of the lips anteriorly and to the pharyngeal mucosa posteriorly. So it exhibits some of the properties of the skin and the gut lining.

FUNCTIONS OF ORAL MUCOUS MEMBRANE

The oral cavity is considered as an organ *per se*, since it performs the functions along with the skin and gastrointestinal tract. It helps to protect the deeper tissues, acts as a sensory organ, and provides a site for glandular secretion. The functions of the oral mucous membrane are as follows:

Initiation: Initiation of tooth development starts from the oral ectoderm. The primary epithelial band, the primordium of the dental lamina forms in the primitive oral epithelium due to induction from the underlying ectomesenchyme.

Development of salivary glands occurs by the ingrowth of the oral epithelium.

Protection: The oral mucosa protects the deeper tissues and organs from the mechanical stresses or forces of mastication, and the external environment. It prevents the entry of bacteria and their toxins by forming a physical barrier and antibodies secretion. The commensal organisms of the oral cavity become pathogenic if the host defense is compromised.

> Membrane-coating granules, which contain lipids, are believed to be responsible for the formation of the permeability barrier in superficial layer of the stratified squamous epithelium. Apart from the superficial layer, the basement membrane also plays a role in controlling the passage of materials across the junction between epithelium and connective tissue.

Sensation: Receptors in the oral cavity respond to touch, pain, temperature, and proprioception, and also enable reflexes like swallowing, gagging, retching, and salivation. The taste buds on the tongue help to perceive taste sensation. The olfactory and taste sense complement each other. The act of chewing helps to release odor of the food and enable it to reach the olfactory nerve endings, which supplement the taste receptors on the tongue.

Secretion: Oral mucosa contains minor salivary glands in its submucosal part. Saliva secreted by major and minor salivary glands is discharged onto the surface of the oral cavity through the ducts and contributes to the moistness of the oral mucosa, which keeps the oral environment in a healthy state.

Thermal regulation: The oral mucosa might not have an important role of thermal regulation in humans but in some animals like dogs, some of the body heat is dissipated through panting.

Absorption: Oral mucosa absorbs fluids, electrolytes, and drugs by various mechanisms (transcellular pathway and paracellular transport through cell junctions). Drugs kept in direct contact with the oral mucosa are more readily absorbed than those dissolved in saliva. The absorption potential of oral mucosa is greater than the skin.

Excretion: Some metabolites are excreted through oral mucous membrane.

Esthetics: Color and amount of visibility of the gingiva and color of the lip mucosa enhance facial esthetics.

> **Points to Remember**
> - The oral cavity is anatomically located between the skin on the exterior and the gastrointestinal tract on the interior.
> - It exhibits some of the properties of the skin and the gut lining.
> - The functions of the oral cavity are:
>   - Initiation
>   - Protection
>   - Sensation
>   - Secretion
>   - Thermal regulation
>   - Absorption
>   - Excretion
>   - Esthetics

BOUNDARIES OF THE ORAL CAVITY

Since the oral mucosa covers the entire oral cavity, it is imperative to know the boundaries of the oral cavity. Though the term "oral cavity" is commonly used to denote the mouth, it is divided into two specific parts namely—vestibular cavity and the oral cavity proper.

❖ The vestibule is that part of the mouth bounded by the lips and cheeks on the outer aspect and facial surface of the teeth, gingiva, and the alveolar process on the inner aspect.

❖ The oral cavity proper is that portion of the mouth, which lies interior to the palatal or lingual aspect of the teeth, and the gingiva. It is bounded superiorly by the hard and soft palate, inferiorly by the tongue and floor of the mouth and posterolaterally by the anterior pillar of fauces and tonsils **(Figure 13-1)**.

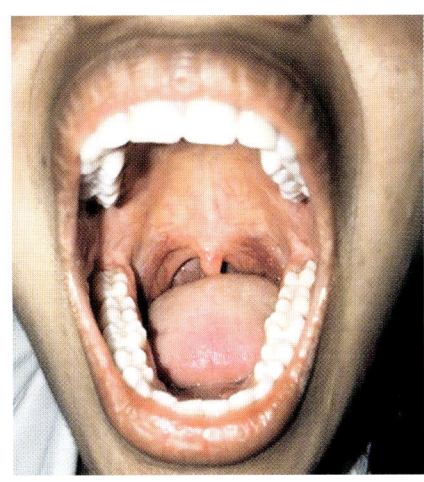

Figure 13-1: Normal oral cavity.

CLINICAL APPEARANCE AND REGIONAL VARIATIONS

The surface area of the oral mucosa in an adult human is around 200 cm^2. Though the entire oral mucosa is moist, it is not smooth and flat throughout. It exhibits variations in color, consistency, mobility, suppleness, thickness, and texture as an adaptation to its function.

The color of the oral mucosa is pinkish, however, this is not uniform. Lips are in lighter pink color than the gingiva and hard palate, where it is darker. The anterolateral part of the hard palate and lateral part of the soft palate appears yellowish since it contains fat in the connective tissue. Buccal mucosa may contain sebaceous glands, which also appear as yellowish bumps. The color of the mucosa depends on thickness of the epithelium, degree of keratinization, vascularity of the underlying connective tissue, and the concentration of melanin pigment in the epithelium.

The consistency of the oral mucosa depends on the degree of keratinization and the nature of the subepithelial tissues. Accordingly, the hard palate and gingival mucosa are firm and rest of the oral mucosa is soft.

Mucosa of the gingiva and hard palate is immobile since it is tightly bound to the bone, whereas the lining mucosa is mobile and distensible.

The suppleness of the oral mucosa depends on the nature of the connective tissue, its solid (epithelium and the fibrous tissue) and fluid components (blood and interstitial fluid) and the structure to which it is attached. The suppleness of the hard palate and gingiva is less than that of the remaining portion of the oral cavity. Mucosa overlying the muscle and mucosa containing elastic fibers are suppler than the mucosa attached to the bone and mucosa that do not contain elastic fibers.

Thickness of the oral mucosa varies over a wide range (0.3 to 6.7 mm). It is thinnest at the cheek, floor of the mouth, and ventral surface of the tongue and thickest at the maxillary tuberosity. The epithelial thickness of the oral mucosa also varies (50 to 500 μm). Epithelial thickness of the nonkeratinized mucosa is usually greater than the keratinized mucosa; however, it is thinnest in the floor of the mouth.

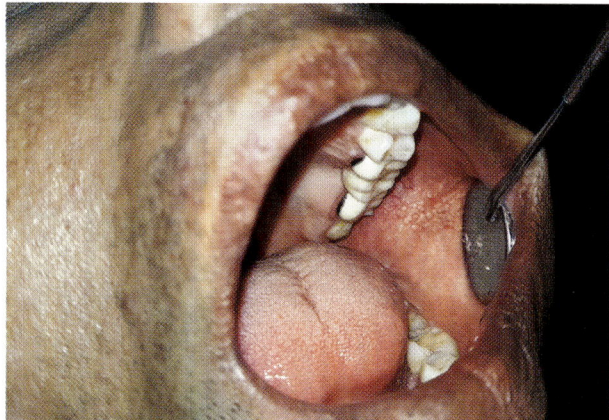

Figure 13-2: Fordyce's spots.

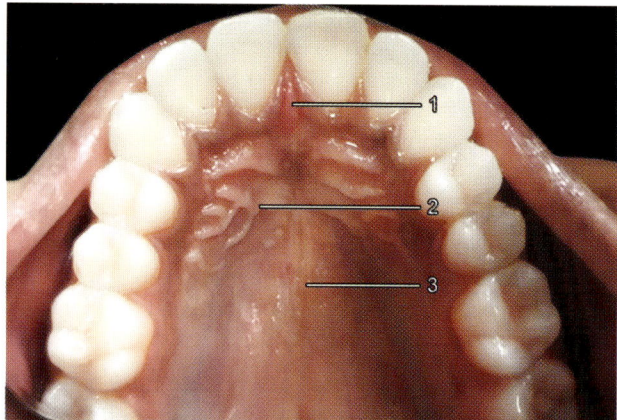

Figure 13-4: Hard palate. 1. Incisive papilla, 2. rugae, and 3. mid palatine raphe.

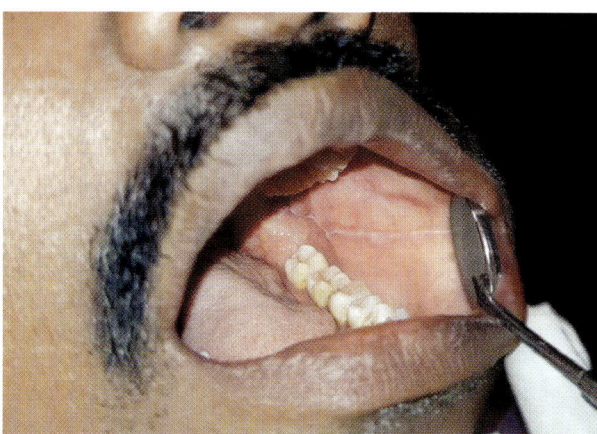

Figure 13-3: Linea alba.

The texture of the oral mucosa varies from one region to another region. In cheek, lips, vestibule, ventral surface of the tongue, floor of the mouth, and soft palate, it is smooth, though not entirely. Buccal mucosa may have multiple yellowish elevations due to the presence of sebaceous glands called "Fordyce's spots" **(Figure 13-2)**. In 10% of the population a horizontal, linear, grayish white elevation corresponding to the occlusal plane of the posterior teeth, called linea alba is seen in the buccal mucosa bilaterally **(Figure 13-3)**. Ventral surface of the tongue exhibits folds on either sides of the lingual frenum, running posterolaterally called as plica sublingualis.

The entire attached gingiva shows surface stippling. The hard palate contains transverse ridges running on either side of the midline known as palatal rugae **(Figure 13-4)**. The dorsal surface of the tongue appears velvety due to the presence of papillae.

Apart from these features, the entire oral mucosa except the anterior part of the hard palate and gingiva is perforated by the openings of the minor salivary glands.

The variations in thickness and texture of the oral mucosa are important to the dental surgeon when giving local injections or when taking oral biopsies. The masticatory mucosa such as the gingiva and hard palate is firm and immovable, where suturing a wound is difficult when compared to the lips and cheeks which are soft, resilient, and pliable.

Oral Frenum

Frenum is a thin band or fold of mucosa with enclosed muscle fibers. It connects the movable part to the rigid portion, *i.e.*, it attaches the lips and cheeks to the alveolar process and limits their movements **(Figures 13-5A and B)**. All the frena are seen in the vestibular cavity except the lingual frenum, which connects the ventral surface of the tongue to the lowest portion of lingual gingiva of the lower central incisors in the midline. The size, shape, and location of the frena may vary. Labial frena are present in the labial vestibule at the midline and in canine region. Upper labial frenum is more prominent than the lower. Buccal frena are located on premolar region. Primary function of the frena is to provide stability for the upper and lower lip and the tongue. Extensive or high frenal attachment at the midline can cause median diastema (space between central incisors) and gingival recession **(Figure 13-5C)**. Short lingual frenum restricts tongue movements, which in turn causes difficulty in pronouncing certain words.

Points to Remember

- The oral cavity is divided into two parts namely- vestibular cavity and the oral cavity proper.
- The color of the oral mucosa is pinkish but not uniform.
- Buccal mucosa may contain sebaceous glands appearing as yellowish bumps and are called Fordyce's granules.
- The color of the mucosa depends on thickness of the epithelium, degree of keratinization, vascularity of the underlying connective tissue, and the concentration of melanin pigment in the epithelium.
- The consistency of the oral mucosa depends on the degree of keratinization and the nature of the subepithelial tissues.
- Ventral surface of the tongue exhibits folds on either sides of the lingual frenum, running posterolaterally called as plica sublingualis.
- The entire attached gingiva shows surface stippling. The hard palate contains palatal rugae and the dorsal surface of the tongue appears velvety due to the presence of papillae.
- Frenum is a thin band or fold of mucosa with enclosed muscle fibers and connects the movable part to the rigid portion.

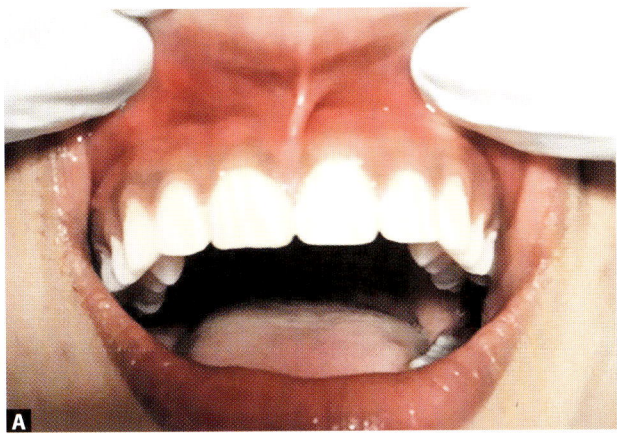
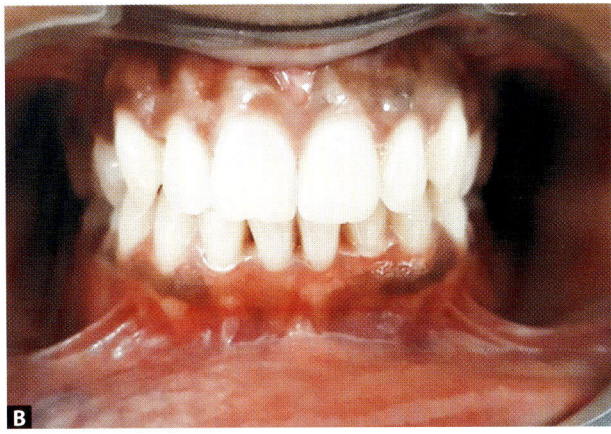
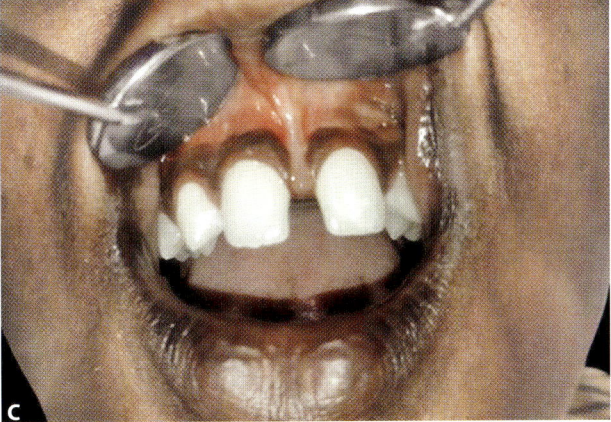

Figures 13-5A to C: (A) Labial frenum; (B) Buccal frena; (C) Diastema caused by high frenal attachment.

CLASSIFICATION OF ORAL MUCOSA

As enumerated above, the regional variations are due to the functional needs. Oral mucosa in different parts of the oral cavity encounters different types and degrees of stress during chewing, swallowing, speech, and facial expression. As an adaptation to the varied functional requirement the structure of the oral mucosa exhibits variation in terms of epithelial thickness, presence or absence of keratinization, the nature of the epithelial-connective tissue interface, composition of the lamina propria, and the presence or absence of submucosa.

Based on the functions, the oral mucosa is classified into three categories; masticatory mucosa, lining or reflecting mucosa, and specialized mucosa **(Figures 13-6A and B)**.

Masticatory Mucosa

It is seen in the areas where the mucosa has to face high compression and friction. The epithelium is keratinized, so it is also called as keratinized mucosa. The lamina propria is thick. Masticatory mucosa is tightly bound to the bone and is immobile. Gingiva and the hard palate are covered by masticatory mucosa.

Lining Mucosa

Also called reflecting mucosa, is not exposed to much masticatory load. It is movable and distensible. The epithelium is nonkeratinized. Collagen fibers in the lamina propria are arranged in such a way that they allow free movement of the mucosa. Lining mucosa covers the musculature and is more resilient, adapting to the contraction and relaxation of the cheeks, lips, and tongue, and to the movements produced by the masticatory muscles. Lamina propria also has elastic fibers. Lining mucosa contains a distinct submucosa. Lips, cheek, vestibular sulcus, alveolus, floor of the mouth, soft palate, and the ventral surface of the tongue are covered by lining mucosa.

Specialized Mucosa

Since this mucosa performs special sensory function, *i.e.*, perception of taste, it is called so. Dorsum of the tongue is covered by specialized mucosa, which contains taste buds. Lining mucosa forms about 60%, masticatory mucosa about 25%, and specialized mucosa about 15% of the oral mucosal lining.

COMPONENTS OF THE ORAL MUCOSA

All the mucous membranes are made up of epithelium and connective tissue. The analogous part in skin is called epidermis and dermis. Similarly, the oral mucosa is made up of epithelium, which develops mainly from the ectoderm except in tongue, where the epithelium develops from endoderm. The connective tissue portion of the oral mucosa is called as the lamina propria **(Figure 13-7)**. As described

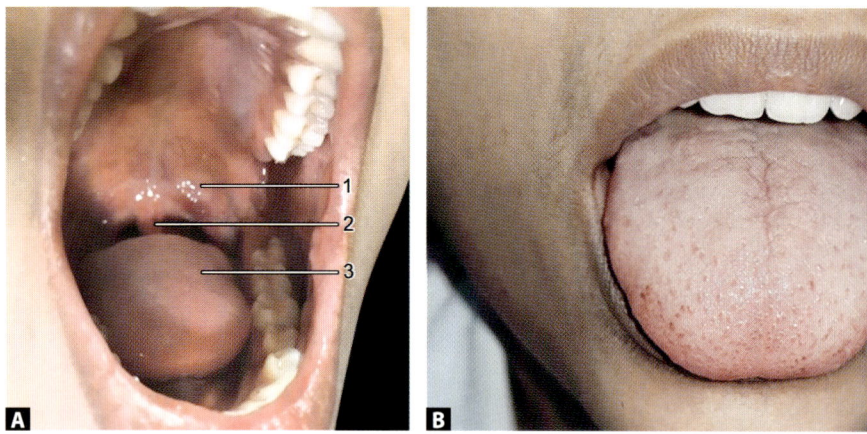

Figures 13-6A and B: (A) Masticatory and lining mucosa: 1. palate (masticatory mucosa), 2. uvula (lining mucosa), 3. tongue (specialized mucosa); (B) Specialized mucosa.

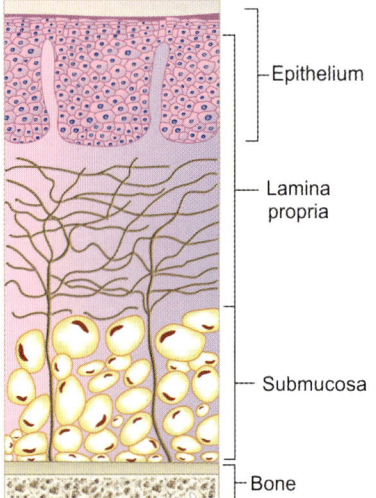

Figure 13-7: Oral mucosa showing epithelium, lamina propria, and submucosa.

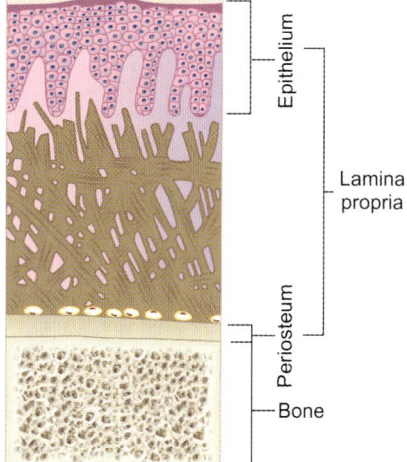

Figure 13-8: Oral mucosa showing epithelium, lamina propria, and no distinct submucosa.

previously the oral mucosa shows regional variations depending on the functional needs. Beneath the lamina propria is the submucosa, which is made up of a loose connective tissue stroma containing blood vessels, nerves, adipocytes, minor salivary glands and muscles. Sebaceous glands are less frequently seen. Though lamina propria is always present, the submucosa may or may not be present. The boundary between the lamina propria and the submucosa is often indistinct.

The submucosa aids in attachment of the mucosa to the underlying structures, the exception being the masticatory mucosa where the mucosa directly attaches to the bone without an intervening submucosa. This is called the mucoperiosteum **(Figure 13-8)**.

The interface between the epithelium and connective tissue is not flat instead it is thrown into folds or corrugations, where the papillae of the connective tissue containing the blood vessels and nerves protrude into the epithelium. The epithelium, as a result, forms intersecting ridges running in various directions. These ridges are called epithelial ridges or rete ridges and they interdigitate with the connective tissue papillae **(Figure 13-9)**. This arrangement increases the surface area of the epithelial-connective tissue junction for better attachment and dissipation of forces exerted on the epithelium to a greater area of the connective tissue. The

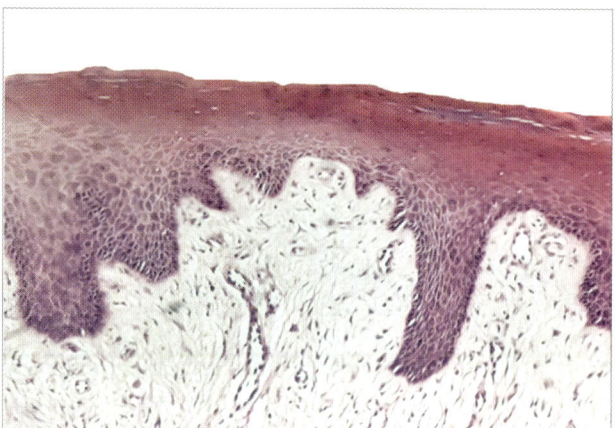

Figure 13-9: Oral mucosa epithelial ridges.

junction provides a mode of exchange of metabolites as the epithelium is devoid of blood vessels. The masticatory mucosa has numerous papillae compared to the lining mucosa.

Epithelium is one of the four basic tissues of the human body. It covers the body surfaces, internal organs, lines the body cavities, vessels, forms glands, and remains as cell rests in fusion lines and after tooth development. By definition they are large cells with little intercellular substance. Epithelium is avascular and supported by the adjacent connective tissue but separated from it by the basement membrane. The epithelial cells are attached to one another by means of cell junctions.

Epithelial cells may be flat (squamous epithelium), cuboidal or columnar and contain tonofilaments in their cytoskeleton. Epithelial cells form a single layer (simple/unilayered epithelium) or multiple layers (stratified epithelium). Pseudostratified epithelium is actually a simple epithelium with the nucleus of the epithelial cells placed at different levels, which gives the false appearance of a multilayer. Surface of the epithelium may be keratinized or nonkeratinized or have cilia. Functions of epithelial cells include protection, secretion, absorption, sensory, and transcellular transport.

Points to Remember

- The oral mucosa is classified into three categories; masticatory mucosa, lining or reflecting mucosa, and specialized mucosa.
- Gingiva and the hard palate are covered by masticatory mucosa.
- Lips, cheek, vestibular sulcus, alveolus, floor of the mouth, soft palate, and the ventral surface of the tongue are covered by lining mucosa.
- Dorsum of the tongue is covered by specialized mucosa, which contains taste buds.
- The mucous membranes are made up of epithelium and lamina propria.
- Beneath the lamina propria is the submucosa which is made up of a loose connective tissue stroma.
- Mucoperiosteum is where the mucosa directly attaches to the bone without an intervening submucosa.
- The interface between the epithelium and connective tissue is thrown into folds or corrugations are called epithelial ridges or rete ridges.

Oral Epithelium

Epithelium of oral mucosa is of stratified squamous type where the polygonal cells are tightly attached to one another and stacked in layers or strata **(Figure 13-10)**. The superficial layer of the epithelium may be keratinized or nonkeratinized. It is keratinized in case of masticatory mucosa (gingiva and hard palate) and nonkeratinized in lining mucosa. In tongue, filiform papillae and circumvallate papillae are keratinized. In masticatory mucosa, the epithelium is tightly bound to the lamina propria and is inflexible, tough, and resistant to mechanical forces. In lining mucosa, the epithelium is thicker and exhibit different rete ridge patterns at the connective tissue interface.

Two types of keratinization may be present in gingiva—orthokeratinization, where there is absence of nuclei or nuclear remnants in the keratin layer **(Figure 13-11)** and parakeratinization, where there is persistence of nuclei or their remnants **(Figure 13-12)**. Stratum granulosum is

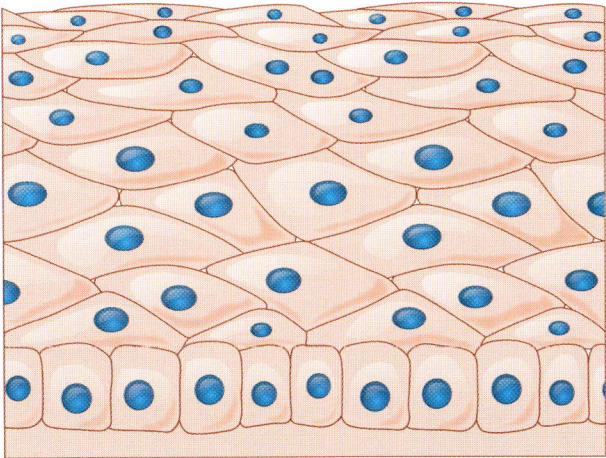

Figure 13-10: Stratified squamous epithelium.

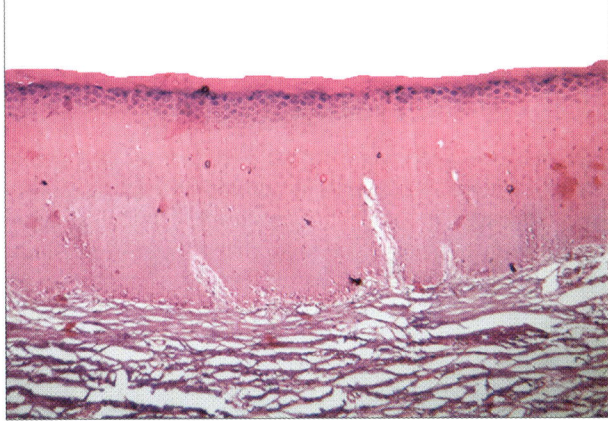

Figure 13-11: Orthokeratinized epithelium.

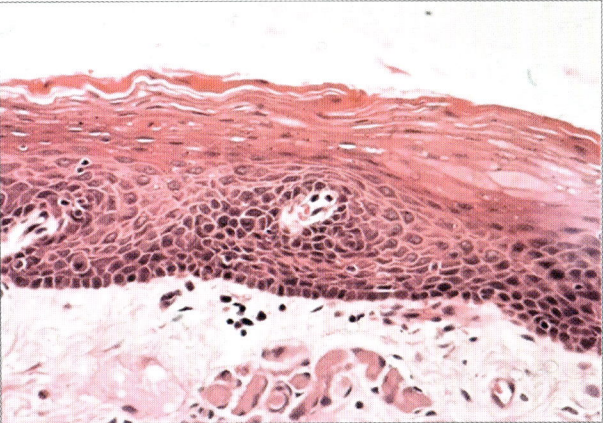

Figure 13-12: Parakeratinized epithelium.

prominent in orthokeratinized epithelium. The thickness and the structural integrity of the epithelium is maintained by moving of cells from the basal layer as a process of maturation and shed as keratinized squames and continuous renewal of cells through mitotic division at the basal layer **(Figures 13-13A and B)**. Mitotic index is the ratio between the number of cells undergoing mitosis to the total number of cells in a population. Nonkeratinized epithelium of the oral cavity has higher mitotic rates than those of the keratinized epithelium.

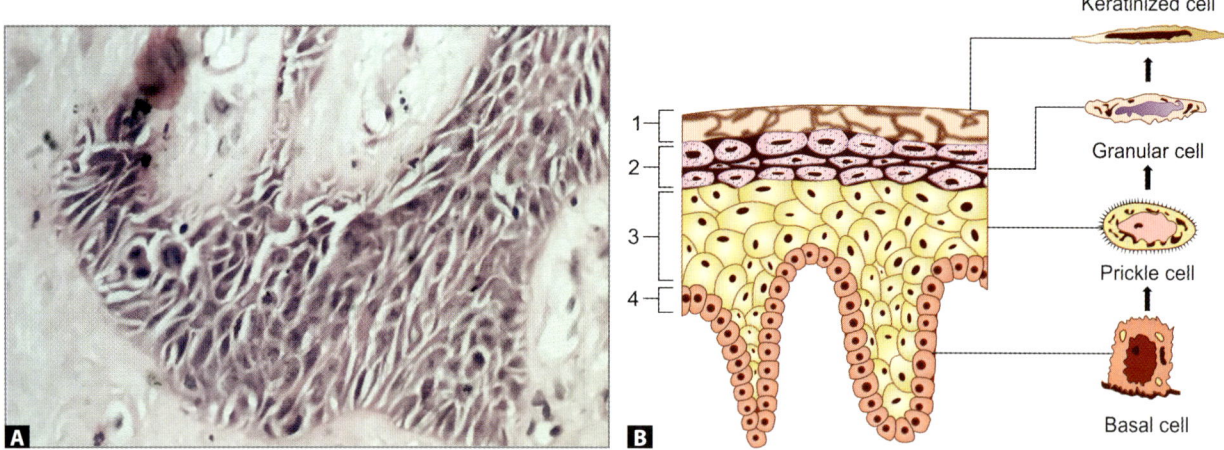

Figures 13-13A and B: Epithelial cell undergoing: (A) Mitosis; and (B) Epithelial maturation; 1. Stratum corneum, 2. Stratum granulosum, 3. Stratum spinosum, 4. Stratum basale.

Epithelial Proliferation and Maturation

It is suggested that there are two cell populations, a progenitor group that provides new cells by continuous mitotic division and a maturing population that continues to differentiate and mature to form a protective layer. The progenitor cells are situated in the basal and parabasal layers when the epithelium is thick and at the basal layers when it is thin. Proliferating cells occur in clusters and are usually seen at the bottom of rete ridges than at the top. This progenitor population is further divided into two functional subtypes of cells, one small population and one large population.

The small population of the cells is the stem cells that divide slowly to produce basal cells thereby maintaining the proliferative potential of the tissue. The larger amplifying population, on the contrary, divides rapidly and functions to provide more number of cells available for subsequent maturation.

After each cell division, the resultant daughter cells either recycle in the progenitor population or enter the maturing compartment to differentiate further. However, it is not possible to morphologically distinguish this population of stem cells or amplifying cells. The time taken for a cell to divide, mature, and pass through the entire epithelium gives the turnover time of the epithelium. It is different for nonkeratinized and keratinized epithelium where the former turns over faster than the latter. It is estimated to be 41–57 days in the gingiva and 25 days in the cheek. Studies have suggested that the growth factors and cytokines control the epithelial proliferation. These include epidermal growth factor, keratinocyte growth factor, interleukin-1, and transforming growth factor alpha and beta.

After the cells enter the maturation compartment, they differentiate as they move up the surface of the epithelium. The matured cells form a specialized protective layer at the surface called the cornified cell envelope that contains keratins embedded in a combination of proteins and surrounded by lipids **(Figure 13-14)**.

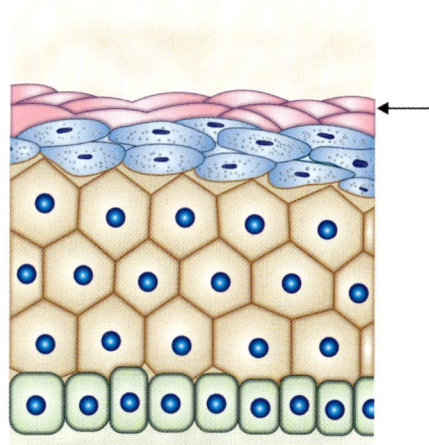

Figure 13-14: Cornified layer at top.

Epithelial Cells and their Cohesiveness

Important function of the surface epithelium is to protect the underlying structures by forming a barrier. This is achieved by the tight placement or close contact of the adjacent cells. The oral epithelial cells are attached to one another by means of cell junctions. The most common one is the desmosome. It is a spot adhering type of cell junction known as macula adherens. It is made up of an attachment plaque of the cell membrane, to which bundles of tonofilaments are inserted. Epithelial cells are attached to the connective tissue by means of hemidesmosomes through basal lamina. Hemidesmosomes also possess intracellular attachment plaques with tonofilaments that are inserted into them. Tonofilaments, hemidesmosomes, and the basal lamina as a unit help to distribute the mechanical stress exerted on the epithelium over a wide area. Apart from acting as structural adhesive complexes, hemidesmosomes also transduce signals from extracellular matrix that may critically affect cell behavior in terms of proliferation, differentiation, and apoptosis.

The epithelial cells of both the keratinized and the nonkeratinized mucosa are called keratinocytes as they contain keratin filaments. Also called as cytokeratin (CK) and tonofilaments, these keratin filaments are categorized as intermediate filaments, since their diameter (7–11 nm) lies between the microfilament (4–6 nm) and macrotubules (25 nm). Cytoskeleton of the epithelial cell is formed by tonofilaments along with the microfilaments. They provide mechanical linkages and function as stress-bearing structures thereby maintaining the shape of the cell.

Cytokeratin
They are the family of water-insoluble intracytoplasmic structural proteins and are the dominant intermediate filament proteins of epithelial cell. They act as the cytoskeleton by forming a dense network of radiating filaments from the nucleus to the plasma membrane within a cell. Cytokeratin is considered as an epithelial marker since it is present in almost all the epithelial cells. 20 types of cytokeratins are recognized and are broadly categorized into the acidic (type I) cytokeratins and the basic or neutral (type II) cytokeratins and are numbered in order of decreasing molecular weight, from high molecular weight to low **(Flowchart 13-1)**. They occur in pairs with combination of type I with type II that makes them stable and in the absence of the pair, they are susceptible to degradation by proteases.

Lowest weight (40 kDa) is found in glandular and simple epithelia, intermediate in stratified epithelia, and highest (67 kDa) in keratinized stratified epithelia. The cytokeratins determine the cell type and differentiation in different epithelia. For example, the ventral surface of the tongue expresses CK 5, 6, and 14 and the dorsal surface expresses CK 7, 8, and 19 (taste buds). However, the best CKs associated with epithelial stratification are pairs 5 and 14, 1 and 10, and 4 and 13. Nonkeratinized epithelium has keratin 4, 13, and 19 **(Table 13-1)**.

Other intercellular attachment such as gap junctions and tight junctions are also seen between the epithelial cells. Gap junctions also called communicating junctions are seen in the oral epithelial cells and allow electrical and chemical communication between cells.

TABLE 13-1: Cytokeratin distribution in oral epithelium, salivary epithelium and odontogenic tissues.

Oral epithelium	
CK-5 and 14	Basal keratinocytes (all stratified squamous epithelium)
CK-1, 2, 3, 10, 11	Supra basal layer of keratinized mucosa
CK-4 and 13	Supra basal layer of nonkeratinized mucosa
CK-6 and 16	Rapidly proliferating epithelium
CK-5,6,14	Epithelium of the ventral surface of the tongue
CK-7, 8,18,19	Epithelium of soft palate
CK-4	Superficial layer of gingival crevicular epithelium
CK-5,14,13,19	Gingival junctional epithelium
CK-9	Basal keratinocytes of gingival and buccal mucosal stratified squamous epithelium
CK-19	Rapid cell proliferation
CK-7,8,19	Taste buds
CK-8,18,19,20	Merkel cells
Salivary epithelia	
CK-14	Myoepithelial cells and basal cells (ductal non-luminal cells)
CK-18, 19	Epithelial elements of salivary gland
CK-7,8,18,19	Luminal duct cells
CK-8,18	Epithelium of striated and intercalated ducts
Odontogenic tissues	
CK-7,13,14,19	Enamel organ
CK-14	Most cells of enamel organ (odontogenic epithelial marker)
CK-7	Stellate reticulum and HERS
CK-19	Preameloblasts and secretory ameloblasts (secretory differentiation)
CK-5 /19	Cell rests of Malassez

Desmosomes
Also known as intercellular bridges, these are macula adherens type of cell junctions enabling cell to cell adhesion, usually seen in tissues that experience great mechanical stress **(Figures 13-15A and B)**. Desmosome is made up of desmosome–intermediate filament complexes, which in turn are composed of the extracellular core region, or desmoglea, the outer dense plaque, and the inner dense plaque. The extracellular core region contains desmoglein and desmocollin, which belong to the cadherin family of cell adhesion proteins. The outer dense plaque contains the intracellular ends of desmocollin and desmoglein, the N-terminus side of desmoplakin, plakoglobin, periplakin, envoplakin, and plakophilin. The inner dense plaque contains the C-terminus end of desmoplakin and their attachment to tonofilaments. Desmoplakin is the most abundant part of the desmosome, as it operates as the mediator between the cadherin proteins in the plasma membrane and the keratin filaments.

Hemidesmosomes look like half desmosomes, and are similar type of cell junctions that help in the attachment of basal cells to the basement membrane, thereby to the connective tissue **(Figure 13-16)**. They are not merely an adhesive complex; instead they also transduce signals that may critically affect the cell behavior. They help to prevent cell migration and displacement. Their functional activity is modulated by growth factors and extracellular matrix protein. Regulation of the hemidesmosome–basement membrane adhesive interaction is necessary for various biological processes such as tissue morphogenesis and wound healing.

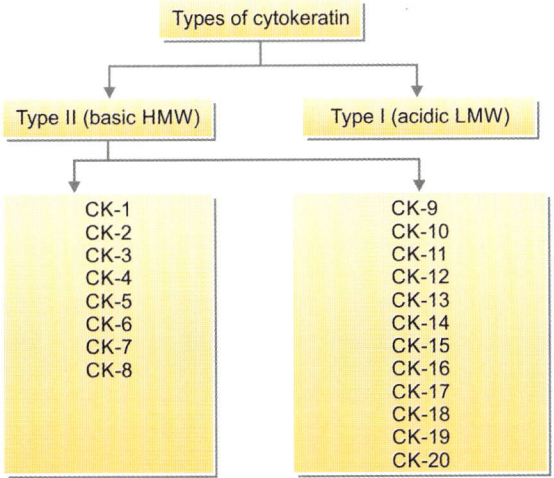

Flowchart 13-1: Cytokeratin.

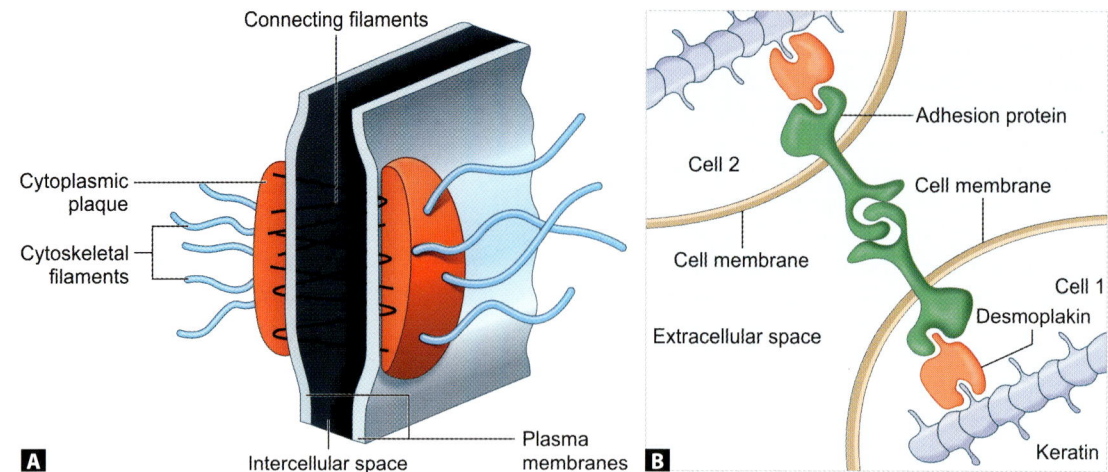

Figures 13-15A and B: Desmosome showing attachment plaque and inserted tonofilaments.

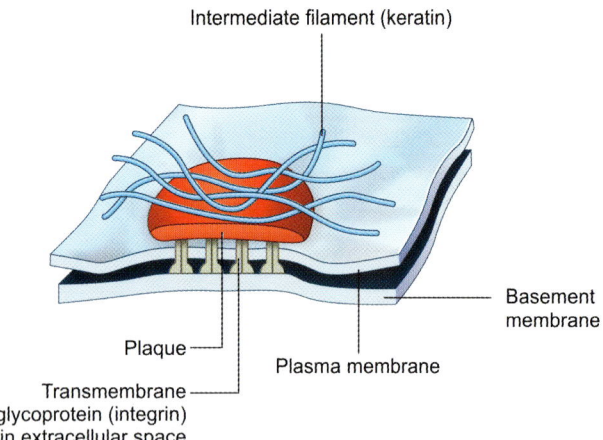

Figure 13-16: Hemidesmosome.

Keratinized Epithelium (Figures 13-17A to C)

The keratinized stratified squamous epithelium of the oral mucosa consists mainly of four distinct layers, and from the bottom to the surface is called:
- Stratum basale
- Stratum spinosum
- Stratum granulosum
- Stratum corneum.

Stratum Basale

The stratum basale or the basal cell layer is present adjacent to the basement membrane and consists of cuboidal or columnar cells along with progenitor cells **(Figures 13-18A and B)**. The basal and the parabasal layer together are called as the stratum germinativum but only the cells of the basal layer can divide. Not all cells of the progenitor population are stem cells; however, the expression of antiapoptotic factor (bcl-2 protein) allows them to remain as stem cells. The cells are least differentiated with limited intracellular organelles associated with protein synthesis and some tonofilaments. The basal cells also synthesize some of the basal lamina proteins.

The dividing stem cells of the basal layer are nonserrated, whereas the amplifying cells are serrated and heavily packed with tonofilaments. The serrated cells are cuboidal cells with protoplasmic process projecting towards the connective tissue. The basal surface of these cells contains hemidesmosomes that provide attachment to the basement membrane. The hemidesmosomes are made up of single attachment plaque, adjacent plasma membrane, and an extracellular structure that appears to attach the epithelium with the connective tissue. Laterally, these cells have desmosomes that aid in the attachment of one cell to adjacent cells. These have a pair of attachment plaques, adjacent cell membranes, and intervening extracellular structures.

Stratum Spinosum

This layer, otherwise called the prickle cell layer is located adjacent to the stratum basale and consists of irregular, polyhedral cells that are larger than the basal cells. Parabasal layer is referred to the deepest layer of prickle cells that lies close to the basal layer. They are elongated cells but show some features of the basal cells. The stratum basale and stratum spinosum together form two-thirds to half of the epithelial thickness.

The intercellular bridges between the cells are evident in light microscope. The intercellular bridges are more obvious and are more in number. The shrinkage of cells during routine histological processing causes the cells to separate except at points of desmosomal attachment giving rise to the "spiny" or prickle appearance and hence this layer is called the stratum spinosum or prickle cell layer **(Figures 13-19A and B)**.

A soluble protein called involucrin first appears in this layer, which is a precursor protein of the cornified layer.

The presence of cytokeratins contributes to the formation of tonofilaments that are thicker and conspicuous.

The upper part of the prickle cell layer consists of membrane-coating granules measuring approximately 25 μ in length and are rich in phospholipids. Presence of lamellae is seen along with these granules in keratinized epithelium. These granules are said to have originated from the Golgi apparatus.

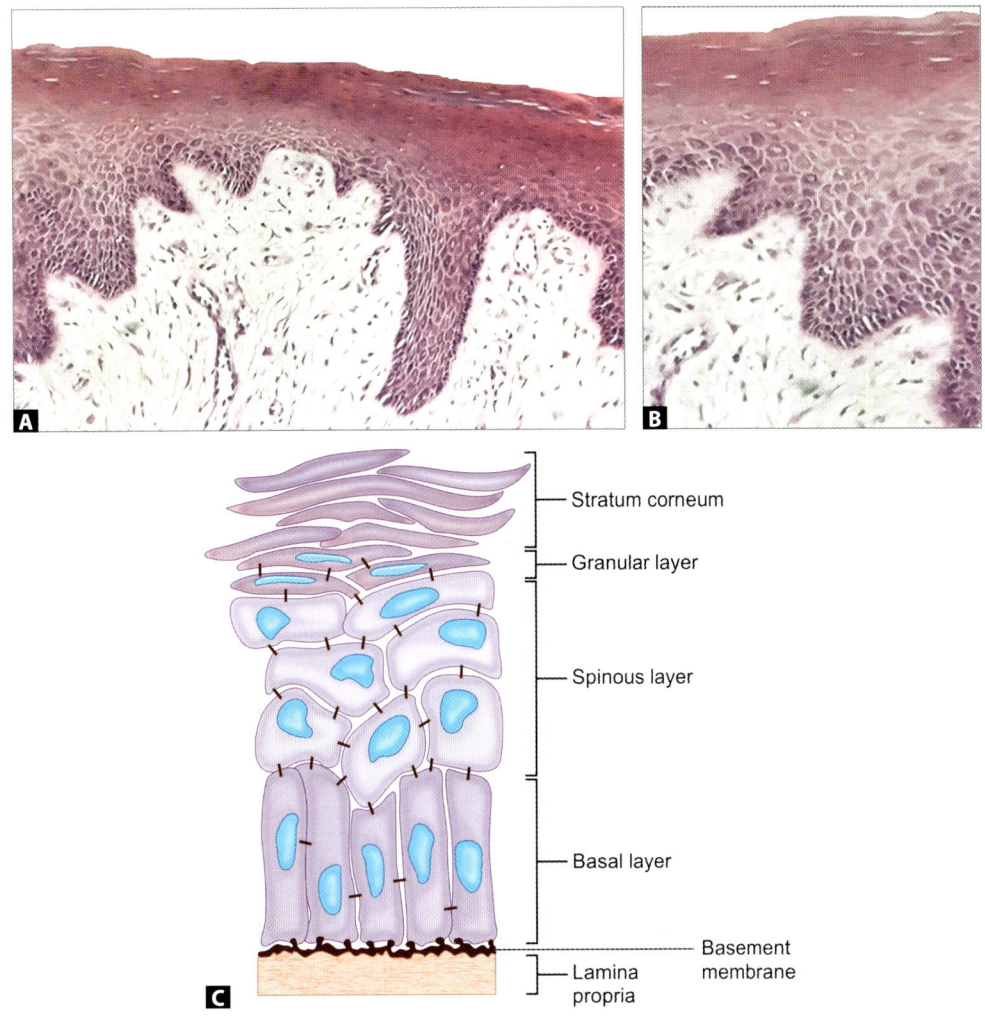

Figures 13-17A to C: Keratinized epithelium: (A) Low power; (B) High power; and (C) Pictographical representation.

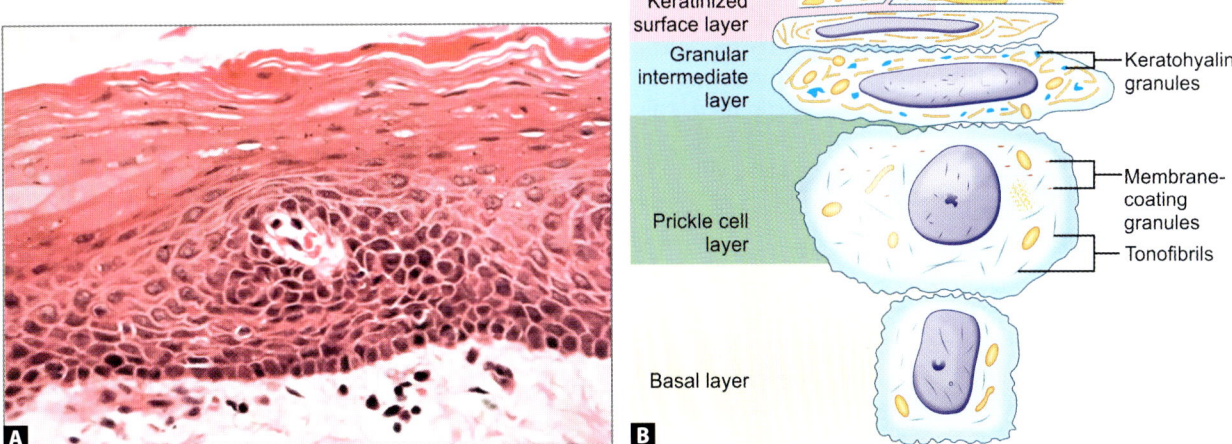

Figures 13-18A and B: Keratinized epithelium showing cuboidal basal cells.

Stratum Granulosum

This layer is situated next to the prickle cells and consists of flatter and wider cells with prominent basophilic keratohyalin granules and hence named as stratum granulosum or granular cell layer **(Figure 13-20)**. These granules are 0.5–1.0 μ in diameter and contain profilaggrin, which is a precursor to the protein filaggrin that binds the keratin together to form a stable network. Protein synthesis, though reduced, is present and nuclei show signs of degeneration and pyknosis. Dense networks of tonofilaments are present and are seen associated with keratohyalin granules.

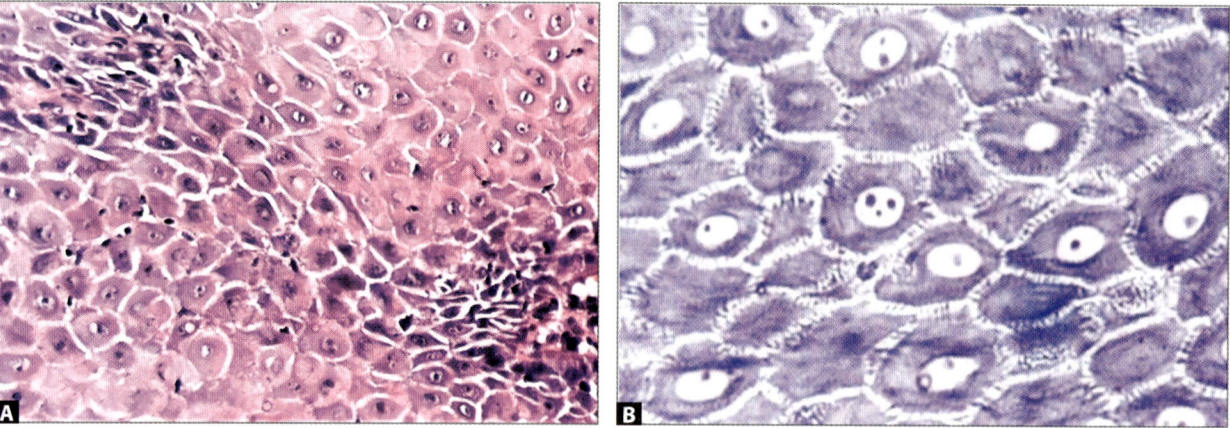

Figures 13-19A and B: Spinous cell layer: (A) Low power; and (B) High power.

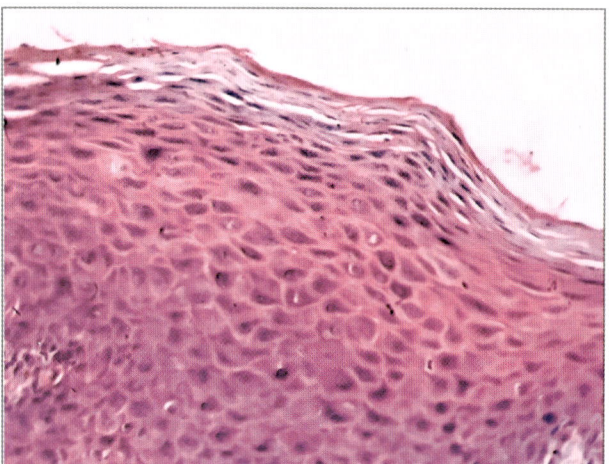

Figure 13-20: Granular cell layer.

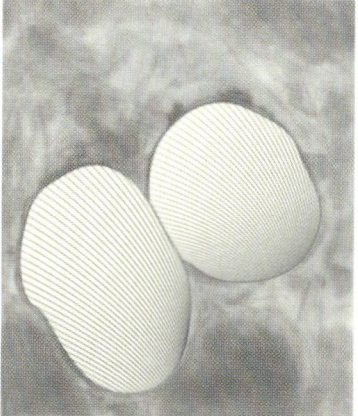

Figure 13-21: Schematic representation of Odland bodies.

The membrane-coating granules that are present in the upper part of the spinous layer and the granular layer are called the keratinosomes or Odland bodies **(Figure 13-21)**. These lamellar bodies contribute to the formation of the permeability barrier between the granular and cornified layer. Additional proteins like loricrin and involucrin that help in the formation of a resistant cell envelope are also evident in this layer.

Stratum Corneum

This layer is also called keratin layer. The final stage of maturation shows larger and flatter epithelial cells with loss of their organelles. The release of proteases results in the autolysis of the cell. The cells are closely packed with tonofilaments that are cross-linked with disulfide bonds and surrounded by the protein filaggrin (which is derived from a precursor in keratohyalin granules) **(Figure 13-22)**.

This mixture of proteins is called keratin **(Figure 13-23)**. The cross-linked disulfide bonds in the keratin layer provide both chemical and mechanical resistance to the epithelium. The protein involucrin becomes cross-linked and binds to loricrin to form a highly resistant and electron dense, cornified layer. This could be due to cell death and the influx of calcium ions.

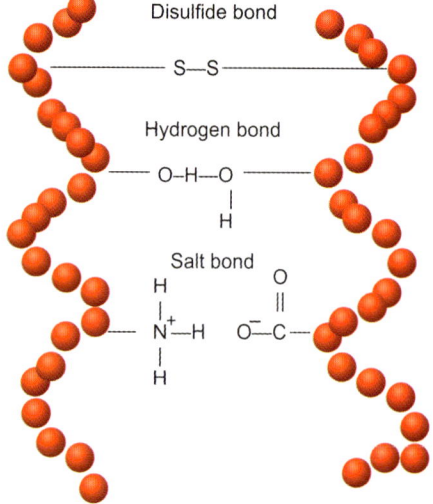

Figure 13-22: Tonofilaments cross-linked by disulfide bonds.

The cells of this layer are called epithelial squames which are shed by the process of desquamation by the weakening of desmosomes and this plays a role in the constant turnover of epithelial cells. The function of this layer is to provide mechanical protection to the mucosa. It varies in thickness.

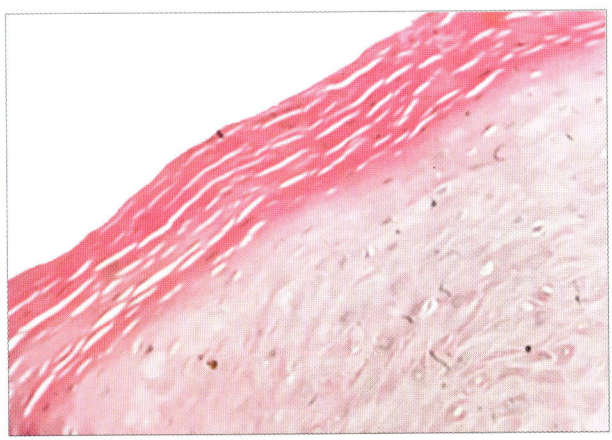

Figure 13-23: Stratum corneum forming the top-most layer.

Nonkeratinized Epithelium

The lining mucosa of the oral cavity that comprises the lips, alveolar mucosa, buccal mucosa, soft palate, ventral surface of the tongue, and floor of the mouth is covered by nonkeratinized epithelium. The epithelium does not produce a cornified surface layer, with only three layers of epithelium present unlike the keratinized mucosa **(Figures 13-24A and B)**. The epithelium is similar to that of keratinized epithelium at the basal and prickle cell layer but have large cells with less prominent intercellular bridges and the term prickle cell layer is not much used. The remaining epithelium is divided into two zones, an intermediate zone (stratum intermedium) and a superficial zone (stratum superficiale). The granular cell layer and the keratin layer are absent and does not stain with eosin like a keratinized epithelium. The cells of the stratum intermedium are nucleated and contain less tonofilaments and keratohyalin granules. These superficial cells desquamate and the rate of cell turnover is more than the keratinized epithelium.

> These nonkeratinized areas become keratinized as a protective mechanism against any chronic irritation and the term "keratosis" and "parakeratosis" is used for such pathological states.

Keratinocytes and Nonkeratinocytes

Keratinocytes

Oral epithelium contains 90% of keratinocytes. As described previously, they are epithelial cells that contain cytokeratin filaments and synthesize keratin. In keratinized epithelium, keratin production is a physiological event. If nonkeratinized epithelium is subjected to chronic irritation, it may also produce keratin. Keratin is a protein, which forms a protective layer and acts as a barrier against the external factors. Nonkeratinocytes are a smaller population of cells (about 10%) that do not synthesize keratin on any account, as they lack these protein filaments. Keratinocytes undergo mitotic division, mature, and desquamate. They increase in volume from basal to superficial layer covering a large area as they move upward. On the contrary, the nonkeratinocytes do not undergo cell division, maturation or desquamation. These

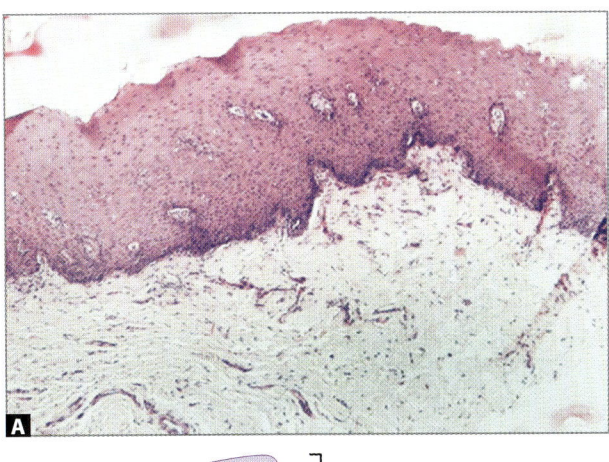

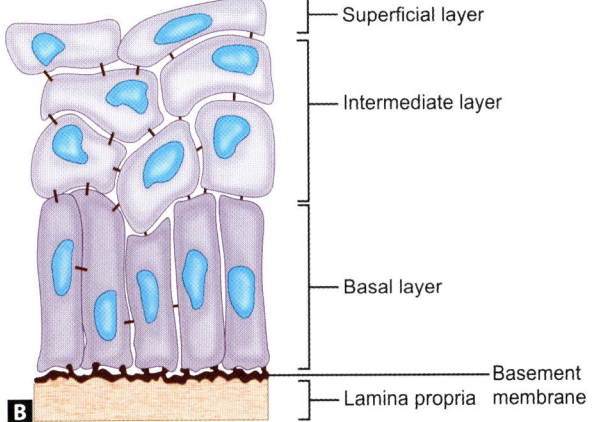

Figures 13-24A and B: Nonkeratinized epithelium: (A) Hematoxylin and eosin stained section; (B) Schematic representation.

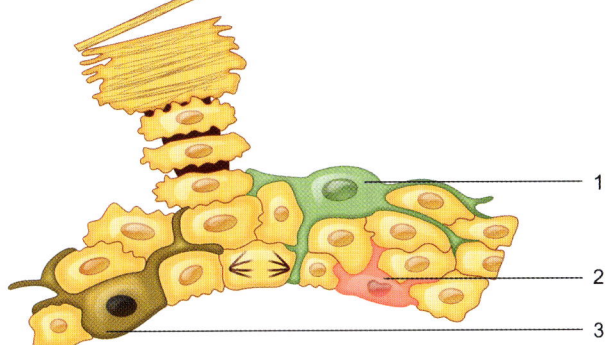

Figure 13-25: Nonkeratinocytes of the oral epithelium: 1. Langerhans cell, 2. Merkel cell, and 3. Melanocyte.

cells migrate from the neural crest cells or the bone marrow. They are not arranged in layers or connected via desmosomes (except Merkel cell) with the adjacent cells. They are clear or unstained cells that possess dendritic process. These cells are identified by special stains or immunohistochemistry. Melanocytes, Merkel cells, and Langerhans cells are the nonkeratinocytes found in the oral epithelium but sometimes lymphocytes are also considered to be nonkeratinocytes **(Figure 13-25)**.

Ebstein Barr virus (EBV) receptors are recognized on keratinocytes of the normal oral mucosa and are confined to middle and upper spinous layer cells of the parakeratinized epithelium.

Angiotensin Converting Enzyme II (ACE 2) is considered to be the cell receptor for the COVID-19 virus and SARS-CoV and HCoV-NL63. Expression of ACE 2 receptor on the oral mucosa, particularly their high expression in the epithelial cells of the tongue, may pose a high risk route for COVID-19 infection.

Nonkeratinocytes of the Oral Epithelium

Melanocytes: Melanocytes are melanin-producing cells that are derived from neural crest cells and enter the oral epithelium at around 11 weeks of gestation. Melanin absorbs UV rays and prevents DNA damage to the keratinocytes of the skin. Melanoblasts, the precursor of melanocytes, differentiate from the neural crest cells, proliferate, and colonize in the basal layer of the epithelium during embryonic stage. These cells are present in the basal layer of the epithelium **(Figures 13-26A and B)**. There are 7–9 melanocytes per 100 epithelial cells. The number of melanocytes per unit area is same for all the individuals and only their activity differs, which gives the color **(Figure 13-27)**. Each melanocyte has dendritic process by which it communicates to about 30–40 keratinocytes. Melanin is produced inside the cell as small melanin-containing membrane bound granules. These are called melanosomes, which are transferred to the keratinocytes through their dendritic process for storage **(Figure 13-28)**. Macrophages phagocytose the melanin pigment that is dispersed in the connective tissue. These phagocytic cells are called melanophages **(Figure 13-29)**.

A variation in pigmentation is due to the number, size, distribution of melanosomes, quantity of the pigment, and the rate of degradation of the pigment. Melanocytes appear as clear cells in routine hematoxylin and eosin stained section, so they are called as low level clear cells. Silver stains, color the dendritic process and the melanin pigment. The pigment can also be demonstrated histochemically by dihydroxyphenylalanine (DOPA) reaction or Fontana-Masson silver stain.

Langerhans cell: This is another clear dendritic cell that is present in the spinous cell layer of the epithelium that appears, may be at the same time as the melanocyte.

Langerhans cells originate from the bone marrow and can move in and around the epithelium in response to chemotactic factors released by keratinocytes to the surface receptors of Langerhans cells **(Figure 13-30)**. Small rod or flask-shaped, trilaminar granules, called Birbeck granules, are present inside the cells which can be seen under electron microscope. These granules are 50 nm long and 4 nm wide resembling tennis racquet with a swelling at one end of the vesicle **(Figure 13-31A)**.

They function as antigen-presenting cells, where they pick up the antigen and present it to the T lymphocytes either locally or at lymph nodes and can probably migrate to the regional lymph nodes. Since they are present in the higher layers of epithelium they are called as high level clear cells. They can be demonstrated by special stains such as gold

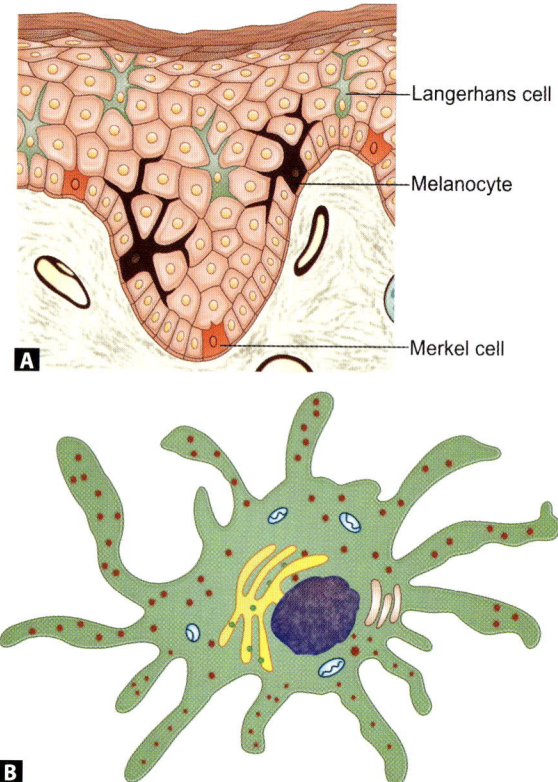

Figures 13-26A and B: Melanocytes.

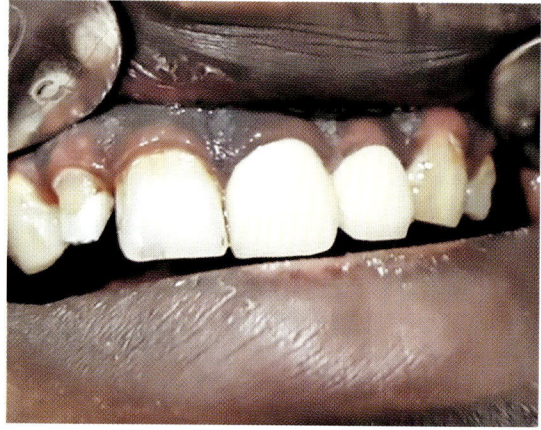

Figure 13-27: Dark colored gingiva due to melanin pigmentation.

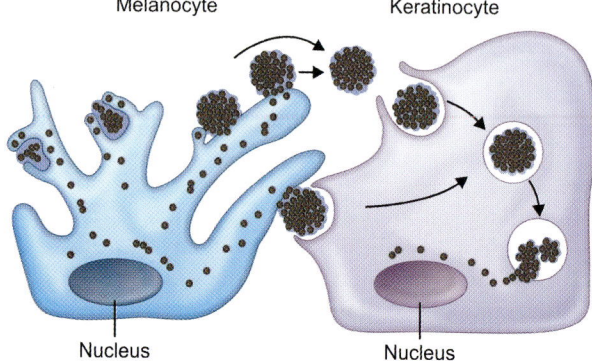

Figure 13-28: Melanin is transferred to keratinocyte.

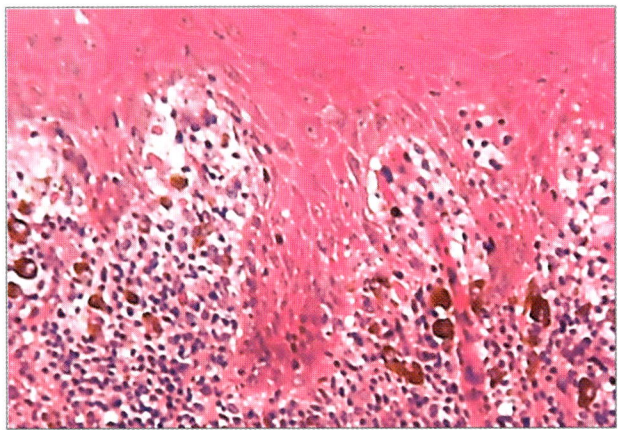

Figure 13-29: Melanophages in the lamina propria.

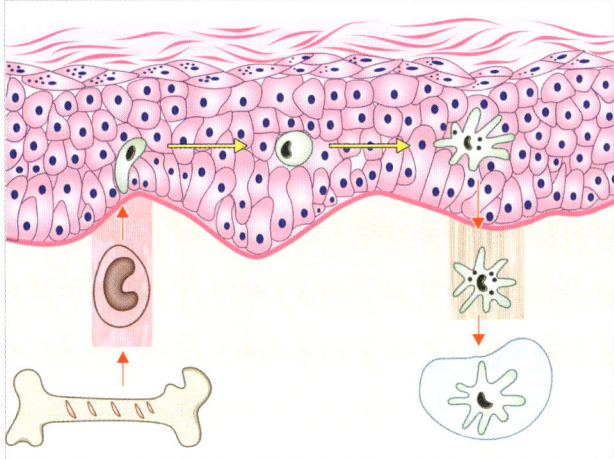

Figure 13-30: Origin of Langerhans cell.

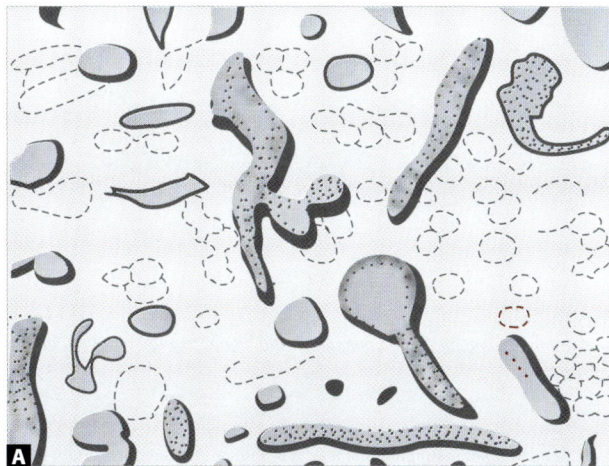

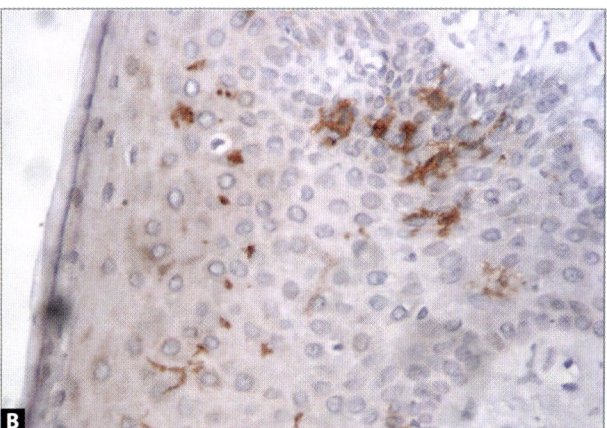

Figures 13-31A and B: (A) Schematic representation of Tennis racquet-shaped Birbeck granules of Langerhans cell; (B) S100 immunohistochemical stain positive Langerhans cells in spinous layer.

chloride, osmium zinc iodide and ATPase method. They are also positive for immunohistochemical stains such as OKT4 and S100 **(Fig. 13-31B)**.

> Langerhans cell population is reduced in oral hairy leukoplakia, a lesion caused by Ebstein Barr virus in immune compromised patients particularly HIV patients. This occurs in the lateral border of the tongue.

Merkel cells: These nonkeratinocytes are situated in the basal cell layer and do not possess dendritic process like the other nonkeratinocytes, however, short cytoplasmic processes are seen. They have been thought to arise from epidermal progenitors but were initially thought to be from the neural crest cells. They contain keratin filaments and sometimes desmosomes linking it with the adjacent cells. These cells are most commonly seen in masticatory epithelia like gingiva than lining epithelia and are sometimes seen situated next to a nerve axon **(Figure 13-32)**. Small membrane-bound cytoplasmic vesicles are characteristic of this cell. In addition, the cytoplasm also contains mitochondria, free ribosomes, and electron dense granules (80–180 nm diameter), and these granules might release a neurotransmitter between the Merkel cell and the nerve fiber to trigger an impulse for

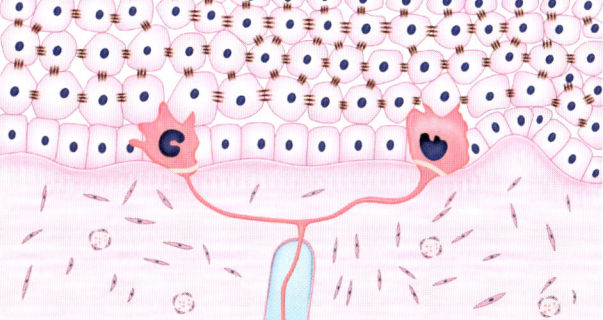

Figure 13-32: Schematic representation of Merkel cell.

sensory functions. Nucleus of Merkel cell is deeply invaginated and contains a characteristic rodlet. Merkel cells act as sensory receptor for the perception of touch and pressure, thus they are referred to as touch cells. They are identified by immunohistochemical staining techniques using antibodies CK 8, 18, and 20.

Inflammatory cells: Inflammatory cells are also seen in the cellular layers and do not undergo mitotic division. The most common cells found are the lymphocytes, which are seen in close association with Langerhans cells, which can activate

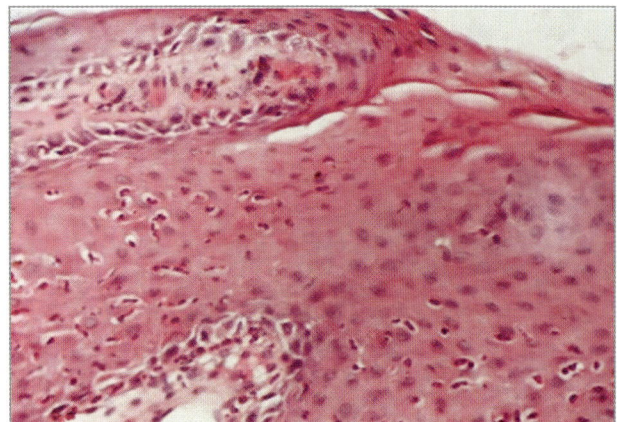

Figure 13-33: Polymorphonuclear leukocytes and mast cells in the epithelium.

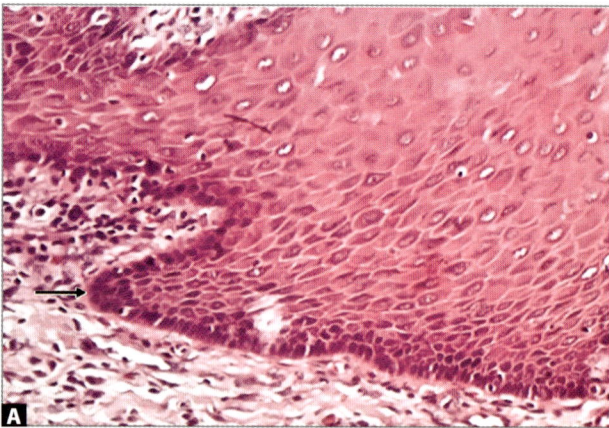

Figures 13-34A and B: Basement membrane.

these T lymphocytes. Sometimes even neutrophils and mast cells may also be seen **(Figure 13-33)** in the epithelium.

Basement Membrane and Basal Lamina

The epithelium is separated from the connective tissue by basement membrane. This is about 1–2 µm in thickness and can be seen by light microscope **(Figures 13-34A and B)**. Basal lamina is somewhat a similar structure, but much thinner and can be demonstrated only by electron microscope. This is a product of epithelium. Along with the subepithelial collagen fibers, it appears as basement membrane in light microscope.

Basal lamina has two layers namely-an electron lucent "lamina lucida" adjacent to the basal epithelial layer and an electron dense "lamina densa" closer to the connective tissue **(Figure 13-35)**. Lamina lucida is thinner (20–40 nm) than lamina densa (20-120 nm) and appears as clear zone. Some consider this as an artefact of tissue processing. Lamina densa is connected to types I and III collagen of the lamina reticularis of the connective tissue with anchoring fibrils. These anchoring fibrils are made up of type VII collagen, which forms loops with the lamina densa, to which the collagen fibers of the connective tissue interlock **(Figure 13-36)**. Basal lamina is composed of type IV nonfibrillar collagen and a number of proteoglycans and glycoproteins. These include fibronectin, laminin, perlecan (heparan sulfate-rich proteoglycan), and transmembrane molecules such as integrins and bullous pemphigoid antigens namely— BP 180 and BP 230. They are also called BPAG1 and BPAG 2, which have molecular weight of 180 kD and 230 kD respectively. They are hemidesmosomal proteins present at the basal keratinocyte-basement membrane interface.

Basal epithelial layer is attached to the basement membrane by means of hemidesmosomes **(Figure 13-37)**. Hemidesmosomes are specialized junctional complexes that contribute to the attachment of epithelial cells to the underlying basement membrane (cell junctions are dealt in detail in the chapter on "Development of tooth"). The cytoplasmic keratin filaments insert into the hemidesmosomes.

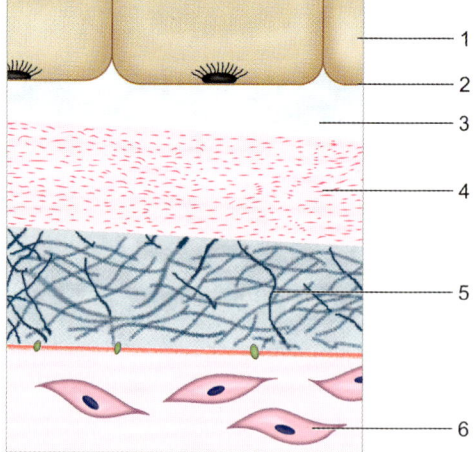

Figure 13-35: Basal lamina: 1. Epithelial cell, 2. cell membrane, 3. lamina lucida, 4. lamina densa, 5. lamina reticularis, and 6. Fibroblast of the lamina propria.

Connective Tissue

Connective tissue of the oral mucous membrane is made up of lamina propria and submucosa. Lamina propria is the superficial portion of the connective tissue. Submucosa lies adjacent to it and serves to attach the mucous membrane to the deeper structures. Lamina propria is always present in the oral mucous membrane. In some regions of the mouth, a

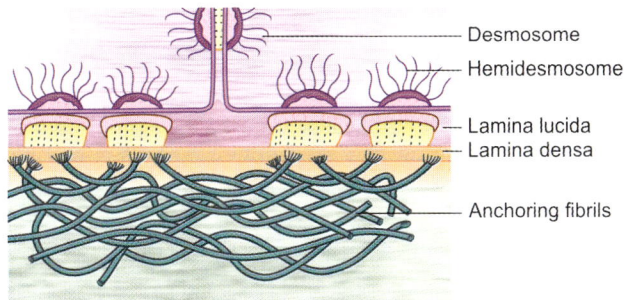

Figure 13-36: Anchoring fibrils.

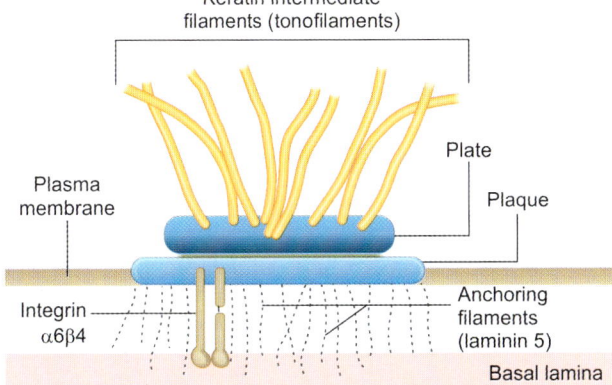

Figure 13-37: Hemidesmosome. Attachment of the basal lamina to the basal epithelial layer by hemidesmosomes.

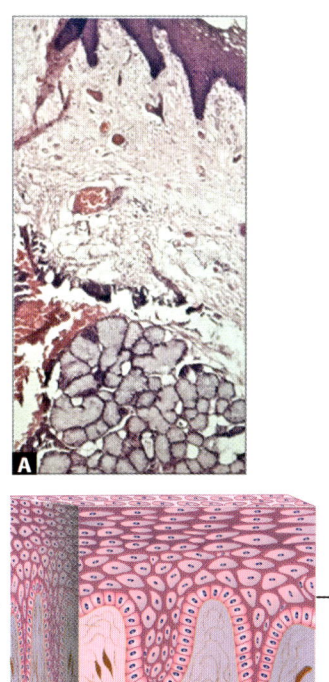

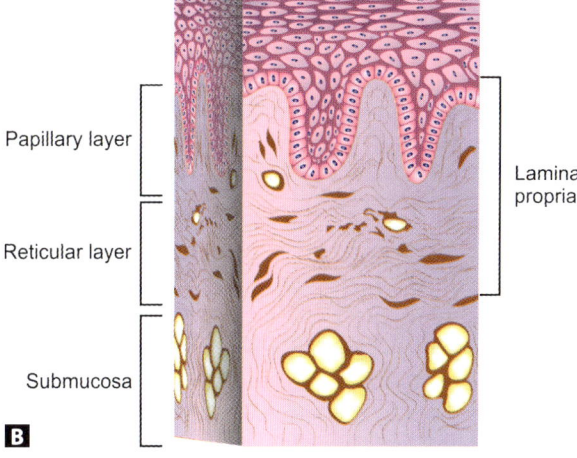

Figures 13-38A and B: Epithelium, lamina propria, and submucosa.

distinct submucosa may be absent and the lamina propria is directly attached to the periosteum.

Lamina Propria

Lamina propria is the connective tissue that supports the oral epithelium. Similar to other connective tissues, it is made up of cells and extracellular matrix. The lamina propria of the oral mucous membrane is divided into two layers:
- Superficial papillary layer associated with the epithelial ridges
- Deeper reticular layer present below the papillary layer **(Figures 13-38A and B)**.

Papillary layer extends from the basal lamina to the edge of the rete ridge. Thus, it is made only of the connective tissue peg or papilla. The collagen fibers of the papillary layer are thin and loose with many capillaries.

Reticular layer extends from the edge of the rete ridge to the submucosa. In contrast to the papillary layer, the collagen fibers in this layer are in thick bundles parallel to the surface and arranged in a netlike fashion and hence the name reticular.

While reticular layer is always present in the oral mucosa, the presence of papillary layer shows regional variations, since the connective tissue papilla may be short or absent in some lining mucosa. The lamina propria provides mechanical support and nutrition to the epithelium.

The connective tissues contain nerves, blood vessels, lymph vessels, and minor salivary glands. Regional variations of vascular concentration, along with the rate of blood flow, causes change in temperature in different parts of the mucosa. For example, alveolar mucosa shows a higher temperature than the attached gingiva.

The principal cell type of the lamina propria is the spindle-shaped fibroblasts. The cell contains abundant cytoplasmic organelles as they play an important role in continuous production of ground substance and extracellular fibers of the connective tissue **(Figure 13-39)**. Keratinocyte growth factor is produced by the gingival fibroblasts for the continuous growth and maintenance of the overlying epithelium. Apart from fibroblasts, macrophages, mast cells, and other inflammatory cells are also seen in the lamina propria **(Figure 13-40)**.

Cells of the Lamina Propria

The cells present in the lamina propria include:
- Fibroblasts
- Macrophages
- Mast cells
- Inflammatory cells:
  - Neutrophils
  - Lymphocytes
  - Plasma cells
- Endothelial cells.

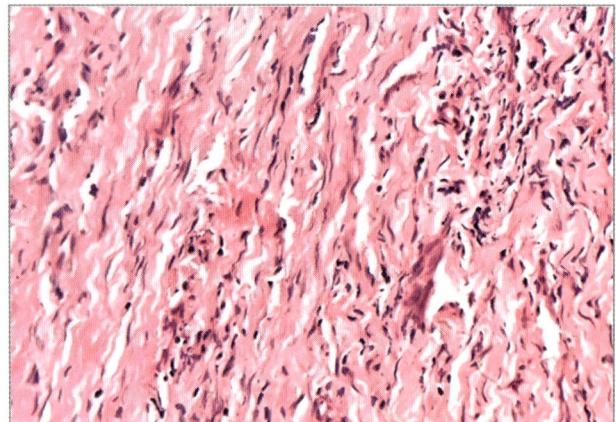

Figure 13-39: Fibroblasts and collagen fibers.

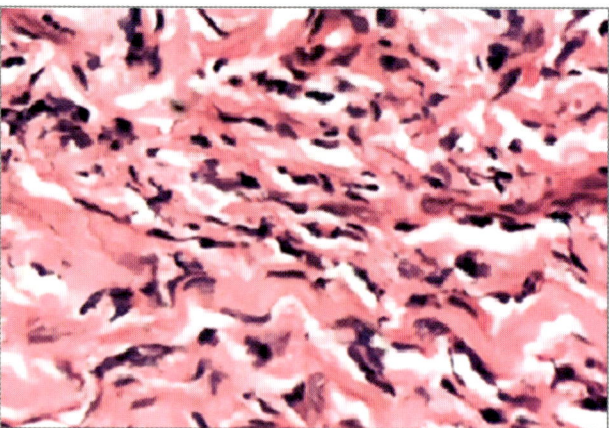

Figure 13-41: Fibroblasts.

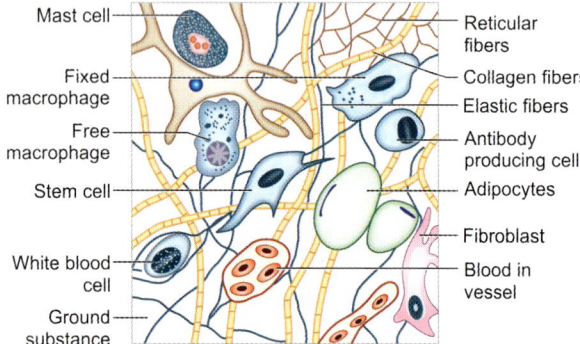

Figure 13-40: Components of lamina propria.

Fibroblasts: Fibroblasts are specialized cells in secreting and providing a supporting framework for collagenous extracellular matrix and functioning in repair mechanisms. These are the principal cells seen throughout the lamina propria and are responsible for maintaining the structural integrity of the connective tissues. Fibroblasts exist functionally and morphologically as heterogeneous subpopulations at different anatomical sites. This is due to the highly divergent patterns of gene expression. This "positional memory" is maintained by the distribution of Hox genes (a subset of homeobox genes). These cells are stellate-shaped or elongated with abundant rough endoplasmic reticulum. They have a low rate of proliferation, which is increased during wound healing. They also show a contractile action during wound healing where the actin content increases **(Figure 13-41)**.

The fibroblasts or their progenitor cells are induced to migrate and proliferate; secrete collagen and other connective tissue molecules; adhere to, contract, and remodel the extracellular matrix; secrete growth factors, cytokines, and chemokines; express surface receptors, and differentiate into apoptosis-resistant myofibroblasts in response to various extracellular signals.

Proliferating capacity of oral mucosal fibroblasts is more than the dermal fibroblasts. Exposure to Transforming growth factor-β_1 (TGF-β_1), more collagen is synthesized by the oral mucosal fibroblasts.

Scarless Oral Healing
Healing of oral mucosal wound is clinically different from healing of skin wounds in terms of rapidity and lack of scar formation. This is attributed to various reasons. These include the following:
- Phenotypic differences between human adult oral and skin fibroblasts in terms of wound contraction, myofibroblast differentiation, and growth factor expression.
- Differences in the composition and reorganization of extracellular matrix by fibroblasts.
- Enhanced growth factor secretion, as well as increased amount, potency, and proliferation capacity of oral keratinocyte stem cells.
- An altered inflammatory response, more specifically a decreased intrinsic inflammatory response, may be an important factor in rapid oral healing, and provide a possible explanation for the altered repair response in oral mucosa. The other factor that might be involved in the reduction of inflammation in oral wounds is secretory leukocyte protease inhibitor, an anti-inflammatory factor found in mucosa.

Macrophages: Macrophages are antigen-presenting and phagocytic cells that are seen in the lamina propria. In their inactive state, they resemble fibroblasts and are called histiocytes. They have a small dark nucleus compared to the fibroblasts, with lysosomes and less endoplasmic reticulum. Found throughout the lamina propria, these cells are stellate-shaped **(Figure 13-42)**. It is difficult to differentiate these cells from fibroblasts unless they contain phagocytic debris. The inactive precursor of these cells is called the histiocyte **(Figure 13-43)**. The main function is phagocytosis where the damaged tissue is ingested in vacuoles that fuse with lysosomes, which initiate the breakdown of these materials. Two specialized macrophages are seen in the lamina propria of the oral mucosa—melanophage that ingests extruded melanin granules from the melanocytes and siderophage that ingests hemosiderin extravasated in the tissues during injury. If the material is present within the cell for some time, it appears clinically as a brownish bruise.

Mast cells: The mast cell is a large mononuclear cell that is spherical or elliptical in shape with a small nucleus and intensely staining granules (histamine and heparin) in the cytoplasm **(Figures 13-44A and B)**. They have been suggested to play a role in vascular homeostasis because of

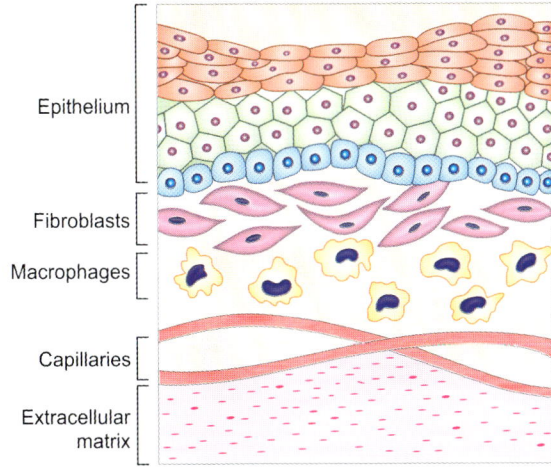

Figure 13-42: Macrophage in the lamina propria.

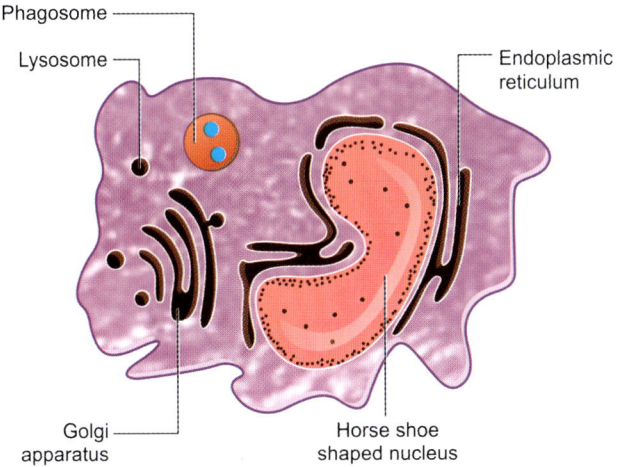

Figure 13-43: Histiocyte with phagosome.

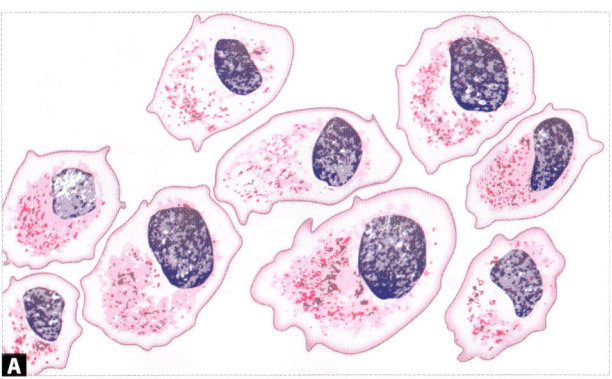

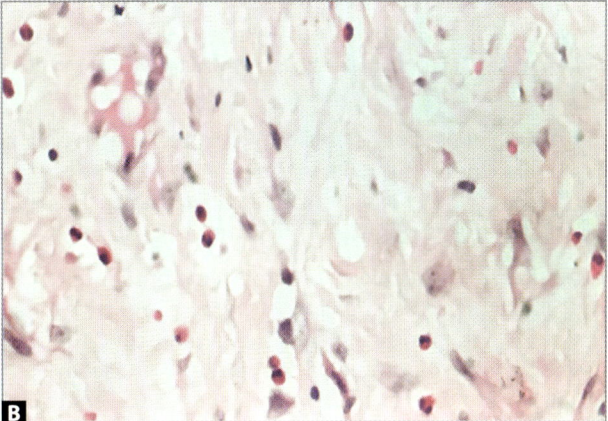

Figures 13-44A and B: (A) Mast cell; (B) Mast cells in tissue section.

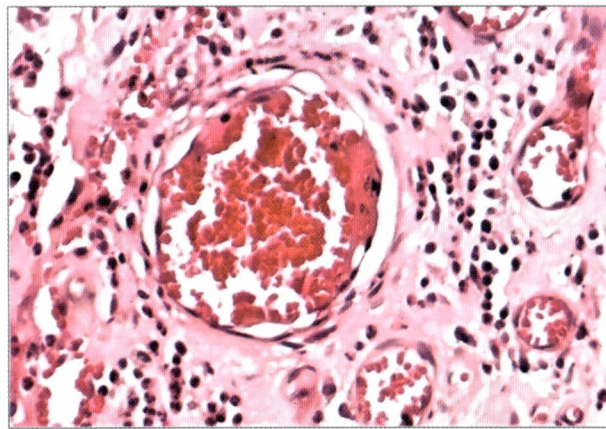

Figure 13-45: Lymphocytes, plasma cells, and polymorphonuclear leukocytes in tissue section.

their close association with small blood vessels. The histamine that is released is important during the vascular stage of inflammation. Mast cells also take part in cell-mediated immunity.

Inflammatory cells: Inflammatory cells such as lymphocytes and plasma cells are seen in less numbers in the lamina propria. However, other inflammatory cells may be seen in significant numbers following a tissue injury and will alter the nature of the overlying epithelium by releasing cytokines.

In acute conditions, neutrophils (polymorphonuclear leukocytes) dominate and in chronic conditions, lymphocytes, plasma cells, monocytes, and macrophages are most commonly seen **(Figure 13-45)**.

Endothelial cells: They are seen lining the vascular and lymphatic channels that are present throughout the lamina propria **(Figure 13-46)**. These cells contain numerous pinocytic vesicles and are associated with a basal lamina probably because the basement membrane is important for the development of new blood vessels and the basement membrane proteins may accelerate the differentiation of endothelial cells.

Extracellular Matrix

The extracellular matrix contains collagen, oxytalan, and elastin fibers and ground substance made up of proteoglycans and glycoproteins (*see* **Figure 13-40**).

Fibers: The connective tissue adjacent to the epithelium contains cells and extracellular matrix. The extracellular matrix supports and binds the cells and regulates a number of cellular functions, such as adhesion, migration, proliferation, signaling, and differentiation. The extracellular matrix is composed of fibers and ground substance.

Collagen: Connective tissue of the oral mucous membrane predominantly contains collagen fibers. Type I collagen fibers

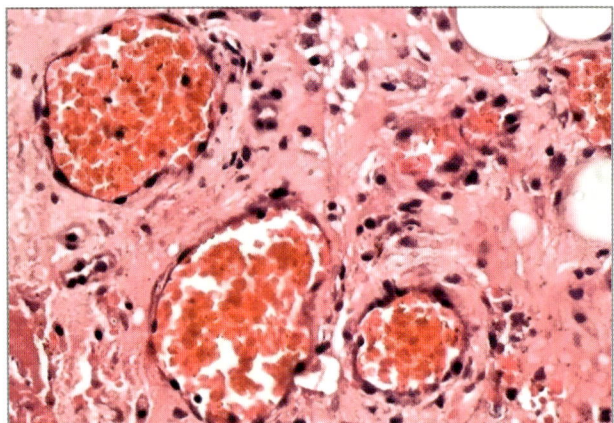

Figure 13-46: Endothelium-lined capillaries containing RBCs in their lumen.

(about 90%) make up the bulk of the matrix. Type III (about 8%) are also found but in lesser quantities. In addition, type IV, VII, V, and VI are also found in small amounts. These are present in bundles **(Figures 13-47A and B)**.

Elastic fibers: Elastic fibers are important component of the extracellular matrix assemblies that endow connective tissues with resilience, permitting long-range deformability, and passive recoil without energy input. These are secreted by fibroblasts and can stretch up to 1.5 times their length, and snap back to their original length when relaxed. They are made up of elastin core surrounded by a mantle of fibrillin-rich microfibrils. Elastic fibers are present in lining mucosa. Unlike collagen, they are branching and run separately. They cannot be seen in hematoxylin and eosin stained sections and can be demonstrated by special stains, such as Verhoeff's stain, orcein and aldehyde fuchsin.

Ground substance: Ground substance is elaborated mainly by the fibroblasts. It is made up of glycosaminoglycans and proteoglycans and the intercellular matrix that contains collagen and elastin that embed in the ground substance along with fibronectin. The proteoglycans of the oral mucosa are the heparan sulfate, hyaluronan, versican, decorin, biglycan, and syndecan. They have a polypeptide core, where the glycosaminoglycan attaches. However, the glycosaminoglycans have only a polypeptide chain.

Submucosa

This portion of the oral mucous membrane is also made up of connective tissue of varying density. Submucosa serves to attach the mucous membrane to the underlying structures. The nature of the attachment is firm in hard palate and loose in areas like alveolar mucosa, floor of the mouth, etc. A distinct submucosa is absent in gingiva and a portion of hard palate. The submucosa mainly consists of large vessels, muscles, nerves, clusters of minor glands, and adipose tissue along with the usual fibrous matrix of the connective tissue. The larger vessels divide and give branches in the submucosa. The vascularity of the oral mucous membrane, particularly the gingiva, is more when compared to the skin. The myelinated nerve fibers lose their myelin sheath as they leave to lamina propria, where they give terminal branches and some of them enter into the epithelium.

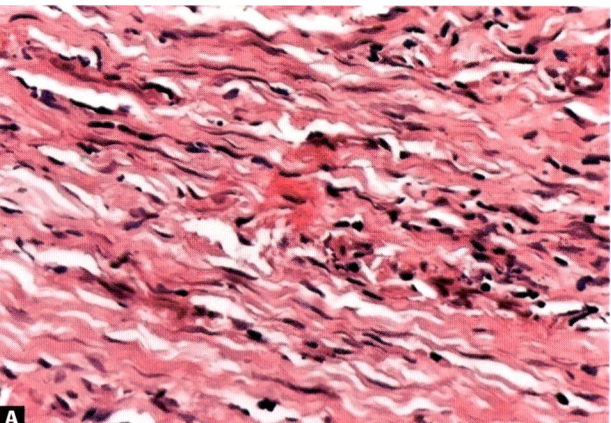

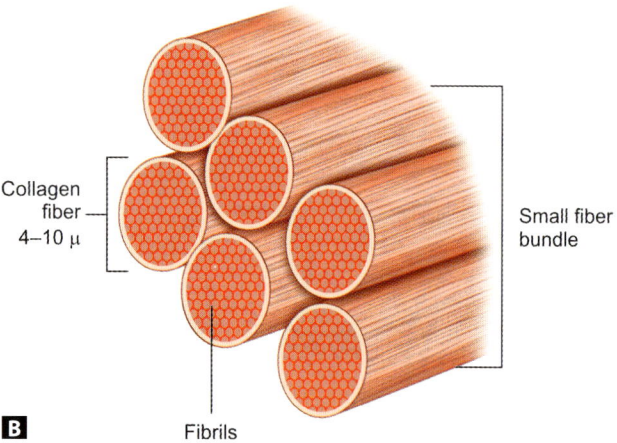

Figures 13-47A and B: (A) Collagen fiber bundles in hematoxylin and eosin stained section; (B) Schematic representation.

Points to Remember

- The stratified squamous epithelium of oral mucosa consists of polygonal cells, tightly attached to each other.
- The superficial layer of the epithelium may be keratinized or nonkeratinized.
- Masticatory mucosa is keratinized and lining mucosa is nonkeratinized.
- In tongue, filiform papillae and circumvallate papillae are keratinized.
- Gingiva consists of orthokeratinization and parakeratinization.
- Keratinized epithelium has 4 disctinct layers in contrast to the nonkeratinized epithelium that lacks the stratum granulosum and keratin layer.
- Keratinocyte are the majorly found cells whereas nonkeratiniocytes comprise of melanocytes, Merkel cells and Langerhans cells.
- Basement membrane separates the epithelium from the connective tissue.
- Basal lamina seen through the electron microscope consists of lamina lucida and lamina densa.
- Connective tissue of the oral mucous membrane is made up of lamina propria and submucosa.
- Lamina propria is the superficial portion of the connective tissue. Submucosa lies adjacent to it and serves to attach the mucous membrane to the deeper structures.
- The connective tissues contain nerves, blood vessels, lymph vessels and salivary glands and their principal cell type are the fibroblasts along with inflammatory cells, mast cells, macrophages and endothelial cells.

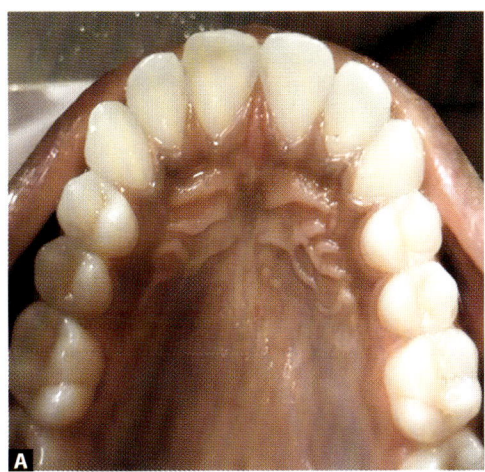
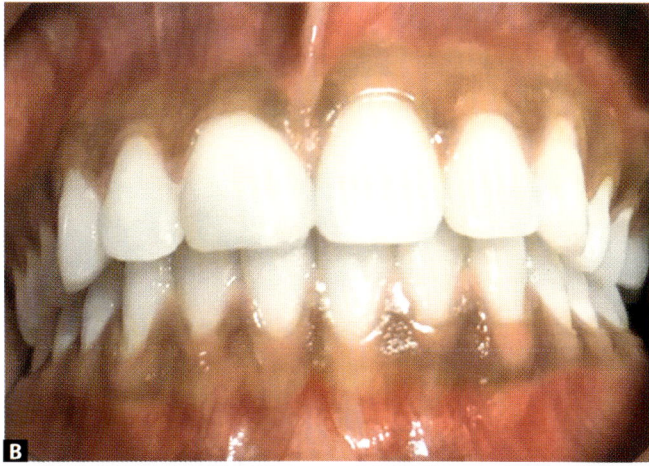

Figures 13-48A and B: (A) Hard palate; and (B) Gingiva.

■ MASTICATORY MUCOSA

Mucosa of the hard palate and the gingiva are covered by masticatory mucosa. This mucosa on both the regions has similar characteristics with respect to keratinization, thickness, and density of lamina propria but, however, varies in their submucosa **(Figures 13-48A and B)**. It is exposed to stress and abrasion during mastication. The tongue is a specialized structure and though it functions as masticatory mucosa it is considered as a separate entity, since it performs taste perception in addition.

Hard Palate

Hard palate is formed by the palatine process of maxilla and the horizontal plates of palatine bones **(Figure 13-49)**. It is concave and forms the roof of the oral cavity proper. The mucosa of the hard palate is dark pink in color, immovable, and fixed to the underlying periosteum. At the level of the maxillary tuberosity, it continues as soft palate. The surface of the anterior part of the hard palate has transverse ridges running on either side of the midline, which are known as palatine rugae **(Figure 13-50)**. They are irregular and asymmetric and made up of dense connective tissue core. Their number, length, width, height, and pattern vary from individual to individual.

The epithelium is uniformly orthokeratinized stratified squamous type and contain nonkeratinocytes such as melanocytes, Langerhans cells, Merkel cells, and lymphocytes. Epithelium of the hard palate is continuous with that of the soft palate and demarcation is indistinct. The connective tissue papillae are long, thick with dense collagenous tissue mostly under the rugae area. The lamina propria varies in thickness and is found to be thicker in the anterior than the posterior region. The capillary loops are short with moderate vascular supply.

The submucosa varies in the different regions of the hard palate. Based on the nature of the submucosa, hard palate can be categorized into four zones, namely, gingival zone, palatine raphe or the median area, anterolateral or fatty zone, and posterolateral or glandular zone **(Figure 13-51)**.

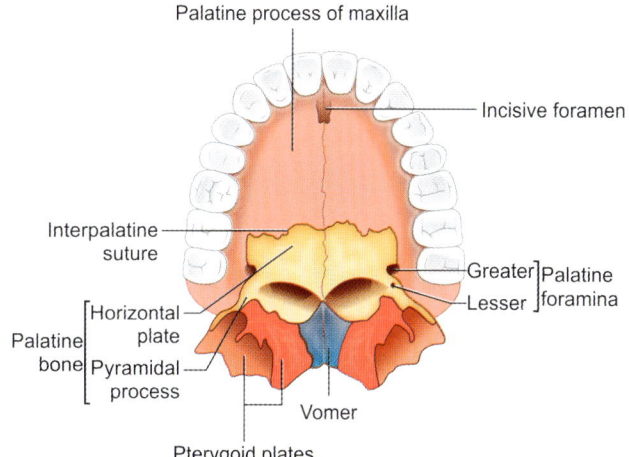

Figure 13-49: Palatine bone and palatine process of maxilla.

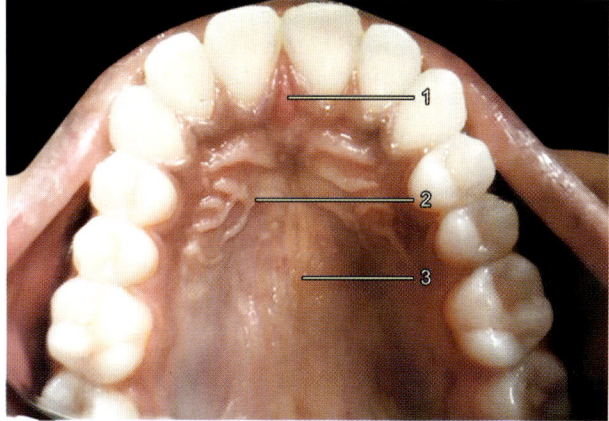

Figure 13-50: Hard palate showing: 1. incisive papilla, 2. rugae, and 3. mid-palatine raphe.

At the area where the palate joins the alveolus, submucosa is present with neurovascular bundles. Despite the submucosa present in other parts of the hard palate, the mucosa is immovably attached to the periosteum of the maxillary and palatine bones by fibrous connective tissue. These fibrous tissue bands run at right angles to the surface thus dividing

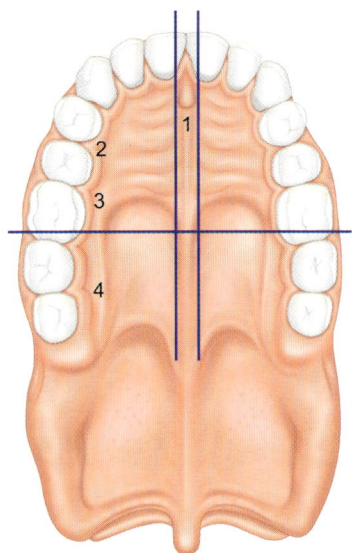

Figure 13-51: Hard palate. 1. mid-palatine raphe, 2. gingival zone, 3. fatty zone, and 4. glandular zone.

the submucosa into irregular intercommunicating spaces at the lateral areas of the hard palate. These spaces contain fat in the anterior region and glands in the posterior region **(Figure 13-52)**. The fatty or the glandular zone provides a cushioning effect to the palate. The mid-palatine raphe region is devoid of the submucosa and the lamina propria is directly bound to the underlying mucoperiosteum. This is similar to the attached gingiva.

The anterior palatine vessels and nerves are found in the wedge-shaped area between the horizontal process and horizontal plate of hard palate. This area is more in the posterior aspect than anterior.

Incisive Papilla

Incisive papilla otherwise called palatine papilla is a small (about 3 mm width), ovoid mucosal prominence located at the anterior end of the palatine raphe, posterior to the upper central incisors **(Figure 13-53)**. This covers the opening of the incisive canal and is made up of dense connective tissue.

During the development of palate, premaxilla contains incisive canal at the midline, which serves as a communication between the oral and the nasal cavity. Through this canal course the terminal branches of the descending palatine and sphenopalatine arteries and the nasopalatine nerve. The nasopalatine duct, or its remnants, may be found within or adjacent to this canal.

Nasopalatine duct remains patent in postnatal life in many lower mammals. These ducts connect the oral cavity with the vomeronasal organs of Jacobson along the anterior septum, which serve as accessory olfactory organs. In humans, these ducts may remain patent in the intrauterine life but degenerate and later obliterated by mucous membrane at their terminal ends prior to birth or within the first year of life. Thus, only vestigial epithelial remnants and/or blind ducts may be found. These blind ducts of varying length are lined by simple or pseudostratified epithelium and contain numerous goblet cells with a dense connective tissue. Mucous glands present in that region open into the duct lumen.

Epithelial pearls are epithelial remnants seen in the region of the incisive papilla or midline, which are formed during fusion of palatine processes. They are sometimes keratinized and arranged concentrically.

The nasal surface of the hard palate is lined by respiratory epithelium with ciliated columnar cells and goblet cells unlike the oral surface that has masticatory mucosa. There is a vascular submucosa with mucous and serous cells below the respiratory epithelium.

Gingiva

Gingiva forms a part of periodontium and is known as marginal periodontium. It surrounds the teeth like a collar, covers the alveolar bone, and extends from the gingival margin to the alveolar mucosa. As a part of the oral mucous membrane, it forms a cuff around the neck of the teeth and maintains the continuity of the oral mucosa. The gingiva is usually pink to red in color and the presence of melanin pigmentation gives it a brown or black hue which is more evident in the interdental areas. Under pathological states, the melanin pigmentation increases. The color of the gingiva depends on the degree of

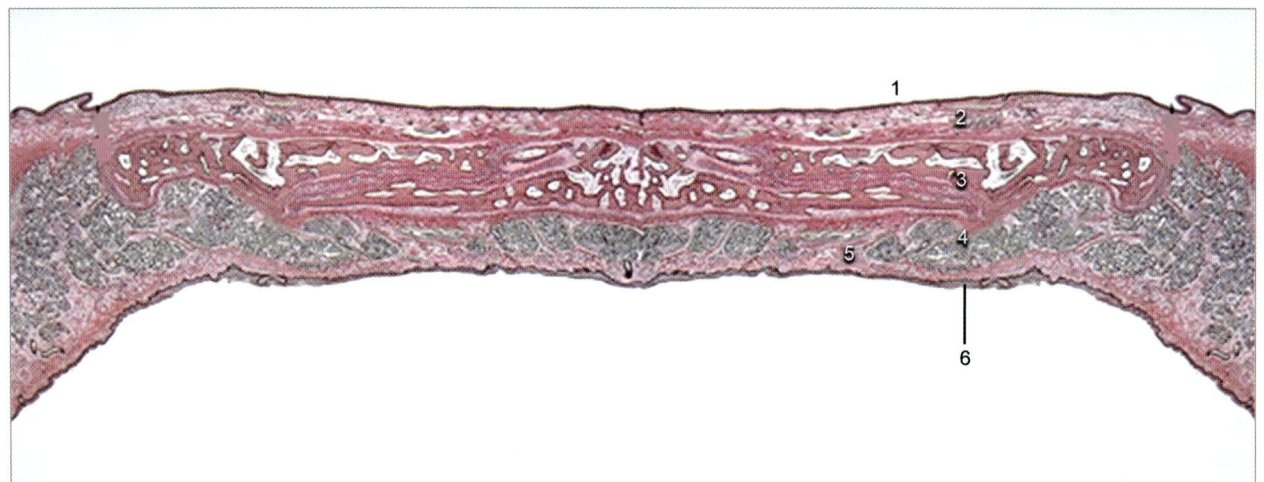

Figure 13-52: Section of hard palate. From above: 1. pseudostratified ciliated columnar epithelium of the floor of the nasal cavity, 2. connective tissue, 3. bone, 4. palatine glands, 5. connective tissue, and 6. keratinized stratified squamous epithelium of the oral cavity.

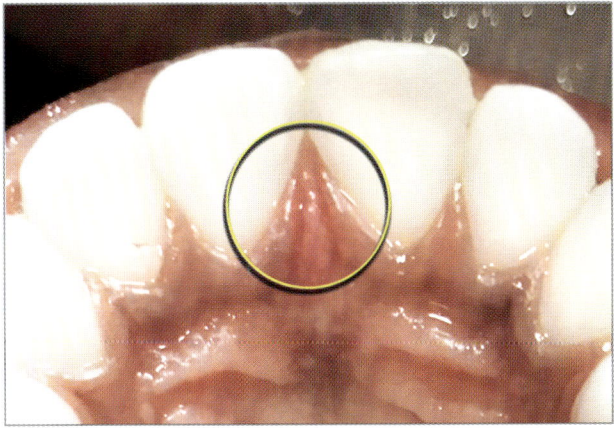

Figure 13-53: Incisive papilla.

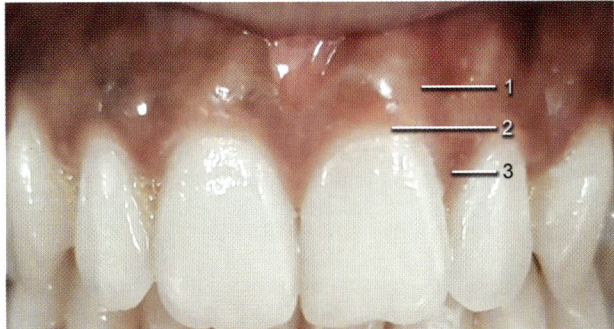

Figure 13-54: 1 Attached gingiva, 2. free gingiva, and 3. interdental papilla.

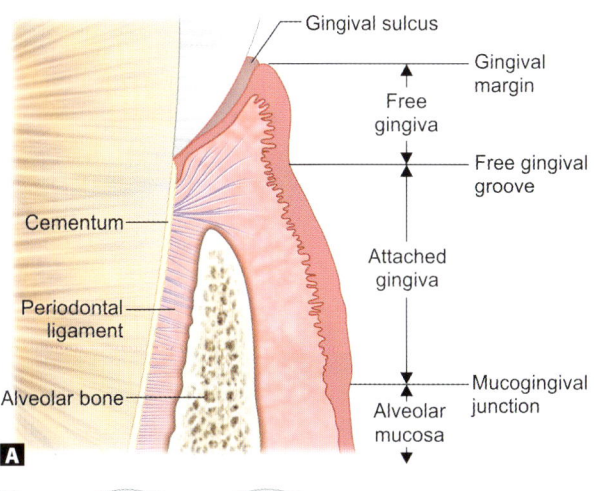

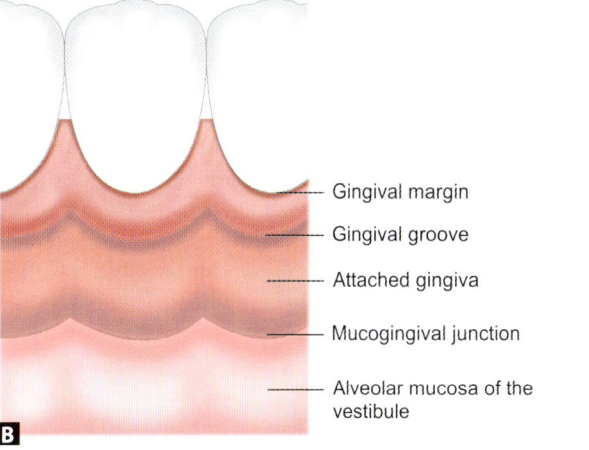

Figures 13-55A and B: Gingival sulcus, free gingiva, free gingival groove, and attached gingiva.

keratinization, thickness of the epithelium, vascularity of the lamina propria, and the pigmentation.

Gingiva is broadly categorized into free gingiva, attached gingiva, and interdental papilla **(Figure 13-54)**. The attached gingiva is the main component and is directly bound to the underlying alveolar bone. Part of gingiva not attached to the bone and seen above the attached gingiva is the free gingiva.

On the vestibular surface, the mucogingival junction separates the attached gingiva from the alveolar mucosa and in the inner aspect, a distinct line is seen between the gingiva and floor of the mouth. In the palatal aspect no such demarcation exists. Here the gingiva is continuous with the palatal mucosa.

❖ *Free gingiva*: The free gingiva also referred to as marginal gingiva is a narrow band of oral mucosa, which follows the scalloped contour of the cervical line of the teeth. It is termed as free gingiva, since it can be moved mechanically toward and away from the tooth. It is demarcated from the attached gingiva by free gingival groove that runs parallel at 0.5–1 mm to the gingival margin **(Figures 13-55A and B)**. This groove follows the contour of cementoenamel junction and is more pronounced in the vestibular aspect. It is not evident clinically in most individuals but appears as a "V"-shaped notch in histological sections. It is produced by bundles of collagen fibers that cross as they radiate from the surface of the cementum to the lamina propria of the gingiva. In some individuals, when the free gingival groove is absent, the demarcation between the attached and the free gingiva is marked by aligned stippling marks. The height of the free gingiva is about 1.5 mm.

> Free gingiva is that portion of the gingiva which lies coronal to the imaginary line connecting the free gingival groove and the cementoenamel junction.

Gingival sulcus or crevice is the space located between the tooth surface and the inner aspect of the free gingiva **(Figure 13-55A)**. It extends from the gingival margin coronally to the coronal portion of the junctional epithelium apically. It is present on the entire circumference of the tooth. The depth of the gingival sulcus ranges from 0.5 to 2 mm. Depth more than 3 mm is known as periodontal pocket and is a manifestation of periodontal diseases. The base of the sulcus is approximately at the level of the free gingival groove on the outer aspect. The epithelium lining the sulcus is known as sulcular or crevicular epithelium. *Sulcular epithelium* is nonkeratinized, thinner than the other regions of the gingiva, and varies in cytokeratin profile **(Figure 13-55A)**. Unlike the junctional epithelium, the sulcular epithelium does not express the epidermal growth factor. It stains positively for CK4 as other lining epithelium. The epithelial-connective tissue interface is smooth. Apical to the gingival sulcus, is the portion of the gingiva attached to the underlying tooth by the junctional epithelium. This is termed as dentogingival junction or epithelial attachment.

- *Attached gingiva*: The attached gingiva is tightly attached to the alveolar bone and is immovable. It extends from the free gingival groove to the mucogingival junction. On the palatal side there is no attached gingiva, since the palatal mucosa extends till the free gingiva. The height of the attached gingiva ranges from 4 to 6 mm. The height is maximum at the maxillary lateral incisors and minimum at the mandibular canine and first premolars. The surface of the attached gingiva shows numerous irregularly distributed ovoid or elongated indentations. This is called stippling **(Figure 13-56)**. This is more pronounced in the maxillary anterior region.

The depth of the indentation varies between 30 and 500 μm and corresponds to the crossing points of the rete ridges. Stippling represents a functional adaptation to mechanical stress and the absence of which may indicate a disease process such as gingivitis. However, gingival stippling is absent in children younger than 6 years of age. The stippling varies among healthy individuals especially based on the age and gender; women tend to have less prominent and fine stippling compared to males.

Between adjacent teeth, the gingiva shows depressions at the eminence of the sockets forming folds called as interdental grooves. These grooves correspond to the depressions of the alveolar sockets.

- *Interdental papilla:* The interdental papilla is a part of gingiva present between two adjacent teeth filling up the space apical to the contact area. It adheres to the shape of contact between two adjacent teeth **(Figure 13-57)**. It is triangular or wedge-shaped from the labial view and from a three-dimensional view it varies for the anterior and posterior teeth. The interdental papilla is pyramidal in shape in the anterior teeth and valley or tent-shaped in the posteriors with high vestibular corners. The center concavity is below the contact area and is called the col **(Figures 13-58A and B)**. This area has been suggested to be more susceptible to periodontal disease as it is not easy

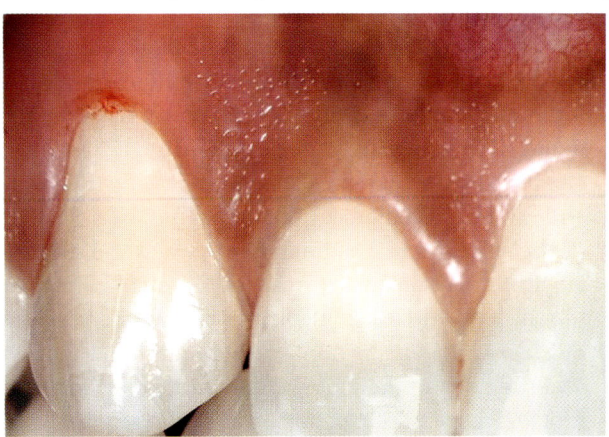

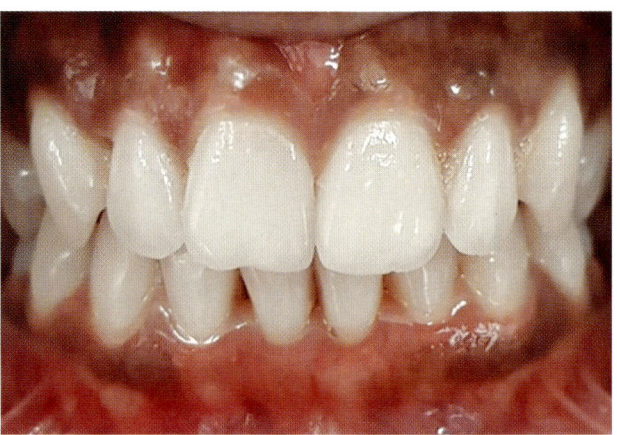

Figure 13-57: Interdental papilla.

to keep this zone plaque free and hence inflammatory cells infiltrating the lamina propria can be seen.

The col is continuous with the junctional epithelium. It is derived from the reduced enamel epithelium and is nonkeratinized. However, if the teeth are spaced, the col is absent with a flat gingiva that is keratinized.

Points to Remember

- Hard palate is formed by the palatine process of maxilla and the horizontal plates of palatine bones. The anterior hard palate has palatine rugae and at the level of the maxillary tuberosity, it continues as soft palate.
- The epithelium is orthokeratinized stratified squamous type. Hard palate can be divided into four zones, namely, gingival zone, palatine raphe or the median area, anterolateral or fatty zone, and posterolateral or glandular zone. The mid-palatine raphe region is devoid of the submucosa and the lamina propria is directly bound to the underlying mucoperiosteum.
- Incisive papilla covers the opening of the incisive canal and is made up of dense connective tissue.
- Gingiva extends from the gingival margin to the alveolar mucosa and is broadly categorized into free gingiva, attached gingiva, and interdental papilla.
- The free/marginal gingiva follows the scalloped contour of the cervical line of the teeth and is demarcated from the attached gingiva by free gingival groove.
- Gingival sulcus or crevice is the space located between the tooth surface and the inner aspect of the free gingiva. Sulcular epithelium is nonkeratinized.
- Dentogingival junction is the portion of the gingiva attached to the underlying tooth by the junctional epithelium.
- Attached gingiva is tightly attached to the alveolar bone and is immovable.
- Between adjacent teeth, the gingiva shows depressions at the eminence of the sockets forming folds called as interdental grooves.
- Interdental papilla is a part of gingiva present between two adjacent teeth and is triangular or wedge-shaped from the labial view. The center concavity is below the contact area and is called the col.

Figure 13-56: Gingival stippling.

Epithelium and Lamina Propria of the Gingiva

Gingiva falls under the category of masticatory mucosa, since it encounters abrasion and friction of the masticatory process.

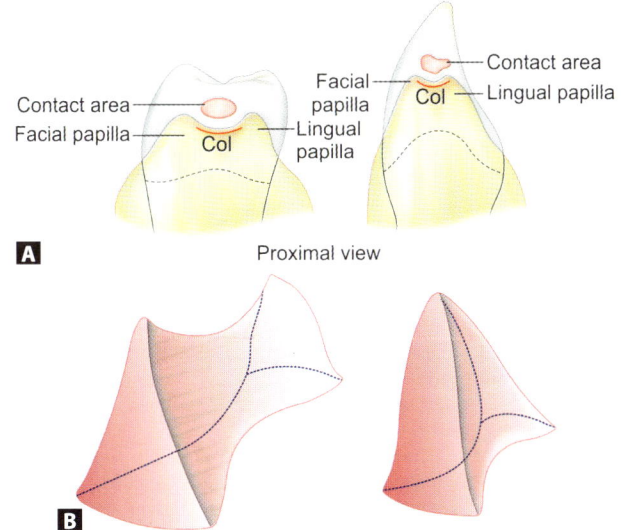

Figures 13-58A and B: Col. Tent-shaped in posterior teeth and pyramid-shaped in anterior teeth.

This is enabled by the keratinized epithelium and dense and immobile connective tissue, which is firmly attached to the alveolar bone.

The gingival epithelium is ortho or parakeratinized. In 75% of the individuals it is parakeratinized, in 15% it is orthokeratinized, and in 10% it is nonkeratinized. A highly keratinized tissue appears white and less translucent. Inflammatory conditions interfere with the keratinization process. In orthokeratinized epithelium, there is a sharp boundary between the stratum granulosum and stratum corneum. In case of parakeratin, there is smooth transition between the stratum granulosum and stratum corneum. Gingival epithelium free from inflammation does not contain glycogen in its cytoplasm, but in case of inflammation it does.

The nonkeratinocytes present in the gingival epithelium include melanocytes, Langerhans cell, Merkel cells, and T lymphocytes. Though they are present in the epithelium, they do not have desmosomal contact with the neighboring epithelial cells except Merkel cell.

The epithelial-connective tissue interface is dove-tailed with one another through rete ridges and connective tissue pegs. The connective tissue papillae are long and slender and roughly parallel to each other. The basal surface of the epithelium has many depressions in between the irregularly running rete ridges.

Junctional Epithelium

The junctional epithelium surrounds the tooth like a collar and attaches the connective tissue to the tooth surface. It extends for about 2–3 mm from the cementoenamel junction to the bottom of the gingival crevice. It is derived from the reduced enamel epithelium and may explain the reason for the cytokeratin profile which resembles the odontogenic epithelium than the stratified squamous epithelium.

Junctional epithelium is nonkeratinized, stratified squamous, and lacks the stratum corneum and granulosum.

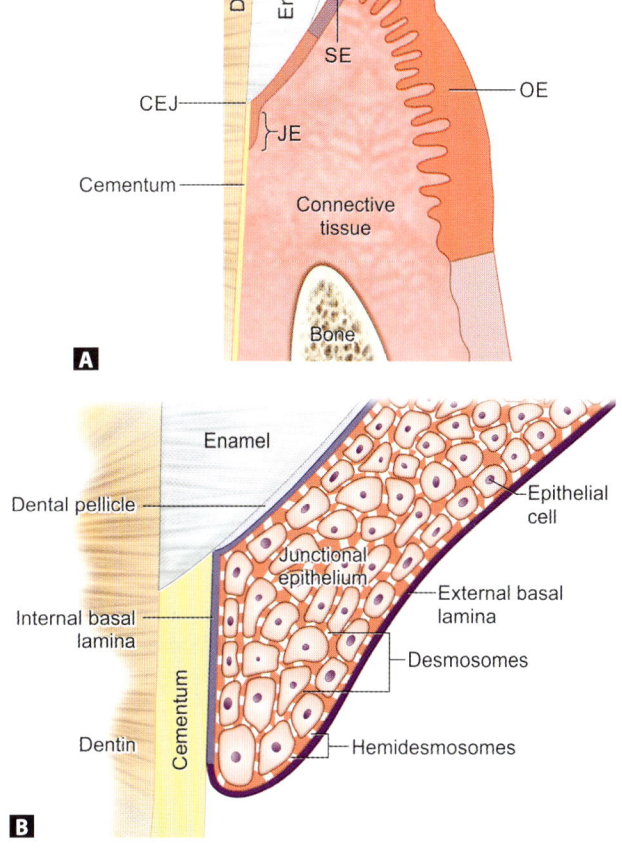

Figures 13-59A and B: Junctional epithelium.
(CEJ: Cementoenamel junction; OE: Oral epithelium; SE: Sulcular epithelium; JE: Junctional epithelium)

The epithelium is thick coronally (15–30 cells) and as it moves apically, it narrows to 1–3 cell layer thickness. The junctional epithelium has two layers of cells, a single layer of cuboidal cells called the stratum germinativum below and several layers of flattened cells above the cuboidal cells similar to stratum spinosum. Unlike the masticatory mucosa, the epithelium connective tissue interface is flat **(Figures 13-59A and B)**.

The dentogingival attachment is continuously renewed throughout the life. The turnover rate of the junctional epithelium is high (5-6 days) with cells exfoliating into the gingival crevice. The rate of turnover depends on the functional demands of the tissue and the degree of inflammation.

The cells of the junctional epithelium are held together by desmosomes and gap junctions with less tight junctions. Though the desmosomes are less in number, the intercellular spaces are large making up 5% volume of tissue. This allows the movement of crevicular fluid and defense cells across the epithelium. Presence of neutrophils is also seen in healthy gingival tissues indicating a protective role. There is a lack of membrane-coating granules that also helps in permeability of the cell layer. The cells contain free ribosomes, rough endoplasmic reticulum, and a Golgi apparatus for synthesis and transport of basal lamina components. The cells lack the keratohyalin granules and contain less cytokeratin filaments. Junctional epithelium lacks CK4 and, being a nondifferentiating tissue, is positive for basal keratinocytic markers like CK5, 14, and 19. Along with the fibroblasts and endothelial cells, the cells express intercellular adhesion molecule-1 (ICAM-1). This helps in the migration of neutrophils to the junctional epithelium.

The cells of the junctional epithelium attach to the tooth through hemidesmosomes and basal lamina. This combination is called the epithelial attachment or the attachment apparatus. These hemidesmosomes have an attachment plaque, which is a thickening on the inner part of the plasma membrane and opposite to that is a dense line similar to the lamina lucida of the epithelium-connective tissue interface. The basal lamina is divided as internal and external basal lamina. The internal basal lamina is the part of the basal lamina attached to the tooth and the part that is in contact with the lamina propria of the attached gingiva is the external basal lamina. The internal basal lamina also has two zones, an electron lucent zone that is adjacent to the cell and an electron dense zone against the tooth surface. This basal lamina lacks the type IV collagen, anchoring fibrils, and laminin unlike the external basal lamina. Under light microscope, this basement membrane appears thicker due to the reticular component of the connective tissue.

Enamel cuticle or dental cuticle is an intervening structure present between the internal basal lamina and the tooth surface. Its thickness may vary from 0.5 to 1 μm. It may be formed over any of the hard tissue of the tooth. It is a nonmineralized, probably an amorphous proteinaceous structure and ultrastructurally different from the basal lamina. It is not considered to be a part of the epithelial attachment, but its role in providing a milieu for attachment, its derivation, and its ultimate fate are yet to be established thoroughly.

The lamina propria consists of dense connective tissue fibers, fibroblasts with less inflammatory cells such as lymphocytes, plasma cells, and neutrophils for defense and repair. Collagen fibers are predominantly seen and are mostly type I. But type III, V, and VI are also seen. Reticulin fibers are dispersed within the framework of collagen fibers and form a subepithelial network. Elastic fibers are less and are usually seen around blood vessels in contrast to alveolar mucosa.

Apart from the fibers, the gingiva varies from the other parts of the mucosa in the composition of the matrix and in the nature of fibroblasts. The matrix has less of type III collagen and releases more of prostaglandin. The fibroblasts lack alkaline phosphatase and have less contractile protein.

The gingiva is firm and immovably attached to the periosteum of the alveolar bone and hence the term mucoperiosteum is applied to denote its connective tissue. Here, coarse collagen fiber bundles run from the bone to the connective tissue whereas the submucosa of the alveolar mucosa is loosely textured with thin and regularly woven bundles. Gingival fibers from the periodontal ligament attach the gingiva to the teeth.

> **Points to Remember**
> - The gingival epithelium is ortho or parakeratinzied. The nonkeratinocytes present in the gingival epithelium include melanocytes, Langerhans cell, Merkel cells, and T lymphocytes. Though they are present in the epithelium, they do not have desmosomal contact with the neighboring epithelial cells except Merkel cell.
> - The epithelial-connective tissue interface is dove-tailed with one another through rete ridges and connective tissue pegs.
> - The junctional epithelium surrounds the tooth like a collar and is derived from the reduced enamel epithelium. It is nonkeratinized, stratified squamous and has two layers of cells, a single layer of cuboidal cells called the stratum germinativum below and several layers of flattened cells above the cuboidal cells similar to stratum spinosum. The dentogingival attachment is continuously renewed throughout the life.
> - The cells of the junctional epithelium are held together by desmosomes and gap junctions with less tight junctions.
> - The cells of the junctional epithelium attach to the tooth through hemidesmosomes and basal lamina. This combination is called the epithelial attachment or the attachment apparatus.
> - Enamel cuticle or dental cuticle is an intervening structure present between the internal basal lamina and the tooth surface.

Gingival Fibers

Collagen fibers of the gingiva support the free gingiva, bind the attached gingiva to the teeth and bone, thereby withstand the masticatory load and connect the teeth to one another. Based on the orientation and attachment, gingival fibers are divided into following groups as mentioned below (**Figure 13-60**):

❖ *Dentogingival fibers:* These fibers are the most in number and extend from the cervical cementum to the lamina propria of gingiva. The superficial fibers lie below the crevicular epithelium, middle fibers lay horizontally, and deep fibers course between gingiva and alveolar bone.
❖ *Alveologingival:* Arise from the alveolar crest and interdental septum, radiates coronally and extends to the lamina propria of gingiva.
❖ *Circular:* These are a small group of fibers that encircle the tooth around the marginal and interdental gingiva and interlace with other fibers of adjacent teeth.

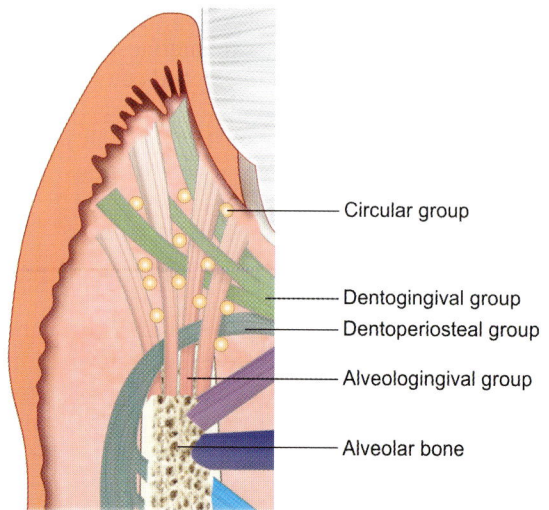

Figure 13-60: Gingival fibers.

- *Dentoperiosteal:* Present on the labial or buccal and lingual gingiva and extends from the cementum to the periosteum of the alveolar crest and to the vestibular and oral surfaces of alveolar bone.
- *Transseptal fibers:* These fibers extend horizontally above the alveolar crest and get inserted into the root of adjacent teeth and have been implicated in the mesial drift mechanism.

Apart from these fibers described, other fiber groups such as the following are also seen:

- *Longitudinal fibers:* Extend within the free gingiva and may be present in the whole of arch.
- *Interdental fibers:* Connect horizontally the buccal and lingual papilla.
- *Vertical fibers:* Run vertically from the alveolar mucosa or attached gingiva to the marginal gingiva or interdental papilla.
- *Semicircular fibers:* These course through the free gingiva and connect cementum on one side of tooth to the other side.
- *Transgingival fibers:* Pass from cementum of one tooth to the marginal gingiva of adjacent teeth and merge with circular and semicircular fibers.

Points to Remember

- Collagen fibers of the gingiva support the free gingiva, bind the attached gingiva to the teeth and bone.
- Dentogingival fibers are the most in number and extend from the cervical cementum to the lamina propria of gingiva.
- Alveologingival fibers arise from the alveolar crest and interdental septum, radiates coronally and extends to the lamina propria of gingiva.
- The small group of circular fibers encircle the tooth around the marginal and interdental gingiva and interlace with other fibers of adjacent teeth.
- The dentoperiosteal fibers extend from the cementum to the periosteum of the alveolar crest and to the vestibular and oral surfaces of alveolar bone.
- The transseptal fibers extend horizontally above the alveolar crest and get inserted into the root of adjacent teeth.
- The other fiber groups are longitudinal, interdental, vertical, semicircular and transgingival.

Development of the Dentogingival Junction

Once the ameloblasts form the enamel matrix, they leave a thin membrane called the enamel cuticle on the surface of the enamel, which is connected to the ameloblasts and the interprismatic enamel substance. Once this cuticle has been formed, the ameloblasts shorten and the epithelial enamel organ is reduced to a few layers of cuboidal cells called the reduced enamel epithelium. During eruption, when the tip of the tooth approaches the mucosa, the reduced enamel epithelium fuses with the oral epithelium. The remnant of this enamel cuticle after eruption is called the Nasmyth's membrane. Once the tip has emerged, the reduced enamel epithelium is called the primary attachment epithelium which is continuous with the oral epithelium at the gingival margin. Eventually the primary attachment epithelium gets replaced by the junctional epithelium. As the tooth eruption progresses, this reduced enamel epithelium shortens and shallow gingival sulcus may develop around the tooth circumference between the gingiva and the tooth. With tooth eruption this sulcus deepens. The gingiva around the sulcus becomes the free or marginal gingiva **(Figures 13-61A and B)**.

Attachment of the junctional epithelium and shift of the dentogingival junction: Based on the stage of eruption of the tooth, the length of the junctional epithelium varies. When the tooth first erupts into the oral cavity, it is completely covered with junctional epithelium. When the tooth reaches the occlusal plane, most of the junctional epithelium is lost and only a quarter of the enamel is covered with this epithelium. Later, it moves apically and lies close to the cementoenamel junction. Sometimes, the junctional epithelium can move even apically and establish a contact with the root surface. The process of separation of the primary attachment epithelium from the enamel is termed passive eruption. When this happens in the absence of an inflammatory process, it could relate to a physiological age change. However, there is an associated loss of collagen fibers at the cervix of the tooth, providing a potential passage for periodontal diseases. The primary attachment epithelium is replaced by the cells from the gingival epithelium and is called the secondary attachment epithelium.

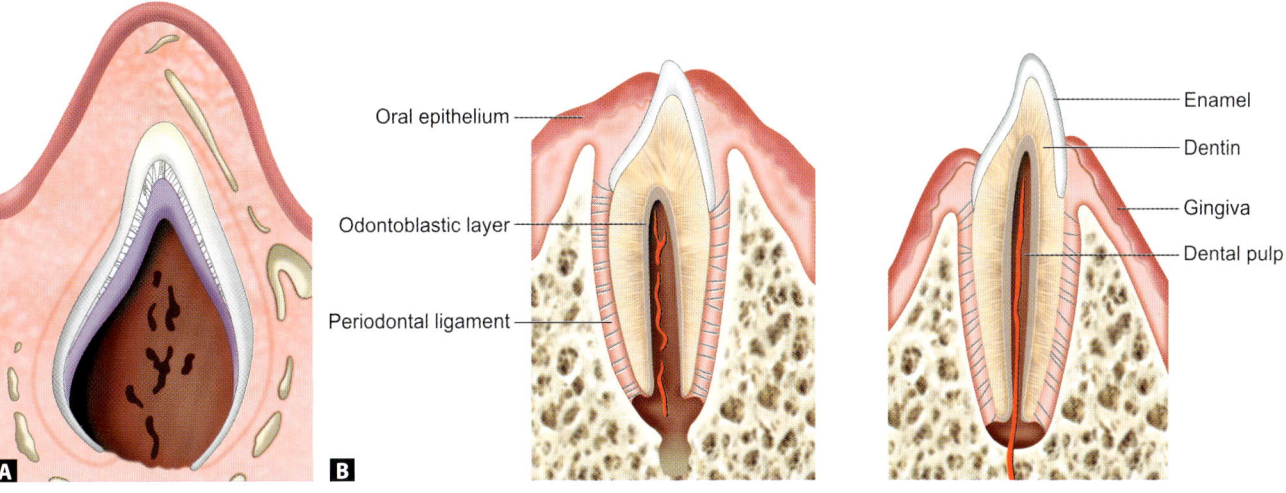

Figures 13-61A and B: Development of dentogingival junction.

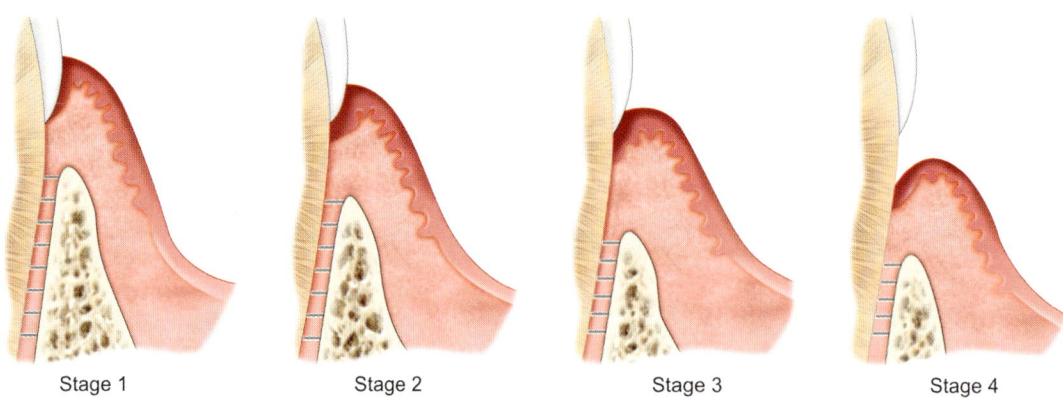

Stage 1　　Stage 2　　Stage 3　　Stage 4

Figure 13-62: Shift of dentogingival junction.

The exposure of crown through passive eruption and the following recession has been described in four stages (**Figure 13-62**).

First stage	Bottom of the gingival sulcus is at the enamel covered crown and apical end of the attachment epithelium at the cementoenamel junction. This relation is present in deciduous teeth till 1 year before shedding and for 20–30 years in permanent teeth.
Second stage	Gingival sulcus is at the same position as stage one and apical end of the attachment epithelium has moved to the surface of cementum due to dissolution of fibers at the cervical region of cementum brought about by enzymes formed by epithelial cells and also due to apical shift of the gingival and transseptal fibers. In case of periodontal diseases, the destruction of fibers is brought about by the dental plaque metabolites.
Third stage	The enamel covered crown is exposed. The bottom of the gingival sulcus is at the cementoenamel junction and epithelial attachment on the cementum. This process is more physiological and body's attempt to maintain an intact dentogingival junction.
Fourth stage	Here the entire gingival attachment is on the cementum, due to pathological recession. Gingiva may appear normal but represents a receded gingiva.

The crown exposure and recession may vary with every individual. It can also vary with different teeth on the same jaw or different surfaces of the same tooth. The exposure is important to distinguish the anatomic crown from the clinical crown.

The part of the tooth covered by enamel is called the anatomic crown and that part seen in the oral cavity clinically is called the clinical crown.

During the first two stages, the clinical crown is smaller than the anatomic crown but as recession progresses the clinical crown is equal and larger than the anatomic crown. Careful examination must be made to distinguish this exposure from the exposure due to periodontal disease, loss of attachment, and pocket formation.

The lamina propria is more cellular and shows anastomosing network of postcapillary venules. This crevicular plexus is separated from the surrounding looping vessels. This plexus is the source for gingival crevicular fluid and upon the slightest stimulation shows vasodilation. Therefore, in response to plaque, there is an increased production of the crevicular fluid. There is a rich network or plexus of nerves close to the basal layer of the junctional epithelium with the nerve endings penetrating into the gingiva itself.

The entire dentogingival unit that comprises the gingival margin, sulcular epithelium, junctional epithelium, and connective tissue attachment, acts as a sealant between the periodontal and the oral environment. The strength of the seal is brought about not only by the junctional epithelium but also by the periodontal fibers and the tissue fluid of the connective tissue. A weak dentogingival junction provides a pathway for bacterial colonization therefore exposing the epithelium to toxic products.

Gingival Crevicular Fluid

It is the fluid present in the gingival sulcus and is different from that of saliva. It was discovered in the nineteenth century, and its composition and defense mechanism were described as early as in 1959. Although the importance of gingival crevicular fluid (GCF) has been recognized for decades, the origin and functions of this fluid have been a matter of controversy. This controversy mainly centered on whether this fluid is the result of a physiological or pathological process.

The GCF originates from the gingival plexus of blood vessels and flows through the basement membrane and the junctional epithelium to reach the gingival sulcus. It has been shown that it is even present in healthy sulcus, although only in small quantity.

There is evidence to suggest that GCF from clinically normal periodontium is an altered serum transudate, which only becomes an inflammatory exudate when disease is clinically present. But the fact that neutrophils migrate into the periodontal crevice even in healthy state tends to maintain the controversy, whether GCF is an inflammatory exudate or a physiologic transudate.

Regarding the origin of GCF, it is postulated that its production is governed by the passage of fluid from the capillaries into the tissues and removal of this fluid by the lymphatics. When the rate of capillary filtrate exceeds that of lymphatic clearance, tissue fluid accumulates as edema and/or gingival crevicular fluid. Since the junctional and sulcular epithelium is permeable, the excess tissue fluid of the inflammatory reaction passes through the permeable junctional epithelium into the gingival crevice and presents as GCF.

Gingival crevicular fluid is essentially composed of local breakdown products, the tissues, inflammatory mediators, immunoglobulins, serum transudate (found in gingival sulcus), subgingival microbial plaque, extracellular proteins, neutrophils, and epithelial cells. However, this composition varies between healthy and diseased periodontium.

The nature and composition of the fluid can indicate the periodontal health including the gingival tissues. This fluid can be used as a diagnostic tool, as the analysis of GCF can help in assessing severity of the periodontal disease.

Vasculature of the Gingiva (Figure 13-63)

Vessels from the periosteum of the alveolar process supply the gingiva. Gingival branches from the periosteal vessels are perpendicular to the surface and form loops in the connective tissue papillae. These loops extend till the epithelium and end as postcapillary venules. Interdental alveolar arteries pierce the alveolar crest and supply the interdental papilla, buccal and lingual gingiva, and the dentogingival junction. Those supplying the dentogingival junction are parallel to the sulcular epithelium. Subepithelial vascular plexus is present lateral to the junctional epithelium. These plexuses of capillary network extend from the apical portion of the epithelial attachment to the base of the gingival sulcus region. These plexuses are extremely permeable because of the presence of numerous venules. The exudate can pass through the vessel wall and seep into the gingival sulcus as GCF.

Branches from the alveolar arteries anastomose with the superficial branches of the arteries that supply the oral and vestibular mucosa and marginal gingiva.

Fine network of lymph vessels permeate the gingival connective tissue. The efferent vessels run along the venous network. Lymph vessels of the gingiva chiefly drain into the submandibular and submental lymph nodes.

Innervation of Gingiva

Gingiva is richly innervated. Branches from the trigeminal nerve are responsible for the sensory and proprioceptive functions. Different types of nerve endings are present in the gingiva. These include Meissner's corpuscles, Krause end bulbs, and intraepithelial terminal fibers.

LINING MUCOSA

The lining mucosa is nonkeratinized with a loose connective tissue stroma and a submucosa. It is mobile and not subjected to friction. The lamina propria has collagen fibers as a network and elastic fibers that help in the resiliency of the mucosa.

The ventral surface of the tongue, inner surface of the lips, floor of the mouth, alveolar process up to the gingiva, along with the soft palate comprise the lining mucosa.

The epithelium and the lamina propria are usually thicker than the masticatory mucosa. The lamina propria has less collagen fibers and has an irregular course enabling the fibers to be stretched to an extent. In addition, there are elastic fibers contributing for the elasticity of the mucosa. When the mucosa covers a muscle, it is attached via the combination of collagen and elastic fibers. During mastication, the elastic fibers retract the mucosa toward the muscle thereby preventing the mucosa from being bitten between the teeth.

Lips

Lip is bounded by the skin on the outer surface and labial mucosa on the inner surface. Between the two tissues is the vermilion zone, which is otherwise called the transitional zone. The lips contain striated muscles which are part of the muscles of facial expression. Beneath the oral mucosa is the submucosa with minor salivary glands. The skin overlying the lip is made up of, a keratinized layer of epidermis and an underlying lamina propria with a flat epidermis-dermis interface. The dermis contains sweat glands, sebaceous glands, and hair follicles.

Vermilion Zone

The vermilion zone, unique for human, is present between the skin and the labial mucosa **(Figure 13-64)**. It lacks skin appendages and salivary glands and needs constant moistening by tongue. Sometimes, sebaceous glands are seen especially near the corner of the mouth. The epithelium is thin, keratinized, and appears translucent. The underlying lamina propria shows long and narrow rete pegs with capillary loops. The vascularity and the thin nature of the epithelium give the red appearance and hence it is called the vermilion (bright red) zone. The surface of the vermilion zone is not smooth; instead it contains many wrinkles or folds that may vary from person to person. Vermilion zone meets the skin at vermilion border **(Figure 13-64)**. The junction between this zone and the labial mucosa is parakeratinized but lacks the granular layer and is called the intermediate zone.

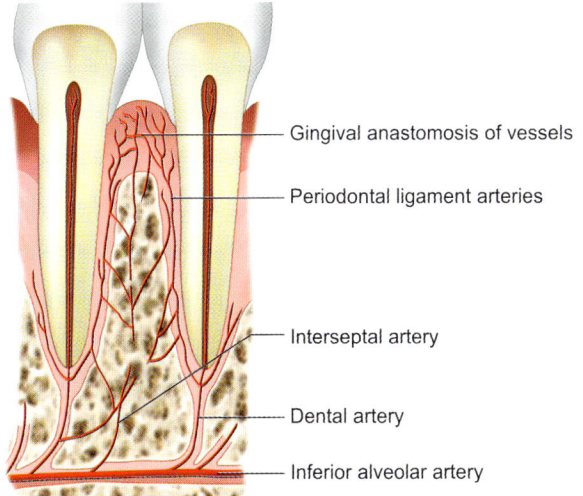

Figure 13-63: Blood supply to the gingiva.

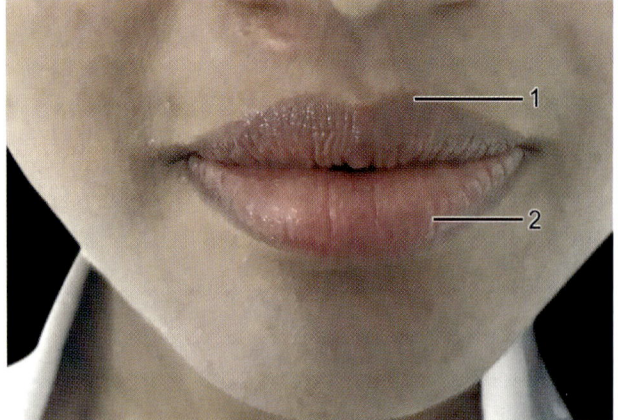

Figure 13-64: 1. Vermilion border, 2. vermilion zone of the lips.

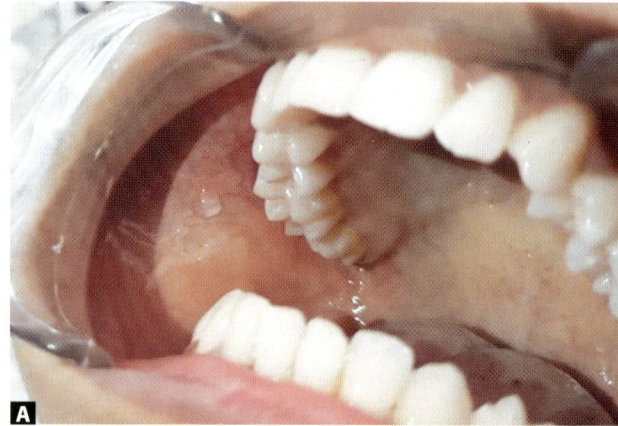

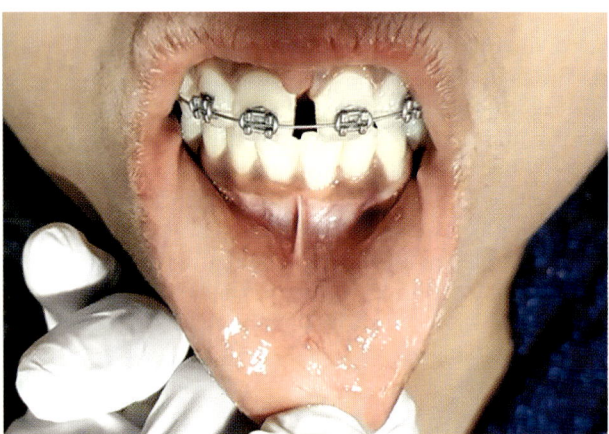

Figure 13-65: Labial mucosa.

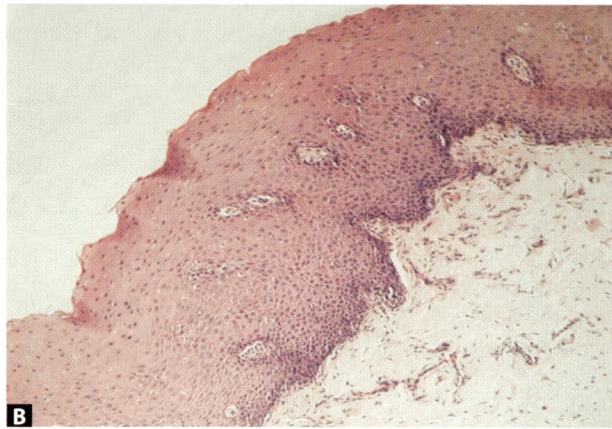

Figures 13-66A and B: Buccal mucosa: (A) Clinical appearance; and (B) Histological appearance (Hematoxylin and eosin stained section).

Labial Mucosa

The vestibular portion of the lip is covered by labial mucosa. The epithelium of the labial mucosa is nonkeratinized and is relatively thick. The underlying connective tissue is wide with short and irregular papillae. The submucosa has many minor mixed salivary glands and adipose tissue. Dense connective tissue holds the mucosa to the underlying orbicularis oris muscle and limits the mobility of the mucous membrane. This prevents the mucous membrane from lodging between the teeth during mastication **(Figure 13-65)**.

Buccal Mucosa

The lining mucosa of the cheek is called the buccal mucosa **(Figure 13-66A)**. The epithelium is nonkeratinized, thicker than the epithelium of the masticatory mucosa. The lamina propria is also thick and contains less collagen fibers. The thicker epithelium (about 500 μm), fewer irregular collagen fibers along with the elastic fibers make this mucosa flexible and withstand stretching. The connective tissue papillae are short and irregular **(Figure 13-66B)**. The submucosa has minor salivary glands, which are usually found between bundles of buccinator muscle and sometimes on its outer surface. The collecting ducts of the minor salivary glands open into the vestibule of the mouth. Linea alba and sebaceous glands (Fordyce spots) may be seen in some individuals.

> In comparison with the masticatory mucosa, the buccal mucosa has thicker epithelium in contrast to the thinner and keratinized epithelium of the masticatory mucosa. The cells of the masticatory mucosa are smaller with an angular shape. It contains many tonofibrils, wide intercellular spaces, and intercellular bridges. The appearance of the keratinized tissue is heightened by the presence of the prickle cell layer. The lamina propria also differs by the presence of more reticular fibers and high and narrow papilla in masticatory mucosa.

Alveolar Mucosa

The alveolar mucosa covers the alveolar bone apical to the attached gingiva and is pink to red in color with numerous blood vessels **(Figure 13-67)**. It contains the submucosa that is loose and allows movement. The mucogingival junction separates the attached gingiva from alveolar mucosa and the difference in these two regions is brought about by keratinization and translucency.

The alveolar mucosa has a thin, translucent, and nonkeratinized epithelial covering. Lamina propria is thicker in the portion where it joins the attached gingiva. The blood vessels are present superficially, which can be seen readily through the thin epithelium. Submucosa contains minor salivary glands, mostly mucous and near the vestibular sulcus contains elastic fibers aiding in free movement.

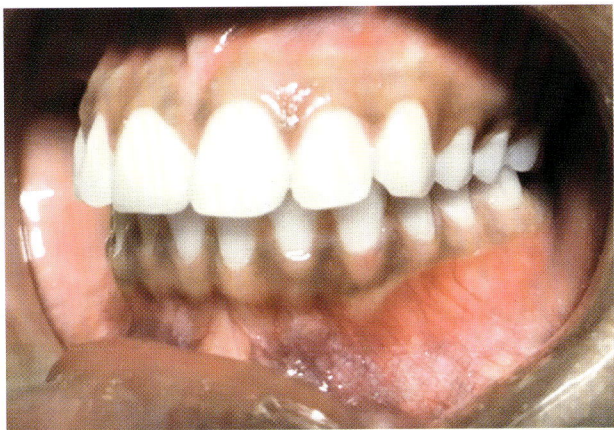

Figure 13-67: Clinical appearance of alveolar mucosa. Note the capillaries seen through the thin epithelium.

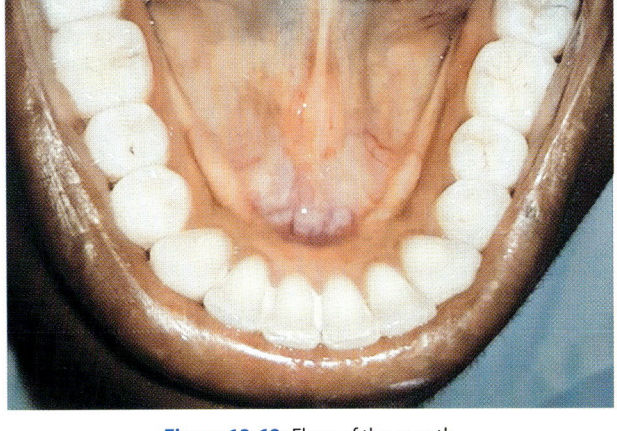

Figure 13-68: Floor of the mouth.

Vestibular Fornix

The mucosa of the lips and the cheeks reflects from the vestibular fornix to the alveolar mucosa. Though the mucous membrane of the buccal mucosa is attached firmly to the underlying muscles, at the fornix, the mucosa is loosely connected to the underlying structures. The alveolar mucosa is loosely attached to the periosteum. It is continuous with the gingiva, which is firmly attached to the periosteum. Labial and buccal frena are present at the midline and the lateral sides.

Floor of the Mouth

The mucous membrane of the floor of the mouth comes under the category of lining mucosa. It is loosely attached to the underlying structure by means of a thick submucosa. This allows free mobility of the tongue. Epithelium is nonkeratinized and extremely thin. The lamina propria has short papillae and contains elastic fibers, which help to restore the mucosa to its original position after distension. Collagen fibers are less. Submucosa contains adipose tissue. The mucosa of the floor of the mouth and the lingual gingiva meet at a junction, which is analogous to the mucogingival junction of the vestibular surface. Floor of the mouth is not flat and smooth. It has a linear elevation running posterolaterally from the sublingual caruncle on either side of the inferior attachment of the lingual frenum. This is called sublingual fold or plica sublingualis and is caused by the superior margin of the sublingual gland, since it lies closer to the mucosa of the floor of the mouth **(Figure 13-68)**.

Soft Palate

The soft palate is movable and forms the distal extension of the hard palate. It has a conical projection in the midline called uvula. The palatal mucosa is covered by nonkeratinized epithelium containing taste buds. Connective tissue papillae are short and broad. The mucosa is intermediate between the reflecting mucosa and the lining mucosa. The connective tissue contains thin bundles of collagen fibers and abundant elastic fibers. It is also highly vascular contributing to the red color in contrast to the hard palate. Small mucous salivary glands are seen in the broad submucosa **(Figure 13-69)**. Nasal part of the soft palate is lined by ciliated columnar epithelium of the respiratory mucosa type.

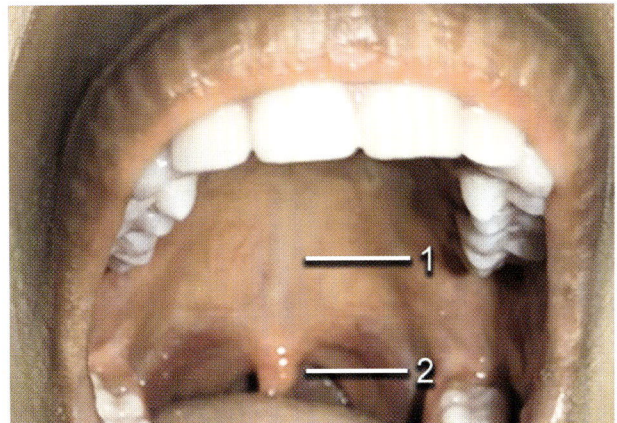

Figure 13-69: 1. Soft palate, and 2. uvula.

Points to Remember

- The lining mucosa comprising of the ventral surface of the tongue, inner surface of the lips, floor of the mouth, soft palate and alveolar process upto gingiva is nonkeratinized with a loose connective tissue stroma and a submucosa.
- Lip is bounded by the skin on the outer surface and labial mucosa on the inner surface. Between the two tissues is the vermilion zone which is otherwise called the transitional zone.
- The lips contain striated muscles which are part of the muscles of facial expression.
- The vermilion zone is present between the skin and the labial mucosa. It lacks skin appendages. The vascularity and the thin nature of the epithelium give the red appearance and hence it is called the vermilion (bright red) zone.
- The vestibular portion of the lip is covered by labial mucosa. The epithelium of the labial mucosa is nonkeratinized and is relatively thick. The underlying connective tissue is wide with short and irregular connective tissue papillae.
- The lining mucosa of the cheek is called the buccal mucosa and the epithelium is nonkeratinized, thicker than the epithelium of the masticatory mucosa. The lamina propria is also thick and contains less collagen fibers.

- The lining mucosa of the cheek is called the buccal mucosa and the epithelium is nonkeratinized, thicker than the epithelium of the masticatory mucosa. The lamina propria is also thick and contains less collagen fibers.
- The alveolar mucosa covers the alveolar bone apical to the attached gingiva and is pink to red in color with numerous blood vessels. It has a thin, translucent, and nonkeratinized epithelial covering.
- The mucosa of the lips and the cheeks reflects from the vestibular fornix to the alveolar mucosa. The alveolar mucosa is loosely attached to the periosteum and is continuous with the gingiva, which is firmly attached to the periosteum.
- The mucous membrane of the floor of the mouth is loosely attached to the underlying structure by means of a thick submucosa allowing free mobility of the tongue. Epithelium is nonkeratinized and extremely thin. The lamina propria has short papillae and contains elastic fibers, which help to restore the mucosa to its original position after distension. It has a linear elevation running posterolaterally from the sublingual caruncle on either side of the inferior attachment of the lingual frenum and it is called the sublingual fold or plica sublingualis and is caused by the superior margin of the sublingual gland, since it lies closer to the mucosa of the floor of the mouth.
- The soft palate is movable and forms the distal extension of the hard palate. It has a conical projection in the midline called uvula. The palatal mucosa is covered by nonkeratinized epithelium containing taste buds. Connective tissue papillae are short and broad. Nasal part of the soft palate is lined by ciliated columnar epithelium of the respiratory mucosa type.

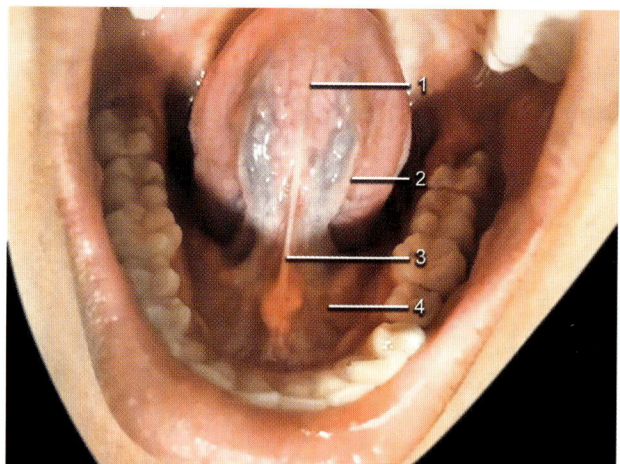

Figure 13-70: Ventral surface of the tongue and floor of the mouth: 1 and 3. lingual frenum, 2. plica fimbriata, and 4. plica sublingualis of the floor of the mouth.

SPECIALIZED MUCOSA

The tongue is considered as a specialized tissue because it not only has mechanical functions but also the special sensory functions for taste. It is a muscular organ covered by mucous membrane all around. But there is difference in the mucosa of the dorsal surface and the ventral surface.

Ventral Surface of Tongue

Ventral surface of the tongue is covered by lining mucosa, which has thin nonkeratinized epithelium and an indistinct submucosa. The mucosa of the ventral surface of the tongue is firmly attached to the intrinsic muscles of the tongue. Similar to the plica sublingualis of the floor of the mouth, the ventral surface of the tongue has plica fimbriata. It is a thin fold of the mucous membrane that runs laterally on either side of the frenum. The free edge of the fold occasionally exhibits a series of fringe-like processes **(Figure 13-70)**.

The thinner epithelium and highly vascular connective tissue allows the easier absorption and diffusion of drugs into the bloodstream when placed in that region. This is known as sublingual administration. Close to covering mucosa of the sublingual folds, lies the sublingual gland.

Dorsal Surface of Tongue

The tongue is divided into anterior two-thirds, otherwise known as body of the tongue and posterior one-third called lymphoid portion, by an indistinct V-shaped groove called the sulcus terminalis. The mucosa of the posterior one-third also contains numerous mucous glands. At the angle of this sulcus is the foramen cecum, which is the former orifice of the

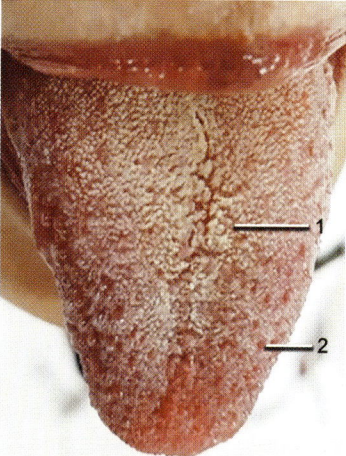

Figure 13-71: Papillary part of the tongue: 1. filiform papilla, and 2. fungiform papilla.

thyroglossal duct. The dorsal surface of the tongue is divided into two equal halves at the midline by a sulcus.

Since the anterior part is derived from the first pharyngeal arch, it is supplied by the lingual nerve, a branch of the trigeminal nerve. The posterior part is supplied by the glossopharyngeal nerve. The anterior two-thirds of the tongue contain filiform, fungiform, foliate, and circumvallate papillae, thus it is also known as papillary part **(Figure 13-71)**. The posterior one-third contains lymphatic nodules or follicles with germinal centers and is called lymphoid part **(Figure 13-72)**.

Papilla of the Tongue

The mucosa of the anterior part can also be categorized as masticatory mucosa since the most numerous cone-shaped or hair-shaped *filiform papillae* have keratinized epithelium with a thick connective tissue core **(Figure 13-73)**. Presence of these papillae gives the dorsal surface a velvety appearance. The regions in between these papillae are nonkeratinized supported by secondary branch of connective tissue core

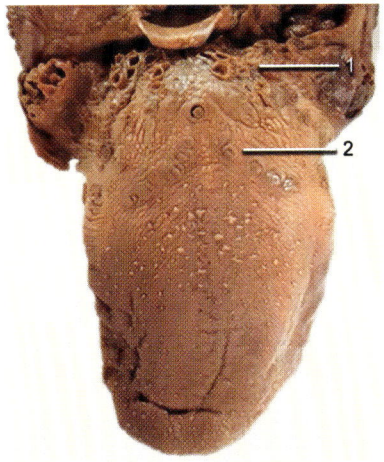

Figure 13-72: Lymphoid part of the tongue: 1. lingual tonsil, and 2. circumvallate papilla.

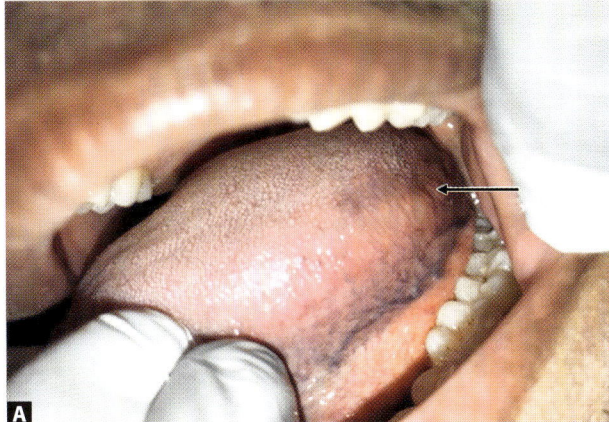

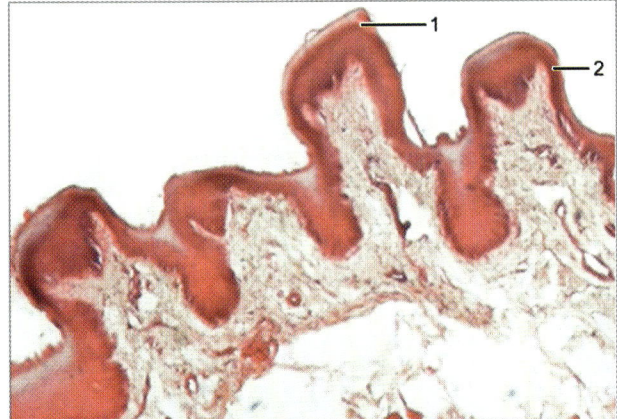

Figure 13-73: Hematoxylin and eosin stained section of 1. filiform, and 2. fungiform papillae.

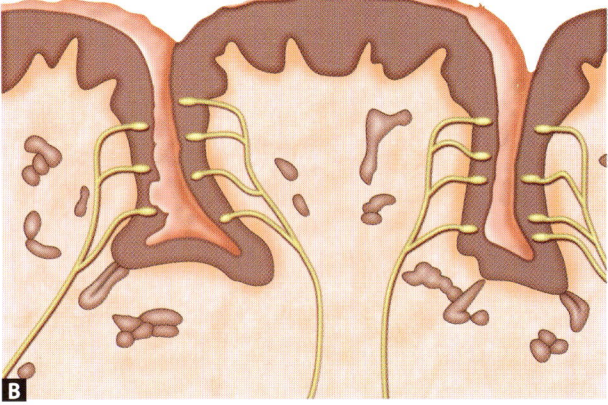

Figures 13-74A and B: (A) Foliate papilla in the lateral border of the tongue; (B) Foliate papilla showing taste buds.

coming out from the central core of the filiform papilla. The dorsal part of the tongue takes active part in mastication by compressing and breaking the food against the palate.

Fungiform papillae are elevated, mushroom-shaped, and present between the filiform papillae, on the anterior part of the dorsal portion of the tongue. They are mostly present at the tip of the tongue and are approximately 150–400 μm in diameter. The epithelium is thin and nonkeratinized with a highly vascular lamina propria and hence these papillae appear red in color. The taste buds are present on the superior surface **(Figure 13-73)**.

Foliate papillae are leaf-like papillae or vertical and parallel ridges present on the lateral border of posterior part of the tongue. They are seldom distinct in humans compared to other mammals. These parallel ridges are separated by deep grooves and have few taste buds on their lateral wall **(Figures 13-74A and B)**. The epithelium is nonkeratinized.

Circumvallate (walled–around) papillae are largest, round papillae that are around 8–12 in number present adjacent or anterior to the sulcus terminalis (an indistinct groove, which separates the anterior two-thirds and posterior one-third of the tongue). Each papilla is around 1 mm in height and 2–3 mm in diameter. They are not raised above the surface and have deep grooves or valley-like depression around them into which the minor serous salivary glands called the von Ebner glands open their ducts. The epithelium is keratinized on its superior surface with a connective tissue core. Taste buds are present along the lateral wall and they perceive the bitter taste. There are around 250 taste buds in the circumvallate papilla. The epithelium is keratinized in the superior surface and nonkeratinized in the lateral wall **(Figure 13-75)**.

> von Ebner glands are also seen in foliate papillae. They secrete digestive enzymes like lipase and amylase, which start to break down the ingested food. Further they aid in taste perception particularly bitter taste by secreting a protein similar to the odorant-binding proteins of the nasal glands.

Taste Buds

They are chemoreceptive intraepithelial organs with a rich plexus of nerves found below them. They are mainly present around the walls of the circumvallate papillae **(Figure 13-76)**. They are also found on the surface of the fungiform papillae, lateral walls of the foliate papillae, soft palate, and epiglottis in small numbers. They are ovoid or barrel-shaped, approximately 30–80 μm in length and 50–80 μm in diameter.

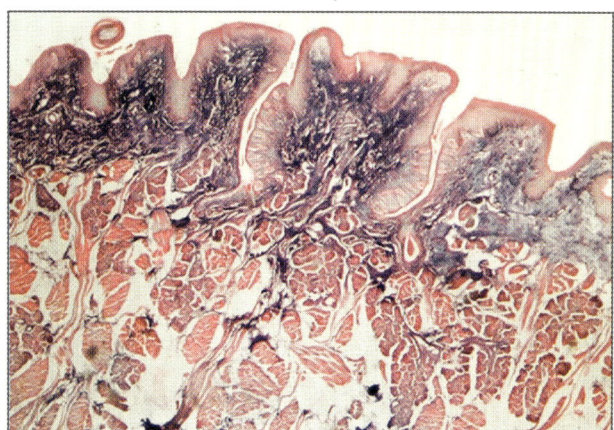

Figure 13-75: Hematoxylin and eosin stained section showing circumvallate and fungiform papillae showing taste buds.

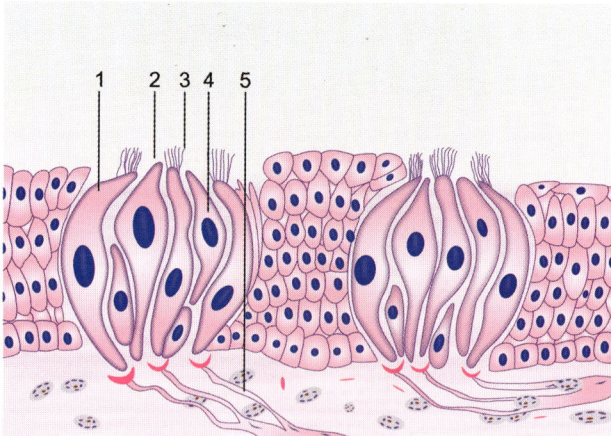

Figure 13-77: Structure of a taste bud: 1. taste cell, 2. taste pore, 3. villi, 4. supporting cell, and 5. afferent nerves.

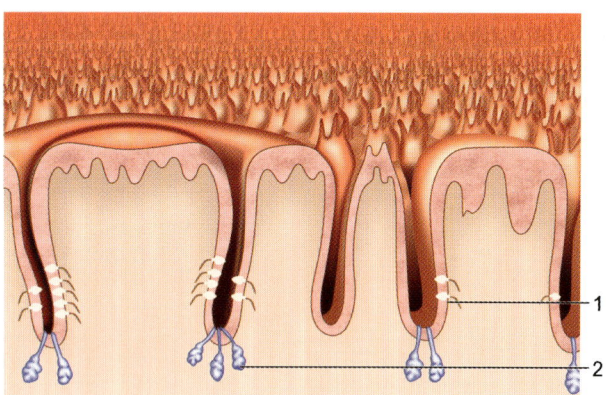

Figure 13-76: 1. Taste bud in fungiform papilla, and 2. serous salivary gland opening at the circumvallate papilla.

Taste bud is inverted onion-shaped and is made up of 30–100 cells. It contains two types of cells, a taste receptor cell and a supporting cell. All the cells of the taste bud are in contact with the basement membrane. The outer surface of these buds is covered by flat epithelial taste receptor cells, which extend from the basal lamina to the surface surrounding a small opening called taste pore. A taste bud can have more than one taste pore. This opens into a narrow space lined by supporting cells.

These supporting cells are arranged as staves of a barrel with inner and shorter ones spindle in shape. Between these shorter cells are 10–12 neuroepithelial cells which contain receptors for taste stimuli. The cells are dark staining and carry a finger-like process at the superficial end **(Figure 13-77)**.

Ultrastructurally, four types of cells have been described. Type I (dark) is the most common type and represents half of the cells of the taste bud. Type II (light), contain vesicles and are adjacent to the intraepithelial nerves and the apical portions are joined by junctional complexes and type III are intermediate cells. Type IV cells are undifferentiated and located at the basal region.

Myelinated nerve fibers enter the taste bud through basement membrane. They lose their myelin sheath within the taste bud and become free nerve endings. These nerve endings form a synaptic contact with the taste cells. Thus the taste bud acts like an intermediary between the tastant and the special sensory nerve endings.

The surface of the taste bud cells has membrane receptors. Once the molecules are adsorbed by these receptors, it activates a signaling cascade mediated by proteins like transducin and gustducin. This causes a change in membrane polarization and there is release of transmitted substances and stimulation of the unmyelinated afferent fibers of the glossopharyngeal nerve. This surrounds the lower half of the taste cells. This is the process of taste stimulation.

Taste bud cells and the Merkel cells are the only true specialized sensory cells of the oral mucosa. The taste buds are positive for CK 7, 8, and 19 and sometimes positive for CK 18.

The primary taste sensations like salt, sweet, bitter, and sour are perceived by different regions of the palate and tongue such as sweet at the tip, salt at the lateral borders, bitter in the middle, and sour in the lateral areas of the tongue. Bitter and sour is also perceived on the palate and posterior tongue **(Figure 13-78)**. Bitter and sour sensations are mediated by the glossopharyngeal nerve and sweet and salty by the chorda tympani nerve.

However, some people believe that these taste sensations consist of stimuli that form a spectrum of these sensations making up the taste senses. Taste happens when a chemical substance contacts the taste receptor, which fires the nerve fiber.

Lingual Tonsil

Posterior one-third of the tongue consists of lymphoid follicles, which form the component of the Waldeyer's ring. They are also associated with the foliate papillae and appear as bilateral red, glistening papules and nodules on the posterolateral border of the tongue. These prominences or nodules have a lingual crypt, which is a small pit at the center and is lined by stratified squamous epithelium. The lingual tonsil is composed of 30–100 lymph follicles beneath the epithelium and open onto the surface of the tongue. From the epithelial surface numerous lymphocytes enter these crypts **(Figure 13-79)**.

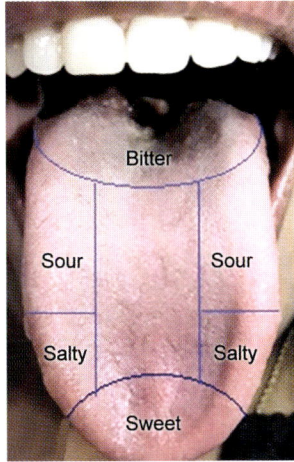

Figure 13-78: Distribution of taste sensation.

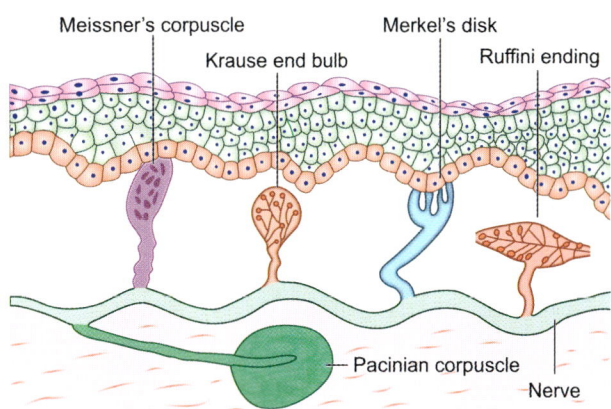

Figure 13-80: Different types of nerve ending of oral mucosa.

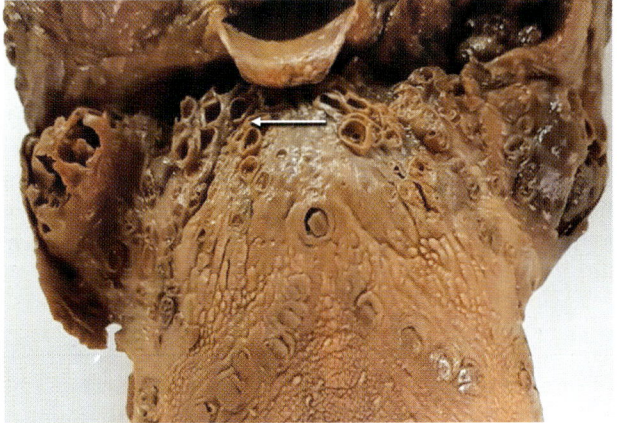

Figure 13-79: Lingual tonsil.

nerve. The sensory fibers lose their myelin sheath and form a subepithelial plexus in the reticular layer.

The sensory fibers end as organized and free nerve endings, where the latter are found in the lamina propria and the epithelium associated with Merkel cells. Apart from these, there are intraepithelial nerve endings too with a sensory function, which run between the keratinocytes and end as simple endings in the middle layers. They are not surrounded by Schwann cells.

The organized nerve endings are found in the papillary region of the lamina propria as groups of coiled fibers surrounded by a connective tissue capsule. These have been grouped as Meissner's or Ruffini corpuscles, Krause's bulbs, and mucocutaneous end organs **(Figure 13-80)**.

Touch, pain, temperature, proprioception, and taste are the various sensations perceived by these specialized nerve endings. However, there is no evidence that states one receptor is capable of detecting one type of stimulus.

The sensory receptors are more dense and developed in the anterior region than the posterior parts of the oral cavity and even denser with prominent connective tissue papillae. For example, touch is most acute in the anterior part of the tongue and hard palate, whereas in the posterior part it is important for swallowing, gagging, and retching.

Temperature is more acute in the anterior regions like the tip of tongue, anterior hard palate, and vermillion border of lip.

Blood Supply

Oral mucosa is richly vascularized. The blood supply is derived from arteries running parallel to the surface in the submucosa. When submucosa is absent these arteries are present in the deeper part of the reticular layer. Smaller branches arise from these vessels, which anastomose with adjacent vessels in the reticular layer forming a network. Capillary loops from this network pass into the connective tissue papillae and come to lie closer to the basal layer of the epithelium. Extensive anastomoses of arterioles and capillaries contribute to the quick healing of the oral mucosal wounds.

In the oral mucosa, the gingiva has the greatest blood flow and in the lips and where the connective tissue undergoes extension and flexibility, the arterioles follow a tortuous course with extensive branching.

Nerve Supply

The nerve supply to the oral mucosa is sensory to initiate and maintain various activities like mastication, swallowing, speaking, salivation, and gagging. The efferent fibers are autonomic (innervate blood vessels and salivary glands) and modulate sensory activity. They arise from the second and the third division of the trigeminal nerve and the afferent fibers arise from the facial, glossopharyngeal, and vagus

> **Points to Remember**
> - The tongue is a muscular organ covered by mucous membrane all around.
> - Ventral surface of the tongue is covered by lining mucosa, which has thin nonkeratinized epithelium and an indistinct submucosa. The mucosa of the ventral surface of the tongue is firmly attached to the intrinsic muscles of the tongue.
> - The dorsal surface of the tongue is divided into anterior two-thirds, and posterior one-third by an indistinct V-shaped groove called the sulcus terminalis.
> - At the center of this sulcus is the foramen cecum, which is the former orifice of the thyroglossal duct.
> - The anterior part of the tongue is supplied by the lingual nerve. The posterior part is supplied by the glossopharyngeal nerve. The anterior two-thirds of the tongue contain papillae and the posterior one-third contains lymphatic nodules or follicles with germinal center.

- Presence of the filiform papillae gives the dorsal surface a velvety appearance. The regions in between these papillae are nonkeratinized supported by secondary branch of connective tissue core coming out from the central core of the filiform papilla.
- Fungiform papillae are elevated, mushroom-shaped, and present between the filiform papillae, on the anterior part of the dorsal portion of the tongue. They are mostly present at the tip of the tongue. The epithelium is thin and nonkeratinized with a highly vascular lamina propria and hence these papillae appear red in color.
- Foliate papillae are leaf-like papillae or vertical and parallel ridges present on the lateral border of posterior part of the tongue and are rarely distinct in humans compared to other mammals. They may contain von Ebner glands and lymphoid follicles.
- Circumvallate papillae are largest, round papillae present adjacent or anterior to the sulcus terminalis. They have deep grooves or valley-like depression around them into which the minor serous salivary glands called the von Ebner glands open their ducts. The epithelium is keratinized on its superior surface with a connective tissue core. Taste buds are present along the lateral wall and they perceive the bitter taste. There are around 250 taste buds in the circumvallate papilla.
- Taste buds are ovoid/barrel shaped, chemoreceptive intraepithelial organs with a rich plexus of nerves below them. They are mainly present around the walls of the circumvallate papillae, surface of the filiform papillae, lateral walls of the foliate papillae, soft palate, and epiglottis in small numbers.
- Posterior one-third of the tongue consists of numerous mucous glands and lymphoid follicles, which form the component of the Waldeyer's ring. These prominences or nodules have a lingual crypt and the lymphoid follicles open onto the surface of the tongue.

The circumvallate and foliate papillae appear around 7 weeks of gestation followed by the fungiform papillae. Later the filiform papillae develop at about 10 weeks. Evidence of stratification of the masticatory and the lining mucosa is seen around 10–12 weeks.

The areas that will become the future keratinized areas show darkly stained columnar cells with a prominent basal lamina and an adjacent connective tissue, whereas the lining mucosa shows cuboidal cells with a flat epithelial-connective tissue interface. Keratohyalin granules appear around 13–20 weeks making it easy to differentiate prickle cell and granular cell layer. At the same time, melanocytes and Langerhans cells also appear. Until the tooth erupts into the oral cavity, orthokeratinization of the masticatory mucosa does not occur.

The underlying ectomesenchyme shows spaced stellate cells, and the extracellular matrix is amorphous. By 6 weeks, reticular fibers appear. Collagen fibers and capillaries can be detected by 8–12 weeks, and as the number of fibers increases, they form bundles and those adjacent to the epithelium are perpendicular to the basal lamina. Around 17–20 weeks, elastic fibers become prominent.

Cells of the taste bud develop from the epithelium of the tongue and it starts at 7–11th week of intrauterine life. There is an inductive link between the gustatory nerve fibers and the development of taste buds. A fully formed taste bud can be recognized between 15th and 20th week of intrauterine life.

DEVELOPMENT OF THE ORAL MUCOSA

After the rupture of the buccopharyngeal membrane, the primitive oral cavity continues with the foregut and the boundary between these two becomes indistinct. Epithelium covering the palate, cheeks, and gingiva is derived from the ectoderm and the epithelium of the tongue, epiglottis, and pharynx from endoderm **(Figure 13-81)**.

At around 5–6 weeks of gestation, single layered lining of the primitive oral cavity becomes five to six cell layers thick. Around 7–8 weeks, a thickening arises at the region of future vestibular lamina. Around 10–14 weeks, the cells at the center of this thickening undergo degeneration and form the oral vestibule. At the same time around 8–11 weeks, the palatine shelves elevate and fuse with each other resulting in the establishment of a rough morphology of the future oral cavity.

AGE CHANGES

As age advances, the oral mucosa becomes thin and atrophic, friable, and drier. This could be the result of physiological process or effects of systemic diseases or medications. The epithelium becomes thinner and the epithelial-connective tissue interface is flat. In the tongue, papillae become less in number and the reduction in the filiform papillae makes the fungiform papillae more prominent and the dorsal surface appears glossy. There is reduction in cell-mediated immunity due to decrease in Langerhans cells. Varicose veins become prominent on the ventral surface of the tongue and it is called caviar tongue and these are commonly seen in patients with varicose veins.

The connective tissue shows more collagen content with decreased cellularity. Sebaceous glands are more prominent

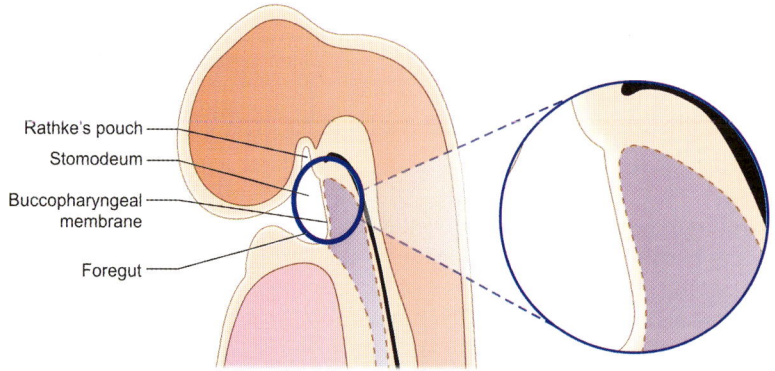

Figure 13-81: Buccopharyngeal membrane.

with age and minor salivary glands show fibrous changes and reduction in salivary secretion.

Changes in the nerve function include progressive loss of general sensation and taste perception. Burning sensation, dysgeusia, and dryness of the mouth are seen in postmenopausal women and elderly patients.

CLINICAL CONSIDERATIONS

Numerous disease processes involving the oral mucosa, ranging from developmental disturbances to malignancies can occur.

There is a saying that—"Mouth is the mirror of the body". Systemic disorders may have or proceeded by oral manifestations. These manifestations may be in the form of discolorations, thinning of epithelium (erosion), discontinuity of the epithelium (ulcers) or pain or burning sensation of the mouth. Drugs used for the treatment of certain systemic diseases can affect the oral health.

Oral cavity harbors a number of microorganisms. Any breach in the oral epithelium or imbalance in the oral microbial flora can cause infections. For example, candida is a normal commensal fungus in a healthy mouth. When intake of antibiotics suppresses the oral bacteria, this fungus will overgrow and cause oral candidiasis.

Fordyce spots are heterotopic collections of sebaceous glands in any mucosal surfaces including oral mucosa. In the oral cavity, they appear as elevated yellowish spots; occur singly or in groups, measuring about few millimeters in diameter. They are more common in buccal mucosa but may also occur in the inner aspect of the lips, retromolar region **(Figure 13-82)**. They are thought to arise from inclusion in the oral cavity of ectoderm having potentialities of the skin during the formation of maxillary and mandibular process. Occurrence of sebaceous glands is considered as normal variation of oral mucosa.

White sponge nevus is a white lesion that can present as thick, white plaques on the nonkeratinized areas. This is due to the mutation of CK 13 and/or CK 4. The epithelium is thick with parakeratinization and vacuoles in the suprabasal layers.

Pigmented cellular nevi are hamartomas in which proliferations of nevus cells occur either in the epithelium or connective tissue. This may manifest at birth or later in life. It may be seen in skin as well as in any mucosal surfaces. Oral nevi are common in hard palate, buccal mucosa, and labial mucosa. Clinically they appear as brown to dark brown or black pigmented spots of few millimeters in diameter. They may be flat or elevated but asymptomatic.

Oral melanotic macule is flat pigmented lesion caused by the accumulation of melanin pigmentation. This is more common in females. The frequent sites of involvement include lower lip, buccal mucosa, gingiva, and hard palate **(Figure 13-83)**.

Oral pigmentations may occur in smokers (smoker's melanosis), many systemic conditions, and intake of certain drugs.

Malignant melanoma is a malignant tumor arising from melanocytes.

Benign migratory glossitis, otherwise known as wandering rash of the tongue, is characterized by irregular areas of redness due to depapillation of the filiform papillae, bordered by grayish white line occurring in the dorsal surface of the tongue **(Figure 13-84)**. It remains in one area for some time, then disappear only to reappear in another area. This condition

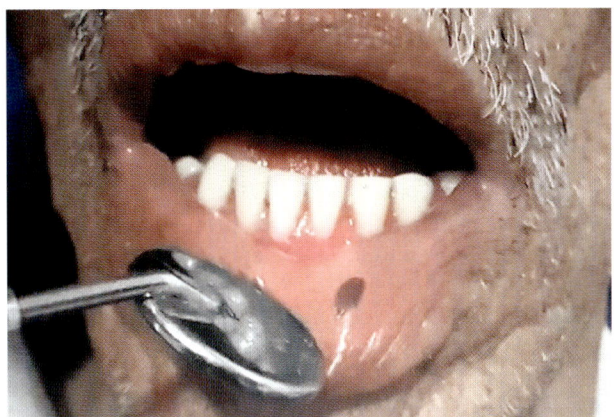

Figure 13-83: Melanotic macule in the lip.
Source: Dr S Rohini, GRM Dental Clinic, Ambattur, Chennai, Tamil Nadu, India.

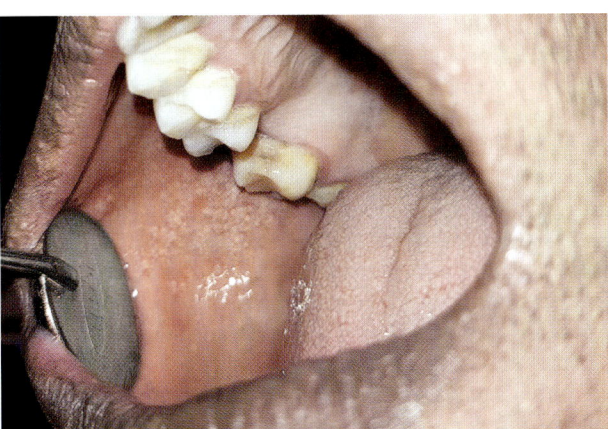

Figure 13-82: Fordyce spots on buccal mucosa.
Source: Dr Raguganesh, Meenakshi Ammal Dental College, Chennai, Tamil Nadu, India.

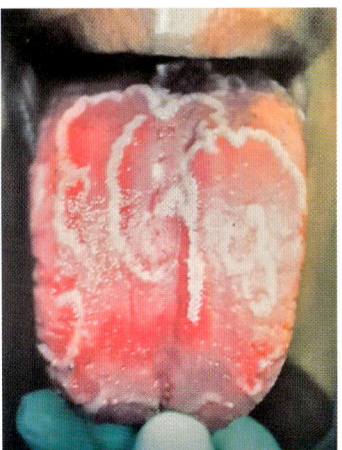

Figure 13-84: Benign migratory glossitis.
Source: Dr Spencer Lilly, Chennai, Tamil Nadu, India.

is asymptomatic but patients may sometimes complain of burning tongue; most commonly seen in adults.

Hairy tongue is characterized by hypertrophy of filiform papillae. This condition is also called as black hairy tongue, as use of tobacco, coffee, and tea causes discoloration and gives hair-like appearance to the elongated filiform papillae **(Figure 13-85)**.

Lingual thyroid is a developmental anomaly seen on the dorsal surface of the tongue at the site of foramen cecum, as a midline swelling and is due to the thyroid tissue that has failed to migrate to their functional position.

Loss of moistness of the oral mucosa due to insufficient saliva results in dry mouth known as xerostomia. This condition is characterized by soreness, burning sensation, and pain in oral mucosa. The oral mucosa appears pale, translucent, dry, atrophic or inflamed. Fissuring and cracking may be seen in severe cases. Tongue appears shiny due to atrophy of the papillae.

Recurrent mechanical trauma such as those caused by sharp tooth or sharp portion of a restoration causes localized retention of keratin layer as a protective measure and is known as traumatic keratosis. Removal of the etiological factor results in disappearance of the lesion.

Leukoplakia is a nonscrapable white patch of the oral mucosa caused by chronic tobacco usage. The whiteness is due to the retention of keratin **(Figure 13-86)**. This lesion is considered as potentially malignant, since there may be dysplasia in the epithelium. More common in males and buccal commissure is the most common site of involvement.

Oral submucous fibrosis is another potentially malignant condition caused by chronic betel nut use. This condition is characterized by atrophy of the epithelium and fibrosis of the subjacent connective tissue that leads to restricted mouth opening and limitation of tongue movements. Clinically the oral mucosa appears pale and blanched due to the atrophic epithelium, fibrosis of the underlying connective tissue, and obliteration of blood vessels **(Figure 13-87)**. Palpable fibrous bands are present in the involved areas.

Squamous cell carcinoma is the most common of all oral cancers and is a malignant neoplasm arising from the

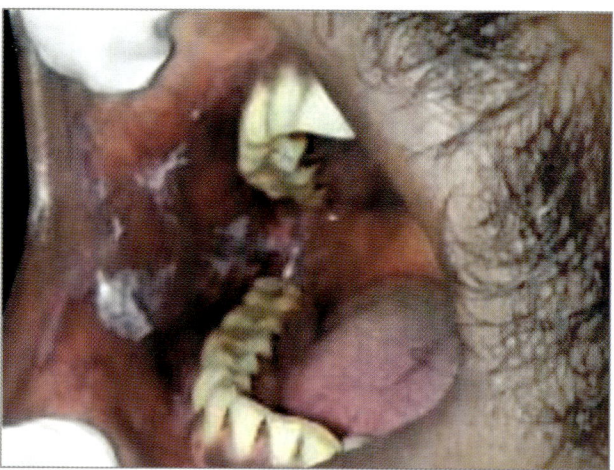

Figure 13-86: Leukoplakia of buccal mucosa.

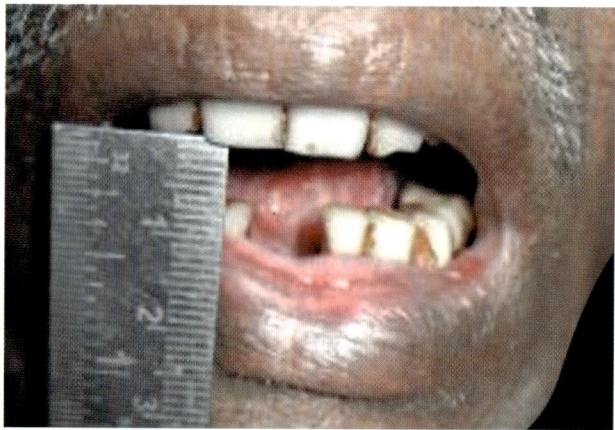

Figure 13-87: Oral submucous fibrosis. Blanched lips and restricted mouth opening mucosa.
Source: Shafer's Textbook of Oral Pathology, 8th ed. Elsevier India.

epithelium. It is more common in males than in females and often associated with chronic tobacco use. It may present itself clinically as chronic nonhealing ulcer, exophytic mass or verrucous growth **(Figure 13-88)**.

Periodontal pockets occur as a result of plaque accumulation and subsequent alveolar bone loss and apical migration of epithelial attachment. This is a characteristic feature of chronic periodontitis **(Figure 13-89)**.

Autoantibodies targeted against the desmosomes may result in a skin disease associated with oral mucosal lesions called pemphigus. There is a suprabasal split evident histologically. When the autoantibodies are targeted against BP 180 and 230, they weaken the bond between the epithelium and connective tissue. This results in a subepithelial split and these lesions present as blisters and ulcers clinically.

Mutation of genes encoding for cytokeratin may cause various skin lesions like epidermolysis bullosa where the mutation affects CK 5 and CK 14. Various genes like *p53*, *p16*, *p21*, and *bcl-2* when altered may result in oral cancer.

Epithelial cells which are exfoliated, scrapped or abraded can be studied microscopically after smearing on a glass slide and staining. This procedure is known as exfoliative cytology. This is used in cancer detection and follow-up.

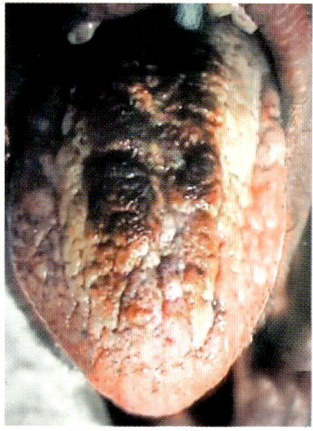

Figure 13-85: Black hairy tongue.
Source: Dr S Rohini, GRM Dental Clinic, Chennai, Tamil Nadu, India.

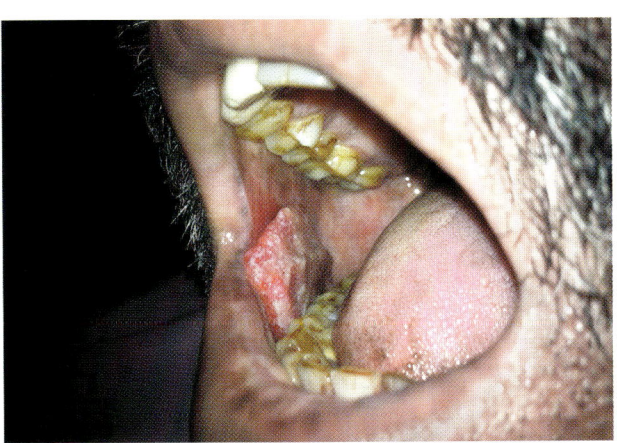

Figure 13-88: Squamous cell carcinoma of right buccal mucosa.
Source: Dr H Srinivasan, Sparks Dental Center, Chennai, Tamil Nadu, India.

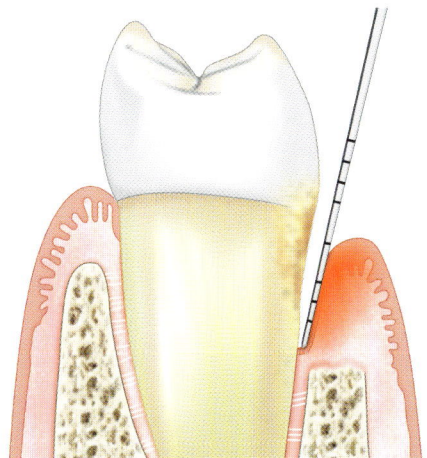

Figure 13-89: Periodontal pocket.

PRACTICE QUESTIONS

1. Write notes on the functions of oral mucosa.
2. Write in detail about the types of oral mucosa.
3. Write notes on non-keratinocytes.
4. Write notes on desmosome and hemidesmosome.
5. Write in detail about the lamina propria and submucosa of the lining mucosa.
6. Write notes on the architecture of the gingiva.
7. Write notes on junctional epithelium.
8. Write in detail about the papillae of the tongue.
9. Write notes on taste buds.
10. Write notes on lingual tonsil.
11. Write notes on age changes in oral mucosa.

MULTIPLE CHOICE QUESTIONS

1. **Masticatory mucosa develops from:**
   a. Ectomesenchyme
   b. Ectoderm
   c. Endoderm
   d. Mesoderm
2. **Function of the oral mucosa does not include:**
   a. Protection
   b. Sensory
   c. Mineralization of the alveolar bone
   d. Secretion
3. **Which part of the oral cavity appears yellowish due to the presence of fat:**
   a. Gingiva
   b. Floor of the mouth
   c. Anterolateral part of the hard palate and lateral part of the soft palate
   d. Inner aspect of the lip
4. **Which part of the oral mucosa immobile and tightly bound to the bone?**
   a. Alveolar mucosa
   b. Gingiva
   c. Floor of the mouth
   d. Lining mucosa
5. **Minor gland are seen in:**
   a. Lamina propria
   b. Epithelium
   c. Submucosa
   d. Papillary portion of the connective tissue
6. **Type of epithelial covering of the oral mucosa is:**
   a. Simple epithelium
   b. Stratified squamous
   c. Pseudostratified ciliated columnar
   d. Stratifies columnar
7. **Specialised mucosa is seen in:**
   a. Hard palate
   b. Soft palate
   c. Gingiva
   d. Tongue
8. **Minor salivary glands are not seen in:**
   a. Soft palate
   b. Gingiva
   c. Buccal mucosa
   d. Circumvallate papilla

9. Suppleness of the oral mucosa is depends on the following, *except:*
   a. Nature of the connective tissue
   b. Its solid (epithelium and the fibrous tissue) and fluid components (blood and interstitial fluid)
   c. The glandular component
   d. The structure to which it is attached
10. Color of the mucosa depends on the following, *except* the:
    a. Thickness of the epithelium
    b. Degree of keratinization
    c. Vascularity of the underlying connective tissue
    d. Presence of taste buds
11. Fordyce spots are:
    a. Minor serous present in the buccal mucosa
    b. Sweat glands present in the buccal mucosa
    c. Dark black spots present in the buccal mucosa
    d. Sebaceous glands present in the buccal mucosa
12. Stippling of the surface is seen in:
    a. Attached gingiva
    b. Interdental gingiva
    c. Free gingiva
    d. Mucogingival line
13. Frenum is:
    a. A thin band or fold of mucosa with enclosed muscle fibers
    b. Other name for ligament
    c. Seen in soft palate
    d. Made up of smooth muscle fibers
14. Masticatory mucosa is seen in:
    a. Gingiva and hard palate
    b. Ventral surface of the tongue
    c. Soft palate
    d. Floor of the mouth
15. Mucosa of the tongue is called specialized mucosa since it contains:
    a. Papilla
    b. Taste buds
    c. Intrinsic muscles
    d. Helps in mastication and speech
16. A distinct submucosa is not seen in:
    a. Tongue
    b. Buccal mucosa
    c. Gingiva and hard palate
    d. Soft palate
17. Mucoperiosteum:
    a. Contains muscles
    b. Characterized by the attachment of mucosa directly to the bone
    c. Contains glands
    d. Is seen in floor of the mouth
18. Keratinization in which there is absence of nuclei and nuclear remnants is called:
    a. Parakeratinization
    b. Orthokeratinization
    c. Partial keratinization
    d. None of the above
19. The membrane coating granules present in the granular layer are called:
    a. Odland bodies
    b. Zymogen granules
    c. Cytoplasmic inclusions
    d. Eosinophilic granules
20. Layers of keratinized epithelium do not include:
    a. Stratum basale
    b. Stratum Spinosum
    c. Stratum granulosum
    d. Stratum intermedium
21. Keratinized squames are seen in:
    a. Stratum corneum
    b. Stratum spinosum
    c. Stratum basale
    d. Stratum granulosum
22. Which of the following is not a nonkeratinocyte?
    a. Merkel cell
    b. Langerhans cell
    c. Melanocyte
    d. Langhans cell
23. Pigment producing cell in the oral mucous membrane is
    a. Hematocyte
    b. Melanocyte
    c. Langerhans cell
    d. Histiocyte
24. The processes by which melanocyte communicates with keratinocytes are called:
    a. Tomes process
    b. Dendritic process
    c. Odontoblastic process
    d. None of the above
25. Lamina lucida and lamina densa are the electron microscopic components of:
    a. Connective tissue
    b. Stratum corneum
    c. Basement membrane
    d. Submucosa
26. Hemidesmosomes are seen in between:
    a. The adjacent epithelial cells
    b. Basement membrane and the basal cells of the oral epithelium
    c. The cell of the granular layer
    d. Keratinocytes and nonkeratinocytes
27. Intercellular bridges is the other name for:
    a. Desmosomes
    b. Hemidesmosomes
    c. Basal lamina
    d. Gap junctions
28. Principal cell population present in the lamina propria are:
    a. Inflammatory cells
    b. Endothelial cells
    c. Fibroblasts
    d. Histiocytes
29. Ground substance is mainly composed of:
    a. Glycoproteins and proteoglycans
    b. Elastic and oxytalan fibers
    c. Collagen fibers
    d. None of the above

30. The time taken for the cell to divide, mature and pass through the entire epithelium is called:
    a. Shedding time
    b. Maturation time
    c. Turnover time
    d. Exfoliation time
31. Which of the following does not contain masticatory mucosa?
    a. Hard palate
    b. Ventral surface of tongue
    c. Gingiva
    d. None of the above
32. The interdental papilla in the posterior teeth below the contact area is called as:
    a. Junctional epithelium
    b. Reduced enamel epithelium
    c. Col
    d. Sulcular epithelium
33. Major intracytoplasmic protein present in the epithelial cell is:
    a. Laminin
    b. Elastin
    c. Cytokeratin
    d. None of the above
34. As age advances, the oral mucosa becomes:
    a. Atrophic
    b. Friable
    c. Drier
    d. All of the above
35. Attached gingiva is separated from the alveolar mucosa by:
    a. Mucogingival junction
    b. Free gingival margin
    c. Sulcular epithelium
    d. None of the above
36. The structure that is present between the skin and labial mucosa is called:
    a. Dark zone
    b. Vermilion zone
    c. Vestibule
    d. Commissure
37. Dentogingival fibers:
    a. Extend from cervical cementum to the lamina propria of gingiva
    b. Encircle the tooth
    c. Extend horizontally above the alveolar crest and get inserted into the root of adjacent teeth
    d. Pass from cementum of one tooth to the marginal gingiva of adjacent teeth
38. Conical projection seen on the midline of soft palate is called:
    a. Midpalatine raphe
    b. Rugae
    c. Palatine tonsil
    d. Uvula
39. The depth of the gingival sulcus ranges from:
    a. 1–3 mm
    b. 0.5–2 mm
    c. 2–4 mm
    d. 1.5–2.5 mm
40. Which one of the following papilla is non-keratinized:
    a. Filiform papilla
    b. Fungiform papilla
    c. Circumvallate papilla
    d. Incisive papilla

ANSWERS

1. b	2. c	3. c	4. b	5. c	6. b	7. d	8. b	9. c	10. d	11. d	12. a	13. a	14. a	15. b
16. c	17. b	18. b	19. a	20. d	21. a	22. d	23. b	24. b	25. c	26. b	27. a	28. c	29. a	30. c
31. b	32. c	33. c	34. d	35. a	36. b	37. a	38. d	39. b	40. b					

BIBLIOGRAPHY

1. Alfano MC. The origin of gingival fluid. J Theor Biol. 1974;47:127-36.
2. Avery JK, Chiego DJ. Essentials of Oral Histology and Embryology: A Clinical Approach, 3rd edition. US: Mosby; 2006.
3. Avery JK. Oral Development and Histology, 3rd edition. New York: Thieme; 2002.
4. Bancroft JD, Gamble M (Eds). Bancroft's: Theory and Practice of Histological Techniques, 5th edition. New York: Churchill Livingston; 2002.
5. Barrandon Y, Green H. Three clonal types of keratinocyte with different capacities for multiplication. Proc Natl Acad Sci USA. 1987;84:2302-6.
6. Barros SP, Williams R, Offenbacher S, et al. Gingival crevicular as a source of biomarkers for periodontitis. Periodontol 2000. 2016;70(1):53-64.
7. Bauer WH. Histogenesis of the so-called secondary enamel cuticle and dental cuticle. Am J Orthod Oral Surg. 1943;29(11):B626-34.
8. Berkovitz BKB, Holland GR, Moxham BJ. Oral Anatomy, Histology and Embryology, 4th edition. US: Elsevier; 2009.
9. Borradori L, Sonnenberg A. Structure and function of hemidesmosomes more than simple adhesion complexes. J Invest Dermatol. 1999;112:411-8.
10. Bosshardt DD, Lang NP. The junctional epithelium: from health to disease. J Dent Res. 2005;84(1):9-20.
11. Bragulla HH, Homberger DG. Structure and functions of keratin proteins in simple, stratified, keratinized and cornified epithelia. J Anat. 2009;214(4):516-59.
12. Carter WG, Ryan MC, Gahr PJ. Epiligrin, a new cell adhesion ligand for integrin a3b1 in epithelial basement membranes. Cell. 1991;65:599-610.
13. Chandra S, Chandra S, Chandra M, et al. Textbook of Dental and Oral Histology with Embryology and MCQ's, 2nd edition. New Delhi: Jaypee Brothers Medical Publishers (P) Ltd; 2010.
14. Chatterjee K. Essentials of dental anatomy and oral histology, 2nd edition. New Delhi: Jaypee Brothers Medical Publishers (P) Ltd; 2014.
15. Chen J, Ahmad R, Li W, et al. Biomechanics of oral mucosa. J R Soc Interface. 2015;12:20150325.
16. Çiçek Y, Ertaş U. The normal and pathological pigmentation of oral mucous membrane: a review. J Contemp Dent Pract. 2003;4(3):76-86.

17. Corso, Eversole, and Hut-Fletcher, Hairy leukoplakia: Epstein-Barr virus receptors on oral keratinocyte plasma membranes, ORAL. SURG ORAL MED ORAL PATHOL 1989;67:416-21
18. Cruchley AT, Williams DM. Langerhans cell density in normal human oral mucosa and skin: relationship to age, smoking and alcohol consumption. J Oral Pathol Med. 1994;23(2):55-9.
19. Culling CFA. Handbook of Histopathological and Histochemical Techniques, 3rd edition. UK: Butterworth-Heinemann; 1974.
20. Cutler CW, Jotwani R. Dendritic cells at the oral mucosal interface. J Dent Res. 2006;85(8):678-89.
21. Dickhuth J, Koerdt S, Kriegebaum U, et al. In vitro study on proliferation kinetics of oral mucosal keratinocytes. Oral Surg Oral Med Oral Pathol Oral Radiol. 2015;120(4):429-35.
22. Egelberg J. Permeability of the dentogingival blood vessels. J Periodontal Res. 1966;1:180-91.
23. Eppley BL, Delfino JJ. Bilateral nasopalatine ducts of the premaxilla. J Maxillofac Surg. 1988;17:360-2.
24. Garlick JA, Parks WC, Welgus HG, et al. Reepithelialization of human oral keratinocytes in vitro. J Dent Res. 1996;75:912-8.
25. Gaunt WA, Osborn JW, Ten Cate AR. Advanced dental histology, 2nd edition. Bristol: John Wright & Sons Ltd; 1971.
26. Haschek W, Bolon B, Rousseaux C, et al. Fundamentals of toxicologic pathology, 3rd edition. Texas: Gulf Professional Publishing; 2017.
27. Herzberg AJ, Raso DS, Silverman JF. Color Atlas of Normal Cytology, 1st edition. USA: Churchill Livingstone; 1999.
28. Hill MW. Epithelial proliferation and turnover in oral epithelium and epidermis with age. In: Squier CA, Hill MW (Eds). The Effect of Aging in Oral Mucosa and Skin. USA: CRC Press; 1994. pp. 75-83.
29. Hirobe T. Keratinocytes regulate the function of melanocytes. Dermatologica Sinica. 2014;32:200-4.
30. Izumi K, Tobita T, Feinberg SE. Isolation of human oral keratinocytes progenitor/stem cells. J Dent Res. 2007;86:341-6.
31. Jones PH. Isolation and characterization of human epidermal stem cells. Clin Sci. 1996;91:141-6.
32. Kakodkar PV, Patel TN, Patel SV, et al. Clinical assessment of diverse frenum morphology in permanent dentition. Internet J Dent Sci. 2009;7:2.
33. Kang MK, Mehrazarin S, No-Hee P. Oral mucosal stem cells: identification, characterization, and clinical and disease implications. Stem Cell Biology and Tissue Engineering in Dental Sciences. US: Elsevier; 2015.
34. Khurshid Z, Mali M, Naseem M, et al. Human gingival crevicular fluids (GCF) proteomics: an overview. Dent J. 2017;5:12.
35. Kumar GS. Orban's Oral Histology and Embryology, 14th edition. India: Elsevier; 2015.
36. Lin JY, Fisher DE. Melanocyte biology and skin pigmentation. Nature. 2007;445 (7130):843-50.
37. Marinkovich MP, Lunstrum GP, Burgeson RE. The anchoring filament protein kalinin is synthesized and secreted as a high molecular weight protein precursor. J Biol Chem. 1992;267:17900-6.
38. Mattson L, Theilade J, Attström R. Electron microscopic study of junctional and oral gingival epithelia in the juvenile and adult beagle dog. J Clin Periodont. 1979;6:425.
39. Mintz SM, Siegel MA, Seider PJ, et al. An overview of oral frena and their association with multiple syndromic and nonsyndromic conditions. Oral Surg Oral Med Oral Pathol Oral Radiol Endod. 2005;99:321-4.
40. Moharamzadeh K, Brook IM, Van Noort R, et al. Tissue-engineered oral mucosa: a review of the scientific literature. J Dent Res. 2007;86(2):115-24.
41. Nanci A. Ten Cate's Oral Histology, 8th Edition. India: Elsevier; 2012.
42. Nanci A. Ten Cate's Oral Histology, 9th edition. US: Elsevier; 2018.
43. Ngo LH, Darby IB, Veith PD, et al. Mass spectrometric analysis of gingival crevicular fluid biomarkers can predict periodontal disease progression. J Periodontal Res. 2013;48:331-41.
44. Odell EW, Morgan PR. Biopsy Pathology of the Oral Tissues, 1st edition. UK: Chapman & Hall; 1998.
45. Park JY, Chung HS, Choi Y, et al. Phenotype and tissue residency of lymphocytes in the murine oral mucosa. Front Immunol. 2017;8:250.
46. Pocket Dentistry. (2015). Oral epithelium. Available from https://pocketdentistry.com/3-oral-epithelium/ [Accessed June 2018].
47. Pocket Dentistry. (2015). Oral mucosa. Available from https:// pocketdentistry.com/9-oral-mucosa/ [Accessed June 2018].
48. Presland RB, Dale BA. Epithelial structural proteins of the skin and oral cavity-function in health and disease. Crit Rev Oral Biol Med. 2000;11:383.
49. Provenza DV, Seibel W. Oral Histology: inheritance and development, 2nd edition. USA: Lea & Febiger; 1986.
50. Rajkumar K, Ramya R. Textbook of Oral Anatomy, Histology, Physiology and Tooth Morphology, 2nd edition. India: Wolters Kluwer Health; 2017.
51. Rathbone MJ, Hadgraft J. Absorption of drugs from the human oral cavity. Int J Pharmaceutics. 1991;74:9-24.
52. Renshaw AA. Aspiration Cytology: A Pattern Recognition Approach, 1st edition. China: Elsevier; 2005.
53. Russo FB, Pignatari GC, Fernandes IR, et al. Epithelial cells from oral mucosa: how to cultivate them? Cytotechnology. 2016;68(5):2105-14.
54. Schroeder HE, Listgarten M. Fine structure of the developing epithelial attachment of human teeth. Monogr Dev Biol. 1971;2:1-134.
55. Schroeder HE. Differentiation of human oral stratified epithelia. Basel, Switzerland: Karger; 1981.
56. Shannon DB, McKeown ST, Lundy FT, et al. Phenotypic differences between oral and skin fibroblasts in wound contraction and growth factor expression. Wound Repair Regen. 2006;14:172-8.
57. Shimura Y, Nakamura A, Michi K. Palatal opening of the nasopalatine duct. A case report. Int J Oral Maxillofac Surg. 1993;22:142-3.
58. Siqueira WL, Custodio W, McDonald EE. New insights into the composition and functions of the acquired enamel pellicle. J Dent Res. 2012;91(12):1110-8.
59. Skalli O, Jones JCR, Gagescu R, et al. IFAP 300 is common to desmosomes and hemidesmosomes and is a possible linker of intermediate filaments to these junctions. J Cell Biol. 1994;125:159-70.
60. Slack JM. Stem cells in epithelial tissues. Science. 2000;287:1431-3.
61. Squier C, Brogden K. Human Oral Mucosa, Development, Structure and Function. Oxford: Wiley-Blackwell; 2011.

62. Squier C, Brogden K. Human Oral Mucosa: Development, Structure, and Function, 1st edition. US: John Wiley & Sons, Inc; 2011.
63. Squier CA, Kremer MJ. Biology of Oral Mucosa and Oesophagus. J Natl Cancer Inst Monogr. 2001;29:7-15.
64. Stern IB. Current concepts of the dentogingival junction: the epithelial and connective tissue attachments to the tooth. J Periodontol. 1981;52(9):465-76.
65. Szpaderska AM, Zuckerman JD, Di Pietro LA. Differential injury responses in oral mucosal and cutaneous wounds. J Dent Res. 2003;82:621.
66. Taylor JJ, Preshaw PM. Gingival crevicular fluid and saliva. Periodontol 2000. 2016;70:7-10.
67. Ten Cate AR, Déporter D. The role of the fibroblast in collagen turnover in the functioning of the periodontal ligament of the mouse. Arch Oral Biol. 1974;19:399.
68. Ten Cate AR. Morphological studies of the fibrocytes in connective tissue undergoing rapid remodeling. J Anat. 1972;112:401.
69. Tenchini ML, Ranzati C, Malcovati M. Culture techniques for human keratinocytes. Burns. 1992;18:S11-6.
70. Thier K, Petermann P, Rahn E, et al. Mechanical barriers restrict invasion of herpes simplex virus 1 into human oral mucosa. J Virol. 2017;91(22):e01295-17.
71. Thosar N, Murak P, Baliga S, et al. Assessment of maxillary labial frenum morphology in primary, mixed and permanent dentitions in Wardha district. Eur J Gen Dent. 2017;6:14-7.
72. Tsai MT, Chen Y:D, Lee CY, et al. Noninvasive structural and microvascular anatomy of oral mucosae using handheld optical coherence tomography. Biomed Opt Express. 2017;8(11):5001-12.
73. Vijayashree RJ, Sivapathasundharam B. The diverse role of oral fibroblasts in normal and disease. J Oral Maxillofac Pathol. 2022;26:6-13.
74. Vitkov L, Hannig M, Nekrashevych Y, et al. Supramolecular pellicle precursors. Eur J Oral Sci. 2004;112:320-5.
75. Vitorino R, Calheiros-Lobo MJ, Williams J, et al. Peptidomic analysis of human acquired enamel pellicle. Biomed Chromatogr. 2007;21:1107-17.
76. *Xu H, Zhong L, Deng J, PenJ, Dan H, Zeng X, LiT, Chen Q.* High Expression of ACE2 Receptor of 2019-nCoV on the Epithelial Cells of Oral Mucosa. *Int J Oral Sci 2020;12(1):8.*
77. Zhou J, Rogers JH, Lee SH, et al. Oral mucosa harbors a high frequency of endothelial cells: a novel postnatal cell source for angiogenic regeneration. Stem Cells Dev. 2017;26(2):91-101.
78. Zumi K, Terashi H, Marcelo CL, et al. Development and characterization of a tissue-engineered human oral mucosa equivalent produced in a serum-free culture system. J Dent Res. 2000;79:798-805.

CHAPTER

Salivary Glands

Pratibha Ramani, Einstein T Bertin, B Sivapathasundharam

Chapter Outline

- Glands 216
- Classification of Glands 216
  - Number of Cells Involved 217
  - Ductal Morphology and Branching 217
  - Mode of Discharge 217
  - Mechanism of Secretion 217
  - Type of Secretions 219
- Salivary Glands 219
- Classification of Salivary Glands 220
  - Major Salivary Glands 220
  - Minor Salivary Glands 220
  - Type of Secretions 220
- Development of Salivary Gland 220
  - Stages in the Development of Salivary Gland 221
  - Branching of the Epithelial Cord 224
  - Role of Extracellular Matrix 224
- Histology of Salivary Glands 224
  - Histology of the Secretory Units 224
- Myoepithelial Cells (Basket Cells) 226
  - Structure 227
  - Function 227
  - Identification of Myoepithelial Cells 228
- Other Cells 229
- Ductal System 229
  - Intercalated Ducts 229
  - Striated Ducts 230
  - Excretory Ducts 230
- Connective Tissue Component of the Gland 231
- Formation and Secretion of Saliva 231
- Ductal Modification of Saliva 232
- Composition of Saliva 232
- Properties of Saliva 233
- Functions of Saliva 233
  - Protection 233
  - Growth Factors 233
  - Antimicrobial Property 234
  - Wound Healing 234
  - Mastication and Deglutition 234
  - Digestion 234
  - Taste and Smell Perception 234
  - Speech 234
  - Excretion 234
- Major Salivary Glands 234
  - Parotid Gland 234
  - Submandibular Gland 235
  - Sublingual Gland 236
- Minor Salivary Glands 236
- Tubarial Glands—The New Salivary Gland Organs? 237
- Clinical Considerations 237

GLANDS

Glands are defined as modified epithelial structures that are specialized to produce, release and transport macromolecules, ions, water into its surrounding environment, to carry out useful body functions, *e.g.*, thyroid gland, salivary glands, etc. The secretory products are synthesized and stored inside the cell as secretory granules and are subsequently released by various mechanisms.

The glandular epithelial cells are usually arranged into secretory units and the associated ductal system, together referred to as the parenchyma. The epithelial component is supported by the connective tissue stroma that penetrates the glands and divides it into lobes and lobules.

CLASSIFICATION OF GLANDS

Though glands share a similar basic architecture and secretory function, they differ from one another in various aspects. Glands can be thus classified based on the following features:
a. Number of cells involved
b. Ductal morphology and branching
c. Mode of discharge
d. Mechanism of secretion
e. Type of secretion.

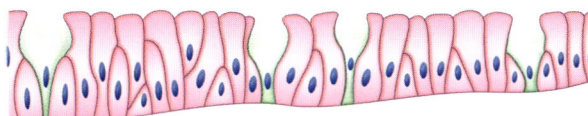

Figure 14-1: Unicellular secreting goblet cells.

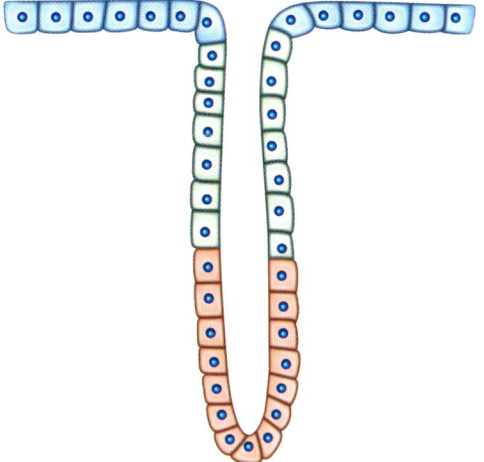

Figure 14-2: Multicellular—salivary glands.

Number of Cells Involved

According to the number of secretory units, they are typed into following:

Unicellular: Mucus-secreting goblet cells are the only example of single-celled glands in humans. These goblet cells secrete mucus and are easily visualized in histological sections of the small intestine **(Figure 14-1)**.

Multicellular: These glands have numerous secretory cells **(Figure 14-2)**, e.g., submandibular gland.

Ductal Morphology and Branching

According to the ductal morphology and branching of ducts, glands are typed as follows **(Figures 14-3A to C)**:
a. Ducts can be *simple* (unbranched) or *compound* (with two or more branches)
b. Secretory portions can be *tubular* (either short or long and coiled) or *acinar* (round or globular)
c. Either type of secretory portion may be branched. Compound glands can have *tubular*, *acinar*, or *tubuloacinar* secretory portions.

Mode of Discharge

According to the mode of discharge of secretions, glands are typed into exocrine, endocrine, paracrine, and autocrine.

Exocrine glands

They are also called ducted glands, these glands maintain contact with the surface through a tube called duct and their secretions are discharged onto the surface through the duct **(Figure 14-4)**, *e.g.*, salivary glands.

Endocrine Glands

These glands do not have a ductal system; instead their products are directly secreted into the blood and are carried by the blood and tissue fluid to the target area **(Figure 14-5)**, *e.g.*, thyroid gland.

Paracrine Glands

These glands secrete products that influence the secretion of another product by a local gland or cell (products act on neighboring cells).

Autocrine Glands or Cells

These glands secrete products that influence the secretion of another product by the same cell (products act on the same cell, which produce them).

Mechanism of Secretion

According to the mechanism of secretion, glands are classified into merocrine, holocrine, and apocrine glands.

Merocrine Glands (Figure 14-6)

The term merocrine is derived from the Greek words "meros", meaning part, and "krinos", meaning to separate. Glandular cells that secrete products via the merocrine method, form membrane-bound secretory vesicles internal to the cell. These vesicles move to the apical surface and coalesce with

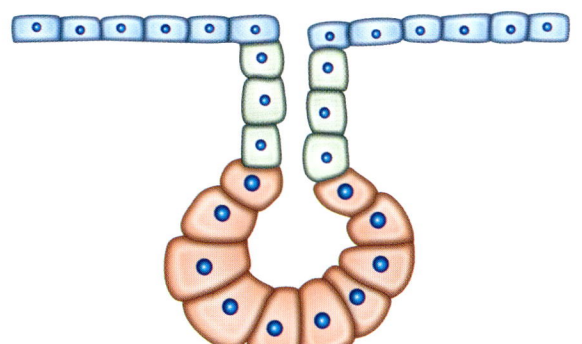
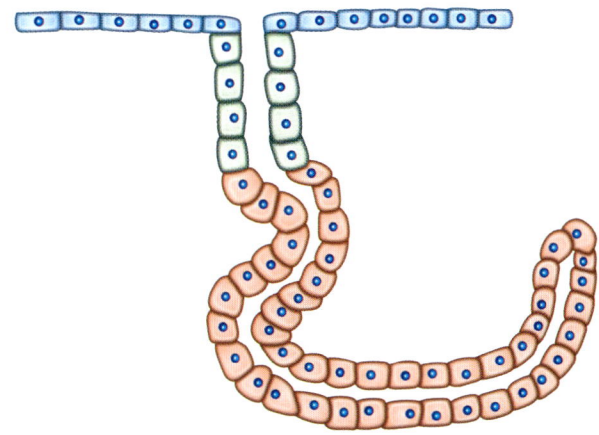

Figure 14-3A: Simple glands.

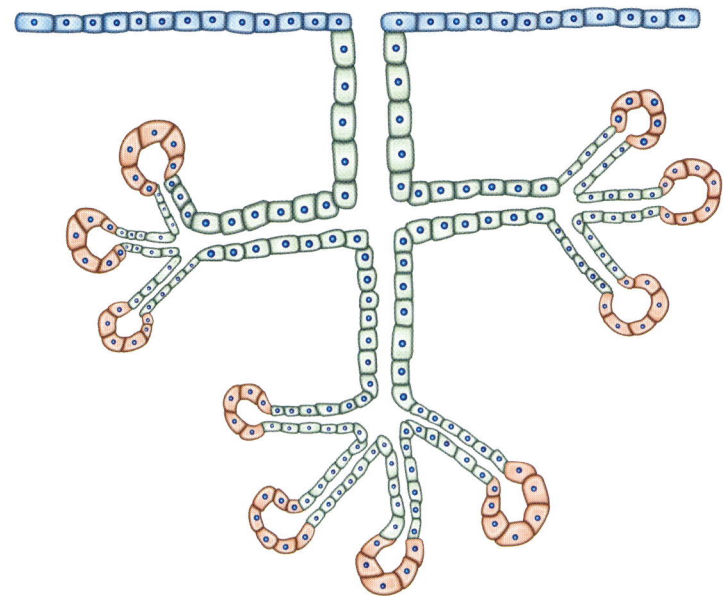

Figure 14-3B: Compound and branched glands.

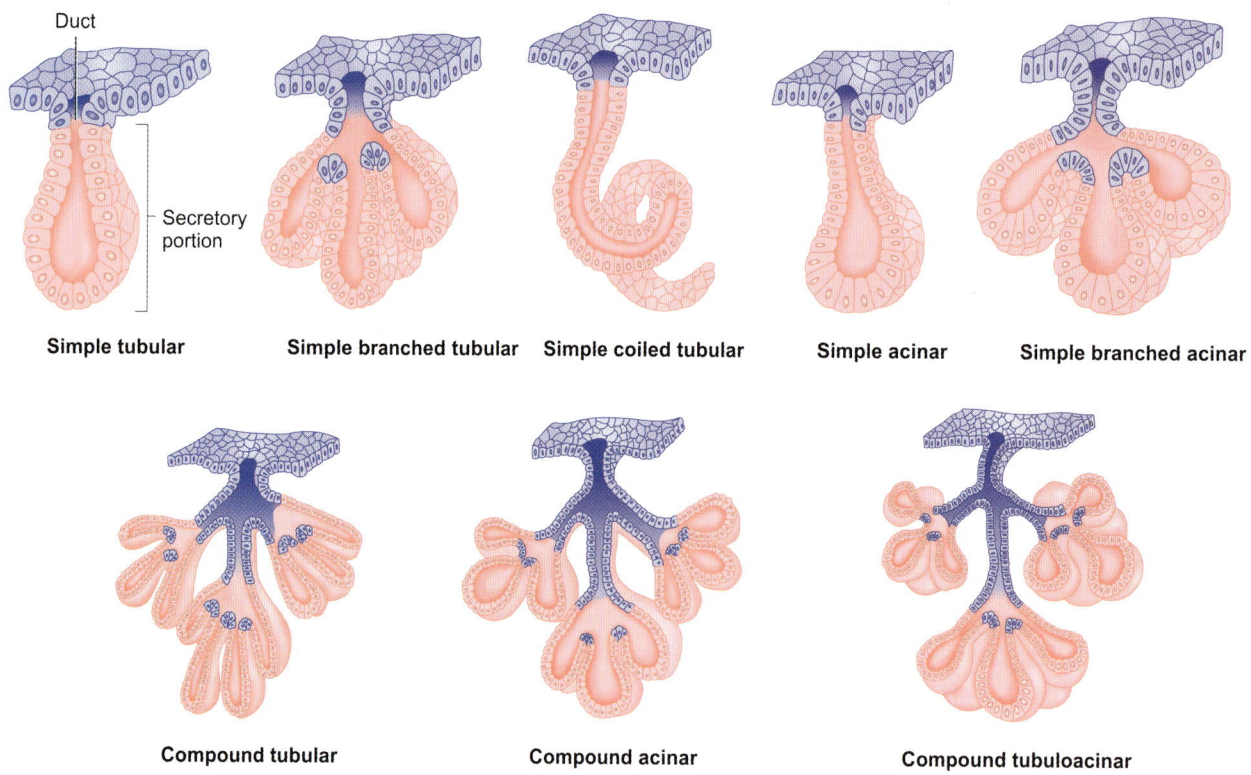

Figure 14-3C: Different types of ducts and acinar units.

the apical part of the cell membrane to release the product by exocytosis, *e.g.*, salivary glands.

The process of storage of secretory product in the membrane-bound vesicles, along with the insertion of vesicular membrane into the apical part of the cell membrane preserves the contents of the vesicles and conserves cell membrane. The vesicular membrane that is added to the apical membrane is later recycled through endocytosis for reutilization in the formation of new secretory vesicles.

Apocrine Glands (Figure 14-7)

In these glands, the secretory product is secreted through apocrine method where the apical portions of the cells are pinched off and lost during the secretory process (a portion of

CHAPTER 14: Salivary Glands

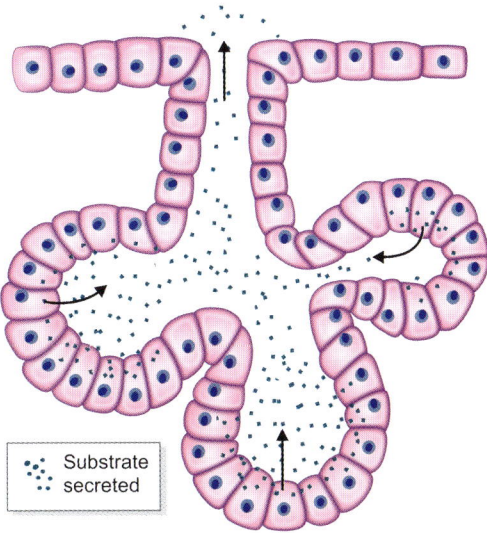

Figure 14-4: Exocrine glands.

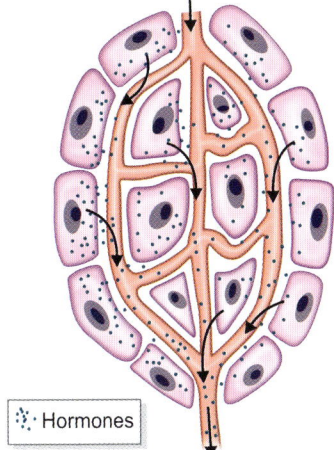

Figure 14-5: Endocrine glands.

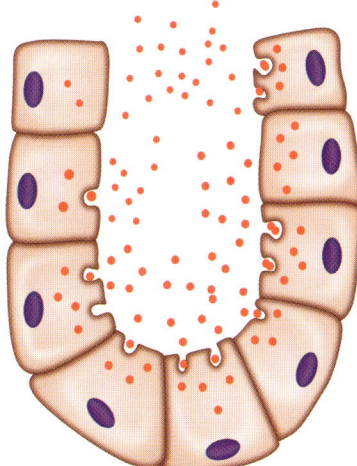

Figure 14-6: Merocrine glands.

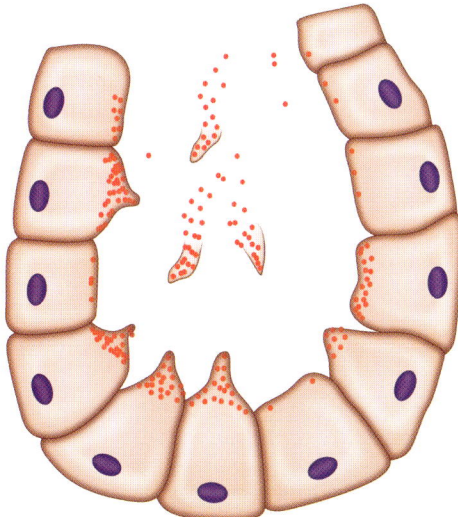

Figure 14-7: Apocrine glands.

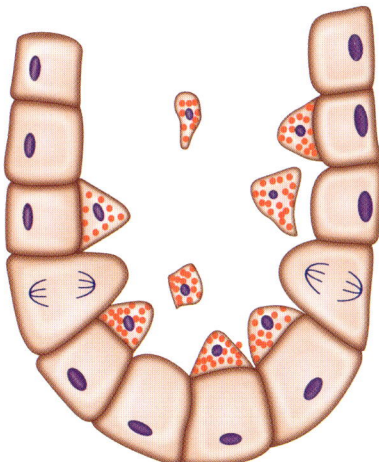

Figure 14-8: Holocrine glands.

Holocrine Glands (Figure 14-8)

Holocrine secretion involves death of the cell. The secretory cell is released and as it breaks apart, the contents of the cell become the secretory product. This mode of secretion results in the most complex secretory product, *e.g.*, some sweat glands located in the axilla, pubic areas, and around the areola of the breasts. Sebaceous glands are also of this type.

Type of Secretions

Glands can differ based on their secretory products that include hormones, enzymes, or sometimes just fluid, though each with specific functions.
- ❖ Endocrine glands secrete hormones
- ❖ Pancreas secretes digestive enzyme like amylase, trypsin, and lipase
- ❖ Sweat glands secrete sweat that regulates body temperature and also excretion
- ❖ Sebaceous glands secrete sebum in the skin and the ear, which keeps the skin oily and protects it
- ❖ Lacrimal glands secrete water to moisten the eye

the cytoplasm is lost). This results in a secretory product that contains a variety of molecular components including those of the membrane (*e.g.* mammary gland and sweat gland).

❖ Salivary glands secrete saliva and the functions of which will be dealt later.

SALIVARY GLANDS

Tissues secreting fluid to facilitate feeding emerge progressively throughout evolution and can be found in very simple organisms (e.g., *Caenorhabditis elegans*) and more complex species (e.g., *Drosophila melanogaster*, placental mammals). In humans, salivary glands produce and secrete digestive fluids or protein-rich fluids.

Salivary glands are multicellular, exocrine, merocrine, and tubuloacinar glands, located inside and outside the mouth. Their main function is to secrete saliva, which is discharged into the oral cavity proper and the vestibular cavity by means of ducts. Saliva plays a major role in digestion in addition to the variety of other functions it performs in the mouth.

CLASSIFICATION OF SALIVARY GLANDS

Salivary glands are classified into major salivary glands and minor salivary glands according to their size. According to the type of secretion, they are classified into serous, mucous and mixed glands.

Major Salivary Glands (Table 14-1)

Major salivary glands are larger in size. There are three pairs of major salivary glands, namely parotid, submandibular and sublingual and they contribute to the most of the saliva secreted. The salient features of the major salivary glands are given in **Table 14-1**.

Minor Salivary Glands

The minor salivary glands are smaller in size and around 600-1000 in number, are distributed throughout the oral cavity except gingiva, anterior most part of the palate and anterior two-thirds of the dorsum of the tongue. The examples of minor salivary glands include buccal, labial, anterior lingual, posterior lingual, palatine, glossopalatine and von Ebner glands. Their location and the type of secretion is given in **Table 14-2**.

TABLE 14-2: Types of minor salivary glands.

Name	Location	Type of secretion
Superior labial and inferior labial glands	Lips	Mixed (Predominantly mucous)
Buccal and retromolar glands	Buccal mucosa and retromolar region	Mixed (Predominantly mucous)
Palatine glands	Hard palate, soft palate, uvula	Purely mucous
Glossopalatine glands	Anterior faucial pillar, Glossopalatine fold	Purely mucous
Anterior lingual glands (Blandin-Nuhn) glands	Anterior tongue	Mixed (Predominantly mucous)
Posterior lingual (von Ebner) glands	Circumvallate papilla	Purely serous
Posterior lingual glands (Tonsil, lingual)	Base of the tongue	Purely mucous

Type of Secretions

According to the type of secretion, salivary glands are classified into serous, mucous, and mixed (**Figures 14-9A to C**).

Serous glands secrete serous fluid that is thin and watery and contains water, enzymes, a variety of salts and organic ions, *e.g.*, parotid gland.

Mucous glands secrete relatively thick fluid that contains mucin, which acts as a lubricant to aid in mastication, deglutition and digestion, *e.g.*, glossopalatine, palatine glands.

Mixed glands otherwise known as seromucous glands, in which the serous cells form demilunes over the mucous acini, *e.g.*, submandibular glands. Their secretion is the combination of serous and mucous fluid.

DEVELOPMENT OF SALIVARY GLAND

The three major salivary glands show variation in their developmental origin.

The parotid glands originate from the ectoderm, near the corners of the stomodeum by the 6th week of prenatal life.

The submandibular glands arise from the endoderm in the floor of the mouth at the end of the 6th week or the beginning of the 7th week *in utero*.

TABLE 14-1: Comparision of major salivary glands.

Features	Parotid gland	Submandibular gland	Sublingual gland
Size	Largest	Intermediate	Small
Location	Anterior to the ear	Beneath the mandible, near the angle	Anterior floor of the mouth
Capsulation	Entire gland	Entire gland	Minimum
Excretory ducts	**Stenson (Parotid) duct:** Opens on the buccal mucosa opposite to the maxillary second molar	**Wharton (Submandibular) duct:** Opens on the floor of the mouth, near the lingual frenum, at sublingual caruncles	**Bartholin (Sublingual) duct:** Opens in same area as submandibular duct; smaller ducts of Rivinus also open directly along the sublingual folds.
Striated ducts	Shorter	Longer	Rare or absent
Intercalated ducts	Longer	Shorter	Absent
Terminal secretory unit (Acini)	Serous acini	Serous acini; also some mucous acini with serous demilunes	Mucous acini; also some serous demilunes
Secretory product	Purely serous	Predominantly serous (mixed)	Predominantly mucous (mixed)

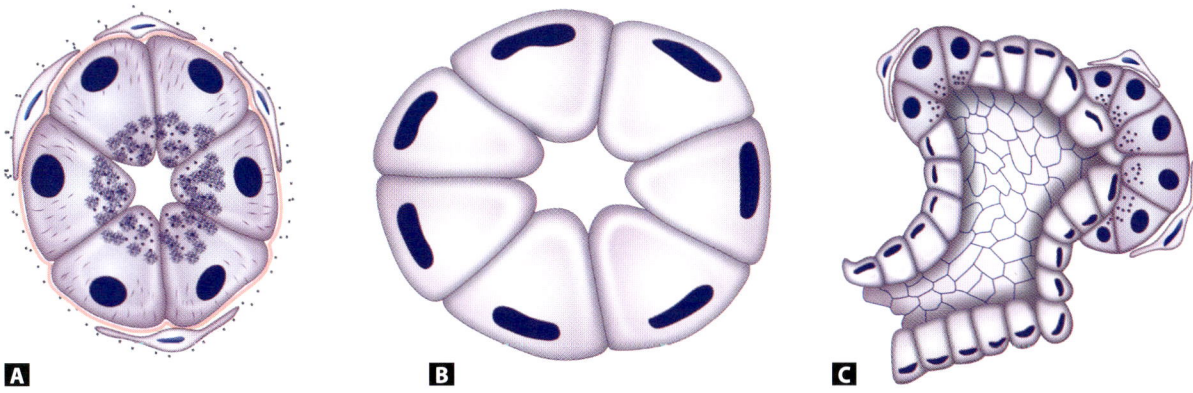

Figures 14-9A to C: (A) Serous; (B) Mucous; and (C) Mixed gland.

The sublingual glands arise from endoderm, lateral to the submandibular primordium at about 8th week *in utero*.

All the minor salivary glands form from the epithelium overlying a specific area of the oral cavity and begin to develop during the 12th week of prenatal life.

Although the site and the time of development differ slightly from the major salivary glands, the processes involved in development are similar.

Stages in the Development of Salivary Gland

Stage 1: Bud Formation (Figure 14-10)

Salivary glands originate from an epithelial placode between 4th and 12th weeks of embryonic development. This bud-shaped epithelial placode, is formed by the proliferation of overlying epithelium, under the inductive influence of the underlying mesenchyme that condenses and surrounds the epithelial bud. A thin layer of basal lamina separates the epithelial bud from the underlying mesenchyme.

Epithelial–mesenchymal interactions: These interactions are referred to as 'secondary induction'. Mesenchyme is the embryonic connective tissue composed of undifferentiated pluripotent connective tissue cells and extracellular matrix. The epithelial-mesenchymal interactions are defined as proximate tissue interactions in which the presence of mesenchyme, in close proximity to the epithelium, is required for the normal development of the epithelium. In salivary glands, epithelial-mesenchymal interactions regulate both the initiation and growth of the glandular tissue and the eventful cytodifferentiation of cells within the glands. Thus, mesenchyme has an essential role in development as well as in forming the supporting part of the gland.

Extracellular matrix: The extracellular matrix consists of basal lamina and the intercellular substance.

Basal lamina: It is composed of type IV collagen, heparan sulfate, and other proteoglycans, as well as laminin and entactin, two glycoproteins that interact with each other and with other components of the extracellular matrix. The basal lamina is secreted by the epithelium and serves for supportive and filtering functions as well as for regulating migration, polarity, and differentiation of epithelial cells.

Intercellular substance or the extracellular matrix: It is synthesized by connective tissue cells. The extracellular matrix is composed of fibers and ground substance. The major fibers are type I and III collagen fibers and the ground substance is made up of glycoproteins, fibronectin, and tenascin, and proteoglycans such as chondroitin sulfate. The components of the basal lamina and surrounding extracellular matrix therefore differ in the types of glycoproteins and proteoglycans present in each location.

The extracellular matrix provides regulatory cues for cell proliferation, cell differentiation, and morphogenesis.

> **Cell proliferation:** Cell proliferation is the increase in number of cells that occurs throughout development as organs enlarge, and also in cell replacement systems throughout life. Proliferating cells enter the cell cycle, replicate their DNA, and subsequently undergo cytokinesis to form two progeny, *i.e.* daughter cells. These cells may either undergo specialization or remain as part of a dividing or stem cell population that continues to proliferate.
> **Differentiation:** Differentiation is defined as the extent to which the daughter cell resembles the parent cell structurally and functionally. Differentiation describes those processes responsible for the development of cell specificity and diversity as observed at the morphological or molecular level. Differentiated cells express a specific portion of the genome that is characteristic of that particular cell type.
> **Morphogenesis:** Morphogenesis describes those developmental processes that are responsible for the formation of the shape and form of an organ. Glandular branching as occurs in the developing salivary glands is one of the best examples of a morphogenetic process.

Morphogenesis and differentiation are independent but concurrent processes required for the development of adult architecture and specificity of cell types, respectively. All salivary glands follow a similar developmental pattern.

The functional glandular tissue, the parenchyma, develops as an epithelial outgrowth of the buccal epithelium that invades the underlying mesenchyme. The connective tissue stroma (capsule and septa) and blood vessels form from the mesenchyme. The mesenchyme is composed of cells derived from both mesoderm and ectomesenchyme.

> Ectomesenchyme is not only essential for the formation of most of the facial structures including the teeth, but also for the normal differentiation of the salivary glands.

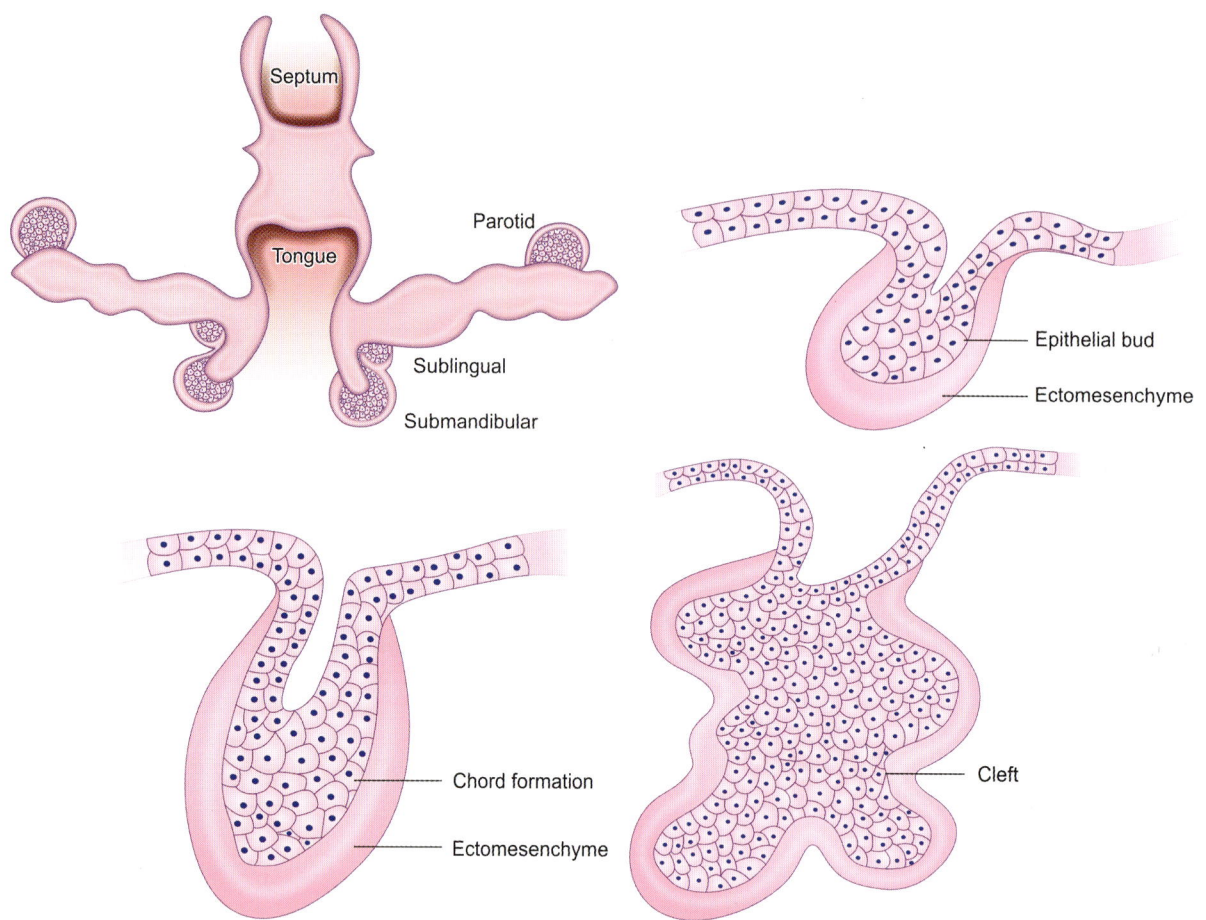

Figure 14-10: Summary of salivary gland development. Stages 1-3.
Source: Department of Oral Pathology, Saveetha Dental College, Chennai, India

It is the extracellular matrix components, synthesized by mesenchymal connective tissue cells that provide important signals. These signals direct the morphogenesis and differentiation of the glandular bud.

As the epithelial bud forms during development, those portions of the bud closest to the ectodermal lining of the primitive oral cavity eventually differentiate into the main excretory duct of the gland. The most distal portions arborize to form the terminal portions of the duct system, the secretory end pieces or acini.

> The origin of the epithelial buds is believed to be **ectodermal** in the parotid and minor salivary glands and **endodermal** in the submandibular and sublingual glands.

Stage 2: Formation and Growth of Epithelial Cord

The epithelial bud proliferates to form a solid cord of cells. The underlying condensed mesenchymal cells also proliferate. The basal lamina is believed to play a role in influencing the morphogenesis and differentiation of the salivary glands. A solid cord of cells forms the epithelial bud by cell proliferation. Condensation and proliferation occur in the surrounding mesenchyme, which is closely associated with the epithelial cord. The basal lamina is found between the cord and the mesenchyme, composed of collagen, glycosaminoglycans and glycoproteins.

Stage 3: Initiation of Branching in Terminal Parts of Epithelial Cord

The epithelial cord proliferates and its ends branch into bulbs. This stage denotes the initiation of the branching. The epithelial cord proliferates rapidly and branches into terminal bulbs. Branching is the primary morphogenetic process in salivary gland development. Cleft formation in distal buds initiates the branching process, which is followed by epithelial proliferation. Collagen type III accumulates at the cleft points and appears to be a key substance in the morphogenetic process of branching. Type I and IV collagen appear to be more important for maintenance and support of established branches. Local release of acetylcholine induces proliferation of epithelial progenitor, which positively regulates epithelial branching.

Stage 4: Dichotomous Branching of Epithelial Cord and Lobule Formation (Figure 14-11)

The terminal ends branch extensively, forming numerous bulbs. The connective tissue below the epithelial cord forms

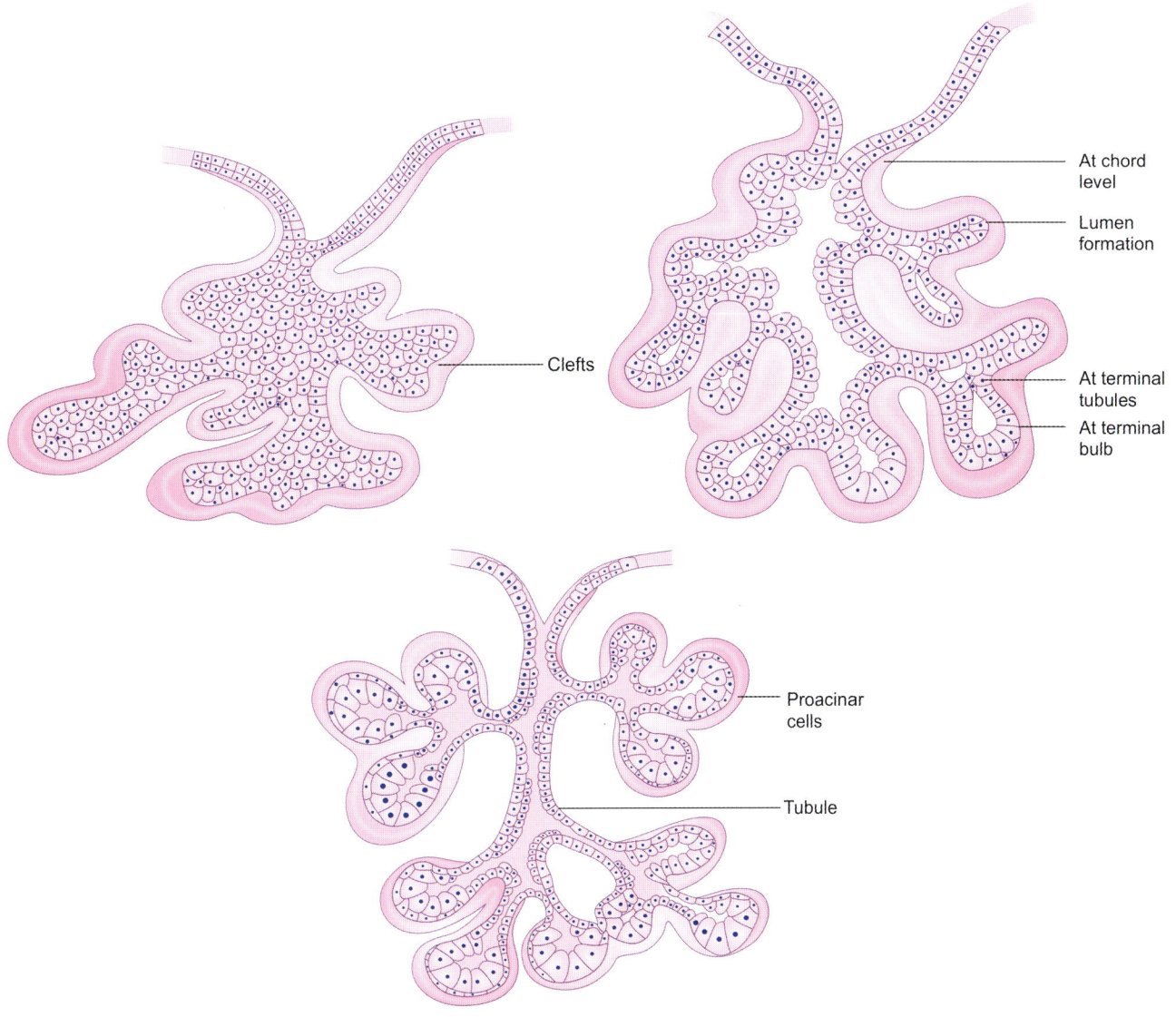

Figure 14-11: Summary of salivary gland development. Stages 4–6.
Source: Department of Oral Pathology, Saveetha Dental College, Chennai, India

a capsule and surrounds the entire glandular structure. The branching continues at the terminal portions of the cord, forming an extensive tree-like system of bulbs. As branching occurs, connective tissue differentiates around the branches, eventually producing extensive lobulation. The glandular capsule forms from mesenchyme and surrounds the entire glandular parenchyma.

Stage 5: Canalization

In this stage, the cord forms a central tube or duct. This canalization is believed to occur due to different rates of cell proliferation between the outer and inner layers of the epithelial cord and fluid secretion by the duct cells, which increases the hydrostatic pressure within to form a canal. In addition, during this stage further branching of the system occurs. Canalization of the epithelial cord, with formation of a hollow tube or duct, usually occurs by the 6th month in all three major salivary glands.

Experimental studies have led to the proposition of two main theories to explain the mechanism of canalization namely–

- The different rates of cell proliferation between the outer and inner layers of the epithelial cord
- The lumen is formed within the cord due to the increased hydrostatic pressure caused by fluid secretion.
- Further branching of the duct structure and growth of connective tissue septa continues at this stage of development.

Stage 6: Cytodifferentiation

Cytodifferentiation is the final stage of salivary gland development, in which the functional acini and intercalated ducts develop. It is initiated by a pre-programmed developmental process, which starts with an epithelial–mesenchymal interaction followed by exocrine cell differentiation without the continued presence of mesenchyme. There is increased mitotic activity in the terminal bulb portions of the epithelial cord. In this last stage of development, the cells of the bulb region differentiate into proacinar and terminal tubule cells.

Proacinar cells form the acinar cells. Maturation of the acinar cells occurs in specific stages, classified according to the morphology of secretory granules and cellular organelles. Acinar development differs for serous and mucous cells. Terminal tubule cells eventually differentiate into the intercalated duct cells of the adult gland. Myoepithelial cells arise from epithelial stem cells in the terminal tubules and develop in concert with acinar cytodifferentiation.

Cytodifferentiation is completed postnatally, and functionally competent after the onset of masticatory stimuli. This postnatal development process includes:
- Acinar cell secretion controlled by the maturation of stimulus-secretion coupling.
- Formation of neural network from the autonomic nervous system.
- The peripheral nervous system participates in directing salivary gland maturation. The primordial epithelial structure is innervated by cholinergic neurons, whose axonal growth follows the ramified pattern of the developing gland.
- A network of capillaries derived from terminal arterioles develops in parallel with the acini-duct systems and has an instructive role in the establishment of the epithelial patterning.

> Various intrinsic factors, which are a predetermined pattern of gene expression for every cell type and extrinsic factors, which are signals given by cell to cell and cell to matrix interactions along with growth factors and cytokines, influence the development of salivary gland and control the cell proliferation, differentiation, and morphogenesis.

Branching of the Epithelial Cord

Branching is the primary morphogenetic process, which is followed by epithelial proliferation. It has been extensively studied by analysis of salivary gland rudiments grown *in vitro*.

Branching and proliferation must be coordinated for the normal development of salivary glands. Mitotic activity is normally localized to the most peripheral regions of the bud. The basal lamina is implicated in the stabilization of the epithelium and the initiation and maintenance of lobular morphology. Destabilization of the basal lamina inhibits cleft development, and also affects subsequent events such as cell proliferation. The regulation of morphogenetic changes by the basal lamina is carried out either directly or by selective filtration or channelling of materials to the epithelium. The basal lamina regulates flow of ions such as calcium to the epithelium that may affect the function of microtubules and microfilaments in cellular proliferation, migration, and differentiation.

Collagenogenic and collagenolytic activity is also important in salivary gland development. Collagen synthesis by the mesenchymal cells provides structural stabilization after branching has occurred. The stabilization appears to be provided by type I and IV collagen, which are associated with maintenance and support of the branched organization of the adult gland. In addition, the collagenolytic activity in the epithelium and mesenchyme may allow for selective breakdown of the basal lamina and communication between the epithelium, basal lamina, and surrounding mesenchyme at key stages of development.

Role of Extracellular Matrix

The extracellular matrix in concert with growth factors appears to regulate the morphogenesis occurring during salivary gland development.

> *Genetics*
> - Embryogenesis: Homeotic and dorsoventral patterning genes
> - Morphogenesis: *Chickadee, rhomboid1, egalitarian, bitesize, and capricious*
> - Ductal formation: *PH4SG1* and *PH4SG2* genes

HISTOLOGY OF SALIVARY GLANDS

Salivary glands consist of two main components; the parenchyma and the stroma. The parenchyma consists of the glandular secretory tissue and the ducts, and the stroma is made up of connective tissue, which supports the parenchyma.

Salivary gland contains the following structures (**Figures 14-12 and 14-13**)
- Secretory end piece/unit (serous/mucous/mixed acini)
- Myoepithelial cells
- Other cells
- Intercalated ducts
- Striated ducts
- Excretory duct
- Connective tissue stroma
- Capsule

Salivary gland is divided into numerous lobes and lobules by the connective tissue stroma (**Figure 14-13**). These lobules contain the secretory units called acini. Each secretory unit consists of acinar cells and branching ducts. Ducts within lobules or intralobular ducts are connected with bigger interlobular ducts found in the connective tissue stroma, which are seen in-between the lobules.

> Salivon is a functioning unit of a salivary gland and forms the basic component of the salivary glands. Each salivon forms one branch in the glandular tree, is composed of acini, intercalated ducts, striated ducts, and intra- and interlobular secretory ducts. Salivons are separated from the interstitial stroma by a continuous basement membrane, which surrounds these tubuloacinar epithelial structures.
>
> Adenomere is the part of a developing salivary gland destined to become responsible for its function (formation and secretion of saliva). Thus, they consist of all the secretory cells that release their products into a single intralobular duct, namely acini, intercalated ducts, and striated ducts.

Histology of the Secretory Units

The functional unit of the salivary gland is called secretory unit, which consists of terminal secretory cells

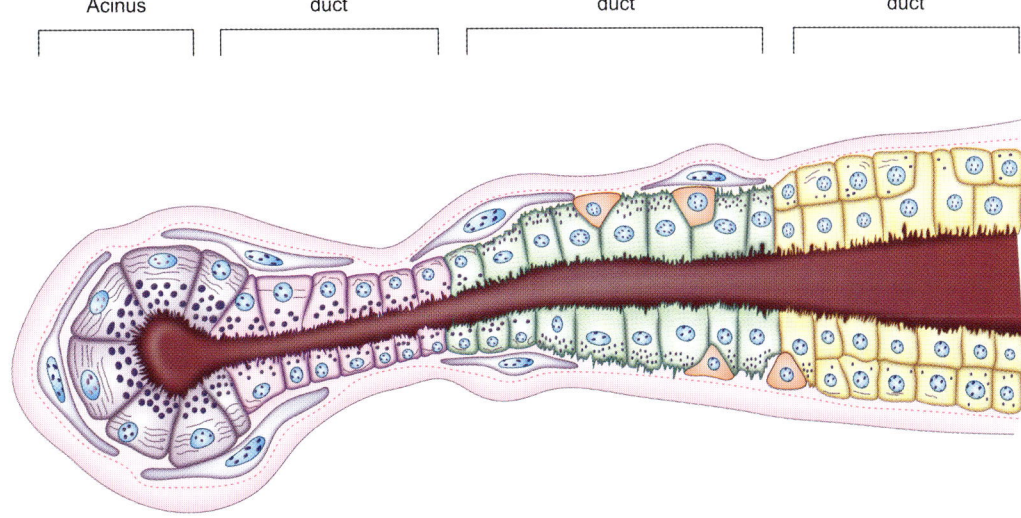

Figure 14-12: Schematic representation of the structure of salivary gland.
Source: Adapted from James Avery.

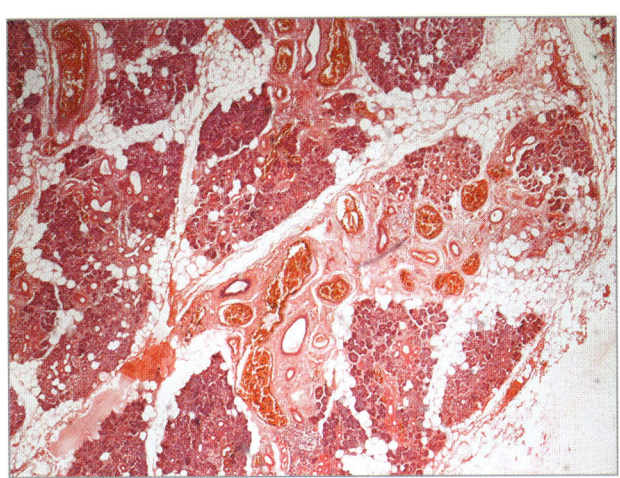

Figure 14-13: Histology of salivary gland.

called acini. They are classified according to the cell types they contain:

Serous acini: Made up of only serous cells and are spherical in shape.

Mucous acini: Made up of only mucous cells and are tubular in shape.

Seromucous (mixed) acini: Contain a mixture of serous and mucous cells and serous demilunes.

Serous Acini

Serous acinus or serous secretory end piece is a spherical structure containing 8–12 acinar cells surrounding a central lumen **(Figures 14-14A to D)**. The cells are typically pyramidal in shape with a narrow apex, forming part of the lumen and a broad base. The lumen usually has intercellular canaliculi, which increases luminal surface area of the cells. The nuclei are spherical in shape and are located basally or suprabasally.

Numerous densely packed secretory granules, housing the macromolecular components of saliva, are seen in the apical cytoplasm. The granules are 1 μm in diameter with a limiting membrane and may present as homogeneously electron-dense to a combination of electron-dense and electron-lucent regions with intricate patterns. These granules are called zymogen granules, since they contain zymogen. Zymogens are an inactive enzyme precursor and are formed in the rough endoplasmic reticulum.

The basal cytoplasm is rich in rough endoplasmic reticulum, which congregates on the large Golgi complex located adjacent to the nucleus. Newly formed secretory granules are seen at the trans-face of the Golgi apparatus, which later convert into mature secretory granules and accumulate at the apical portion of the cells. They are discharged into the lumen by exocytosis. The luminal surface has numerous short microvilli and the lateral and the basal surfaces have interdigitating folds. The secretory cells are attached to the basal lamina by hemidesmosomes. These junctions are vital for salivary homeostasis as they provide the route for macromolecules and neurotransmitters.

BMP6 is positive for the adult serous acini of the parotid and submandibular glands.

Mucous Acini

Mucous acini or mucous secretory end piece typically have a tubular configuration. In cross section, they appear circular surrounding a larger central lumen compared to the serous acini **(Figures 14-15A to D)**. The adjacent acinar cells are attached to each other by a variety of cell junctions. There is accumulation of large amounts of mucus in the apical cytoplasm that compresses the nucleus and endoplasmic reticulum against the basal cell membrane. Their secretions reach the lumen of the end piece through intercellular canaliculi extending between the mucous cells at the end of the tubule.

In routine histological sections, they do not take any stain and thus, the apical cytoplasm appears empty. The secreted mucus can be demonstrated with periodic acid–Schiff stain or Alcian blue due to their affinity for sugar residues.

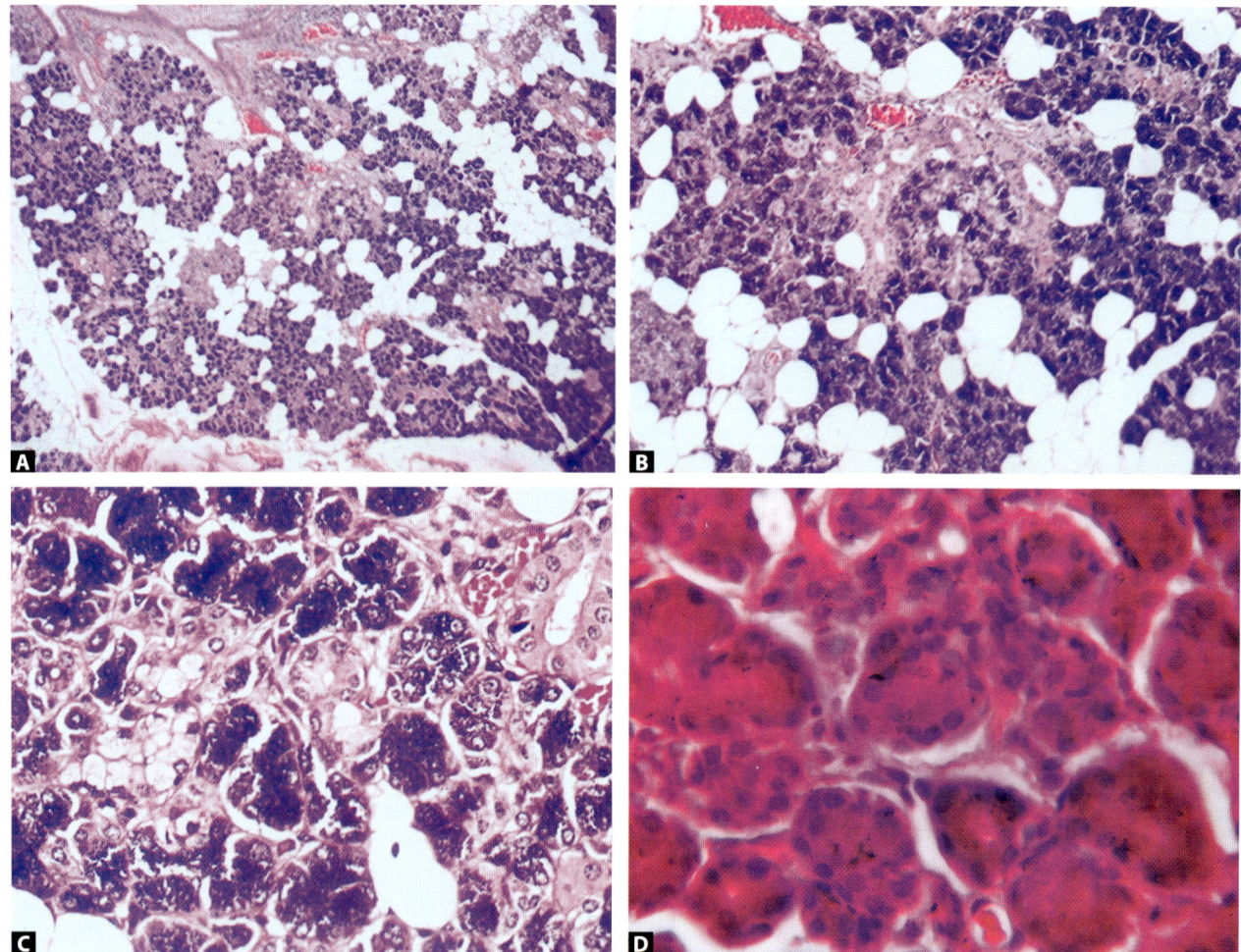

Figures 14-14A to D: Hematoxylin and eosin stained sections of serous gland in different magnifications.

In electron microscopy mucus secretory granules appear distended with a disrupted limiting membrane. This causes fusion of the granules with one another and the content appears electron lucent, which include some filamentous or flocculent material. The nucleus is flattened and pushed to the basal part of the cell. But there is a view that this appearance is caused by artifact due to the chemical fixation.

The features are entirely different when frozen sections are prepared for electron microscope, which reveal small dense mucous secretory granules with intact membrane and lie freely and not fused with one another. Golgi apparatus, endoplasmic reticulum, and organelles are placed at the basal cytoplasm.

Differences between serous and mucous acini are enumerated in **Table 14-3**.

Serous Demilunes

Serous demilunes of Giannuzzi or Demilunes of Heidenhain are half-moon-shaped serous cellular formations on some mucous secretory end pieces of the major and some minor salivary glands. They are the serous acini at the distal end of mucous tubuloalveolar secretory unit of mixed salivary glands **(Figures 14-16A to D)**. These serous cell capping is very much similar to the serous end piece cells present in the same gland. Their secretion is transported to the lumen through the intercellular canaliculi extending between the mucous cells at the end of the tubule. This appearance is seen only in routine sections.

However an alternate view considers the serous demilunes to be caused by the processing artifact of the tissue preserved in formalin. In formalin fixed tissues, mucous cells are distended and displace the serous cells toward the basal portion of the acini, which imparts the "demilune" appearance. When the tissue is frozen and leaving no room for any dimensional change, the serous cells align with the mucous cells surrounding a common lumen and no demilunes were found.

MYOEPITHELIAL CELLS (BASKET CELLS)

Myoepithelial cells, otherwise known as basket cells are contractile in nature, which are seen to lie between basal lamina and the basal membrane of the acinar cells and intercalated duct cells of the salivary gland. Myoepithelial cells are epithelial in origin, since they contain cytokeratin intermediate filaments. They are contractile cells and have functions similar to smooth muscle cells. They also contain large amounts of microfilaments and contractile proteins characteristic of smooth muscle cells. These cells are also seen in lacrimal glands, mammary glands, sweat glands, and prostate.

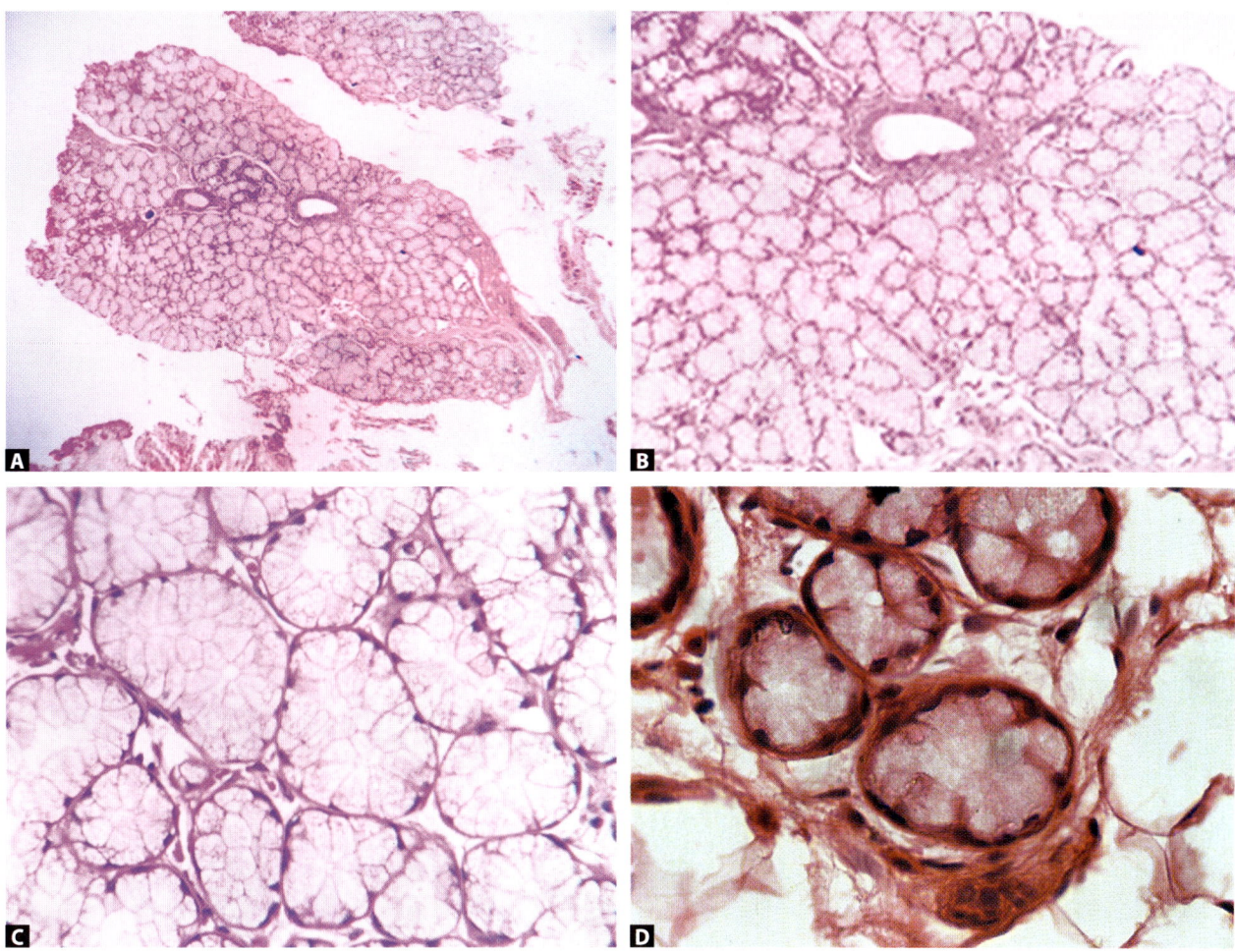

Figures 14-15A to D: Hematoxylin and eosin stained sections of mucous gland in different magnifications.

TABLE 14-3: Differences between serous and mucous acini.

Factors	Serous acini	Mucous acini
Size	Small	Large
Lumen	Narrow	Wide
Number of units in each acini	5–8	More than 8
Shape	Pyramidal or columnar	Pyramidal or low columnar
Shape of nucleus	Round	Flat
Position of nucleus	Central	Toward the base
Apical cytoplasm	Electron-dense zymogen granules	Electron-lucent mucinogen granules
Myoepithelial cells	Less	More
Secretion	Watery and rich in enzymes	Thick or viscous, rich in glycoproteins

Structure (Figures 14-17A and B)

They are predominantly stellate-shaped cells with a flattened nucleus and made of actin filaments and soluble myosin. Nucleus is dark and rounded and the cytoplasm appears vacuolated. Most of the other organelles are located around the nucleus. Myoepithelial cells have numerous caveolae, which are vital in initiating contraction.

The shape of myoepithelial cells depends on their location. Myoepithelial cells associated with acini have a central body and four to eight processes radiating from it with each process subdivided and undergoing several ramifications, surrounding and embracing the secretory end pieces, giving rise to the appearance of an octopus sitting on the rock. On the other hand, myoepithelial cells associated with intercalated ducts are fusiform in shape with few short processes oriented lengthwise along the duct.

In electron microscopy they are seen in two forms, a filamentous form in which the filaments are arranged parallel as bundles, similar to the myofilaments of smooth muscle in their processes and the non-filamentous form containing the nucleus and the organelles.

Function

Myoepithelial cells are controlled by the autonomic nervous system. On stimulation, they contract and expel secretions from the gland. This contraction of myoepithelial cells is thought to provide support for the secretory end pieces during active secretion of saliva, which may help to expel the primary saliva into the ductal system and also help in maintaining their patency. They prevent or reduce the back permeation of fluid by supporting the underlying

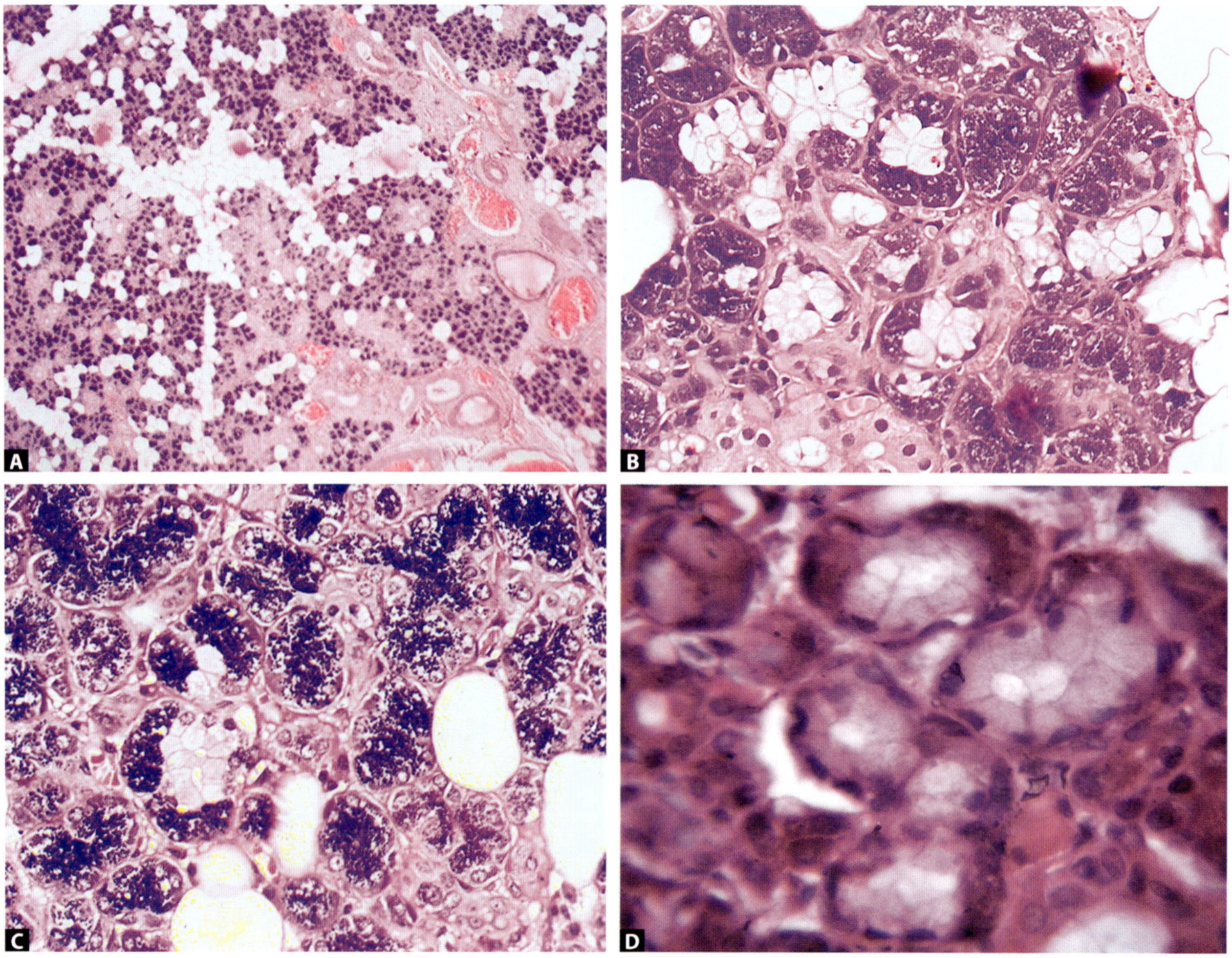

Figures 14-16A to D: Hematoxylin and eosin stained sections of mucous cells with serous demilune in different magnifications.

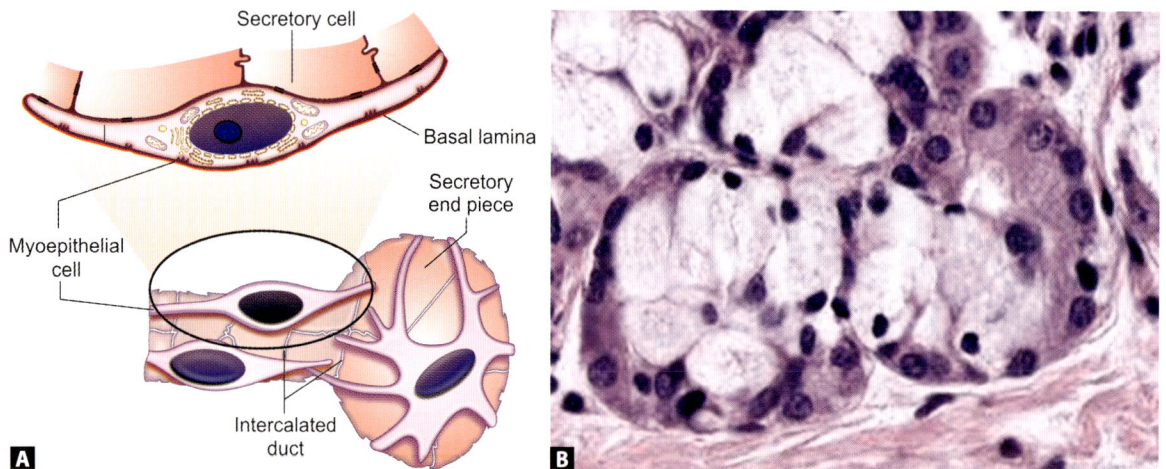

Figures 14-17A and B: Myoepithelial cells: (A) Diagrammatic representation; (B) Hematoxylin and eosin stained section.

parenchyma. Further, they are implicated in signaling the secretory cells and protecting the salivary acinar cells by maintaining cell polarity and the structural organization of the secretory end piece. Since they are located between the glandular epithelial cells and the stroma containing the blood vessels, they may have a role in the transport process and/or control of glandular metabolism.

They also produce a number of proteins that act as a protective barrier to the epithelium.

Identification of Myoepithelial Cells

These cells are inconspicuous in routine hematoxylin and eosin-stained sections and appear as a layer of flat cells running around the acini and ducts. The various special stains used to identify myoepithelial cells are silver stain and tannic phosphomolybdic acid dye. The stains that demonstrate the property of birefringence of myosin and actin filaments are: Thiazine Red R and Levanol Brilliant Red BB and the stains that demonstrate the property of fluorescence are rhodaminephalloidin and nitrobenzoxadiazole phallacidin.

They can be identified by enzyme histochemistry by demonstrating alkaline phosphatase, adenosine triphosphatase, glycogen phosphorylase, and inosine diphosphatase. Immunohistochemical markers for myoepithelial cells include S-100 protein, α-SMA, SMMHC, h-caldesmon, basic calponin, CK5, CK14, CK17, α1β1 integrin, laminin, fibronectin, metallothionein, p63, CD29, and CD109.

OTHER CELLS

Other cells present in the salivary parenchyma include tuft cells and dendritic antigen presenting cells. Rarely melanocytes are present in the interlobular ducts.

The stroma of the salivary gland contains fibroblasts, the essential component of the fibrous stroma, plasma cells, involved in the production of antibodies, fat cells, macrophages, and polymorphonuclear leukocytes.

The inflammatory cells present in the salivary glands help to maintain the normal milieu.

DUCTAL SYSTEM

The ductal system of salivary glands is made up of a wide network of tubular structures that begin at the acini and are then connected to other ducts to end at the oral mucosal surface. The diameter of these ducts increases gradually from inner to outer portion of the gland. The duct system starts as a smallest duct called intercalated duct, which connects to the relatively bigger striated duct. The ducts in the interlobular stroma join with one another, thereby increasing in size, and ultimately reach the biggest excretory duct.

The three types of ducts of the major glands are intercalated, striated, and excretory, which are different from each other in every aspect including their structure and function. Intercalated and striated ducts are intralobular and the excretory ducts are the interlobular.

Minor glands have single ducts that secrete saliva directly into the oral cavity. They are named intralobular and interlobular ducts based on their presence within the lobule or in the interlobular stroma.

Apart from conducting the salivary secretion, ducts play a vital role in the production and modification of saliva. Electrolyte modification is carried out by the different segments of the salivary gland's duct system.

Intercalated Ducts (Figures 14-18A and B)

Intercalated ducts are the smallest and the most distal ducts. The length of the intercalated ducts varies in the different major and minor salivary glands.

The overall diameter of intercalated ductal cell is smaller than the acinus but their lumen is larger. The lumina of acini

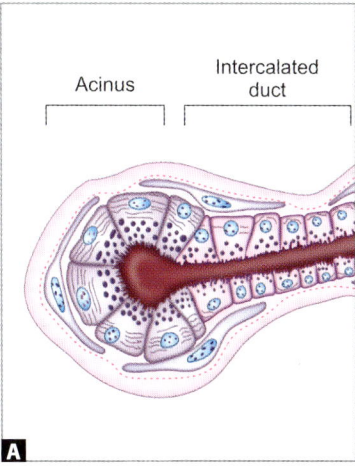

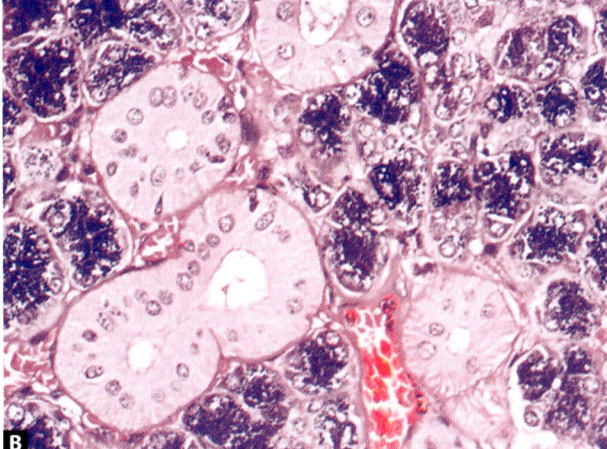

Figures 14-18A and B: Intercalated ducts: (A) Diagrammatic representation; (B) Hematoxylin and eosin stained section.

are continuous with the lumina of the intercalated ducts. The primary saliva from the acini, through small canaliculi, enters the intercalated ducts, which in turn empty it into the striated ducts.

The intercalated ducts are lined by a simple squamous or low cuboidal epithelium. The nucleus is centrally placed and the cytoplasm is scant, which possesses few rough endoplasmic reticulum and Golgi apparatus. Since they are compressed between the secretory units, it is difficult to identify these ducts in light microscopy. Myoepithelial cell layer is irregular with their processes located along the basal surface of the ductal cells. At ultrastructural level, they are similar to serous acini in several aspects. Few secretory granules are seen in the apical cytoplasm, especially among those near the acinus. The apical cytoplasm has very less microvilli. The intercalated duct cells are joined by junctional complexes, desmosomes, and gap junctions with adjacent cells.

Function

The intercalated ducts secrete macromolecular components including lysozyme and lactoferrin along with small quantity of fluid. Bicarbonate is secreted into and chloride is absorbed from the saliva within the intercalated duct segment. Salivary gland stem cells are believed to be present in the intercalated ducts, which replace damaged acini and cells of the striated ducts.

Striated Ducts

The striated ducts receive the primary saliva from the intercalated ducts and form the largest unit of the intralobular duct system **(Figures 14-19A and B)**. The cells are columnar, with a centrally placed nucleus and eosinophilic cytoplasm. At the basal end of the cell, there are numerous striations produced by the infoldings of the plasma membrane to increase the surface area. The diameter and lumen of the striated duct is larger than the acini and intercalated ducts. A basal lamina encloses the striated duct and a capillary plexus is present in the surrounding connective tissue.

Electron microscopy shows numerous active mitochondria present in the narrow cytoplasm separated by highly folded basolateral cell membranes. This combination of plasma membrane infoldings and presence of large amount of vertically oriented mitochondria explains the striations observed at the light microscopic level. Well-developed tight junctions and junctional complexes, which lack gap junctions, connect the adjacent cells.

Functions

The main modification of primary saliva takes place in the striated ducts. These ducts are involved with the reabsorption of sodium and chloride from the primary secretion and the concomitant secretion of potassium and bicarbonate into the primary saliva. They also modify the organic content of the primary saliva. Rarely small secretory granules containing kallikrein, lysosomes, and peroxisomes and other secretory proteins, participate in endocytosis of substances from the lumen. Striated duct cells also secrete epidermal growth factor (EGF). It is to be noted that these ducts along with the excretory ducts are impermeable to water and all the water content enter the saliva at secretory end unit level.

Excretory Ducts

The excretory or collecting ducts are interlobular or extralobular in location and are formed by the joining of the striated ducts **(Figures 14-20A and B)**. These ducts and their surrounding connective tissue stroma gradually increase in size as they leave the interlobular location to reach the oral surface. Excretory ducts predominantly have pseudostratified epithelium with columnar cells extending from the basal lamina to the lumen. The basal cells are short and do not

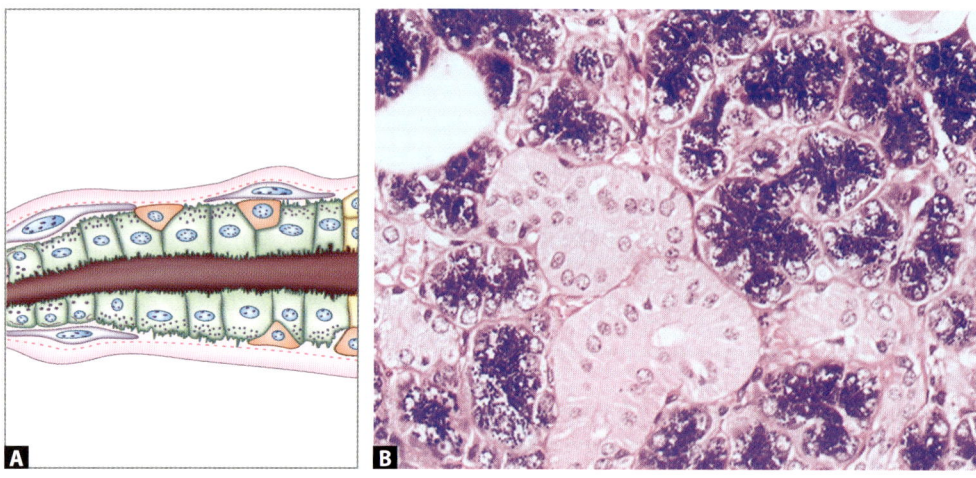

Figures 14-19A and B: Striated duct: (A) Diagrammatic representation; (B) Hematoxylin and eosin stained section.

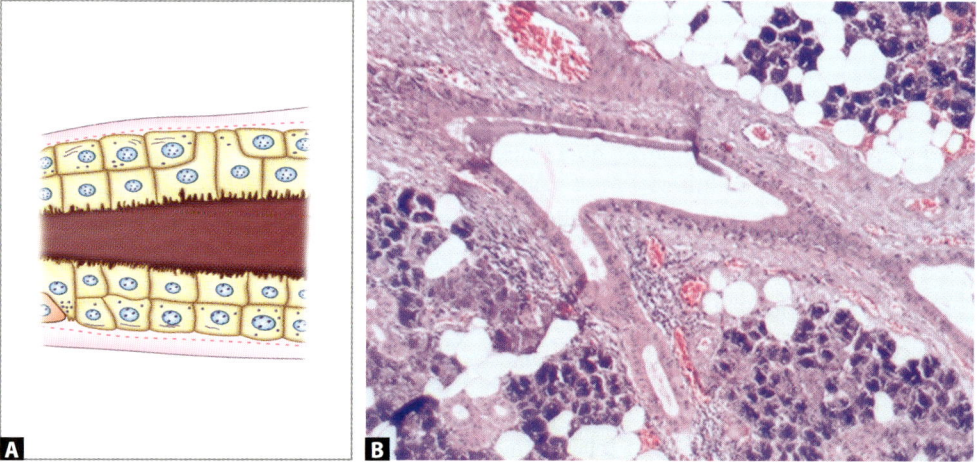

Figures 14-20A and B: Excretory ducts: (A) Diagrammatic representation; (B) Hematoxylin and eosin stained section.

reach the lumen. Number of basal cells increase, as the smaller ducts unite to form larger excretory ducts. The basal cells have tonofilaments and are attached to the basement membrane by means of hemidesmosomes. These cells are also implicated as potential stem cells for turnover and the regeneration of salivary acinar cells. Rarely they have elongated processes similar to myoepithelial cells and contain actin filaments. Few goblet cells and ciliated cells are also seen in the ductal lining. The epithelium may become stratified squamous near the oral opening and merge with the oral epithelium. The cells show several characteristics of the oral epithelium as the duct reaches the opening at the oral surface.

Tuft cells, also called brush cells or caveolated cells are seen in smaller numbers in excretory ducts and to certain extent in striated ducts. These cells are characterized by deep surface invaginations and possess long microvilli and apical vesicles. Their basal portion is closely related to the nerve endings. Thus, they are thought to be some receptor cells. Other cells present in the excretory duct epithelium include dendritic antigen presenting cells, lymphocytes, and macrophages.

CONNECTIVE TISSUE COMPONENT OF THE GLAND

The connective tissue, which supports and protects the salivary gland, comprises capsule and septa. This is separated from the parenchyma by means of basement membrane. The capsule surrounds the entire gland and demarcates it from the adjacent structures whereas the septa extend inward from the capsule and divide the gland into lobes and lobules. The cells of the connective tissue include fibroblasts, macrophages, adipocytes, plasma cells, and mast cells. The extracellular matrix is made up of fibers and ground substance. The fibrous component consists of collagen and elastic fibers embedded in the matrix of ground substance containing glycoproteins and proteoglycans.

The septa contain blood vessels and nerves, which supply and innervate the glandular components and the excretory ducts of the gland. The septa further divide into finer partitions within the lobules of the gland and carry the arterioles, capillaries, venules, and nerve fibers that innervate the secretory and ductal cells.

Plasma cells in the connective tissue produce immunoglobulins, the majority being IgA. It is bound to a receptor on the basolateral membrane of salivary gland epithelial cells. These immunoglobulins are secreted into the saliva by a process called transcytosis. This involves the transport of IgA vesicles in the salivary gland epithelial cells from its basolateral cytoplasm to the apical end. These bound immunoglobulins, along with a portion of receptor called secretory component, are then released at the luminal surface of the cell. Other immunoglobulins like IgG and IgM are also secreted in smaller amounts in saliva.

Around the acini, the density of the nerves is more. The nerve ending and axons are intimately associated with the acinar cells. Similarly they are also seen along the intralobular ducts but are not abundant. Myoepithelial cells are also associated with the nerves, which are parasympathetic motor innervation in nature.

FORMATION AND SECRETION OF SALIVA

The initial fluid or the primary saliva secreted by the acinar cells is similar to the ultrafiltrate of plasma in terms of its osmotic concentration of sodium, potassium, and chloride. Secretion of saliva occurs in two stages, namely formation of the primary saliva and the modified end product, which is released into the oral cavity.

Primary saliva is an isotonic fluid made mainly of water and organic components, which is secreted by the acinar cells and intercalated duct cells. When it passes through the striated and excretory duct, it is modified extensively by addition of electrolyte and reabsorption. The final saliva that is discharged into the oral cavity is hypotonic. Autonomic nervous system controls the salivary secretion and determines the volume and type of saliva secreted.

> The initial fluid or the primary saliva is secreted by the acinar cells and as it passes through the ducts, its composition is altered. Depending on the flow rate, sodium and chloride are reabsorbed and potassium is added by the ductal secretion.

There are two methods by which the protein synthesis occurs in the salivary acini. The first one is called "main regulated pathway" in which the cells, after receiving the appropriate neuronal signal, synthesize and store secretory granules that move toward the apical region where they fuse with the cell membrane and discharge their contents (exocytosis). Similar to any other cells involved in active synthesis, the secretory end pieces of the salivary gland are also studded with rough endoplasmic reticulum, Golgi apparatus, and membrane-bound granules containing secretory products.

The second pathway is called "constitutive pathway". In this pathway, formed proteins are not stored but are released as and when they are formed. The formed proteins after modification in Golgi apparatus, move toward plasma membrane and are released either into the lumen or to the interstitial tissue.

> The organic contents of the saliva are mainly proteins and glycoproteins, which are responsible for its physical properties such as its viscosity and stringy or stretchy property.

When individual cells are stimulated by neurotransmitter substances, calcium ions are released from intracellular stores by inositol triphosphate, which is released into the cell from cell membrane when the transmitter interacts with the receptor. It then passes across the cell and triggers protein and mucin exocytosis and movement of ions. The actual process of secretion of fluid and ions takes place by the activation of co-transporter system carrying sodium, potassium, and chloride ions into the cells on the basal side, which creates a concentration gradient to enable the chloride ions to move to the apical side of the cell. Release of water molecules by the terminal secretory unit is regulated by parasympathetic innervation. The protein and electrolyte secretion by the acinar cells may be affected by other signaling molecules like norepinephrine, substance P, gastrin, cholecystokinin, vasoactive intestinal polypeptide, neuropeptide Y, and nitric oxide. The blood vessels of the stroma are innervated by the sympathetic (vasoconstrictor fibers) and parasympathetic (vasodilator fibers) nerves. So the availability of water, electrolytes, and other metabolic substances are regulated by the vascular response elicited by the autonomic stimulation.

> Parasympathetic stimulation produces abundant watery saliva, which is less in amylase. Sympathetic stimulation produces scant, viscous saliva, which is rich in amylase.

◼ DUCTAL MODIFICATION OF SALIVA

In addition to conveying saliva from the secretory end pieces to the oral cavity, an important function of the striated and excretory ducts is modification of the primary saliva produced by the end pieces and intercalated ducts, through reabsorption and secretion of electrolytes. The luminal and basolateral membranes of the striated ducts and few portions of the excretory duct have abundant transporters that function to produce a net reabsorption of sodium (Na^+) and chloride (Cl^-) ions, resulting in the formation of hypotonic final saliva. The ducts also secrete potassium (K^+) and bicarbonate (HCO_3^-) ions, but little if any secretion or reabsorption of water occurs in the striated and excretory ducts.

The final electrolyte composition of saliva varies, depending on the salivary flow rate. At high flow rates, the contact time of saliva with the ductal epithelial cells decreases, thus reducing the reabsorption of Na^+ and Cl^- and the release of K^+. This explains the higher Na^+ and Cl^- concentrations rise and lower K^+ concentration. At low flow rates the electrolyte concentrations change in the opposite direction.

The HCO_3^- concentration, however, increases with increasing flow rates, reflecting the increased secretion of HCO_3^- by the acinar cells to drive fluid secretion. Electrolyte secretion and reabsorption in the ducts is regulated by the autonomic nervous system and mineralocorticoids of the adrenal cortex. Due to the presence of large number of cyclic adenosine monophosphate (cAMP)-regulated Cl^- channels in the luminal cell membrane, the sympathetic innervation has a more important role in regulating electrolyte transport in the ducts than in the acinar cells.

◼ COMPOSITION OF SALIVA

The whole saliva or the mixed saliva is the mixture of saliva secreted by the major and minor glands and gingival crevicular fluid, contaminated with microorganisms and their products, leukocytes, desquamated epithelial cells, and food particles. Strictly speaking, the composition of saliva depends on the age, gender, gland which secretes, time of secretion, flow rate, whether stimulated or resting nature and the duration of the stimulus, the type of diet, and the plasma composition.

The composition of parotid saliva is different from that of other glands. The composition of unstimulated or the resting saliva is quite different from that obtained when a stimulus is employed. The "unstimulated" secretion usually contains extremely high levels of potassium, chloride, and phosphorus.

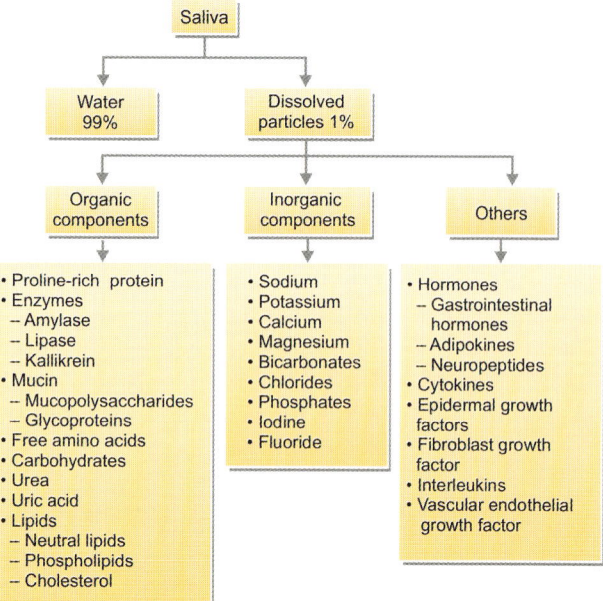

Flowchart 14-1: Composition of saliva.

When parasympathomimetic drug is administered as a stimulus, the saliva produced has high electrolyte levels which are not found in saliva secreted by masticatory or gustatory stimuli.

The whole saliva is composed of 99% of water and the remaining is organic and inorganic substances (**Flowchart 14-1**).

Organic substances mainly comprise wide variety of proteins. As much as 27% of proteins present in the saliva are derived from blood. Many of these proteins contain high levels (35–40%) of proline, and are known as proline-rich proteins (PRP). This PRP are further categorized into acidic, basic, and glycosylated basic PRP. The rest of the protein content is mostly amylase. Apart from amylase, the other enzymes present in the saliva are lingual lipase and kallikrein. Mucin in saliva mainly consists of mucopolysaccharides and glycoproteins. Other minor organic components include lysozyme, lactoferrin, salivary peroxidase, myeloperoxidase, histatin, defensin, cathelicidins, cystatins, agglutinins, and secretory immunoglobulins, mainly IgA (IgG and IgM to smaller extent). Free amino acids, carbohydrates, urea, uric acid, and lipids (neutral, phospholipids, and cholesterol) are also present in minor quantities.

Inorganic constituents of saliva are mainly electrolytes, which include sodium, potassium, calcium, magnesium, bicarbonates, chlorides, phosphates, iodine, and fluoride (concentration of fluoride depends on its level in the drinking water).

Metabolic hormones present in minute quantities in the saliva are gastrointestinal hormones (insulin, vasoactive intestinal peptides, ghrelin and obestatin), adipokines (adiponectin and leptin) and neuropeptides (oxytocin, and nesfatin-1).

In addition, saliva also contains cytokines, EGFs, fibroblast growth factor (FGF), interleukins, and vascular endothelial growth factor (VEGF).

PROPERTIES OF SALIVA

In human adult, saliva produced per day is about 750–1,500 mL. The amount of saliva secreted in females is slightly lesser when compared to males and this is attributed to the female hormonal pattern and smaller glands.

Parotid gland contributes to about 20%, submandibular gland about 65%, sublingual gland 7–8%, and numerous minor glands less than 10% of the unstimulated saliva. As far as the stimulated saliva is concerned, parotid contributes to more than 50% of the total salivary secretions. Stimulated saliva is reported to contribute as much as 80–90% of the average daily salivary production.

Salivary flow rate varies between gland to gland and whether it is stimulated or unstimulated. It also exhibits variation related to the circadian rhythm. The normal salivary flow rate for unstimulated saliva is anything above 0.1 mL per minute. For stimulated saliva, it increases to 0.2 mL per minute. Salivary flow during sleep is almost nil.

pH of resting whole saliva is slightly acidic and varies between 5.75 and 7.05. The pH value increases up to 8 with increasing flow rate. It decreases with decreased salivary flow. Salivary proteins, bicarbonate, and phosphate ions that have considerable buffering capacity also alter the salivary pH.

Viscosity is defined as the resistance to flow. It is related to the thickness. Water has low viscosity but some oils are highly viscous. Viscosity is inversely proportional to diffusion. Though saliva is a watery fluid, its viscosity is not always equal to that of water. The mean viscosity of saliva is about 1.57 ± 0.32 cps at 37°C. It varies from individual to individual and in the same individual at different time periods. Viscosity of the stimulated saliva is lower than that of unstimulated saliva and it decreases with the rate of secretion. Salivary viscosity is related to its mucin content. High-molecular-weight glycoproteins increase the salivary viscosity beyond that of water.

FUNCTIONS OF SALIVA

As enumerated previously, saliva has many important functions to maintain the healthy oral environment, which include protection of the oral cavity, lubrication, aiding in taste perception, mastication and deglutition, digestion, maintenance of tooth integrity, buffering action, antimicrobial action, and speech.

Protection

Saliva protects the oral cavity in number of ways. The continuous flow of saliva keeps the oral mucosa wet and moist, which prevents drying of the oral hard and soft tissues. By its fluid nature, it removes microorganisms, desquamated epithelial cells, leukocytes, and food debris by the swallowing process, and thus prevents halitosis. This flushing action removes the fermentable carbohydrates or reduces their oral retentiveness and thus its availability to the cariogenic microorganisms. By its mucin content, it lubricates the oral soft tissues and prevents their abrasion during movements.

Also it softens the hard food particles, which otherwise would scratch and injure the oral mucosa.

Continuous flow of unstimulated saliva helps to prevent retrograde infection of the salivary glands by preventing the entry of oral microorganisms through the salivary ducts. It safeguards the oral tissues from potentially injurious thermal changes, when very hot or very cold food substance is consumed.

Saliva also has the buffering capacity against acid. But unlike other buffers, after reaction with acid, there is no accumulation of the acidic form of the buffer, because of the presence of carbonic anhydrase VI. Bicarbonate is an ideal buffer present in the saliva. When it reacts with hydrogen ions, it produces carbonic acid. The carbonic anhydrase present in the saliva acts on it and converts it into water and carbon dioxide.

Saliva protects the teeth from attrition, abrasion, and erosion by the salivary pellicle or the acquired enamel pellicle. Salivary pellicle is a thin, acellular, organic film that forms on the tooth surface upon exposure to saliva. It is a protein film formed by selective binding of salivary glycoproteins. Pellicle has been shown to reduce the frictional coefficient between opposing teeth by 20-fold, thus it reduces the damage caused by tooth to tooth contact as well as other mechanical damage caused to the tooth. It helps to prevent erosion (loss of tooth substance caused by chemicals) and acting as a diffusion barrier both to inward movement of hydrogen ions and outward movement of calcium and phosphate ions.

Saliva contains calcium and phosphate ions and is supersaturated with respect to hydroxyapatite. So there would be a tendency for crystals of hydroxyapatite to grow on the tooth surface, which may cause enlargement of the tooth. This is prevented by the salivary pellicle, but at the same time, it is sufficiently permeable to allow calcium and phosphate ions to pass through it and helps in remineralization of early subsurface caries lesions.

Protection against Dental Caries

Calcium, phosphate, and bicarbonate are the major inorganic components present in the saliva, involved in tooth protection. The bicarbonates, phosphates, and other buffers (basic proteins) present in the saliva prevent the fall of salivary pH and initiation of dental caries after the consumption of fermentable carbohydrates. Urea is another important anticariogenic component present in the saliva.

Growth Factors

Saliva contains several signaling molecules, such as EGF, FGF, NGF (nerve growth factor), TGF-α (transforming growth factor- α), trefoil factor, and VEGF that are essential for the regeneration of oral and esophageal mucosa. EGF is in highest concentration in parotid saliva. The esophageal mucosal cells contain luminal receptors for EGF, which can diffuse from the saliva, through the mucous coat of the esophagus, and promote the proliferative activity of the mucosal cells.

Melatonin present in saliva functions as a scavenger of free radicals and acts as an indirect antioxidant.

Antimicrobial Property

Apart from salivary mucins acting as physical barrier, saliva contains a large number of proteins and peptides, which have been shown to possess antibacterial, antiviral, and antifungal effects. Salivary proteins, which possess antimicrobial property, include lysozyme, peroxidase, lactoferrin, and secretory leukocyte protease inhibitor. Apart from IgA, there are a number of bacterial agglutinins in saliva, which agglutinate microorganisms, thereby facilitating their removal by swallowing and possibly inhibiting their attachment to oral surfaces. Histatin, a cationic protein, has been shown to inhibit the growth of *Candida albicans*, an opportunistic fungus. Unstimulated submandibular saliva has been shown to inhibit the HIV-1 virus.

Wound Healing

Saliva plays important roles in the healing of oral wounds. Salivary mucous layer keeps the oral mucosa from becoming desiccated. Antibacterial factors present in saliva are usually sufficient to prevent infection of an oral wound. Various growth factors and biologically active peptides present in the saliva enhance cell growth, differentiation, and repair. VEGF is one of the main angiogenic growth factors and is also involved in reepithelialization and regulation of the extracellular matrix.

Mastication and Deglutition

Saliva wets the food substance and aids in breaking it into smaller particles. These broken down food particles will form a bolus with the help of saliva. By the lubricating property of the saliva, the bolus can easily be swallowed.

Digestion

Saliva contributes to digestion by dissolving the food substances and helps in the formation of bolus to enable swallowing. Presence of digestive enzymes such as α-amylase and lipase starts the digestive process in the oral cavity.

Taste and Smell Perception

To perceive the taste, the substance has to reach the taste buds in a dissolved form. Saliva plays an important role by providing the fluid, which dissolves the solid tastants and takes them to the areas where taste buds are present. The hypotonicity of unstimulated saliva helps in recognizing the taste of salty substances. Some salivary proteins have trophic effect on taste receptors.

The olfactory and taste sense complement each other. Chewing is associated with odor release. Both the chewing process and gustatory stimulation increase salivary flow in an additive manner. The longer chewing period of food bolus extends the time of odor release and the greater will be the incorporation of saliva. A highly liquefied food bolus will also increase the contact area between the bolus and the oral and pharyngeal mucosa, which favors the flavor release.

Speech

Keeping the oral tissues wet and moist, saliva lubricates and helps in speech.

Excretion

Similar to the glands of the pancreas and stomach, salivary glands also have an excretory function, though not to a greater extent. The secreted saliva is not lost but is reabsorbed by the gastrointestinal tract by swallowing. Many substances from the blood reach the saliva since the primary saliva is the ultrafiltrate of the plasma. Saliva excretes the harmful products of bacterial metabolism. It also plays a major role in excretion of drugs hence it can also be used to find the excretion of drugs by using drug monitoring system. Salivary elimination of various compounds, like mercury derivatives, has been known for a long era.

In addition to the above-mentioned functions, saliva helps in creating the thirst sensation, when body is deprived of water. When water level is low, the secretion of saliva stops. This makes the individual feel the dryness of the mouth and creates the desire to drink water.

MAJOR SALIVARY GLANDS

Parotid Gland

The parotid gland, the largest of the salivary glands, is purely serous and weighs about 14.5g. It is wrapped around the mandibular ramus, anterior and inferior to external ear, and occupies parotid space (**Figure 14-21A**). It has a fibrous tissue capsule. The capsule is formed from the investing layer of deep cervical fascia which divides into two laminas to enclose the gland. The superficial lamina is thick and adherent to the gland while the deep lamina is thin. The superficial lamina joins with the epimysium of masseter muscle to create a thick parotid masseteric fascia that is connected superiorly to the zygomatic arch. The thin deep lamina is connected to the tympanic plate and styloid process of the temporal bone; it thickens to form stylomandibular ligament, which divides the parotid from the submandibular gland (**Figure 14-21B**). The gland is divided into lobes and lobules by the connective tissue septa arising from the capsule.

Parotid secretion is released into the oral cavity through Stensen duct, which opens at the buccal mucosa opposite to the maxillary second molar tooth. The length of the duct is about 4–6 cm with a diameter of about 5 mm.

There is abundance of fat in this gland and the amount of fat increases with age. Lymph nodes are found within the gland and its surface, which are not normally seen in other salivary glands. Stromal connective tissue, which divides the parenchyma (secretory portion of the gland) into lobules contain blood vessels, nerves, and large excretory ducts (interlobular). These interlobular ducts are lined by a pseudostratified columnar epithelium. In a well-defined lobule, the secretory acinar cells and ducts are seen. These acinar cells are fairly uniform in size, structure, and staining and produce a watery secretion. The intralobular ducts are in

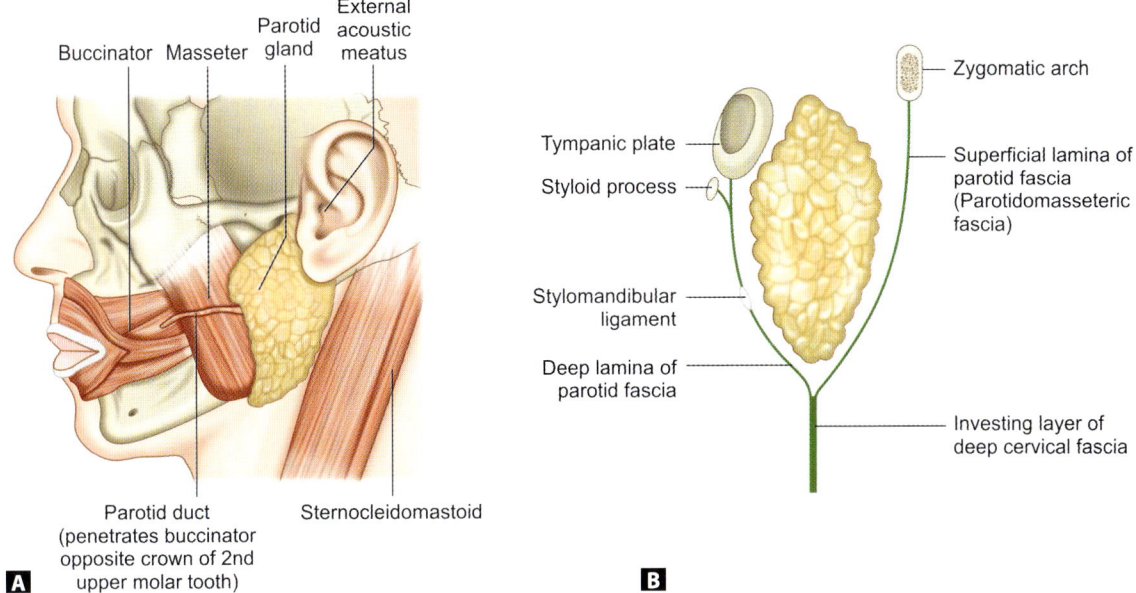

Figures 14-21A and B: Parotid gland and its relations.

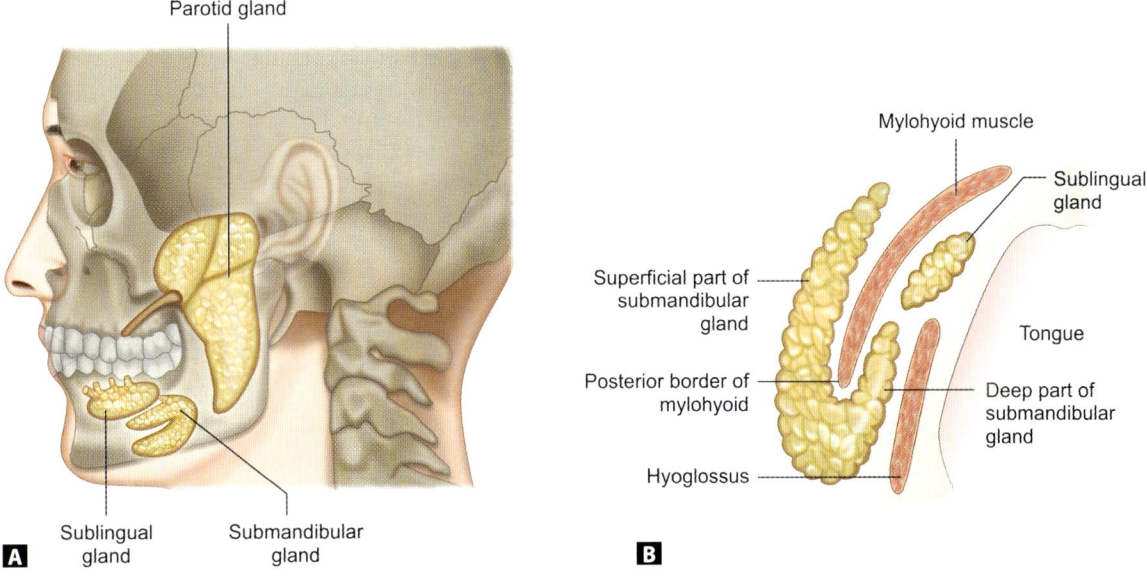

Figures 14-22A and B: Submandibular gland and it relations.

turn, further subdivided into striated and intercalated ducts. The thin, intercalated ducts, which are long and branching, link the secretory acini and striated duct.

In humans, 20% of individuals possess an accessory parotid gland, equipped with its own blood supply, and a secondary excretory duct independent from the main body of the gland.

Submandibular Gland

Submandibular glands, previously referred to as the submaxillary glands, are paired seromucous major glands that lie beneath the floor of the mouth **(Figures 14-22A and B)**. Submandibular gland is 25% of the size of the parotid gland and measures 3–4 cm. The gland is located within the anterior part of the submandibular triangle. Lying superior to the digastric muscles, each submandibular gland is divided into superficial and deep lobes. The superficial portion is large. The deep portion is smaller. The two lobes are continuous with each other and form a "U" shape around the posterior border of mylohyoid muscle. The middle layer of the deep cervical fascia encloses the submandibular gland.

The submandibular gland of humans is predominantly serous. Its mucous acini are frequently capped with a serous demilune, a crescent of serous cells around one or more of their surfaces.

Acinar cells empty their secretion into ductules, which in turn pass it to the submandibular duct (Wharton duct). Wharton duct is the main excretory duct of the submandibular gland, which is approximately 4–5 cm long, running superior to the hypoglossal nerve while inferior to the lingual nerve. It empties the saliva lateral to the lingual frenulum on either side, through a papilla in the floor of the mouth behind the lower incisor tooth, along with the major Bartholin ducts of the sublingual gland.

It is surrounded by a capsule of moderately dense connective tissue, from which septa divide the gland into lobes and lobules. The secretory end pieces consist of a more or less spherical mass of acinar cells.

Acinar cells appear triangular in sections, with their apex directed towards the lumen, and their base resting on a basement membrane. They secrete their product in a merocrine fashion into the lumen. Contractile myoepithelial cells lie between the basement membrane and the plasma membrane of the secretory cells. They are also found in the proximal part of the duct system. Myoepithelial cells possess many actin-containing microfilaments, which squeeze on the secretory cells and move their products toward the excretory ducts.

As mentioned earlier, submandibular gland contains both the serous and mucous acini. Serous cells have a circular nucleus and many secretory granules in their cytoplasm. They are joined near their apical surfaces by junctional complexes. Their secretion is thin, watery, and proteinaceous.

Mucous cells secrete a viscous, glycoprotein-rich product, which is stored as mucinogen granules. They typically look pale and empty in standard histological sections, because their granules get washed away during histological preparation. The nuclei are usually flattened against the base of the cells (unless the cells have just discharged their contents, in which case they look more like serous cells).

Sublingual Gland

They lie anterior to the submandibular gland under the tongue, beneath the mucous membrane of the floor of the mouth **(Figure 14-23)**. They are drained by 8–20 excretory ducts called ducts of Rivinus. The largest duct, the sublingual duct (of Bartholin) joins the submandibular duct to drain through the sublingual caruncle. The sublingual gland consists mostly of mucous acini capped with serous demilunes and is therefore categorized as a mixed gland. Most of the remaining small sublingual ducts open separately into the mouth on an elevated crest of mucous membrane, the plica fimbriata, formed by the gland and located on either side of the frenulum linguae. The chorda tympani nerve is secretomotor to the sublingual glands.

> Three types of ducts in the major salivary glands:
> **Intercalated ducts** are slender ducts continuous with the terminal acini, and lined with flat, spindle-shaped cells.
> **Striated ducts** have eosinophilic cuboidal to columnar cells with basal striations. These result from infoldings of the basal membranes.
> Both intercalated and striated ducts are found within the parenchyma of the gland and are therefore *intralobular ducts*.
> **Excretory ducts** are the largest ducts. They are found in the connective tissue septa, and are therefore *interlobular ducts*. They ultimately open in the oral cavity. Their epithelium is variable, it can be simple cuboidal, stratified cuboidal, stratified columnar or pseudostratified. Near the oral cavity, it becomes stratified squamous.

MINOR SALIVARY GLANDS

The submucosa of the oral cavity and oropharynx is lined extensively by groups of minor salivary glands. The number of minor glands ranges from 600 to 1000 and the size from 1 mm to 5 mm. They are distinguishable from major glands not only in their reduced size and late embryological development but also in their abbreviated ductal systems and paucity of capsular tissues. They contribute to about 8% of the unstimulated and stimulated whole saliva.

Minor salivary glands are classified based on their location. The greatest number of these glands is found in the lips, tongue, buccal mucosa, and palate. They can also be seen along the tonsils, supraglottis, and paranasal sinuses.

- Labial glands are seen in hundreds, lining the upper and lower lips.
- A complex of around 230 palatine salivary glands is seen in the submucosa of posterior hard palate and soft palate.
- The buccal salivary glands include the large molar and retromolar glands.
- The anterior lingual glands include the glands of Blandin and Nuhn, which are seen bilaterally in the anteroinferior part of the tongue on either side of lingual frenum. They are neither lobulated nor encapsulated. Few of them are seen in the tip and anterolateral margins of the tongue.
- The posterior lingual glands are the von Ebner glands, embedded in the lamina propria of circumvallate papillae and to a lesser extent in the foliate papillae on the dorsal

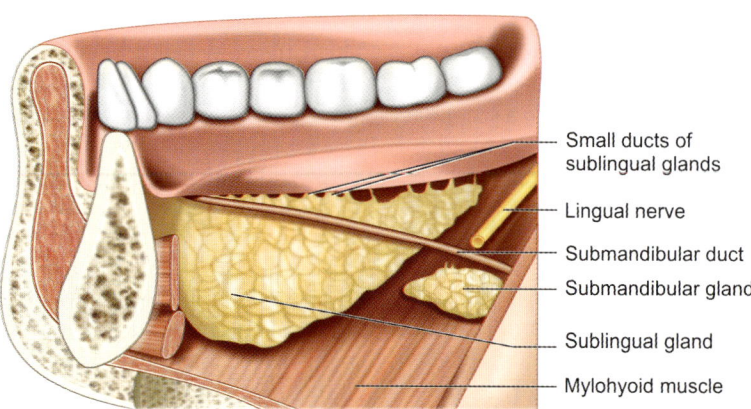

Figure 14-23: Sublingual gland and its relations.

and posterolateral tongue, which drain into the papillary sulci.
- Numerous lingual glands called Weber glands are found in the posterolateral tongue, which drain into the follicular crypts and interfollicular fissures of the lingual tonsil.
- Lastly, incisive salivary gland is seen in the lingual side of the mandibular incisor teeth in the floor of the mouth.

TUBARIAL GLANDS—THE NEW SALIVARY GLAND ORGANS?

Dr. Valstar and his team of researchers have reported in 2020 a new pair of salivary glands in the posterior nasopharynx. These structures were discovered to be present bilaterally in the nasopharynx demonstrating ligand uptake similar to salivary glands, during patient PSMA PET/CT scans. Also, these structures did not fit any known previous anatomical descriptions. Histologically, these glands were made of mucous glandular tissue and draining ducts.

These new salivary gland organs have been named as 'tubarial glands', based on their location above the torus tubarius. It remains to be seen if the glands are classified as minor or major salivary glands.

CLINICAL CONSIDERATIONS

Knowledge of the anatomy and histology of salivary glands and the importance of saliva are essential for a good clinical practice. Pathologies of salivary glands may be developmental, inflammatory, infectious, metabolic, hormonal or neoplastic. Further, salivary glands or the secretion and flow of saliva may be affected in a number of systemic disorders. Salivary glands are present all over the oral cavity except in gingiva, anterior most part of the palate and anterior two-thirds of the dorsum of the tongue. So virtually any part of the oral cavity can develop a salivary gland pathology. However, certain anatomical locations are common for specific lesions. For example, salivary gland neoplasms commonly involve the upper lip and non-neoplastic lesions involve the lower lip.

The most common salivary gland lesion is mucous extravasation cyst **(Figure 14-24)**, caused by the severance of the ducts of the minor salivary glands in the lower lip, resulting in the accumulation of saliva in the submucosal tissue.

Salivary ducts may be blocked by salivary calculi (sialolith), resulting in retention of the formed saliva within the gland, forming a retention cyst or salivary duct cyst. Both extravasation and retention cysts clinically present as soft swellings.

Inflammation of the salivary gland is called sialadenitis, and may be of bacterial or viral origin.

Mumps is a viral infection caused by mumps virus belonging to the paramyxovirus family. It usually affects children and presents as painful swelling of one or both parotid salivary glands. Though highly contagious and can spread rapidly, it is preventable by administrating mumps vaccine.

Oncocytes are eosinophilic cells occurring singly or in groups, in the salivary glands and other glands, the occurrence of which is considered due to aging or degeneration. The eosinophilic granular appearance is due to the increased number of mitochondria.

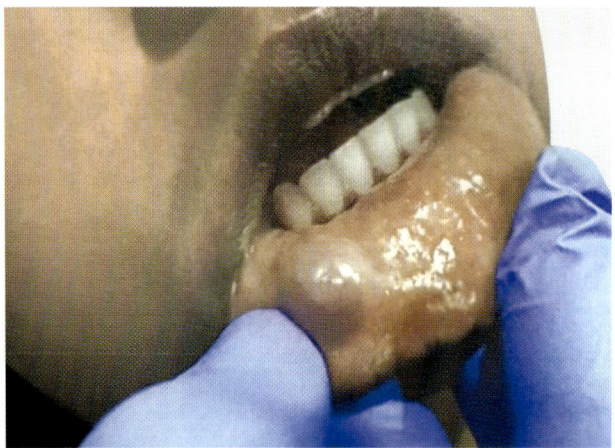

Figure 14-24: Mucous extravasation cyst.
Source: Dr Shyam Sundar, Meenakshi Ammal Dental College, Chennai, India.

Chronic, bilateral, diffuse, non-inflammatory, and non-neoplastic swelling of the major salivary glands is called sialadenosis or sialosis. It primarily affects the parotid glands, but occasionally involves the submandibular glands and rarely the minor salivary glands. This condition is seen in some metabolic disorders.

Enlargement of major salivary glands is common in some autoimmune diseases (Sjögren syndrome and Mikulicz disease).

Normal salivary output per day ranges from 0.75 L to 1.5 L and the major share is contributed by the parotid gland. The amount of saliva secreted in a day depends on many factors, which include psychological status, medication taken, smoking habit, and presence of other systemic disorders. Salivary secretion is usually increased during meal time. Increased salivary secretion is called sialorrhea.

Decrease or absence of salivary secretion and flow results in dry mouth, which is known as xerostomia. This condition may be temporary or permanent. Some common causes for dry mouth include anxiety, stress, chronic smoking, intake of certain medications, aging, radiation therapy for malignant tumors, and autoimmune disorders like Sjögren syndrome and Mikulicz disease. In xerostomia, patient feels dryness or stickiness of the oral mucosa, difficulty in chewing, speaking, and swallowing. Inflammation of the oral mucosa leads to burning sensation and increased incidence of dental caries.

During aging, there is reduction in the salivary secretion due to the gradual replacement of salivary parenchyma with fatty tissue.

Tumors may also affect salivary glands. 65% of the salivary gland tumors are benign. Pleomorphic adenoma is the most common benign salivary gland tumor and mucoepidermoid carcinoma is the common malignant tumor.

Saliva may be used as an important diagnostic tool for variety of systemic diseases. In toxicology, it is used to determine the concentration of lithium, cadmium, and gallium. It is also used to determine the alcohol content.

It has an application in forensic odontology. For example, DNA may be retrieved from the shed epithelial cells from the saliva and may be used for personal identification.

Points to Remember

- Glands are modified epithelial structures specialized to produce, release and transport macromolecules, ions, water into its surrounding environment, to carry out useful body functions. Salivary glands are multicellular, exocrine, merocrine, and tubuloacinar glands, located inside and outside the mouth and secreting saliva. Salivary glands are classified as major and minor, with three pairs of major salivary glands, namely parotid, submandibular and sublingual glands and around 600–1000 minor salivary glands distributed throughout the oral cavity except gingiva, anterior most part of the palate and anterior two-thirds of the dorsum of the tongue.
- According to the type of secretion, salivary glands are classified into serous, mucous and mixed. **Serous glands** secrete serous fluid, which contains water, enzymes, a variety of salts and organic ions, e.g., parotid gland. **Mucous glands** secrete relatively thick fluid that contains mucin, which acts as a lubricant to aid in the mastication, deglutition and digestion, e.g., glossopalatine, palatine glands. **Mixed glands** are those in which the serous cells form demilunes over the mucous acini, e.g., submandibular glands, with a seromucous secretion.
- Salivary glands originate from an epithelial placode between 4th and 12th weeks of embryonic development. The origin of the epithelial buds is believed to be ectodermal in the parotid and minor salivary glands and endodermal in the submandibular and sublingual glands.
- Histologically, salivary glands are well-encapsulated structures containing secretory end pieces/units/acini (serous/mucous/mixed), myoepithelial cells, and other cells, continuous with a ductal system made of striated ducts, intercalated ducts, and excretory ducts, and a connective tissue stroma separating the gland into lobules and lobes.
- The initial fluid or the primary saliva secreted by the acinar cells is similar to the ultrafiltrate of plasma in terms of its osmotic concentration of sodium, potassium, and chloride. In addition to conveying saliva from the secretory end pieces to the oral cavity, an important function of the striated and excretory ducts is modification of the primary saliva produced by the end pieces and intercalated ducts, through reabsorption and secretion of electrolytes. The final electrolyte composition of saliva varies, depending on the salivary flow rate.
- In human adult, saliva produced per day is about 750–1,500 mL. Parotid gland contributes to about 20%, submandibular gland about 65%, sublingual gland 7–8%, and numerous minor glands less than 10% of the unstimulated saliva. Saliva has many important functions to maintain the healthy oral environment, which include protection of the oral cavity, lubrication, aiding in taste perception, mastication and deglutition, digestion, maintenance of tooth integrity, buffering action, antimicrobial action, and speech.
- Knowledge of the anatomy and histology of salivary glands and the importance of saliva are essential for a good clinical practice. Pathologies of salivary glands may be developmental, inflammatory, infectious or neoplastic. Further, salivary glands or the secretion and flow of saliva may be affected in a number of systemic disorders.

PRACTICE QUESTIONS

1. Classify salivary glands. Compare and discuss the histology of major salivary glands in detail, with suitable diagrams.
2. Discuss in detail the development of salivary glands.
3. Compare and contrast the salient features of mucous and serous acini.
4. Discuss the ductal architecture of major salivary glands.
5. Describe the minor salivary glands in detail.
6. Describe the secretion and ductal modification of saliva.
7. Write notes on the composition, properties, and functions of saliva.
8. Discuss in detail the histology of myoepithelial cells.

MULTIPLE CHOICE QUESTIONS

1. **Which of the following correctly describes the structure of the major salivary glands?**
   a. Simple tubular gland
   b. Compound acinar gland
   c. Simple tubuloacinar gland
   d. Compound tubulocinar gland
2. **The crescents or demilunes of the mucous acini of sublingual gland are composed of which of the following cells?**
   a. Mucous cells
   b. Serous cells
   c. Myoepithelial cells
   d. Ductal cells
3. **Which of the following glands is predominantly mucous?**
   a. Parotid gland
   b. Submandibular gland
   c. Sublingual gland
   d. von Ebner glands
4. **Salivary, sweat, sebaceous, and von Ebner's glands all have in common the characteristic of being**
   a. Apocrine glands
   b. Merocrine glands
   c. Holocrine glands
   d. Paracrine glands
5. **The apical cytoplasm of active serous glandular cells is typically filled with which of the following?**
   a. Large amount of DNA
   b. Abundance of ribosomes
   c. Abundance of mitochondria
   d. Abundance of zymogen granules
6. **Striated ducts of major salivary glands are composed of which of the following types of epithelium?**
   a. Simple cuboidal
   b. Simple columnar
   c. Stratified squamous
   d. Pseudostratified ciliated columnar
7. **Which of the following are pure serous glands?**
   a. Glands of Blandin-Nuhn
   b. Glands of Brunner
   c. Glands of von Ebner
   d. Labial glands
8. **The major duct of sublingual salivary gland is**
   a. Wharton duct
   b. Stensen duct
   c. Bartholin duct
   d. Ducts of Rivinus

9. The acid neutralizing substance in the saliva is:
    a. NH_2
    b. Carbonate
    c. Bicarbonate
    d. Chlorides
10. The glands of Blandin and Nuhn are:
    a. Posterior lingual glands
    b. Anterior lingual glands
    c. Glossopalatine glands
    d. Palatine glands
11. After the ductal modification, the salivary secretion, compared to plasma, becomes:
    a. Hypertonic, sometimes
    b. Hypotonic
    c. Isotonic
    d. Hypertonic, always
12. Tuft cells are receptors seen in:
    a. Cell-rich zone
    b. Salivary duct
    c. Sinus lining
    d. TMJ capsule
13. Which of the following are pure mucous glands?
    a. Glossopalatine and palatine glands
    b. Labial and buccal glands
    c. Glands of von Ebner
    d. Lingual glands
14. Which structure listed below is a functional unit in salivary glands?
    a. Adenomere
    b. Lobule
    c. Lobe
    d. Salivon
15. Which of the following salivary gland ducts shows basal cell membrane foldings with radically arranged mitochondria?
    a. Intercalated ducts
    b. Excretory ducts
    c. Striated ducts
    d. Lobar ducts
16. Compressed nuclei pushed towards the basal aspect of the cell is seen in:
    a. Striated ducts
    b. Intercalated ducts
    c. Mucous acinar cells
    d. Serous acinar cells
17. Glands which secrete products that influence the secretion of another product by local gland or cell (products act on neighboring cells) are:
    a. Exocrine glands
    b. Endocrine glands
    c. Paracrine glands
    d. Autocrine glands
18. The epithelial buds are believed to be of ectodermal origin in?
    a. Parotid gland
    b. Submandibular gland
    c. Sublingual gland
    d. Minor salivary glands
19. Which of the following ducts are not usually identified under light microscopy?
    a. Striated ducts
    b. Intercalated ducts
    c. Excretory ducts
    d. Terminal excretory ducts
20. Which of the following salivary gland cells are characterized by the presence of actin filaments and soluble myosin?
    a. Mucous acinar cells
    b. Myoepithelial cells
    c. Serous acinar cells
    d. Intercalated duct cells
21. Decreased salivary secretion is seen in:
    a. Sialorrhea
    b. Xerostomia
    c. Sialosis
    d. Sialadenosis

ANSWERS

1. d 2. b 3. c 4. b 5. d 6. b 7. c 8. c 9. c 10. b 11. b 12. b 13. a 14. d 15. c
16. c 17. c 18. a 19. b 20. b 21. b

ACKNOWLEDGMENTS

Gifrina Jayaraj, Hannah Grace, Sakthi Samyuktha Prabhakaran, Uma Kannan, Sandhya, and Abilasha Ramasubramanian.

BIBLIOGRAPHY

1. Animireddy D, Bekkem VTR, Vallala P, et al. Evaluation of pH, buffering capacity, viscosity and flow rate levels of saliva in caries-free, minimal caries and nursing caries children: an in vivo study. Contemp Clin Dent. 2014;5(3):324-8.
2. Ball WD. Development of the rat salivary glands. III. Mesenchymal specificity in the morphogenesis of the embryonic submaxillary and sublingual glands of the rat. J Exp Zool. 1974;188:277.
3. Barka T. Biologically active polypeptides in submandibular glands. J Histochem Cytochem. 1980;28:836.
4. Bhaskar SN. Synopsis of oral pathology, 5th edition. St. Louis: The CV Mosby Co; 1977.
5. Bradley RM. Essentials of Oral Physiology, 1st edition. USA: Mosby; 1995.
6. Carlson ER, Ord R. Textbook and color atlas of salivary gland pathology: diagnosis and management, 1st edition. Singapore: Willy-Blackwell; 2008.
7. Cawson RA, Odell EW. Essentials of oral pathology and oral medicine, 6th edition. UK: Churchill Livingstone; 1998.
8. Chiappin S, Antonelli G, Gatti R, et al. Saliva specimen: a new laboratory tool for diagnostic and basic investigation. Clin Chim Acta. 2007;383:30-40.
9. Cohen B, Kramer IRH. Scientific Foundation of Dentistry, 1st edition. Great Britain: Letterpress; 1976.

10. Coughlin, M.D. Early development of parasympathetic nerves in the mouse submandibular gland. Dev. Biol. 1975, 43, 123–139
11. Cutler LS, Gremski W. Epithelial-mesenchymal interaction in the development of salivary gland. Crit Rev Oral Biol Med. 1991;2(1):1.
12. de Almeida PDV, Grégio AMT, Machado MÂN, et al. Saliva composition and functions: a comprehensive review. J Contemp Dent Pract. 2008;(9)3:072-080.
13. Dobrosielski-Vergona, K. Biology of the Salivary Glands; CRC Press, Taylor & Francis Group: Abingdon, UK, 1993; ISBN 978-0849388477.
14. Dodds MW, Johnson DA, Yeh CK. Health benefits of saliva: a review. J Dent. 2005;33:223-33.
15. Egdar WM. Saliva: its secretion, composition and function. Br Dent J. 1992;172:305-12.
16. Ferguson DB. Oral Bioscience, 1st edition. UK: Churchill Livingstone; 1999.
17. Ferguson MM, Barker MJ. Saliva substitutes in the management of salivary gland dysfunction. Adv Drug Deliv Rev. 1994;13:151-9.
18. Hand AR, Ball WD. Ultrastructural immunocytochemical localization of secretory proteins in autophagic vacuoles of parotid acinar cells of starved rats. J Oral Pathol. 1988;17: 279-86.
19. Hand AR. Synthesis of secretory and plasma membrane glycoproteins by striated duct cells of rat salivary glands as visualized by radioautography after 3H-fucose injection. Anat Rec. 1979;195:317-39.
20. Hansson HA, Tunhall S. Epidermal growth factor and insulin- like growth factor I are localized in different compartments of salivary gland duct cells. Immunohistochemical evidence. Acta Physiol Scand. 1988;134:383-9.
21. Ichikawa M, Sasaki K, Ichikawa A. Immunocytochemical localization of amylase in gerbil salivary gland acinar cells processed by rapid freezing and freeze-substitution fixation. J Histochem Cytochem. 1989;37:185-94.
22. Kaufman DL, Lamster B. The diagnostic application of saliva. Crit Rev Oral Biol Med. 2002;13:197-212.
23. Khurana A, Khurana I. Human embryology, 2nd edition. New Delhi: CBS Publishers and Distributor (P) Ltd; 2012.
24. Kumar GS. Orban's Oral Histology & Embryology, 14th edition. India: Elsevier India (P) Ltd; 2015.
25. Kusy RP, Schafer DL. Rheology of stimulated whole saliva in a typical pre-orthodontic sample population. J Mater Med. 1995;6:385-9.
26. Kwon HR, Nelson DA, DeSantis KA, Morrissey JM, Larsen M. Endothelial cell regulation of salivary gland epithelial patterning. Development 2017, 144, 211–220.
27. Lamkin MS, Oppenheim FG. Structural features of salivary function. Crit Rev Oral Biol Med. 1993;4(3-4):251-9.
28. Liang T, Cascieri MA. Substance P receptor on parotid cell membranes. J Neurosci. 1981;1:1133-41.
29. Looms D, Tritsaris K, Pedersen AM, et al. Nitric oxide signaling in salivary glands. J Oral Pathol Med. 2002;31:569-84.
30. Mandel ID. Sialochemistry in diseases and clinical situations affecting salivary glands. Crit Rev Clin Lab Sci. 1980;12:321-66.
31. Mandel ID. The diagnostic uses of saliva. J Oral Pathol Med. 1990;19:119-25.
32. Mandel ID. The role of saliva in maintaining oral homeostasis. J Am Dent Assoc. 1989;119:298-304.
33. McVicar AJ, Greenwood CR, Fewell F, et al. Evaluation of anxiety, salivatory cortisol and melatonin secretion following reflexology treatment: a pilot study in healthy individuals. Complement Ther Clin Pract. 2007;13:137-45.
34. Mese H, Matsuo R. Salivary secretion, taste and hyposalivation. J Oral Rehabil. 2007;34:711-23.
35. Miles TS, Nauntofte B, Svensson P. Clinical oral physiology, 1st edition. Copenhagen: Quintessence Publishing Co Ltd; 2004.
36. Nagler RM, Hershkovich O. Relationships between age, drugs, oral sensorial complaints and salivary profile. Arch Oral Biol. 2005;50:7-16.
37. Neville B, Douglas DD, Allen C, et al. Oral and maxillofacial pathology, 1st South Asia edition. India: Elsevier; 2016.
38. Pagella P, Jimeìnez-Rojo L, Mitsiadis TA. Roles of innervation in developing and regenerating orofacial tissues. Cell Mol Life Sci. 2014, 2014;71:2241–51.
39. Pedessen AM, Bandow A, Jensen GB, et al. Saliva and gastrointestinal functions of taste, mastication, swallowing and digestion. Oral Dis. 2002;8:117-29.
40. Percival RS, Challacombe SJ, Marsh PD. Flow rates of resting whole and stimulated parotid saliva in relation to age and gender. J Dent Res. 1994;73:1416-20.
41. Preetha A, Banerjee R. Composition of artificial saliva substituent. Trends Biomater Artif Organs. 2005;18(2):178-86.
42. Schenkels LC, Veerman EC, Nieuw Amerongen AV. Biochemical composition of human saliva in relation to other mucosal fluids. Crit Rev Oral Biol Med. 1995;6:161-75.
43. Schroeder HE. Oral structural biology, 4th edition. New York: Thieme; 1991.
44. Ship JA. Diagnosing, managing, and preventing salivary gland disorders. Oral Dis. 2002;8:77-89.
45. Sivapathasundharam B. Manual of salivary gland diseases, 1st edition. New Delhi: Jaypee Brothers Medical Publishers (P) Ltd; 2014.
46. Sivapathasundharam B. Shafer's Textbook of Oral Pathology, 8th edition. India: Elsevier; 2016.
47. Soames JV, Southam JC. Oral pathology, 3rd edition. New York: Oxford; 1999.
48. Streckfus C. Saliva as a diagnostic fluid. Oral Dis. 2002;8:69.
49. Turner RJ, Sugiya H. Understanding salivary fluid and protein secretion. Oral Dis. 2002;8(1):3-11.
50. Valstar MH, et al The tubarial salivary glands: A potential new organ at risk for radiotherapy. Radiother Oncol. 2021;154: 292-298.
51. Van Nieuw Amerongen A, Bolscher JG, Veerman EC. Salivary proteins: protective and diagnostic value in cariology? Caries Res. 2004;38:247-53.
52. Vigneswaran N, Haneke E, Hornstein OP. A comparative lectin histochemical study of major and minor salivary glands with special reference to the labial glands. Arch Oral Biol. 1989;34:739.
53. Walker JL, Menko AS, Khalil S, Rebustini I, Hoffman MP, Kreidberg JA, Kukuruzinska MA. Diverse roles of E-cadherin in the morphogenesis of the submandibular gland: Insights into the formation of acinar and ductal structures. Dev. Dyn. 2008;23:3128–41.
54. Wang SL, Zhao ZT, Li J, et al. Investigation of the clinical value of total saliva flow rates. Archives of Oral Biology. 1998;43: 39-43.
55. Zolotukhin S. Metabolic hormones in saliva: origins and functions. Oral Dis. 2013;19(3):219-29.
56. Zussman E, Yarin AL, Nagler RM. Age- and flow-dependency of salivary viscoelasticity. J Dent Res. 2007;86(3):281-5.

CHAPTER

15

Temporomandibular Joint

B Sivapathasundharam, Gururaj N

CHAPTER OUTLINE

- Development of Temporomandibular Joint 242
  - » Postnatal Development and Modification 243
- Gross Anatomy and Microscopic Structure of the Temporomandibular Joint 243
  - » Articulating Surfaces 243
- » Ligaments of Temporomandibular Joint 247
- » Otomandibular Ligaments 248
- Blood Supply 248
- Nerve Supply 248
- Functions of Temporomandibular Joint 248
- Clinical Considerations 249

The temporomandibular joint (TM joint or TMJ) is a condyloid variety of diarthrodial joint. It is also known as craniomandibular joint and are anatomically two joints, connecting the lower jaw bone to the skull but function as a single joint. It is classified as compound joint, since three bones are involved in forming the joint. It forms bilateral synovial articulation between the temporal bone of the skull above and the condyle of the mandible below and hence called temporomandibular joint **(Figures 15-1A and B)**.

This joint is unique to mammals, because a single bone, the mandible forms the lower jaw, which articulates with the temporal bone of the skull. In other vertebrates, the lower jaw is a composite one by having teeth bearing bone and articular bone. The compound lower jaw is converted to a single bone as mandible, during the evolution in mammals.

Mandible is one of the earliest bones to develop in the body, having the condyle at articulating surfaces, which lies at the same level on right and left side and articulates with mandibular fossa of temporal bone of the skull. The morphology of the mandible is such that the body bends horizontally back and ascends vertically upward as ramus at the same level on the right and left side and possesses two joints having similar morphology and function **(Figure 15-2)**.

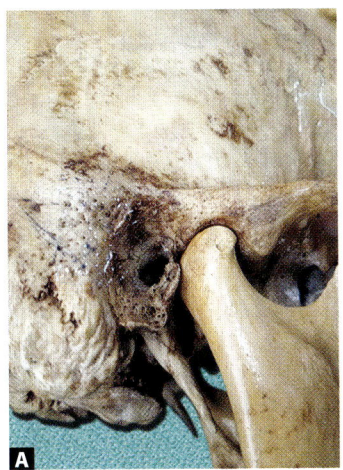
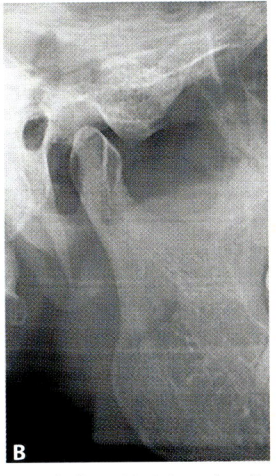

Figures 15-1A and B: (A) Lateral view of the TM joint showing relationship of the mandible to the skull by TM joint; (B) TMJ radiograph showing glenoid fossa, mandibular condyle and the articular eminence.

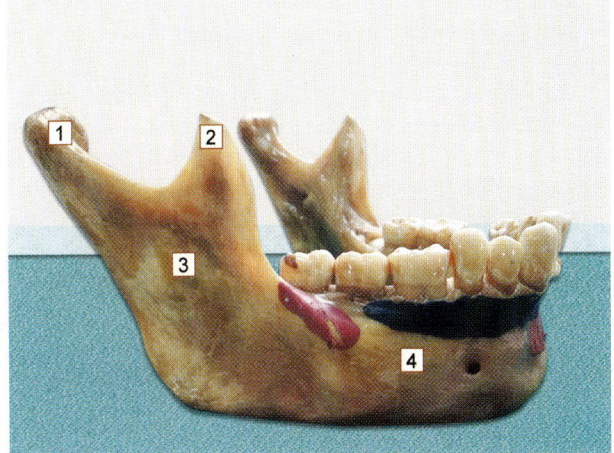

Figure 15-2: Mandible showing its components namely condylar process (1), coronoid process (2), ramus (3), and the body (4).

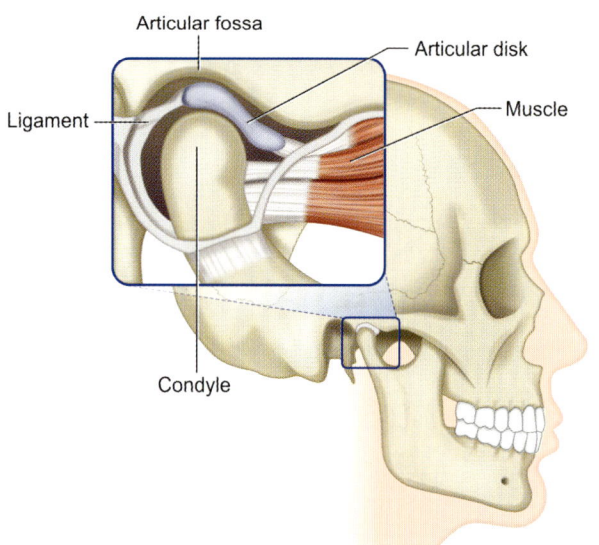

Figure 15-3: Temporomandibular joint showing its upper and lower articulating surfaces with central articular disk.

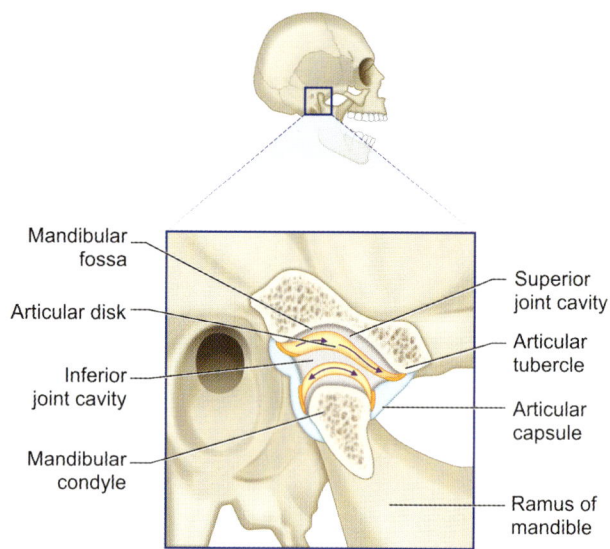

Figure 15-4: Joint cavity with its components.

The movements like protrusion, retrusion, elevation, depression, and side to side movements are possible at both the ends at a time. Between the articular surfaces of the condyle and the mandibular fossa of the temporal bone lies a dense fibrous connective tissue disk, called meniscus or intra-articular disk **(Figure 15-3)**. The TM joint is one of the few synovial joints in the human body with an articular disk.

Mandible has both synarthrodial (teeth in socket-gomphosis) and diarthrodial synovial joints. Thus, there are totally 18 joints in the mandible, i.e., 16 gomphosis and two TM joints. The components of the TM joint include the joint capsule, articular disk, mandibular condyle, mandibular fossa of the temporal bone, temporomandibular ligament, stylomandibular ligament, sphenomandibular ligament, and lateral pterygoid muscle.

Ligaments, muscles, and fibrous capsule associated with the TM joint stabilize it functionally. The synovial fluid, a viscous liquid secreted by the synovial membrane, lubricates the joint surfaces and enables smooth movement. The masticatory movement in humans is not restricted only to the hinge movement as in carnivores, but includes protrusive, retrusive, lateral movements, and combinations of the above three.

Temporomandibular joint differs from other joints by the following features namely, the joint cavity is divided into two (upper and lower) by the intra-articular disk **(Figure 15-4)**, articular surfaces which are not composed of hyaline cartilage, instead by a sturdy avascular fibrous tissue and the secondary condylar cartilage is present in the head of the condyle until adolescence. The shape and the movements of the TM joint are influenced by the presence of teeth.

DEVELOPMENT OF TEMPOROMANDIBULAR JOINT

The TM joint develops by three stages namely blastemic, cavitation, and maturation stages. Development of TM joint takes place between 8th week and 14th week of intrauterine (IU) life.

In the blastemic stage the glenoid fossa and condylar blastema (blastema is a group of undifferentiated cells that proliferate and differentiate to form the required parts of the organs) develops, and in the cavitation stage the lower joint space develops, and in the maturation stage, the upper joint space develops and continue to form till the birth. The contribution of Meckel's cartilage, which is present during this time is nil. The first evidence of TM joint development is the appearance of the glenoid or temporal blastema and condylar blastema, the two distinct mesenchymal condensations, **(Figure 15-5)**.

The temporal blastema appears somewhat earlier than the condylar blastema, and ossification first occurs in the temporal blastema. Condylar blastema develops from the condensation of the mesenchyme at the 8th week of IU life. A slit or cleft appears immediately above the condensed mesenchyme of the condylar blastema, which becomes the inferior joint cavity. At the dorsal end of the ossifying mandibular arch, the condyle develops as a cap of condylar cartilage. It rapidly increases in size posteriorly and laterally during 10th to 12th week. Ossification of the temporal portion of the TM joint begins from the temporal blastema at 8th week of IU life dorsal to the condyle and proceeds in an anterior direction. This forms a primitive temporal fossa at about 10th week. Condylar cartilage grows into it. After 10th week, another slit appears in relation to temporal ossification and forms the superior joint cavity. The intervening mesenchyme becomes the articular disk at about 14th week. Mesenchyme surrounding this area forms the fibrous capsule of the joint.

All the joint structures are formed at 14th week and after that, only topographical modifications occur. After 16th week, the articulating surface of the condyle shows a three-layered structure composed of fibrous connective tissue layer, a cell-rich intermediate layer, and a thick chondroblast layer. Endochondral ossification begins below this chondroblastic layer. The thick chondroblastic layer becomes narrower as the ossification of the condyle progresses outward.

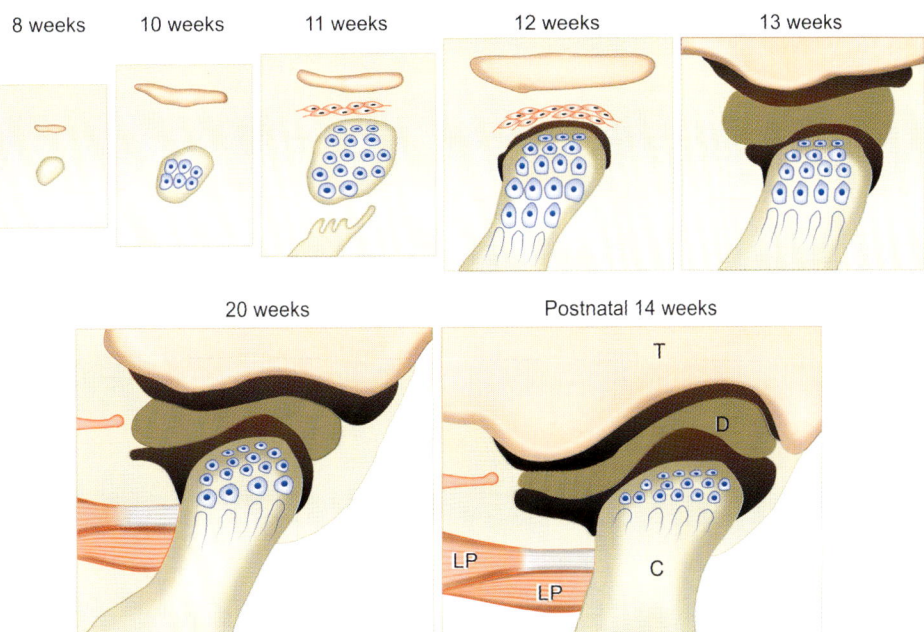

Figure 15-5: Development of temporomandibular joint.
(T: temporal bone, D: disk; C: condyle; LP: lateral pterygoid)

Postnatal Development and Modification

Temporomandibular joint is small and flat at birth. It grows progressively and becomes almost double the size at the age of 20 years and the size remains unchanged till old age. The temporal portion of the joint, which is flat at birth, undergoes considerable modifications between the ages of 12 years and 15 years. The rudimentary articular eminence increases in height and the articular fossa becomes deeper.

The three-layered structure of the condyle is irregular at birth. The cartilage layer is quite thick. The thickness becomes reduced to 0.5 mm in the first 6 months and decreases further to 0.3 mm. The trilayered condylar tissue becomes more regular and remains so till 18 years. After this, the chondroblastic layer disappears completely. The articular disk, which is relatively flat at birth, becomes biconcave shape with the growth of the articular eminence. Further the disk becomes cell-poor and collagen-rich. At birth, the internal parts of the joint are richly vascular. The vascularity decreases rapidly during first 6 months and at a slower rate thereafter.

GROSS ANATOMY AND MICROSCOPIC STRUCTURE OF THE TEMPOROMANDIBULAR JOINT

The components of the TM joint include condyle of the mandible, mandibular fossa or glenoid fossa of the temporal bone, articular disk, TM joint capsule, temporomandibular ligament, stylomandibular ligament, sphenomandibular ligament, and lateral pterygoid muscle (**Figures 15-6A and B**).

Articulating Surfaces

Condyle of the Mandible

The mandible is the largest, strongest, and only movable bone of the skull (other than ossicles of the middle ear) that forms the lower jaw. The mandible is made up of ramus and the body. It has three processes namely alveolar process, coronoid process, and condylar process. Alveolar processes of the body of the mandible hold the teeth. Coronoid process of the ramus of the mandible gives attachment to the fibers of the masseter and temporalis, and the condylar process forms an integral part of the TM joint.

The condyle is that part of mandible that forms the joint and has head and neck portion. The head of the condyle has two poles namely medial and lateral poles. The articular component of the mandible includes head of the mandible, neck of the mandible, and pterygoid fovea (**Figure 15-7**).

The head of the condyle is convex in all aspects and it is wider mediolaterally than anteroposteriorly. When viewed from above it is roughly ovoid in outline. The appearance of the mandibular condyle varies greatly among different age-groups and individuals. The medial surface is wider than the lateral. At the lateral extremity of the condyle is a small tubercle for the attachment of the temporomandibular ligament. The articular surface of the head of the condyle is covered by fibrous tissue and synovial membrane.

The constricted portion, which connects the head of the condyle with the ramus is called neck of the mandible. The TM joint capsule is attached to the entire circumference of the neck of the condyle. Pterygoid fovea is a small depression located on the anterior surface of the neck of the mandible to which the inferior head of the lateral pterygoid muscle is attached.

Histology: Mature TM joint differs from immature joint, since the postnatal development phase is long. The bulk of the condyle is made up of cancellous bone with a thin layer of compact bone covering. The trabeculae of the cancellous bone of the condyle are arranged in such a way that they fan out from the neck of the mandible to reach the surface at

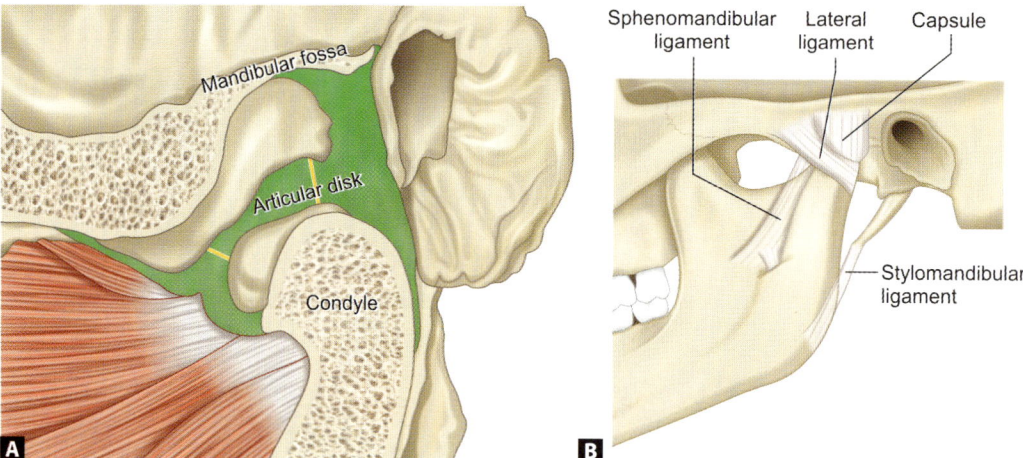

Figures 15-6A and B: (A) Temporomandibular joint showing condyle of the mandible, mandibular fossa or glenoid fossa of the temporal bone and articular disk; (B) Temporomandibular joint showing capsule, temporomandibular ligament, stylomandibular ligament, and sphenomandibular ligament.

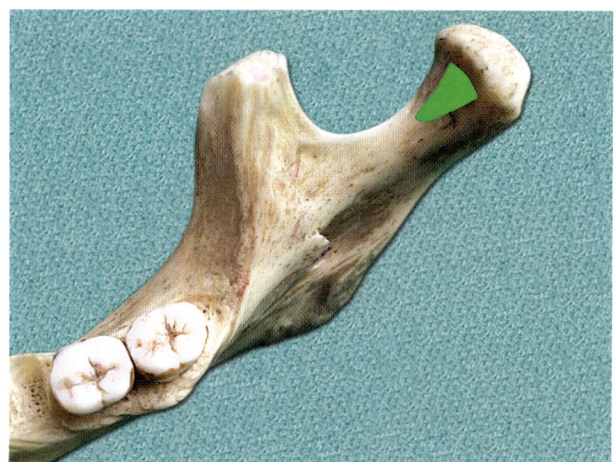

Figure 15-7: Condyle of the mandible showing pterygoid fovea.

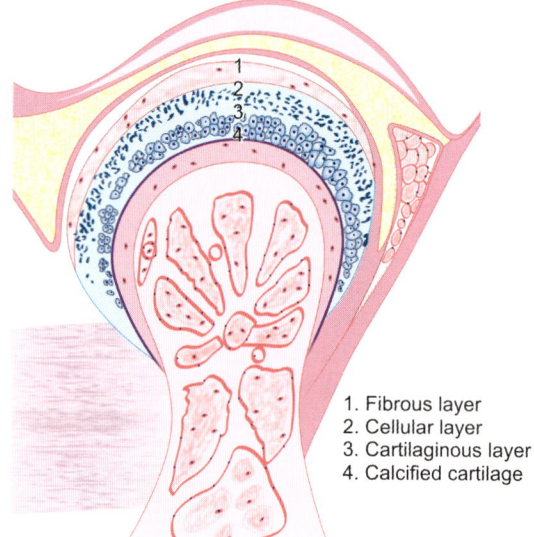

Figure 15-8: Mandibular condyle showing thin compact bone lining with central cancellous region.

right angles. The marrow tissue in between the trabeculae is myeloid or cellular type **(Figure 15-8)**.

In a growing joint, a four-layered structure can be appreciated. This four-layered structure from the lower joint cavity toward the center of the condyle consists of the fibrous connective tissue layer, the cell-rich proliferative layer, a hyaline cartilage layer, and the zone of endochondral ossification **(Figure 15-8)**.

The superficial fibrous layer of the articular surface is uniform in thickness and predominantly composed of collagen fibers and few elastic fibers. The collagen fibers at the superficial portion are wavy and arranged parallel to the surface in anteroposterior direction. In deeper portion they are vertical. Fibroblasts lie in between them and also in the surface. At the periphery, the fiber bundles of this layer are continuous with the periosteum.

The next layer is the cell-rich proliferative layer, which provides source of cells to replenish the adjacent layers. Its superficial portion contains many slender, ovoid, undifferentiated cells with increased mitotic activity. Deeper portion of this layer contains cells that have differentiated into prechondroblasts. This layer provides growth potential for the condyle. In adult condyle, this layer is thin, often incomplete, patchy or even absent.

The third layer is made up of hyaline cartilage and contains chondroblasts and chondrocytes, and is irregular. The same layer in adult condyle is made up of fibrous tissue with rounded cells, which appear like cartilage cells. So this layer in adult is called fibrocartilaginous layer.

In the deeper fourth layer the pericellular matrix of the cartilage layer becomes calcified. This calcified cartilage is the remnant of the secondary condylar cartilage.

Glenoid Fossa or Mandibular Fossa

It forms the cranial component, which is an ovoid depression found in the inferior aspect of base of the skull in the temporal bone immediately anterior to the external acoustic meatus. Similar to the condyle, its mediolateral dimension is more than the anteroposterior one. Into this depression the mandibular condyle fits, however the shape of the mandibular fossa does

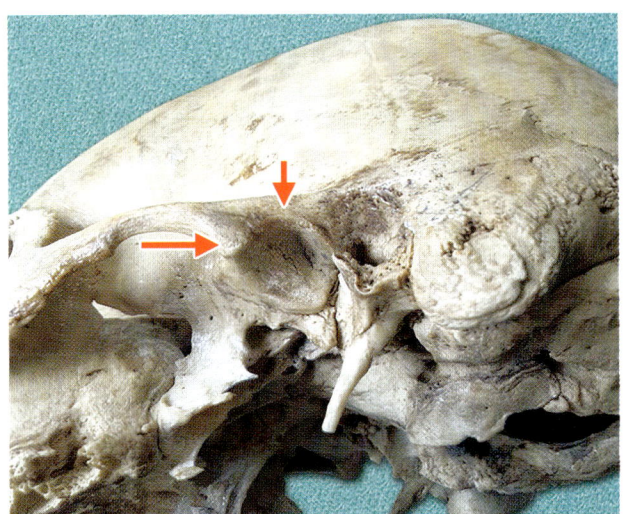

Figure 15-9: Base of the skull. Short arrow showing the mandibular fossa and long arrow showing articular eminence.

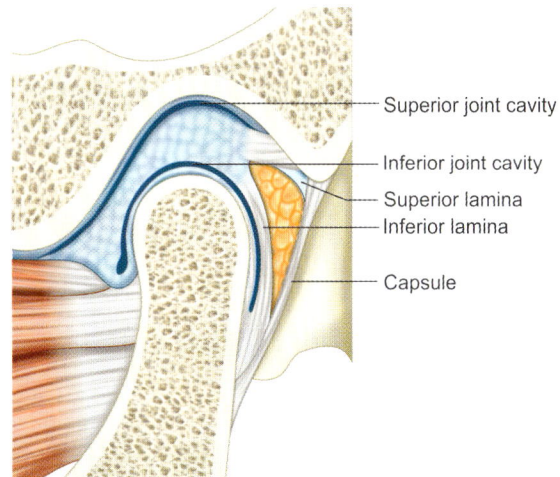

Figure 15-10: Schematic representation showing articular disk and its relations.

not conform to the shape of the condyle. The glenoid fossa has various components and boundaries. It is bounded by the articular eminence anteriorly, zygomatic process laterally, and tympanic plate posteriorly **(Figure 15-9)**. Entire mandibular fossa does not form part of the joint. Mandibular fossa that lies anterior to tympanic plate and the anterior portion of petrotympanic and petrosquamous fissures alone forms the joint.

Anterior or Articular Eminence

It is a small, raised bony protuberance, which forms the root of the zygomatic bone or projection at the anterior part of the mandibular fossa. Sometimes the articular eminence contains air-filled cavities similar to mastoid bone. The lateral ligament of the joint is attached to it **(Figure 15-9)**. The condyle and disk has to ride over this area during opening and closing movements of the jaw. A preglenoid plane is that part of articular surface continuing anteriorly from the anterior eminence. The articulating surface of mandibular fossa and eminence is in the form of an "S".

Postglenoid Process

Anterior to the external acoustic meatus, an elevated bony triangular ridge forms posterior part of glenoid fossa. The structure, which connects the articular tubercle and postglenoid process, forms the lateral margin or border for the glenoid fossa. Toward the medial aspect of the fossa, a bony wall called entoglenoid process narrows the fossa further. The roof of the glenoid fossa is flat and a protruding inferior edge of tegmen tympani divides the tympanosquamous suture into petrosquamosal suture in front and petrotympanic fissure behind.

The glenoid fossa is made up of thin compact bone. The articular eminence is composed of cancellous bone with a compact bony cortex. The covering layer, typical of the adult condyle, is also found in the articulating surface of the temporal bone. The mandibular fossa of the temporal bone is covered by a thin layer of fibrous tissue and synovial membrane. The articular eminence and its posterior slope contain both the fibrous covering and a layer of fibrocartilage. The cell-rich proliferative layer appears in spots.

Articular Disk (Meniscus)

It is also called meniscus, and is made up of a thick fibrous connective tissue that divides the joint into two compartments (*i.e* superior and inferior joint cavities) and acts a s a shock absorber due to its cushioning effect. It lies in between condyle of mandible and glenoid fossa **(Figure 15-10)**. On an average, the TMJ disk in an adult human is 19 mm long and 13 mm wide. It is saddle-shaped or oval-shaped with its concave surface covering the condyle and convex surface in contact to glenoid fossa. When viewed in sagittal section, the upper surface is concavo-convex from anterior to posterior. The thickness of the disk varies. It is thinnest at the center (about 1 mm) and thickest posteriorly (about 3 mm). Also the lateral half is thinner than the medial half. It has anterior and posterior extensions with thin intermediate zone. There is a still posterior bilaminar region, which has two extensions called retrodiscal laminae. The space between the upper and lower laminae is filled with retrodiscal tissue or pad, which is well vascularized and innervated and contains retrodiscal fat. This retrodiscal tissue can elicit pain when loaded.

The margin of the disk is fused to the TM joint capsule peripherally. Anteriorly, the disk is attached to the anterior margin of the articular eminence above and to the anterior margin of the condyle below. The posterior most bilaminar layer is of much importance as the upper layer gets attached to postglenoid process and prevents the joint from slipping when the jaw is wide opened. The interior or lower lamina fuses with capsule covering most of the back of the condyle. It prevents excessive rotation of the disk. When the mouth is in closed position, the condyle is covered by thick posterior band and when the mouth opens, the disk also slides along the condyle and covers it. Thus, during opening and closing of the mandible, both condyle and disk moves together in harmony on either side. The thick border of the disk prevents it from displacement during translation.

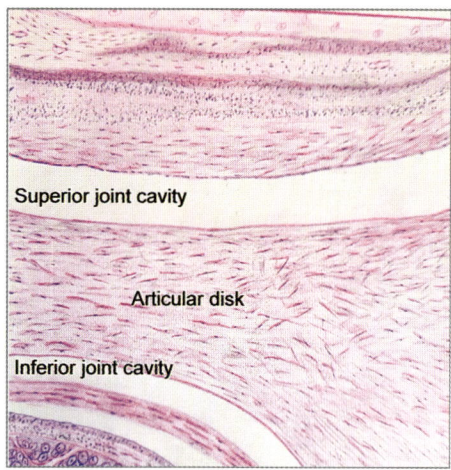

Figure 15-11: Schematic representation of the structure of articular disk.

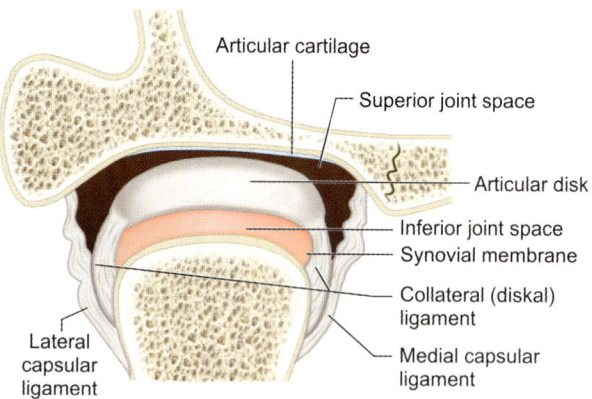

Figure 15-12: Joint capsule and its position.

Histology: The intra-articular disk in young adults is made up of dense fibrous tissue. The fibers which run through the disk vary in direction. In the thick anterior and posterior bands, the fibers run mediolaterally and in the thin intermediate zone, they run anteroposteriorly **(Figure 15-11)**. The disk contains cells embedded in a matrix composed of collagen fibers and ground substance. Upto 80% of the disk's composition is water. At first, the cells are only fibroblasts and later there are also chondroblasts, which will become numerous with age. This produces fibrocartilage. The anterior part of the disk is avascular. Majority of the fibers present are type I collagen. The disk may also have elastic fibers.

Capsule of Temporomandibular Joint

The TMJ capsule is a bilayered structure that consists of fibrous and synovial layers. It is the inner lining of the joint that originates from the border of the mandibular fossa superiorly and encloses the articular tubercle of temporal bone. Inferiorly, it is inserted at the neck of the condyle along its entire circumference above the pterygoid fovea **(Figure 15-12)**.

With regards to the superior attachment, the capsule is attached anteriorly to the crest of the articular eminence, posteriorly to the squamotympanic and petrotympanic fissures, medially to the medial glenoid plane and laterally to the lateral rim of the articular eminence and postglenoid process. The capsule is well-innervated and majority of the collagen fibers run vertically. It is so loose that the mandible can naturally dislocate anteriorly without damaging any fibers of the capsule.

The joint capsule, a metabolically active tissue, is important for the function of a synovial joint. By sealing the joint, it keeps the synovial fluid in position. It provides stability to the joint by limiting the movements and also because of the proprioceptive receptors.

The joint capsule is made up of loose connective tissue, which is well vascularized.

Synovial Membrane

It is a thin highly vascular structure, lining the capsule and covers all the areas other than pressure bearing regions like articulating surface of temporal bone, condyle, and meniscus. The surface exhibits folding to form synovial villi at the anterior and posterior end, which causes distension of the upper and lower joint cavities **(Figure 15-13A)**. The shape of the synovial membrane changes during the joints movements. This folded synovial membrane at rest is flattened out during the movements of the joint. Synovial membrane is made up of a discontinuous layer of flattened endothelial like cells resting on a vascular layer. Plasma filtrate is diffused through the synovial membrane to produce synovial fluid that fills both joint compartments.

The synovial tissue has three layers, namely, the synovial lining (intima) the most intimate part with the functional joint surfaces subsynovial tissue, similar to the intima but with a well-developed connective tissue network and the capsule, a relatively acellular layer with thick bands of collagen, which forms the outer boundary of the joint.

The cells of the synovial membrane are of two types namely, macrophage-like synovial cells or type A cells and fibroblasts-like synovial cells or type B cells **(Figure 15-13B)**. Surface cells have superficial resemblance to the epithelium, but have no basement membrane or junctional complexes as seen normally in any epithelium.

The fibroblast-like cells, derived from mesenchyme, is rich in endoplasmic reticulum, produce a long-chain sugar polymer called hyaluronan, which makes the synovial fluid "ropy" like egg-white, together with a molecule called lubricin. This lubricates the joint surfaces. The water of synovial fluid is not secreted as such but is effectively trapped in the joint space by the hyaluronan.

The macrophage-like synovial cells, rich in Golgi apparatus, derived from monocytes of blood are responsible for the removal of undesirable substances from the synovial fluid. It accounts for approximately 25% of cells of the synovial membrane.

Synovial tissue usually regenerates when damaged.

> Synovial surfaces do not adhere to each other. Continuous movement against opposing surfaces is thought to prevent the formation of crosslinks in the underlying collagenous fibrous tissue. Further secretion of collagenase by the synovial cells prevent the formation of surface adhesions and ensures that fragmented collagen on the tissue surface does not activate the coagulation cascade.

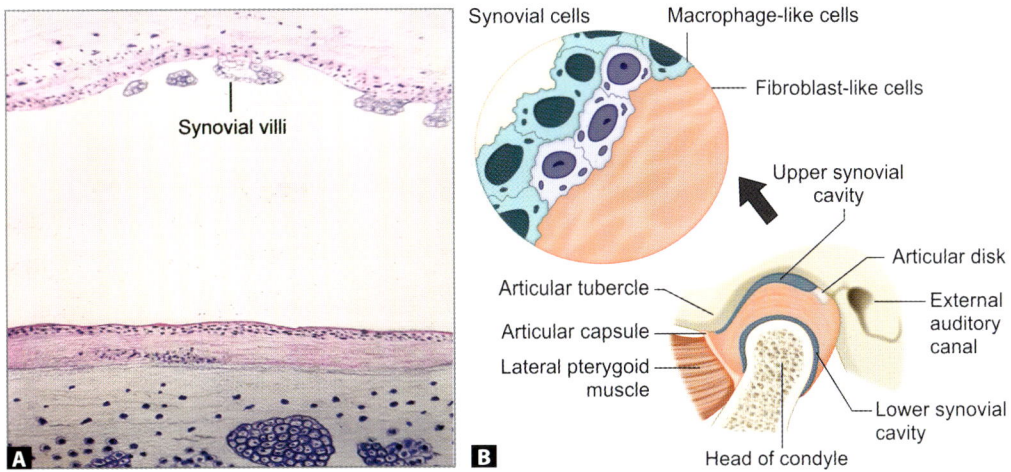

Figures 15-13A and B: (A) Synovial membrane showing synovial villi; (B) Schematic representation of microscopic appearance of synovial membrane.

Synovial Fluid

Synovial membrane produces fluid, which is clear, straw-colored, and viscous. It occupies the joint cavities. The synovial membrane and synovial fluid plays an integral role in normal joint function and inflammation. It is produced by diffusion from the rich capillary network of the synovial membrane and is supplemented with mucin and other products secreted by the synovial cells. Synovial fluid helps in lubrication and reduces friction and also helps in nutrition for the joint structure. Further it removes the debris formed by wear and tear. The important constituents that help in the lubrication are proteoglycans. It also has phagocytic properties. Normal synovial fluid contains various proinflammatory cytokines.

> Tumor necrosis factor (TNF) is consistently detected and interferon-C (IFN-c) and interleukin-2 (IL-2) are sporadically detected in the synovial fluid of TMJ in healthy individuals. Cytokines and growth factors present in synovial fluid are important regulatory factors for the immune and metabolic systems of the joint. Cytokines are secreted by immunocompetent cells of the synovial lining, chondrocytes or may originate from plasma.

Ligaments of Temporomandibular Joint

Temporomandibular joint is associated with three important ligaments—one major ligament, the temporomandibular ligament, and two minor ligaments, namely stylomandibular and sphenomandibular ligaments **(Figure 15-6B)**. The ligaments of this joint do not contribute to the movements of the jaw but in turn help in stabilizing the joint capsule in position.

Temporomandibular Ligament

It is located on the lateral aspect of the capsule and its function includes preventing the lateral or posterior displacement of the condyle. It has two distinct layers, the outer oblique layer and an inner horizontal layer. The outer wide fan-shaped layer arises from the external aspect of articular tubercle and posterior part of zygomatic arch. This ligament runs obliquely downward and backward to insert into the back of the neck of the mandible. A narrow inner deep layer runs horizontally back to the lateral pole of condyle and posterior part of articular disk. It helps in preventing excess opening of jaw.

The sphenomandibular and stylomandibular ligaments are accessory ligaments and do not have any significant role in opening and closing of the mandible.

Sphenomandibular Ligament (Remnants of Meckel's Cartilage)

It arises from spine of sphenoid and petrotympanic fissure and runs downward and outward to get attached to lingula on the medial surface of ramus of the mandible. The ligaments remain passive during movements of mandible and maintain the same degree of tension on both opening and closing of jaws and protects from excess translation. It is believed that this ligament protects the blood vessels and nerves passing through the mandibular foramen from additional tensile stress during jaw opening and closing. The mylohyoid nerves and vessels pierce it.

Stylomandibular Ligament

It arises from apex or tip of the styloid process and passes downward and forward to get attached to the angle on the medial surface and posterior border of the mandible.

It is a dense local condensation of deep cervical fascia and becomes tense when the mandible moves in maximum protrusive position. This ligament can limit excessive protrusive movements.

Apart from these ligaments, the other ligaments associated with the TMJ include collateral ligaments and otomandibular ligaments.

Collateral Ligament

It is also called diskal ligament, and is responsible for dividing the joint into superior and interior compartment. It attaches the medial and lateral aspects of articular disk to medial and lateral pole of condyle. Collateral ligament is made up of dense collagenous fibrous tissue, which prevents stretching. Thus, it helps in gliding the joint anteroposteriorly.

Otomandibular Ligaments

These ligaments connect the malleus, the middle ear ossicle with the temporomandibular joint. The oto-mandibular ligaments are the discomalleolar ligament, which arises from the malleus, the ossicles of the middle ear and runs to the medial retrodiscal tissue of the TMJ, and the anterior malleolar ligament, which arises from the malleus and attached to the lingula of the mandible through the sphenomandibular ligament.

BLOOD SUPPLY

Temporomandibular joint is supplied by three arteries. The main supply comes from the deep auricular artery, a branch of maxillary artery and the superficial temporal artery, a terminal branch of the external carotid artery. In addition, the joint is provided by the anterior tympanic artery, also a branch of the maxillary artery and ascending pharyngeal artery, the smallest branch of external carotid artery.

The venous blood drains through the superficial temporal vein and the maxillary vein. Pterygoid venous plexus is in close relationship with the medial aspect of the joint. The capsule and the posterior attachment of the articular disk have rich vascular plexus.

NERVE SUPPLY (FIGURE 15-14)

Sensory innervation of the TM joint is derived from the auriculotemporal nerve. Masseteric nerve, a motor branch of the mandibular nerve, supplies the masseter muscle and the TM joint.

Free nerve endings have been described in the joint capsule and the periphery of the articular disk but the center portion is not innervated. The proprioceptive receptor of the TMJ includes four receptors. Ruffini endings function as static mechanoreceptors, which position the mandible. Pacinian corpuscles are dynamic mechanoreceptors, which accelerate movement during reflexes. Golgi tendon organs function as static mechanoreceptors for protection of ligaments around the TM joint. Free nerve endings are the pain receptors for protection of the TM joint itself.

FUNCTIONS OF TEMPOROMANDIBULAR JOINT

The movements of TMJ indirectly reflect the basic functions like speaking, mastication, coughing, yawning, and maintain the middle ear pressure. The main function is to open and close, protrusion and retrusion, and lateral deviation of jaw. It is brought about by two basic movements like rotation and translation. Rotation occurs in the infrajoint area and translation occurs at suprajoint area. The muscles of mastication namely, masseter, temporalis, medial pterygoid, and lateral pterygoid help in the movements of the jaw **(Figure 15-15)**.

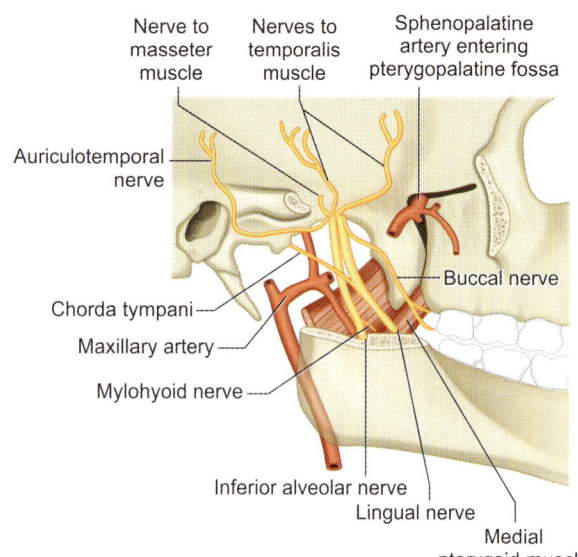

Figure 15-14: Nerve innervations of the temporomandibular joint.

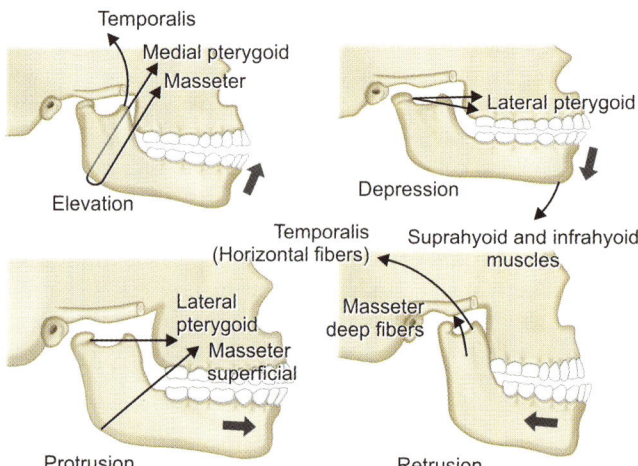

Figure 15-15: Movements of the temporomandibular joint.

Apart from this, the condylar cartilage is an important growth site in the mandible, contributing to the elongation of the mandibular ramus.

Upon opening the jaw, the condyle rotates at the beginning and later on, translatory movement occurs, which permits the condyle to slide forward under the eminence. In closing the jaw, the actions are vice versa.

The muscles, which mainly bring the depression of mandible are inferior head of lateral pterygoid and suprahyoid group of muscles. The superior head of lateral pterygoid along with the masseter, temporalis, and medial pterygoid muscles of both sides help in the elevation of jaw. The posterior fibers of temporalis help in retraction of head of condyle while closing the mouth. Forward or protrusive movement is brought by lateral and medial pterygoids of both sides.

CLINICAL CONSIDERATIONS

Disorders of TMJ have multifactorial etiology. The common symptoms include pain in the joint region (preauricular) or face, clicking sounds, and restricted mouth opening.

Similar to other joints, TMJ is also prone for inflammatory and degenerative disorders.

Clicking of TMJ: Clicking, popping, or grating sounds may be produced in the TMJ, when opening or closing the mouth or during chewing. Though TMJ clicking is most commonly associated with TMJ disorders, it can be present in normal joints also. In about 35% of the population, TMJ produces clicking sound during mouth opening. The articular disk can become displaced forward from its natural position between the end of the head of the condyle and the glenoid fossa. This can occur due to a number of factors. When this disk relocates back to its normal position for completion of the opening movement, a clicking noise is heard. So clicking indicates that there is an issue with the disk position.

Malocclusion, missing teeth, and occlusal disharmony may also predispose to TMJ disorders.

Myofascial pain and dysfunction syndrome is characterized by unilateral pain, muscle tenderness, clicking and popping noise in TMJ, and limitation of jaw function or deviation of jaw. It is caused by tension, fatigue, or spasm in the masticatory muscles (medial and lateral pterygoids, temporalis, and masseter). Diagnosis is based on history and physical examination. Conservative treatment, including analgesics, muscle relaxation, habit modification, and bite splinting, usually is effective.

Synovitis and *capsulitis* are localized inflammatory conditions of the TM joint, which are commonly seen in clinical practice and typically occur following trauma.

TMJ dislocation is an uncommon but debilitating condition. This dislocation is usually bilateral and displacement is anterior. When the mouth is opened unusually wide, for example, during yawning, the condylar head slip forward causing dislocation. The condition may be acute or chronic. Acute TMJ dislocation is common in clinical practice and can be managed easily with manual reduction. Chronic recurrent TMJ dislocation is a challenging situation to manage.

TMJ ankylosis is characterized by fusion of mandibular condyle to the glenoid fossa, by bony or fibrous tissue. This may be unilateral or bilateral. The most common cause for TMJ ankylosis is trauma. The other etiologic factors include arthritis, infection, previous TMJ surgery, congenital deformities, and idiopathic factors. Ankylosis of the growing TMJ results in mandibular deformity **(Figure 15-16)**.

Arthrocentesis is the clinical procedure of using a syringe to aspirate synovial fluid from a joint capsule for diagnosis of certain joint disorders **(Figure 15-17)**. It is also used

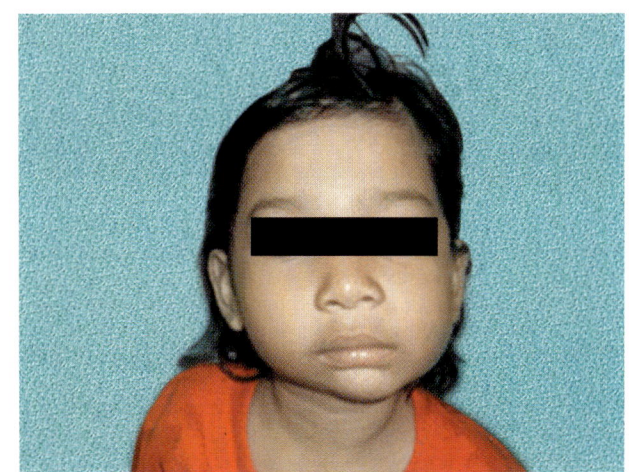

Figure 15-16: Facial deformity due to ankylosis.

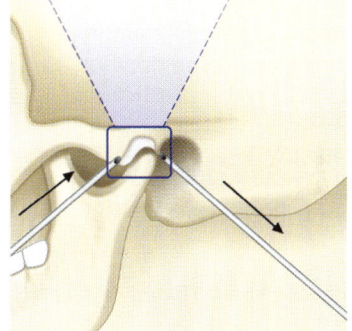

Figure 15-17: Procedure of arthrocentesis.

as a treatment modality, which lies between nonsurgical treatment and arthroscopic surgery. This procedure is applied in TMJ disorders also. It is not an alternative procedure to surgical intervention, but highly efficient procedure with low morbidity. Arthrocentesis could be the best indicated treatment for patients with anterior disk placement. Fibrous adhesions in the upper joint cavity are one of the factors causing limitation of condylar movement. Arthrocentesis involving joint lavage under sufficient pressure can remove adhesions and widen the joint space, thereby restoring the joint physiology. It also gives successful results for pain and dysfunction relief in treating patients with TMJ disorders.

Points to Remember

- The temporomandibular joint (TM joint or TMJ) is a condyloid variety of diarthrodial joint.
- Anatomically two joints but functions as one.
- Located on either side of the skull base, in front of the auditory meatus and posterosuperior to masseter.
- The components of the TM joint include the joint capsule, articular disk, mandibular condyle, glenoid fossa, temporomandibular ligament, stylomandibular ligament, sphenomandibular ligament, and lateral pterygoid muscle.
- Both TMJ have a harmonious coordinated movement while opening and closure of the mandible.
- Condyle can move laterally by rotation and anteriorly by gliding forwards.
- Articulating surfaces are covered by fibrocartilage unlike hyaline cartilage in other joints.
- Mandibular fossa of temporal bone and condyle of the mandible forms the joint.
- TMJ ligaments prevent the lateral or posterior displacement of the condyle.
- TMJ capsule seals the joint to keep the synovial fluid in position and provides stability to the joint by limiting the movements.
- Between the articular surfaces of the condyle and the mandibular fossa of the temporal bone lies a dense fibrous connective tissue disk, called meniscus or intra-articular disk.
- Articular disk acts as shock absorber and separates the joint into upper and lower joint spaces.
- Synovial membrane is a thin highly vascular structure, lining the capsule and covers all the areas other than pressure-bearing regions like articulating surface of temporal bone, condyle, and meniscus.
- Sensory innervation of the TM joint is by auriculotemporal nerve. Masseteric nerve, a motor branch of the mandibular nerve supplies the masseter muscle and the TM joint.
- In about 35% of the population, TMJ produces clicking during mouth opening.
- Fusion of condyle to the glenoid fossa is called TMJ ankylosis.
- Underdeveloped or overdeveloped condyle on any one side results in facial asymmetry.

PRACTICE QUESTIONS

1. Write notes on the development of the temporomandibular joint.
2. Write about ligaments of TMJ.
3. What is interarticular disk and describe its attachment and structure.
4. Write notes on TMJ capsule.
5. Write notes on synovial membrane and synovial fluid.
6. Write short notes on innervations and blood supply of TMJ.
7. Name the muscles of mastication.

MULTIPLE CHOICE QUESTIONS

1. Which of the following types of articulation is present in TMJ?
   a. Fibrous
   b. Cartilaginous
   c. Synovial
   d. Pivot
2. The first formed blastema in tmj development is:
   a. Temporal
   b. Condylar
   c. Coronoid
   d. Articular eminence
3. The layer of condylar tissue which disappears completely by 18 years of age is/are:
   a. Connective tissue layer
   b. Intermediate layer
   c. Chondroblastic layer
   d. All of the above
4. The total number of processes present in the mandible are:
   a. 4
   b. 2
   c. 5
   d. 3
5. A small tubercle at lateral extremity of condyle, gives attachment to which ligament?
   a. Temporomandibular ligament
   b. Sphenomandibular ligament
   c. Stylomandibular ligament
   d. Collateral ligament
6. All the joint structures in tmj are formed at about
   a. 16 Weeks
   b. 12 Weeks
   c. 14 Weeks
   d. 18 Weeks
7. Tmj capsule is attached to the entire circumference of:
   a. Condyle
   b. Coronoid process
   c. Neck of mandible
   d. Coronoid notch
8. The condylar bulk is made up of:
   a. Woven bone
   b. Lamellar bone
   c. Compact bone
   d. Cancellous bone
9. Which layer of adult condyle is thin, often incomplete, patchy/even absent?
   a. Cell-rich proliferative layer
   b. Fibrous layer
   c. Hyaline cartilage layer
   d. Zone of endochondral ossification

CHAPTER 15: Temporomandibular Joint

10. Which of the following structures prevent the joint from slippage during wide opening of the jaw?
    a. Glenoid fossa
    b. Condyle of mandible
    c. Articular eminence
    d. Posterior bilaminar layer
11. Which type of collagen fiber is found in the intra-articular disk?
    a. Type i
    b. Type ii
    c. Type iii
    d. Type iv
12. The synovial membrane of the joint folds to form synovial villi during which jaw movement?
    a. At opening of the jaw
    b. At closure of the jaw
    c. At lateral movements
    d. At rest
13. The ropy egg white tendency of synovial fluid is generated from:
    a. Macrophage-like cells
    b. Fibroblast-like cells
    c. Chondroblast-like cells
    d. Osteoblast-like cells
14. During jaw opening and closure, which ligament protects the blood vessels and nerves passing through the mandibular foramen?
    a. Stylomandibular ligament
    b. Collateral ligament
    c. Temporomandibular ligament
    d. Sphenomandibular ligament
15. Stylomandibular ligament is attached to:
    a. Styloid process and medial surface of the angle and posterior border of the mandible
    b. Styloid process and pterygoid fovea
    c. Styloid process and spine of sphenoid bone
    d. Styloid process and the neck of the mandible
16. The sensory supply to the tmj is by:
    a. Auriculotemporal nerve
    b. Olfactory nerve
    c. Facial nerve
    d. Vagus nerve
17. The ligament which helps in anteroposterior gliding of the joint is:
    a. Stylomandibular ligament
    b. Sphenomandibular ligament
    c. Temporomandibular ligament
    d. Collateral ligament
18. Arthrocentesis is best indicated for patients with:
    a. Posterior disk displacement
    b. Anterior disk displacement
    c. TMJ ankylosis
    d. Synovitis
19. Retraction of condyle is done by:
    a. Lateral pterygoid
    b. Medial pterygoids
    c. Temporalis posterior fibers
    d. Lateral and medial pterygoid
20. The two basic movements aiding in tmj movements are:
    a. Rotation and sliding
    b. Sliding and translation
    c. Sliding and rotation
    d. Rotation and translation
21. The ligament which prevents excessive opening of the jaw is:
    a. Sphenomandibular ligament
    b. Temporomandibular ligament
    c. Collateral ligament
    d. Stylomandibular ligament
22. Unilateral pain, muscle tenderness, clicking and popping noise in TMJ, and limitation of jaw function or deviation of jaw are present in:
    a. Synovitis
    b. TMJ ankylosis
    c. Myofascial pain dysfunction syndrome
    d. Disk displacement

ANSWERS

1. c   2. a   3. c   4. d   5. a   6. c   7. c   8. d   9. a   10. d   11. a   12. d   13. b   14. d   15. a
16. a   17. d   18. b   19. c   20. d   21. b   22. c

BIBLIOGRAPHY

1. Avery JK, Chiego DJ. Essentials of oral histology and embryology- a clinical approach, 3rd edition. St. Louis: Mosby; 2006.
2. Avery JK. Oral development and histology, 3rd edition. New York: Thieme; 2002.
3. Berkovitz BKB, Holland GR, Moxham BJ. Oral anatomy, histology and embryology, 4th edition. US: Elsevier; 2009.
4. Berkovitz BKB, Holland GR, Moxham BJ. The temporomandibular joint. In: Oral anatomy, oral histology and embryology, 3rd edition. St. Louis: Mosby; 2002.
5. Bernick S. The vascular and nerve supply to the temporomandibular joint of the rat. Oral Surg. 1962;15:488.
6. Carini F, Scardina GA, Caradonna C, et al. Human temporomandibular joint morphogenesis. Ital J Anat Embryol. 2007;112(4):267-75.
7. Caruso S, Storti E, Nota A, et al. Temporomandibular joint anatomy assessed by CBCT images. Biomed Research International. 2017;2017:1-10.
8. Chandra S, Chandra S, Chandra M, et al. Textbook of dental and oral histology with embryology & MCQ's, 2nd edition. India: Jaypee Brothers Medical Publishers (P) Ltd; 2010.
9. Chatterjee K. Essentials of dental anatomy and oral histology, 2nd edition. New Delhi: Jaypee Brothers Medical Publishers (P) Ltd; 2014.
10. Choukas NC, Sicher H. The structure of the temporomandibular joint. Oral Surg, Oral Med, Oral Pathol. 1960;13:1203-13.

11. Gaunt WA, Osborn JW, Ten Cate AR. Advanced dental histology, 2nd edition. Bristol: John Wright & Sons Ltd; 1971.
12. Herring SW. TMJ anatomy and animal models. J Musculoskelet Neuronal Interact. 2003;3(4):391.
13. Klineberg I. Structure and function of temporomandibular joint innervations. Ann R Coll Surg Engl. 1971;49(4):268-88.
14. Kumar GS. Orban's Oral histology and embryology, 14th edition. India: Elsevier; 2015.
15. Liang W, Li X, Gao B, et al. Observing the development of the temporomandibular joint in embryonic and post-natal mice using various staining methods. Exp Ther Med. 2016;11(2): 481-9.
16. Moffett B. The morphogenesis of the temporomandibular joint. Am J Orthod. 1966;52:401-15.
17. Nanci A. Ten Cate's Oral Histology, Development, Structure, and Functions, 8th edition. India: Elsevier; 2012.
18. Nozawa IK, Amizuka N, Ikeda N, et al. Synovial membrane in the temporomandibular joint—its morphology, function and development. Arch Histol Cytol. 2003;66:289.
19. Perry HT, Xu Y, Forbes DP. The embryology of the temporomandibular join. Cranio. 1985;3(2):125-32.
20. Piette E. Anatomy of the human temporomandibular joint. An updated comprehensive review. Acto Stomatol Belg. 1993;90(2):103-27.
21. Porto GG, Vasconcelos BC, Andrade ES, et al. Comparison between human and rat TMJ: anatomic and histopathologic features. Acta Cir Bras. 2010;25(3):290-3.
22. Provenza VD, Seibel W. Oral Histology- Inheritance and Development, 2nd edition. USA: Lea & Febiger; 1986.
23. Ramfjord SP, Ash MM. Occlusion. Philadelphia: WB Saunders Co; 1966.
24. Rees LA. Structure and function of the mandibular joint. Br Dent J. 1954;96:6.
25. Sarnat BG. The Temporomandibular Joint, 2nd edition. Springfield, IL: Charles C. Thomas; 1964.
26. Schmolke C. The relationship between the temporomandibular joint capsule, articular disk and jaw muscles. J Anat. 1994;184(2):335-45.
27. Steven R Olmos. Functional anatomy and TMJ pathology, Page 5, https://tmjsnoring.ca/articles/Functional%20Anatomy.pdf, accessed on 10/02/2022.
28. Strauss F, Christen A, Weber W. The architecture of the disk of the human temporomandibular joint. Helv Odont Acta. 1960; 4:1.
29. Ten Cate AR. Temporomandibular joint. In: Nanci A (Ed). Ten Cate's oral histology: development, structure and function, 6th edition. St. Louis: Elsevier; 2003.
30. Thilander B. Innervation of the temporomandibular joint capsule in man. tr Roy Schools Den Stockholm Umea. 1961;7:1.

CHAPTER

Maxillary Sinus

B Sivapathasundharam, Logeswari Jayamani, Govind Rajkumar

CHAPTER OUTLINE

- Anatomy of Maxillary Sinus   253
- Development of Maxillary Sinus   255
- Blood Supply and Nerve Supply   255
- Microscopic Features   257
- Functions   258
- Clinical Considerations   258

The term "sinus" in Latin means "pocket". Sinuses are air-filled spaces located on the skull around the nasal cavity and hence called the paranasal sinuses **(Figure 16-1)**. They are named after the bone, where it is located, namely—frontal sinus, sphenoid sinus, ethmoid sinus, and maxillary sinus. All the paranasal sinuses are paired. These sinuses drain into the nasal cavity through openings called ostia. Though the architecture of the paranasal sinuses appears simple, they are composed of intricate and subdivided air passages and drainage pathways, which connect them to the nasal cavity.

The main purpose of sinuses in the human is to decrease the relative weight of the skull and play an important role in increasing the resonance of the voice. They also act as a buffer against trauma to the face and the brain by serving as a mechanical shock absorber. They insulate and cool down the inhaled air to the body temperature and play a defensive role by filtering the air passage i.e contribute to immune defense of the nasal cavity.

ANATOMY OF MAXILLARY SINUS

Maxillary sinus or maxillary antrum (antrum—a cavity or chamber) is the largest sinus of all the paranasal sinuses located in the body of maxilla and opens in the middle nasal meatus of the nasal cavity with one or multiple openings. They are paired but asymmetrical in size and shape.

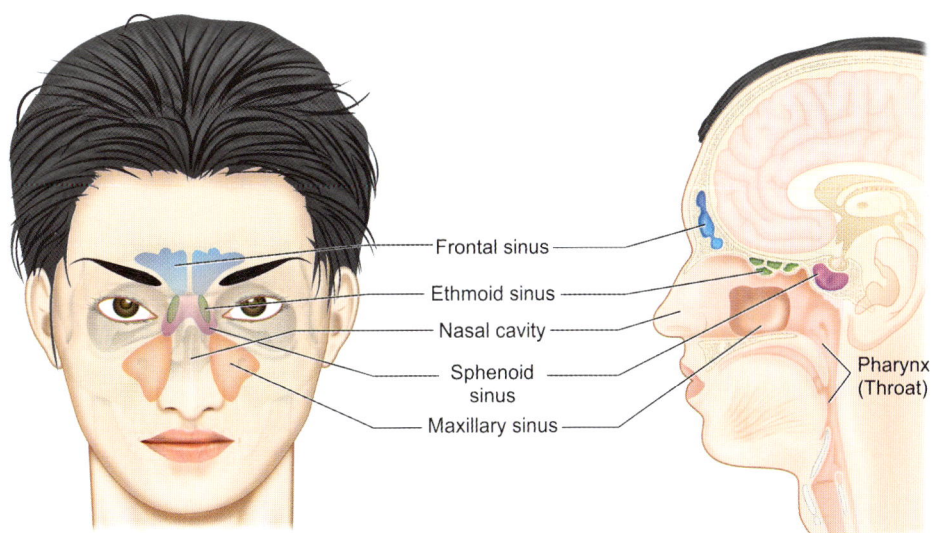

Figure 16-1: Location of paranasal sinuses in the face.

The location may even vary not only in different individuals but also in different sides of the same individual. It is also known as "antrum of Highmore", named after Nathaniel Highmore, a British surgeon and anatomist, who first described the anatomy of the maxillary sinus and the process of pnuematization in detail in the year 1651.

Maxillary sinuses are four-sided pyramidal in shape, located in the maxilla, with its base forming the lateral wall of the nasal cavity, and apex directed laterally towards the zygomatic process of the maxilla. The four sides are walled anteriorly by facial surface of maxilla, posteriorly by the infratemporal surface of maxilla, superiorly by the floor of the orbit and inferiorly related to the palate, alveolar process and posterior teeth of the maxilla **(Figures 16-2A to C)**. The average volume of the maxillary sinus is about 15 mL and it measures about 2.3 cm transversely, 3.4 cm anteroposteriorly, and 3.35 cm vertically. However, the size of the maxillary sinus reduces slowly with age.

None of the maxillary antral wall is flat or smooth except the anterior wall. The superior wall formed by the floor of the orbital cavity may exhibit well-marked ridge extending from the roof to the anterior wall representing the infraorbital canal. Posterior wall presents the alveolar canals, which transmit superior alveolar vessels. The floor of the maxillary sinus may or may not be in level with the floor of the nasal cavity. The maxillary sinus floor shows several conical projections, corresponding to the roots of the first and second maxillary molar teeth and second and first premolar. On rare occasions roots of the teeth may perforate the floor of the sinus. Initially protruding roots are separated from the sinus by a thin bone but later on such bone will get resorbed and the roots protrude extensively into the sinus cavity through openings. This leads to direct contact of antral mucosa with the periodontal ligament of the projecting root apices. In children the deciduous first and second molars are frequently found in proximity with the sinus floor. However, it is not uncommon to notice adaptation of the sinus floor in relation to the neighboring maxillary teeth, like dipping of sinus floor in between the roots of adjacent teeth, areas of elevation to accommodate apices of root, and protrusion of roots into the sinus cavity **(Figures 16-3A and B)**. Similarly compartmentalization of the sinus cavity is noticed periodically **(Figure 16-3C)**. The medial wall is

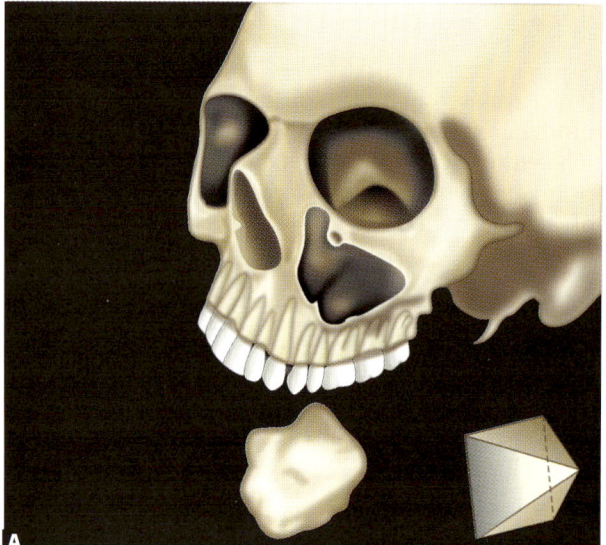
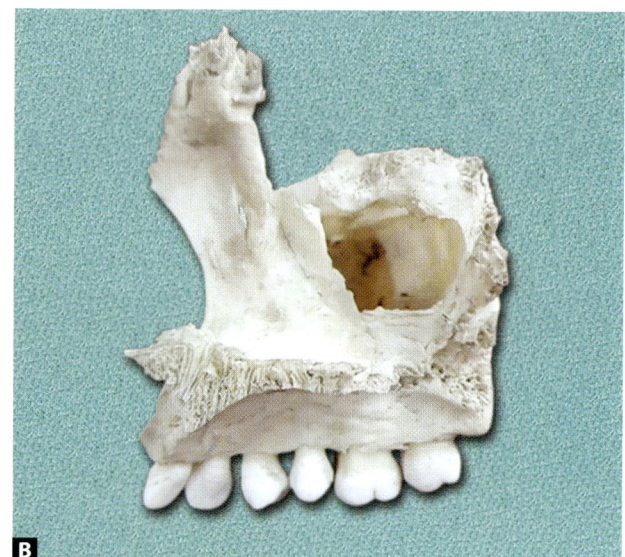
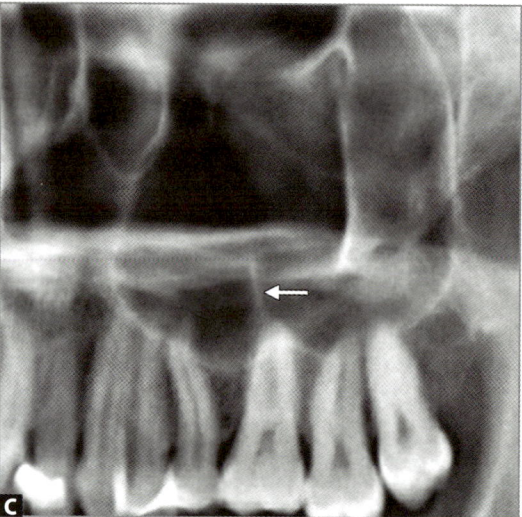

Figures 16-2A to C: (A and B) Anatomy of maxillary antrum; (C) Panoramic radiography, septum showing inside of the left maxillary sinus (white arrow) and also note intimate association of apices of roots of the premolars and molars to the floor of maxillary sinus.

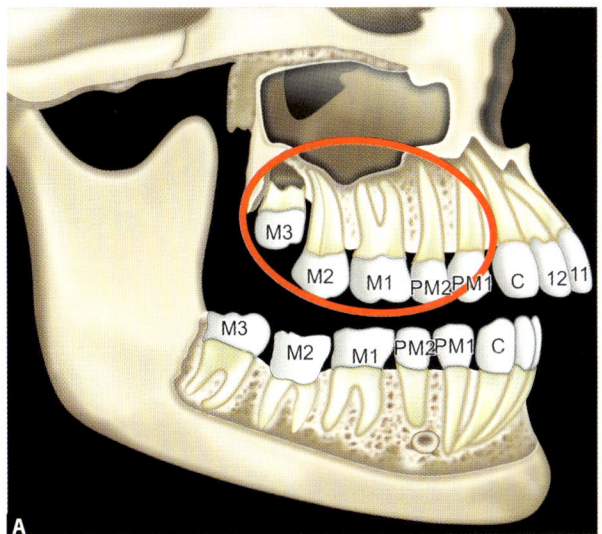
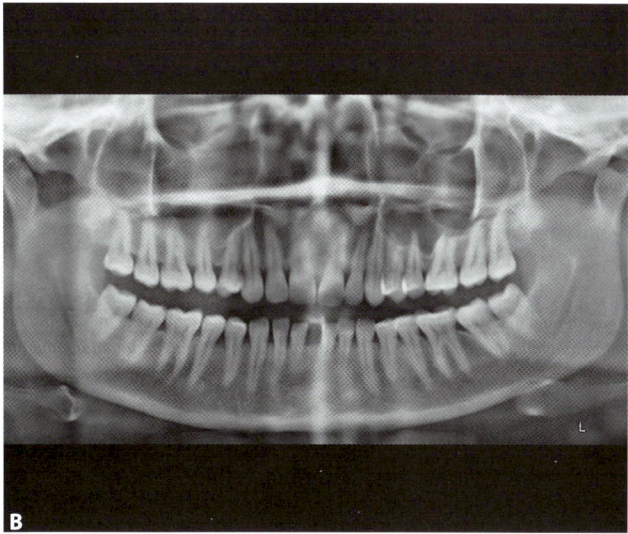

Figures 16-3A and B: (A) Proximity of roots of the maxillary teeth to the floor of antrum; (B) Orthopantomograph showing the same.

composed primarily of cartilage, which exhibits one or more openings for the sinus contents to drain.

The sinus lining produces mucus, which is moved by the action of cilia in a synchronized pattern around the sinus often against the gravity. The maxillary sinus is well-competent by the presence of ciliated columnar epithelium that facilitates the expulsion of bacteria by mucociliary system. It is not entirely dependent on the regular drainage via the opening called "the ostium". The ostium is located high on the lateral wall of the nose in a crescent-shaped or semicircular groove, where frontal sinus, maxillary sinus, and anterior ethmoidal sinus open. The ostium of the maxillary sinus may be a two-dimensional orifice with a diameter of about 2.5 mm or may be a canal with the length of about 5 mm. Accessory openings may also be present. Since the opening is placed high above the floor of the sinus, the role of gravity in draining the mucus is less when the head is in erect position **(Figures 16-4A to C)**.

DEVELOPMENT OF MAXILLARY SINUS

The first sign of the paranasal sinuses development is the appearance of a series of folds called ethmoturbinals on the lateral nasal wall at approximately the eighth week of intrauterine life. Though six to seven folds form initially, only three to four persist through regression and fusion during development.

Maxillary sinus is the first sinus to develop amongst all the paranasal sinuses. Development of maxillary sinus begins as a small lateral evagination of the middle meatus on the lateral nasal wall between the oral cavity and floor of the orbit. Prior to the development of palate and nasal cavity, there is formation of ridges and furrows in the lateral nasal wall for three (superior, middle, and inferior) nasal conchae and meatus. Initially, the superior and inferior meatus remain as a shallow depression, while the middle meatus expands inferiorly into the maxilla as an extension. Thus, the development of sinus begins at the 12th week of intrauterine life as an extension of mucous membrane on the middle meatus of the lateral wall. It remains tubular at birth and continues to grow anteroposteriorly, becomes ovoid in childhood, and further grows in all three directions, *i.e.* anteroposteriorly, superoinferiorly, mediolaterally into pyramidal by adulthood **(Figures 16- 5A and B)**. This process of enlargement of sinus spaces is called pneumatization, which occurs mainly by the bone remodeling (resorption of the internal walls except the medial wall and apposition at the outer surface). Enlargement of the maxillary sinus corresponds with the facial growth. As the face grows forward and downward and with eruption of deciduous and permanent dentition, the sinus enlarges. In young age, pneumatization is proportional to the maxillary growth. As the age advances pneumatization exceeds maxillary growth. Thus the antrum expands at the expense of the maxillary process. Consequently, the expansion of maxillary sinus continues to invade the other processes of maxilla, namely alveolar process, palatine process, zygomatic process, and frontal process. This extension of maxillary sinus into various processes of maxilla is known as recess. Most commonly the recess is noticed in alveolar process (50%), followed by zygomatic process (41.5%), frontal process (40.5%), and palatine process (1.75%) **(Figure 16-6)**.

BLOOD SUPPLY AND NERVE SUPPLY

Sensory innervations are by the maxillary nerve (second division of trigeminal nerve), infraorbital nerve and greater palatine nerve. The sympathetic innervation is from superior cervical ganglion and parasympathetic innervation from sphenopalatine ganglion **(Figure 16-7)**.

The infraorbital, alveolar, greater palatine and sphenopalatine arteries, and branches of the internal maxillary artery give the arterial supply, while either by a single trunk continuation of the sphenopalatine vein, or by three venous plexus—the anterior and posterior pterygoid plexus and the alveolar plexus cover the venous drainage of the maxillary sinus **(Figures 16-8A and B)**. The lymph from the sinus drains into the submandibular lymph nodes.

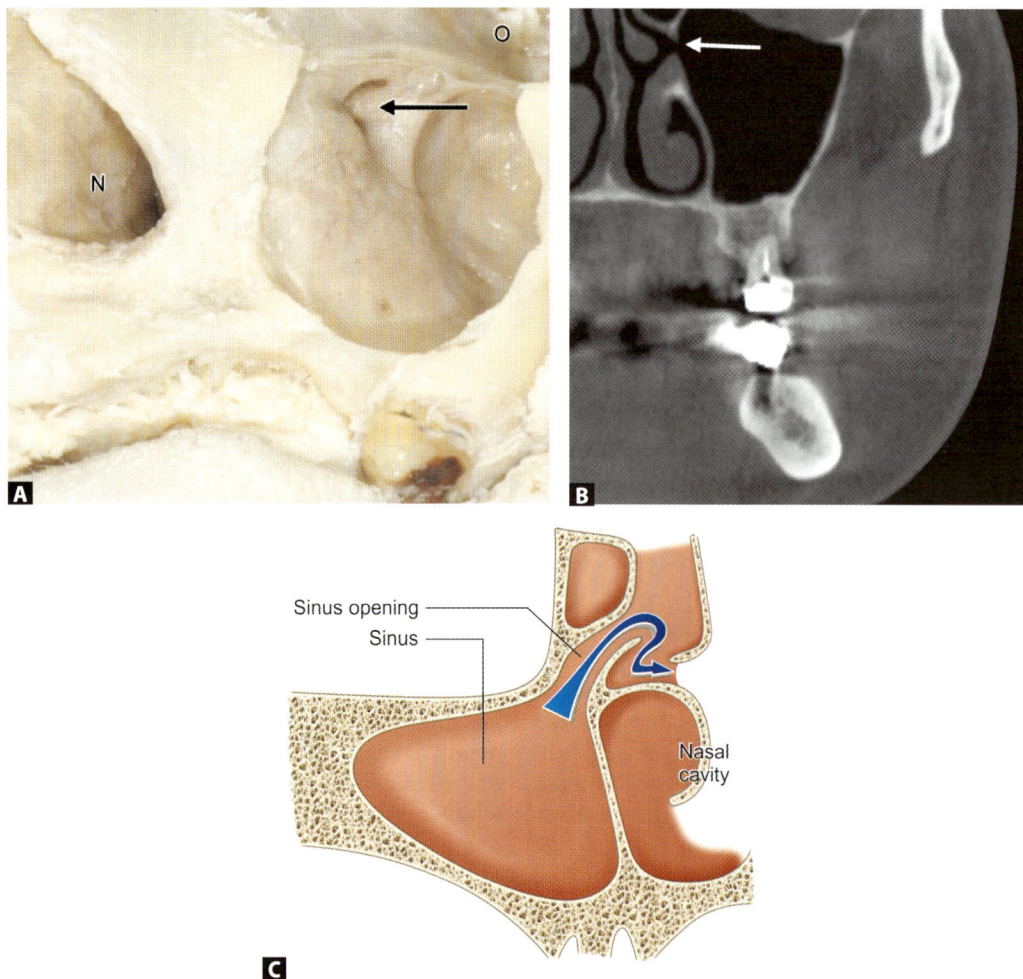

Figures 16-4A to C: (A and B) Ostium on the left maxillary sinus (arrows): (A) Cadaveric dissection (anterolateral view); (B) Computed tomography (coronal image); (C) Schematic representation of the location of the maxillary sinus opening above the floor of the maxillary sinus. N, nasal cavity; O, orbit.

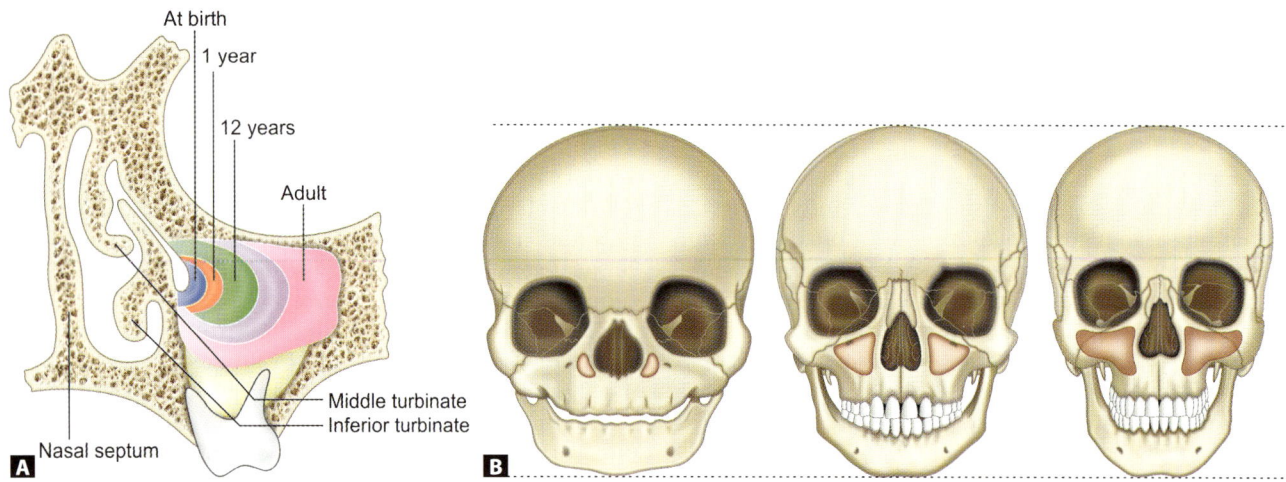

Figures 16-5A and B: Development of maxillary sinus with age.

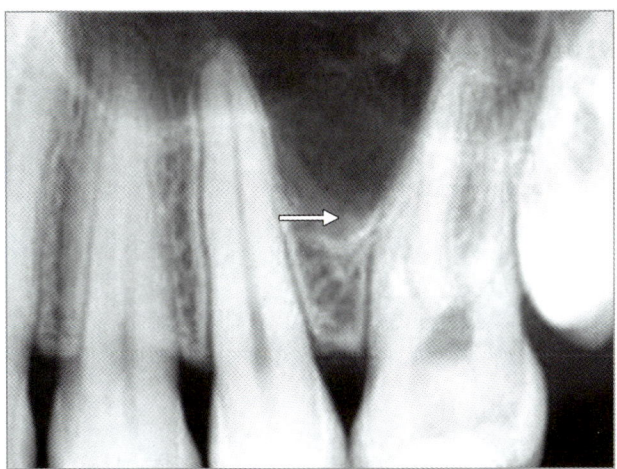

Figure 16-6: Arrow mark in the radiograph shows the invasion of maxillary sinus into the alveolar process, the alveolar recess.

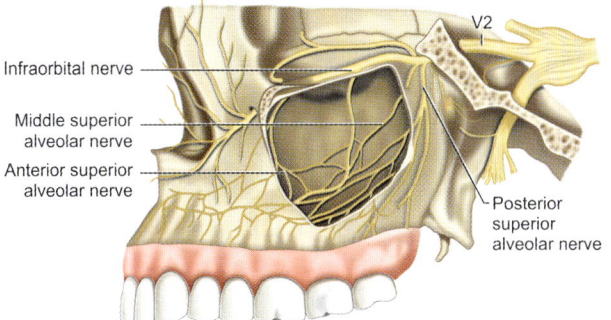

Figure 16-7: Innervations of maxillary antrum.

MICROSCOPIC FEATURES

The maxillary sinus is lined by respiratory mucosa that lines the nasal cavity and the other paranasal sinuses. The mucosa lining the maxillary sinus is a mucoperiosteum, because of its direct connect to the periosteum of the bony walls of the sinus. This sinus lining is also known as "Schneiderian membrane", referring to bilaminar membrane with ciliated columnar epithelium on one side and periosteum on the osseous side **(Figures 16-9A to D)**. Epithelium is thinner than that of the nasal cavity and consists of three distinct layers surrounding the sinus space, *i.e.* epithelial layer, basal lamina, and subepithelial layer or the lamina propria.

The epithelial layer is made up of pseudostratified ciliated columnar epithelium, a derivative of olfactory epithelium of the middle nasal meatus. Three types of cells are noticed within the epithelium, predominately ciliated columnar cells, less commonly nonciliated basal cells and mucous producing goblet cells.

Ciliated cells are specialized cells, with centrally placed nucleus with numerous mitochondria within the cytoplasm. Cilia facilitate the motility and propel the mucus and other substances over the epithelial surface by their rhythmic beatings. The cilium at the basal body (where it is attached to the cell body) is made up of peripherally placed 9 triplets of microtubules and as it extends, exhibits 9 doublets and 2 centrally placed singlets. These cells play a key role in keeping the nasal cavity moist. Basal columnar cells are evident toward the basal membrane with centrally placed nucleus. Goblet cells, which are flask-shaped cells, located in between

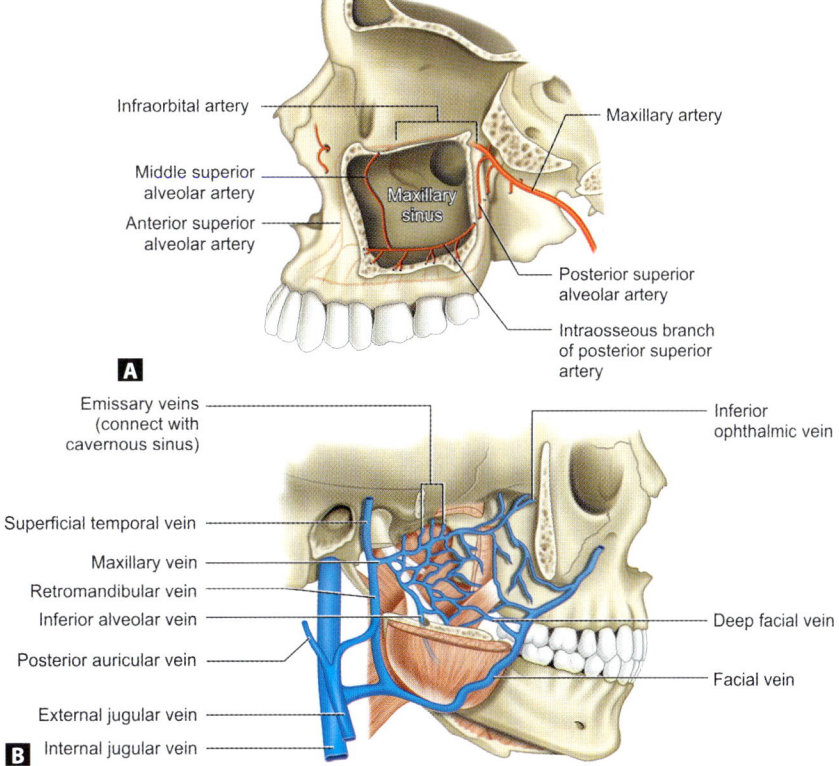

Figures 16-8A and B: Arterial supply.

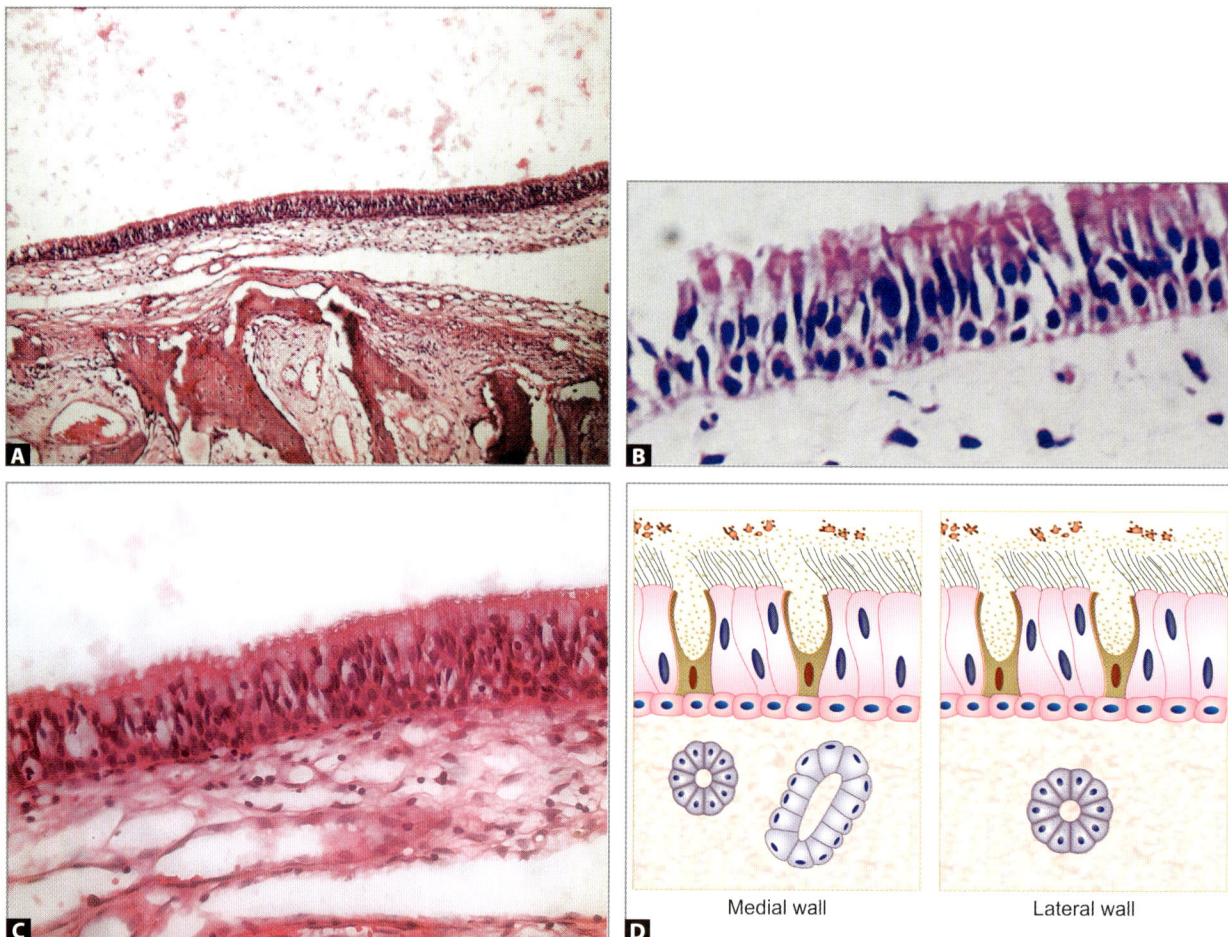

Figures 16-9A to D: Epithelial lining of the maxillary antrum: (A) Low power showing the epithelial lining, connective tissue and bone; (B and C) High power showing pseudostratified ciliated columnar epithelium with Goblet cells; (D) Schematic representation.

the ciliated cells, secrete mucus and appear similar to any protein secreting cells. The rough and smooth endoplasmic reticulum, Golgi apparatus, and cytoplasmic granules are noticed within the cytoplasm. The microvilli are located at the apical part of the cell to expel the secreted mucin by exocytosis. Thus it acts similar to an apocrine gland (both as a synthesizing and secretory cell). This provides protection. The basal lamina separates the epithelium from the submucosal region. The lamina propria fused with periosteum consists of loose collagen bundles, few elastic fibers, subepithelial glands (serous and mucous glands), fibroblasts, vessels, and nerves **(Figures 16-9C and D)**.

In addition to the epithelial secretions, mixed secretions from the subepithelial layers provide additional moisture and are transported to the surface epithelium via excretory ducts after piercing the basal lamina. The serous secretion consists of water, carbohydrates, neutral lipids and proteins, while the mucous secretion consists of glycoprotein and mucopolysaccharides. The mucous cells show positivity to special stains such as Alcian blue, mucicarmine etc.

■ FUNCTIONS

Similar to other paranasal sinuses, the maxillary sinus reduces the weight of the facial skeleton, moistens and humidifies the inspired air, and imparts resonance to the voice. Unique microciliary transport filters the debris from the inspired air. Secretions from the goblet cells and subepithelial glandular secretions facilitate mucous production and storage. It provides thermal insulation to the vital organs located in the skull by assisting in maintaining the intracranial pressure. Prevents and limits the extent of injury to the facial trauma. The shape and structure of the face and paranasal sinuses may act as a crumple zone in severe trauma and thus protect the brain injury. It also serves as an accessory olfactory organ.

■ CLINICAL CONSIDERATIONS

Developmental anomalies of the maxillary sinus like agenesis (complete absence of maxillary sinus) and hypoplasia (defective formation of maxillary sinus) may result in

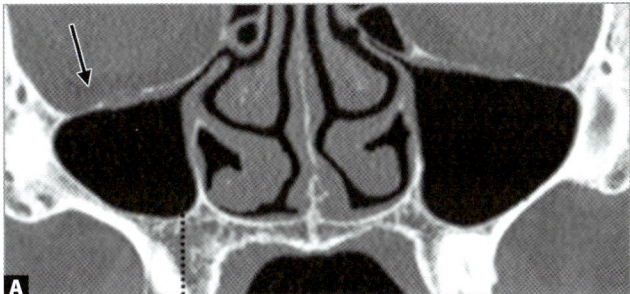
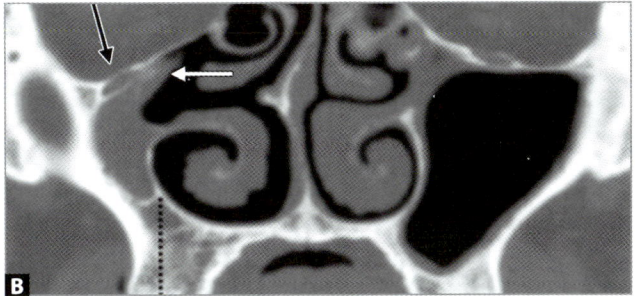

Figures 16-10A and B: (A) Radiograph demonstrating hypoplasia (defective/reduced size in comparison to the counterpart); (B) Radiograph demonstrating agenesis (complete absence of left maxillary sinus with white arrow))

development of small maxillary sinuses in conditions like Crouzon's and Apert's syndrome. These developmental anomalies are rare and may result in headache and voice alteration **(Figures 16-10A and B)**.

The supernumerary maxillary sinus is another developmental condition, wherein two completely separated maxillary sinuses are developed, either by formation of two primordia from the middle meatus or from middle and superior meatus, or middle and inferior meatus, respectively.

Enlarged or large sinuses with larger internal volume are noted in pituitary gigantism. Inversely, smaller sinuses are known to be associated with some congenital infections (*e.g* congenital syphilis).

The maxillary nerve supplies both the maxillary sinus and maxillary teeth and the roots of the maxillary molars and premolars are in proximity to the maxillary sinus lining. This leaves frequent diagnostic dilemmas; the inflammation of the sinus lining may mimic the dental pathology or vice versa.

Since paranasal sinuses have communication with the nasal cavity, an upper respiratory tract infection can spread to the sinuses and cause inflammation (particularly pain and swelling) of the mucosa, and is known as sinusitis.

Oroantral fistula is an iatrogenically created communication between the oral cavity and the maxillary antrum, as a consequence of a difficult extraction of upper posterior teeth **(Figures 16-11A and B)**. Accidental fractures of the maxillary tuberosity while extraction of upper third molars or forcing of root apices into the antral cavity, or any disturbances or removal of sinus lining during surgical procedures, could possibly cause the development of fistulas. This communication may lead to chronic sinusitis as consequence

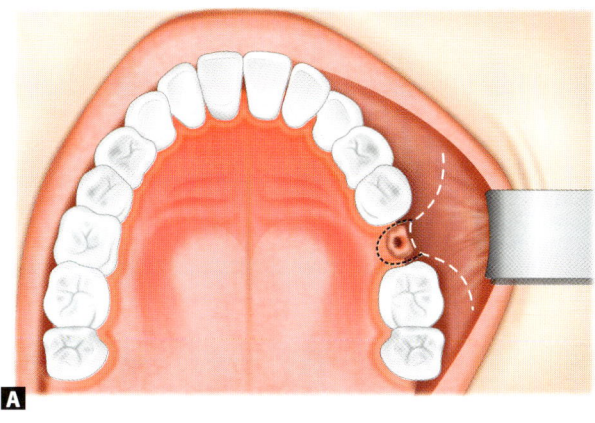
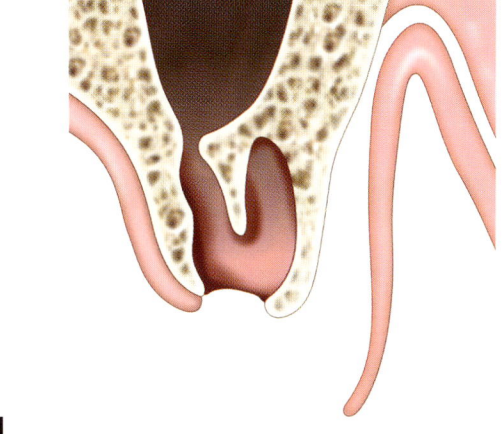

Figures 16-11A and B: Oroantral fistula in relation to maxillary antrum.

of contaminations from the food and saliva and has to be sorted for complete healing.

Sinus polyps are small, painless, benign, tear drop or mushroom-shaped growths that occur due to chronic irritation, recurring infections, allergies or drug sensitivity. These are common in the lining of the nose and maxillary sinus. These are present as solitary or multiple lesions. Larger polyps or clusters may interrupt with breathing and require surgical removal.

Antroliths, of the maxillary sinus are calcified masses (stone) found in the antral cavity infrequently. Previous inflammation and presence of fractured root tips or bone chips are possible causes. Usually asymptomatic, increase in size or occurrence of symptoms warrants a surgical removal.

Cysts of the maxillary antrum are occasionally reported. It can be either extrinsic, from the adjacent areas, that may invade the thin sinus lining and occupy the antral cavity or intrinsic, originating from the sinus lining itself. Most frequent would be sinus mucocele.

Malignancies of maxillary antrum are extremely rare, however loose teeth, bleeding gums, and occasional pain may be the early symptoms, which need to be addressed for early diagnosis and treatment.

Points to Remember

- Sinuses are air-filled spaces in the skull bones around the nasal cavity and are called paranasal sinuses.
- They are named after the bone, where it is located, namely—frontal sinus, sphenoid sinus, ethmoid sinus, and maxillary sinus.
- Maxillary sinus is the largest sinus of all the paranasal sinuses located in the body of maxilla.
- It is also called as antrum of Highmore and it opens in the middle nasal meatus.
- Maxillary sinus is pyramidal in shape, with its base forming the lateral wall of the nasal cavity, and apex directed laterally toward the zygomatic process of the maxilla. The four sides are walled anteriorly by facial surface of maxilla, posteriorly by the infratemporal surface of maxilla, superiorly by the floor of the orbit and inferiorly related to the palate and alveolar process and posterior teeth of the maxilla.
- The process of enlargement of sinus spaces is called pneumatization, which occurs mainly by the bone remodeling .
- Maxillary sinus is lined by pseudostratified ciliated columnar epithelium. This sinus lining is also known as "Schneiderian membrane".
- Three types of cells are noticed within the maxillary sinus epithelial lining, predominately ciliated columnar cells, less commonly nonciliated basal cells and mucus-producing goblet cells. **Ciliated cells** are specialized cells that facilitate the motility and propel the mucus and other substances over the epithelial surface by their rhythmic beatings. These cells play a key role in keeping the nasal cavity moist. **Basal columnar cells** are evident toward the basal membrane with centrally placed nucleus. **Goblet cells** are flask-shaped cells, located in between the ciliated cells and secrete mucus. The basal lamina separates the epithelium from the submucosal region. The lamina propria fused with periosteum consists of loose collagen bundles, few elastic fibers, subepithelial glands (serous and mucous glands), fibroblasts, vessels, and nerves.
- The maxillary sinus reduces the weight of the facial skeleton, moistens and humidifies the inspired air, and imparts resonance to the voice. Unique microciliary transport filters the debris from the inspired air. Secretions from the goblet cells and subepithelial glandular secretions facilitate mucus production and storage and provide thermal insulation to the vital organs located in the skull by assisting in maintaining the intracranial pressure. Prevents and limits the extent of injury to the facial trauma. The shape and structure of the face and paranasal sinuses may act as a crumple zone in severe trauma and thus protect the brain injury. It also serves as an accessory olfactory organ.

PRACTICE QUESTIONS

1. What are sinuses and name the paranasal sinuses?
2. Describe the boundaries of maxillary sinus.
3. Write a note on development of maxillary sinus.
4. List the functions of maxillary antrum.
5. Write notes on the lining of maxillary antrum.
6. What is oroantral fistula?

MULTIPLE CHOICE QUESTIONS

1. **The largest paranasal air sinus is**
   a. Ethmoid sinus
   b. Sphenoid sinus
   c. Maxillary sinus
   d. Frontal sinus
2. **Teeth roots associated with maxillary sinus floor and appear as projections are**
   a. Mandibular premolars and molars
   b. Deciduous canines
   c. Maxillary premolars and molars
   d. Maxillary anteriors
3. **The paranasal sinuses are drained into the nasal cavity via opening / foramen called**
   a. Recesses
   b. Antral fistula
   c. Ostia
   d. Meatus
4. **The process of enlargement of sinus spaces during development is called**
   a. Fusion
   b. Agenesis
   c. Pneumatization
   d. Recesses
5. **Maxillary sinus is also known as**
   a. Antrum of Highmore
   b. Antrum of Tomes
   c. Meckel's antrum
   d. Hopewell–Smith sinus
6. **The superior wall of the maxillary sinus is formed by the**
   a. Floor of the orbit and palate
   b. Medial wall of the nose and palate
   c. Floor of the orbit
   d. Zygomatic process
7. **Motility and propulsion of the mucus and other substances over the epithelial surface is enabled by the presence of**
   a. Stratified epithelium
   b. Ciliated epithelium
   c. Keratinized epithelium
   d. Non-keratinized epithelium
8. **Extension of maxillary sinus into alveolar process or frontal process is called as**
   a. Bone remodelling
   b. Invasion
   c. Recess
   d. None of the above
9. **The lining of maxillary sinus is known as**
   a. Schneiderian membrane
   b. Buccopharyngeal membrane
   c. Nasmyth's membrane
   d. Intermediate membrane
10. **The lymph from the sinus drains into the**
    a. Submental lymph nodes
    b. Submandibular lymph nodes
    c. Preauricular lymph nodes
    d. Post auricular lymph nodes

11. **The epithelial layer of maxillary sinus is made up of**
    a. Stratified squamous epithelium
    b. Keratinized epithelium
    c. Pseudostratified columnar epithelium
    d. Stratified columnar epithelium
12. **The flask-shaped cells of the maxillary sinus epithelium, located in between the ciliated cells and secrete mucus are called**
    a. Acinar cells
    b. Goblet cells
    c. Defence cells
    d. Myoepithelial cells
13. **Below are the functions of maxillary sinus, *except***
    a. Reduces the skull weight
    b. Maintains the resonance of voice
    c. Moistens and humidifies the inspired air
    d. Salivary secretion
14. **Calcified masses present in the antral cavity are called**
    a. Antroliths
    b. Sialoliths
    c. Denticles
    d. Polyps
15. **Bacterial infections associated with smaller sinus formation are**
    a. Congenital syphilis
    b. Tuberculosis
    c. Leprosy
    d. Mumps
16. **Iatrogenically created communication between the oral cavity and the maxillary antrum is known as**
    a. Orocutaneous fistula
    b. Oroantral sinus
    c. Oroantral fistula
    d. Antral fistula

ANSWERS

1. c   2. c   3. c   4. c   5. a   6. c   7. b   8. c   9. a   10. b   11. c   12. b   13. d   14. a   15. a
16. c

BIBLIOGRAPHY

1. Andrew Whyte, Rudolf Boeddinghaus. The maxillary sinus: physiology, development and imaging anatomy. Dentomaxillofacial Radiology 2019;48:20190205.
2. Available from http://dentfac.mans.edu.eg/files/english/pdf/ handouts/Maxillary_Sinus.pdf. [Accessed May 2018].
3. Available from https://www.kau.edu.sa/Files/0004509/ Files/61626 _THE%20M A XILLAR Y%20 SINUS%20 2010(students).pdf. [Accessed May 2018]
4. Avery JK, Chiego DJ. Essentials of oral histology and embryology: a clinical approach, 3rd edition. US: Mosby Elsevier; 2006.
5. Avery JK. Oral Development and Histology, 3rd edition. New York: Thieme; 2002.
6. Bell GW, Joshi BB, Macleod RI. Maxillary sinus disease: diagnosis and treatment. Br Dent J. 2011;210:113-8.
7. Cappello ZJ, Minutello K, Dublin AB. Anatomy, Head and Neck, Nose Paranasal Sinuses. [Updated 2021 Oct 7]. In: StatPearls [Internet]. Treasure Island (FL): StatPearls Publishing; 2022 Jan. Available from: https://www.ncbi.nlm.nih.gov/books/NBK499826/
8. Chandra S, Chandra S, Chandra M, et al. Textbook of dental and oral histology with embryology & MCQ's, 2nd edition. New Delhi: Jaypee Brothers Medical Publishers (P) Ltd; 2010.
9. Chatterjee K. Essentials of dental anatomy & oral histology, 2nd edition. New Delhi: Jaypee Brothers Medical Publishers (P) Ltd; 2014.
10. Gaunt WA, Osborn JW, Ten Cate AR. Advanced dental histology, 2nd edition. Bristol: John Wright & Sons Ltd.; 1971.
11. Hu Z, Sun D, Zhou Q, et al. Radiographic study of maxillary sinus associated with molars in adult. Lin Chung Er Bi Yan Hou Tou Jing Wai Ke Za Zhi. 2014;28(23):1863-5.
12. Jacob S. Human anatomy. UK: Elsevier; 2008.
13. Jafari-Pozve N, Sheikhi M, Ataie-Khorasgani M, et al. Aplasia and hypoplasia of the maxillary sinus: a case series. Dent Res J (Isfahan). 2014;11(5):615-7.
14. Joelwanaga, Charlotte Wilson, Stefan Lachkar, et al. Clinical anatomy of the maxillary sinus: application to sinus floor augmentation. Anat Cell Biol 2019;52:17-24.
15. Kumar GS. Orban's oral histology and embryology, 14th edition. India: Elsevier. 2015.
16. McGowan DA, Baxter PW, James J. The maxillary sinus and its dental implication, 1st edition. Boston: Wright; 1993.
17. Mogensen C, Tos M. Quantitative histology of the maxillary sinus. Rhinology. 1977;15(3):129-40.
18. Nanci A. Ten Cate's oral histology: development, structure, and function, 8th edition. St. Louis Missouri: Mosby Elsevier; 2014.
19. Rajkumar K, Ramya R. Textbook of oral anatomy, histology, physiology and tooth morphology, 2nd edition. India: Wolters Kluwer Health; 2017.
20. Schroeder HE. Oral structural biology, 4th edition. New York: Thieme; 1991.
21. Simon E. Anatomy of the opening of the maxillary sinus. Arch Otolaryngol. 1939;29(4):640-9.

CHAPTER

Lymphatics of Orofacial Region

B Sivapathasundharam, Doddabasavaiah Basavapur Nandini

Chapter Outline

- Lymphatic Organs 262
  - » Primary Lymphatic Organs and Tissues 263
  - » Secondary Lymphatic Organs and Tissues 263
  - » Tertiary Lymphoid Tissue 263
- Development of Lymphatic System 263
- Lymph 264
- Structure of Lymphatic System 264
  - » Lymph Capillaries 264
- » Lymph Vessels 264
- » Lymph Nodes 265
- Lymph Circulation 266
  - » Course of Lymph within the Node 266
  - » Course of Lymph from the Node to the Circulation 267
- Lymphatics of the Head and Neck 267
- Clinical Considerations 267

The lymphatic system is a well-organized uninterruptedly communicated circulatory system, composed of small capillaries to large lymph vessels and regional lymph nodes. This continual system of lymphatic vessels carries a clear fluid called lymph (from Latin, *lympha* meaning "water") toward the heart.

The lymphatic system is a specialized connective tissue that constitutes a group of lymphatic organs, lymph vessels, lymph nodes, and circulatory lymph that together monitors the immune system of the body. The functions include lymphocyte production by the lymph nodes, antibody production and stimulation, filtration of microorganisms and foreign body substances such as toxins, etc., and also aids in transport of larger molecules such as enzymes, and hormones from the site of production to the blood stream. In addition slight gaseous and nutrient exchange, draining of excess fluid, draining proteins and metabolic wastes in tissues back into blood, helping in absorption of digested lipid and fat-soluble vitamins in lacteals, which are specialized lymphatic vessels seen in the villi of the intestine.

Thus, the lymphatic system forms a prime component of immune surveillance of the body and also serves as an accessory return route of the blood into the circulation **(Flowchart 17-1).**

LYMPHATIC ORGANS

These are the sites for lymphocyte production and activation. They are categorized as primary (or central) and secondary

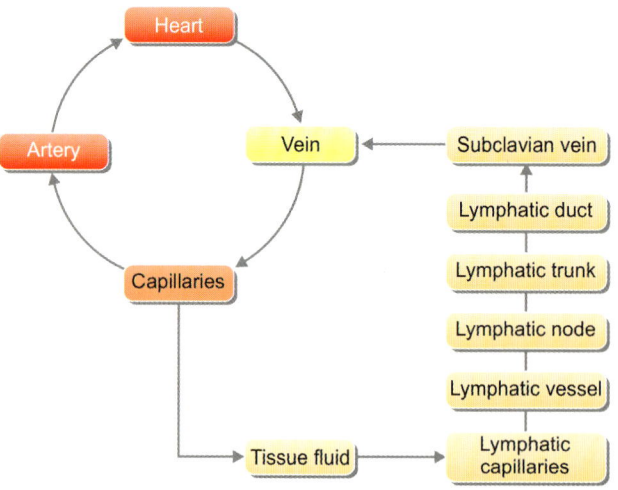

Flowchart 17-1: Components of lymphatic system.

(or peripheral) lymphatic organs based on their function. In general, the primary lymphatic organ generates lymphocytes from immature progenitor cells, while secondary lymphoid organs maintain the mature naive lymphocytes and play an active role in initiating immune response.

Primary Lymphatic Organs and Tissues

These include thymus, bone marrow, and lymphocytes, which undergo antigen-independent proliferation and

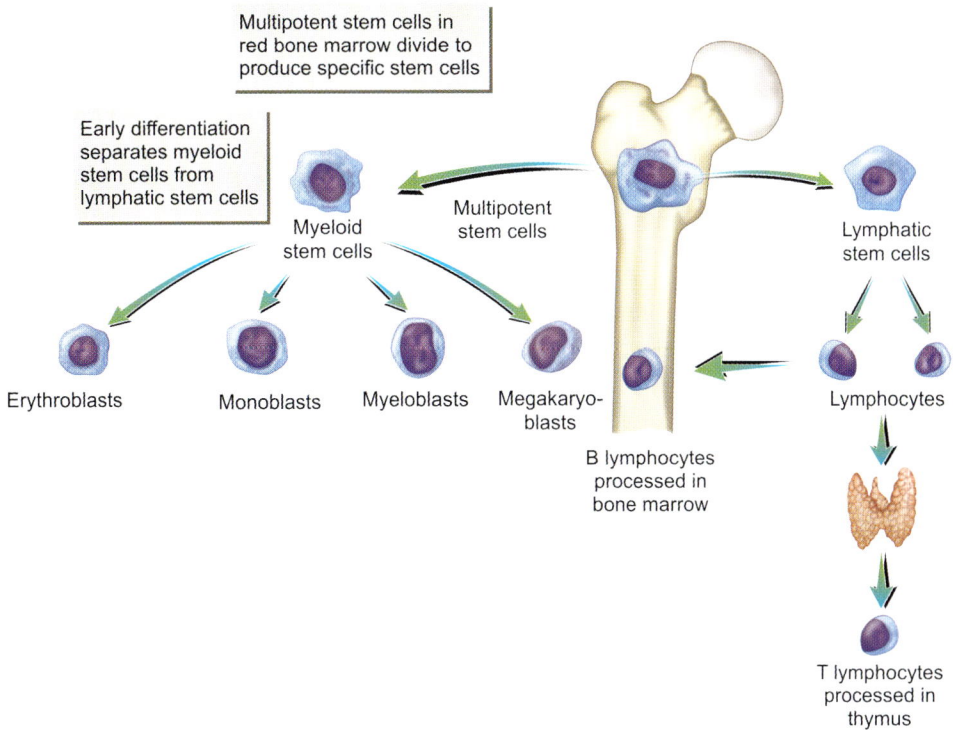

Figure 17-1: Lymphocytes production lineage in bone marrow and thymus.

differentiation. Thymus and bone marrow serve as preliminary organs of lymphoid production **(Figure 17-1)**. The thymus has lymphoid and endocrine function and plays a crucial role in immune system development. Immune function includes processing of T lymphocytes, while endocrine function includes production of thymosin and thymine. The pluripotent stem cells of bone marrow produce two streams of cell lines, myeloid trilineage stem cells and lymphoid stem cells. The myeloid trilineage stem cells further divide to form progenitor cells of erythrocytes, megakaryocytes, and granulocyte–monocytes. Lymphoid stem cells are responsible for the production of both T cells and B cells and maturation of B cells. The matured B cells directly join the circulatory system and eventually enter into the secondary lymphoid organs. Besides, the T cells travel to the thymus and further get matured. Consequently the mature T cells and B cells begin their defensive role on exposure to pathogens.

Secondary Lymphatic Organs and Tissues

Include spleen, tonsils, lymph nodes, lymphatic nodules, and adenoids. Adenoids are frequently referred as nose-associated lymphoid tissue (NALT). In addition, the other lymphoid cells concentration or lymphoid tissues distributed in body include Peyer's patches and other mucosa-associated lymphoid tissue (MALT) a collective term used for lymphoid tissues of the gastrointestinal, respiratory, and genitourinary tracts, bronchus-associated lymphoid tissue (BALT), gut-associated lymphoid tissues (GALT) and skin-associated lymphoid tissue (SALT), together form an integral part of lymphatic system.

Exposure to foreign or altered native molecules (antigens) in the secondary lymphatic tissue or during the recirculation of lymphocytes between the blood and peripheral lymphoid organs, activates and expands the mature lymphocytes. Progressively, lymphocytes assume the immune role.

Tertiary Lymphoid Tissue

Abrupt accumulation of lymphoid cell aggregates in a nonlymphoid tissue occurs as a response to chronic infection. Also accounts for small number of lymphocytes present in the blood and lymph. Tertiary lymphoid tissues are similar to secondary lymphoid tissue in composition, cell population, and presume an immune role only in case of inflammation.

DEVELOPMENT OF LYMPHATIC SYSTEM

Lymphatic system development starts from the formation of a series of endothelium-lined sacs called the lymph sac. These sacs are found at the junction of embryonic veins. Exact origin is not clear; however, it is considered to be originated either from these veins or independent formation from the mesenchyme.

Around 5th week of intrauterine life, six lymph sacs are identified as right and left jugular sacs at the future junction between jugular vein and subclavian veins, right and left posterior (or iliac) sacs lie around common iliac vein, the unpaired retroperitoneal sac in relation to the root of mesentery and another single cisterna chyli in the midline, caudal to the retroperitoneal sac. Soon all the lymphatic sacs except the cisterna chyli are invaded by the lymphocytes and connective tissue stroma to develop into lymph node.

The lymphatic vessels or plexuses develop either by extension of lymphatic sacs or may form *de novo* and extend into various tissues.

LYMPH

Lymph is a product of the blood, wherein approximately 50% of the lost fluids and serum protein are returned to the circulation through the lymph node in the form of lymph and prevent the fall of total blood volume. The lymph vessels facilitate the return of blood plasma that escaped the capillary filtration as the interstitial fluid. Both lymph and interstitial fluid are similar in composition; however lymph is slightly more diluted and is found inside the closed lymph vessels while tissue fluid is found outside the vessel in the tissue spaces.

Lymph is transparent, colorless or slightly yellow in color, and composed of lymphocytes, cellular debris, and waste products with bacteria and proteins. The specific gravity of lymph is 1.015 and has protein concentration of 3–5 g/dL. Lymph differs from blood in many aspects as shown in **Table 17-1**.

The course of lymph begins in the small capillaries, where it absorbs the interstitial fluid from the tissues and moves forward into the larger collecting vessels. Further lymph opens up into the right lymphatic duct and left lymphatic duct (thoracic duct) on either side. Eventually, the lymph vessels are emptied into the subclavian veins and return to the blood stream. Thus lymphatic system serves as an accessory return route of the blood into the circulation **(Figure 17-2)**.

The transport of lymph within the lymph vessels is driven either by the intrinsic contractions of the lymphatic passages or by the extrinsic compressions of the lymph vessels through tissue forces without any central pump. The flow of lymph is unidirectional and the backflow within the vessels is restrained by presence of numerous valves. The valves are noticed in the larger vessels and ducts except in smaller capillaries.

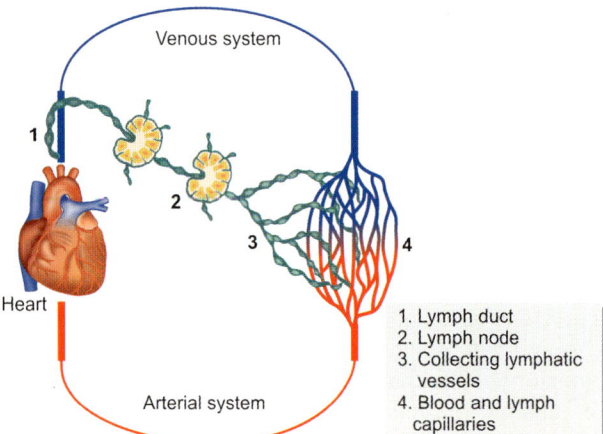

Figure 17-2: Components of lymphatic system and formation of lymph.

STRUCTURE OF LYMPHATIC SYSTEM

Lymph Capillaries

The lymph capillaries are the terminal lymphatics, where the lymph first enters. The tissue fluid which has escaped the capillary filtration is expelled into the connective tissue spaces as an interstitial fluid. The complex capillaries form a plexus and absorb the tissue fluid as lymph and drain into lymph vessels **(Figures 17-3A and B)**. Lymph capillaries are slightly larger than the blood capillaries and are found in every part of the body except the central nervous system, meninges, eyeball (except the conjunctiva), orbit, internal ear, within striated muscle, liver lobule, spleen pulp, kidney parenchyma and entire cartilage.

Structure of Lymph Capillaries

Microscopically these terminal capillaries appear similar to vascular counterpart, the blood capillaries, however differ in function. Ultrastructurally, these capillaries lack definite basement membrane, and it is poorly developed if present. Unlike arterial and venous ends, lymph capillaries lack definitive ends. This prevents the direct re-entry of the lymph into the circulation. The endothelial cells around the lumen are attached to the surrounding connective tissues by means of small bundles of filaments called anchoring filaments. These fibers hold up the lumen, open and prevent vessel collapse even when the hydrostatic pressure is raised outside. The pericytes (the cells which are seen in the outer aspect of the blood capillaries and help in contraction and dilatation of the capillaries) are absent around these capillaries.

Lymph Vessels

The lymph vessels are thin-walled and valved structures that carry lymph to all parts of the body. They are the second collecting unit of the lymph. The vessels are transparent and their contents are visible. The network of lymph vessels begins as tiny capillaries and continues as larger vessels as it enters the lymph node. The lymph vessels, which carry lymph to the lymph node are called the afferent lymph vessels and those that carry the lymph from the node are called as the efferent lymph vessels. Consecutively lymph can be either carried to other lymph node or to the larger ducts and terminally drained into the subclavian vein thus the lost tissue fluid re-enters into circulation, to maintain the blood volume.

Structure of Lymph Vessel

Microscopically, lymph vessels are also very similar to the blood vessels and can be distinctly differentiated by the presence of small lymphocytes within the vessels instead of erythrocytes as in the blood vessels. Occasionally noted pericytes are rudimentary. Greater permeability and presence of numerous vessel valves to prevent the backflow are in contrast to the blood vessels.

Ultrastructurally, the larger lymph vessels are composed of three coats **(Figure 17-4)** similar to blood vessels.
- ❖ Internal coat
- ❖ Middle coat
- ❖ External coat.

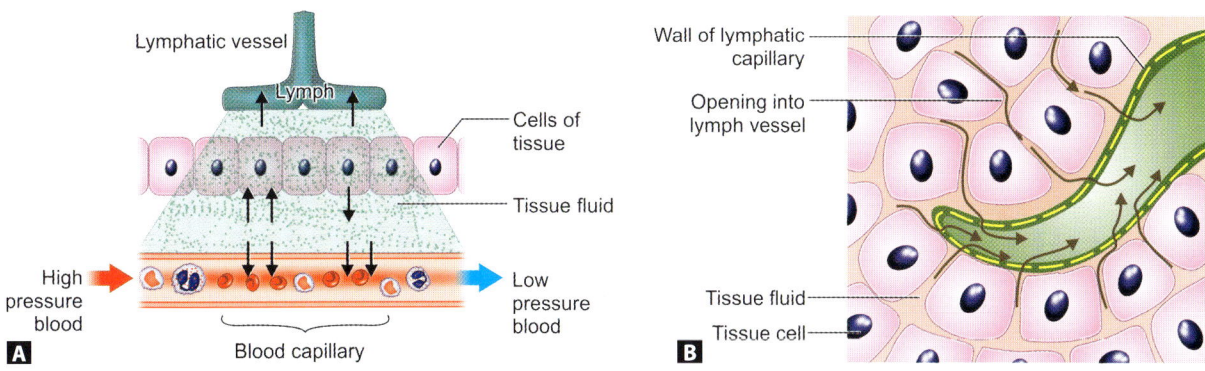

Figures 17-3A and B: Relation of tissue fluid and lymphatic capillaries.

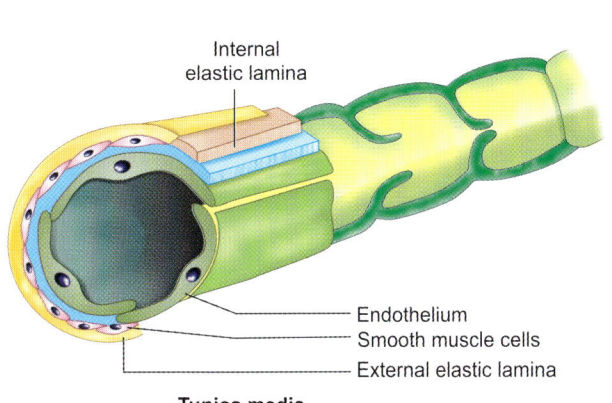

Figure 17-4: Structure of lymph vessel.

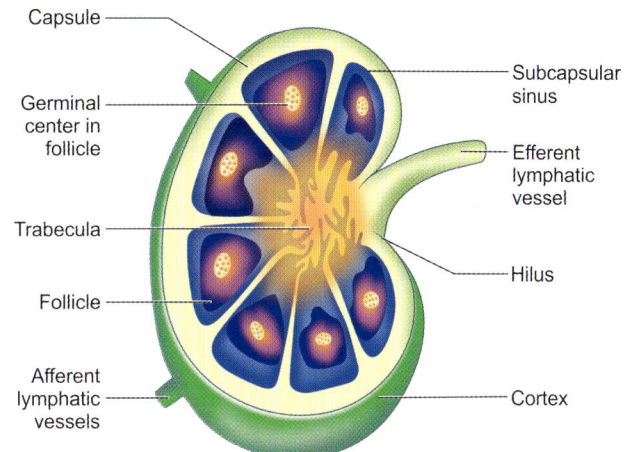

Figure 17-5: Cut section of the lymph node showing the entry of afferent vessels at the periphery of the gland and exit of efferent vessel at the hilus.

Inner Coat

It is the thin layer that lines the interior surface of lumen. It is formed by a single layer of flat endothelial cells that separates the outer membranes by a firm basement membrane. The gap between the endothelial cells and the permeable basement membrane permit the transport of the lymph within the vessel wall, however the backflow is prevented by the valves present within the vessel.

Middle Coat

It is the second coat and is made up of smooth muscles arranged in a circular fashion. The contraction and relaxation of smooth muscles contribute to the pumping of lymph throughout the body.

Outer Coat

It is the third coat, similar to that seen in blood vessels, composed of fibrous tissue, formed by collagen fibers. This layer primarily supports and adds to the stability of the vessel. This layer is noticed only in larger vessels and ducts and is absent in lymph capillaries.

Lymph Nodes

The lymph nodes also called lymph glands are the next lymph collecting unit of the lymphatic system after the lymphatic vessels. The lymph nodes are seeded throughout the body in the form of small clusters and serve a major role in the immunity by acting as a filter against the foreign bodies and tumor cells. The distribution of lymph nodes is wide and it is the major residing site for B and T lymphocytes and other white blood cells. There are around 600 lymph nodes in the body and are dense around the pharynx and neck, chest, armpits, groin, and around the intestines. Interestingly the complete lack of lymph vessels is noticed in the upper central nervous system; conversely tissue fluid is drained into the cerebrospinal fluid rather as lymph.

Structure of the Lymph Nodes

Lymph nodes are small, oval, and bean-shaped bodies found in clusters and approximately 0.5–2.5 cm in size. On longitudinal section, lymph node displays a capsule covering the outer cortex and the inner, dark region called the medulla. The medullary spaces continue to the outer surface through a central depression called the hilus. Thus efferent vessels from the medullary structures leave the node via hilus, while the afferent vessels enter the node on the opposite side through cortical coverings **(Figure 17-5)**.

The capsule of the lymph node is made up of dense fibrous connective tissue. The subsequent cortical space (cortex) is divided into outer or superficial cortex and inner or paracortical area **(Figure 17-6A)**. The outer cortex contains lymphoid follicles, hence called as follicle compartment, while

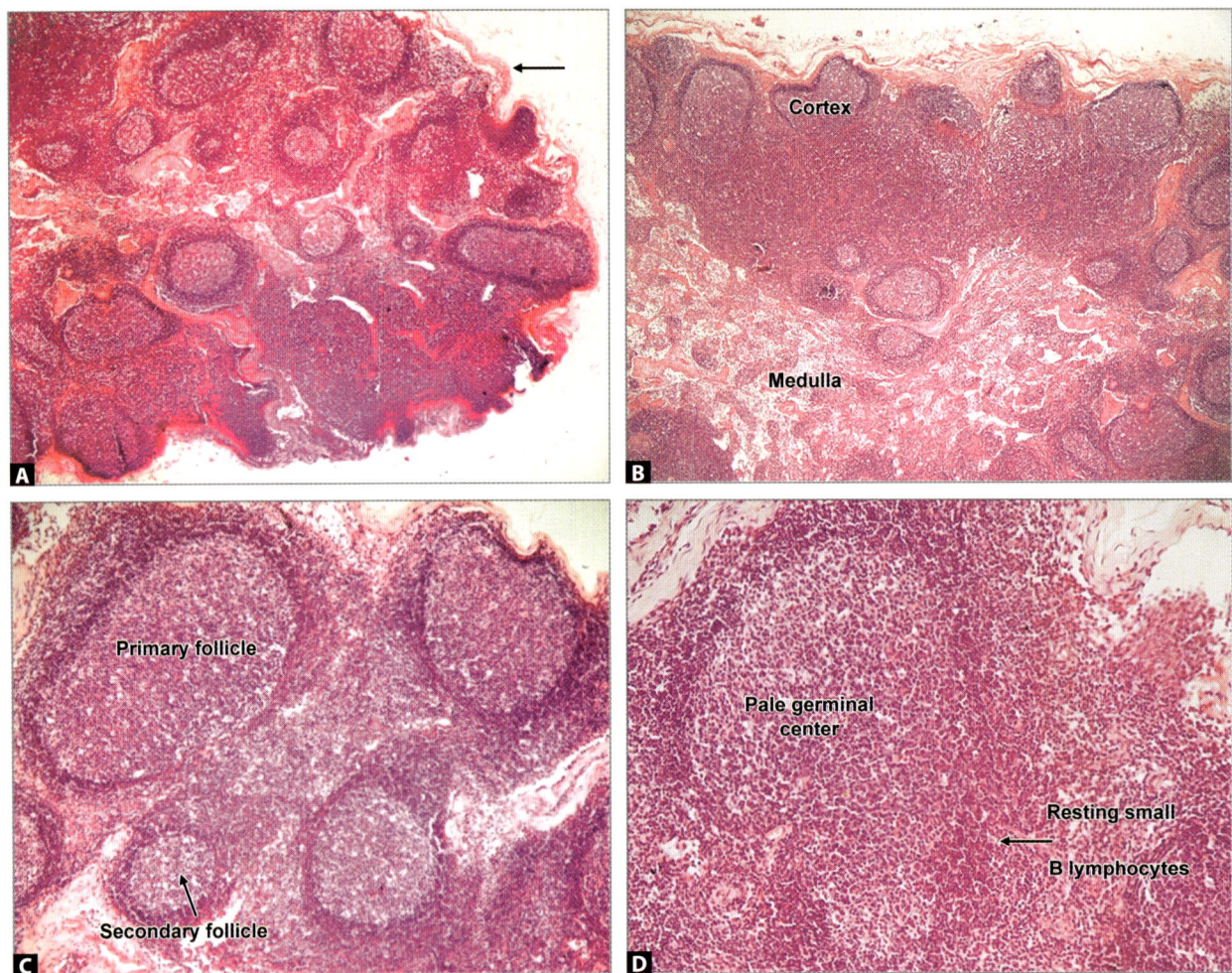

Figures 17-6A to D: Hematoxylin and eosin stained section of a lymph node: (A) Capsule of the lymph node is made up of dense fibrous connective tissue; (B) Lymphoid cells of the inner cortex continue with the medullary compartment; (C) Primary follicles and secondary follicles; (D) Primary follicle with pale germinal center surrounded by resting small B lymphocytes.

the inner cortex comprises lymphoid cells and continues with the medullary compartment **(Figure 17-6B)**. The cortical spaces are divided into irregular compartments by a capsular extension called trabeculae supported by an intricate reticular meshwork. This forms the framework and provides the free spaces for the cells and the blood vessels within the gland. Trabeculae divide the lymph node into compartments known as lymph nodules. Each lymph nodule is composed of B cells in the cortical region and T cells in the paracortical region.

The follicle compartments of the outer cortex consist of primary follicles and secondary follicles **(Figure 17-6C)**. Primary follicles are spherical and composed of small resting B lymphocytes that cluster around specialized antigen presenting cells. The secondary lymphoid follicles are derived from the primary follicles in response to the antigenic stimuli. After antigenic challenge, *i.e.* soon after birth, primary follicles develop into secondary follicles through progressive generation of a mitotically hyperactive population of B cells, which form an area called the germinal center. This is surrounded by a mantle zone of transient small resting B lymphocytes **(Figure 17-6D)**. The follicles also contain other accessory cells namely—follicular dendritic cells, macrophages, some T lymphocytes and other lymphoid cells, in various developmental stages. The inner cortex contains mostly T cells, and some dendritic cells. Distinct venules with plump endothelial cells are noticed in this region, which are essential for homing and distribution of lymphocytes.

The deep cortical and medullary cords contain B cells and plasma cells predominately, along with macrophages, and occasional mast cells, supported by dense reticular meshwork. The plasma cells produce antibodies, while the macrophages filter the antigen from the lymph. The sinuses and blood vessels are noticed intervening the cells of medullary and cortical region and are supported by loose network of reticular fibers.

LYMPH CIRCULATION

Course of Lymph within the Node

The unfiltered tissue fluid is subsequently modified within the lymph node before it enters into the circulation as lymph. The tissue fluid, containing microorganisms, soluble antigens, antigen-presenting cells, and a few B cells, enters the lymph

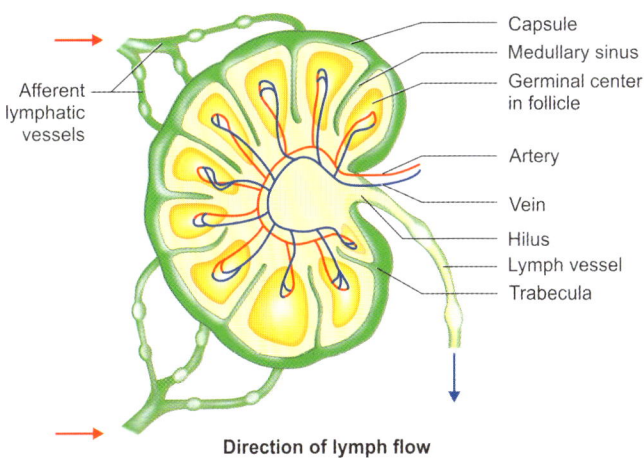

Figure 17-7: Schematic representation of the course of lymph within the gland. The modified lymph enters the gland at capsule, subsequently transported to the cortical sinuses, then to the medullary sinuses, and finally exits the gland at the hilum to enter into the circulation.

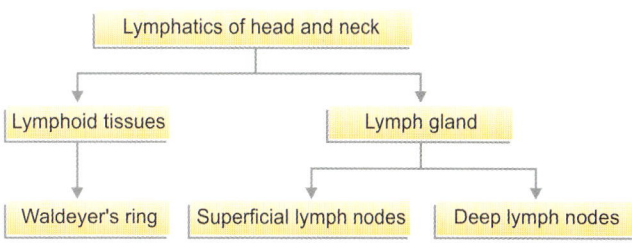

Flowchart 17-2: Categorization of the lymphatic system of the head and neck.

TABLE 17-1: Head and neck lymph nodes.	
Superficial lymph nodes	**Deep lymph nodes**
• Submental nodes • Submandibular nodes • Buccal nodes • Preauricular • Postauricular • Occipital • Anterior cervical • Superficial cervical	• Prelaryngeal and pretracheal • Paratracheal • Retropharyngeal

node via afferent lymph vessels at the capsule and pass into the subcapsular sinus. The sinuses in the lymph nodes are vessel-like spaces, which occur below the capsule and in between the follicles. It then runs into the cortical areas through cortical sinuses and continues through the trabecular sinuses in the deep cortical region. Finally it drains into the medullary sinuses, which are continuation of trabecular sinuses. The medullary sinuses from different lobules converge into the medulla and leave the gland as one single collecting duct, (efferent lymphatic vessel) at the hilus and continue in the circulation as lymph **(Figure 17-7)**.

Course of Lymph from the Node to the Circulation

After the conversion of the tissue fluid into lymph at the nodes, the efferent vessels return the lymph back into the circulation by the lymph trunks and ducts. These are the two terminal large lymphatic structures at the end of the lymphatic system that recirculate the lymph as plasma of the blood stream and replace the tissue fluid loss.

Many of the efferent vessels converge into lymphatic trunk, the large lymph vessel. Lymphatic trunks then drain lymph fluid into the lymph ducts, the final part of the lymphatic system, which in turn opens into respective subclavian veins and join the circulation.

> Lymphatic system lacks a central pumping mechanism like the heart of cardiovascular system. Instead it has its own active pumping system driven by segments that have a function similar to peristalsis. Smooth muscle contractions help to move lymph along the vessels; however skeletal muscle contractions also move lymph through the vessels.

LYMPHATICS OF THE HEAD AND NECK

Lymphatic system is the site for many key immune system functions. The prime function of the lymphoid organs is to guard the body since they are the first site for many pathological processes to present. The knowledge of the regional lymph nodes and course of lymphatics is cardinal in diagnosis and treatment of inflammatory and infectious diseases and malignant tumors of the head and neck region, since they may spread via lymph vessels.

The lymphatic system of the head and neck is widely communicated and highly developed in children and younger adults and starts slowing down with age. This can be categorized broadly into lymph node and lymphoid tissue **(Flowchart 17-2)**.

The lymph nodes in the head and neck region are categorized into superficial and deep nodes based on their relation to deep fascia of neck **(Table 17-1)**. The lymph from scalp, face, and neck drains into superficial group of lymph nodes at the junction of head and neck. The head and neck region comprises a group of lymphoid tissue arranged in the form of a ring, called the Waldeyer's ring **(Figures 17-8A and B)**. It extends from the chin to posterior aspect of the neck and ultimately drains into the deep cervical lymph nodes along the left and right jugular lymphatic trunks. The pharyngeal tonsil at the roof of the pharynx, the two palatine tonsils between the anterior and posterior palatine pillars, and lingual tonsil at the base of the tongue together forms a ring. It monitors at the entrance and prevents the entry of pathogens into the deeper parts of digestive and respiratory tract.

The list and diagram of head and neck lymph nodes are given in **Figure 17-9 and Table 17-2**.

CLINICAL CONSIDERATIONS

Healthy nodes are usually not palpable, but infection or malignancies may cause them to become enlarged. The enlarged node can be felt by passing the sensitive fleshy part of the fingertips over the location of each group of nodes. The evaluation of lymph nodes during clinical examination is

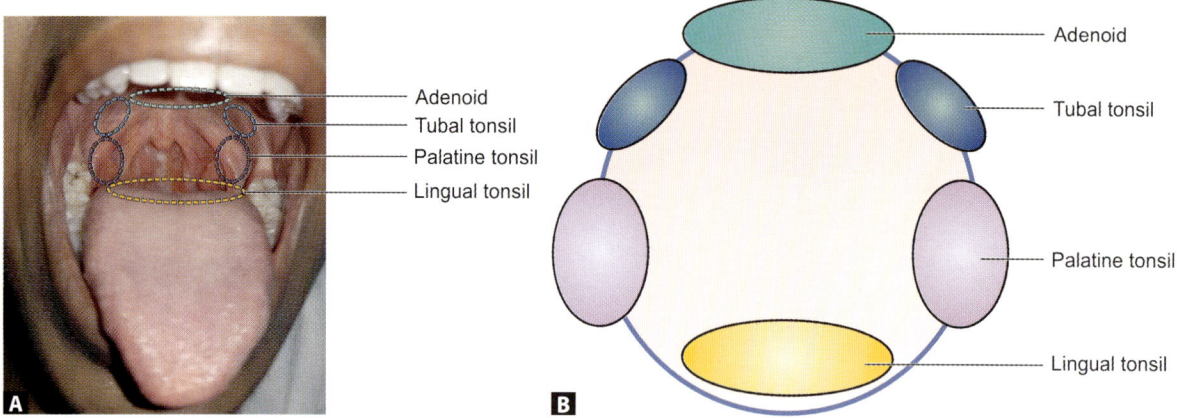

Figures 17-8A and B: (A) Waldeyer's ring, arrangement of lymphoid tissue in the form of a ring; (B) Schematic representation of Waldeyer's ring.

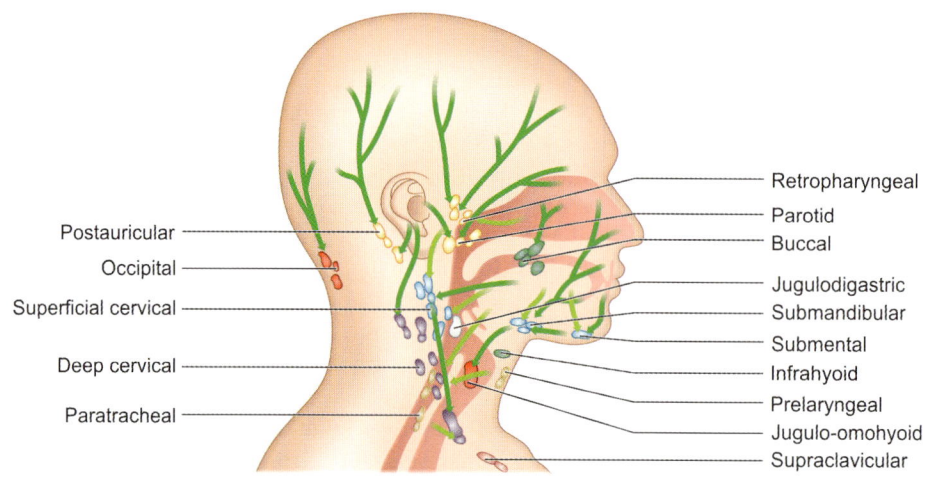

Figure 17-9: Schematic representation of lymph nodes of head and neck.

important, since enlarged nodes may indicate inflammation or infection from sites that drain into them or may be an indicator of the spread of cancer **(Table 17-3)**.

Lymph nodes are generally less than 1 cm in diameter and vary slightly in different regions and age-groups. Lymphadenopathy refers to enlargement of lymph nodes and may be noticed in cases of infection, malignancy, autoimmune diseases, and drug reactions. A lymph node more than 2 cm should be investigated. Jugulodigastric lymph nodes (often the largest of cervical lymph nodes) > 1.5 cm are considered abnormal.

The lymphadenopathy can be classified as localized and generalized. Localized lymphadenopathy is well-confined and involves the localized regional lymph node into which it drains. For example, the submandibular lymph nodes are enlarged in case of any infection in the head and neck region; in particular the dental infections. Inflammation of lymph node is known as lymphadenitis and is characterized by an increase in the size of node. However, lymphadenopathy simply means lymph node enlargement, which may be due to inflammation or other causes. Most often this delineation is not made and both terms are used synonymously.

In contrast, the enlargement of more than two noncontiguous lymph nodes is referred as generalized lymphadenopathy. Generalized lymphadenopathy may be seen in many systemic diseases ranging from minor illness to life-threatening conditions such as leukemia or acquired immunodeficiency syndrome (AIDS).

Lymph nodes may be enlarged and tender in case of inflammation caused usually by an infection. Firm, tender, enlarged, warm lymph nodes and reddened overlying skin may correlate with local infection. Infection origin can be either from the organs that the nodes drain or primarily within the lymph node itself, and are referred to as lymphadenitis.

In malignancies, lymph nodes are painless, hard on palpation, nontender and may be fixed and relatively immovable (due to infiltration into the adjacent tissues) and will continue to get larger. Lymph nodes involvement is evident in both, the primary cancer of lymph node or lymph tissues itself as in lymphomas, or in cases of tumors of other region due to metastasis of tumor cells to the nodes.

Enlarged lymph nodes in the absence of any infection or malignancy may represent a fibrosed node, the result of a previous inflammation.

TABLE 17-2: Anatomical sites and their draining group of lymph nodes.

Anatomical site	Draining lymph node	
	Primary	Secondary
Forehead	Superficial and deep parotid lymph nodes	Deep cervical
Eyelids, conjunctiva		
Lateral part of cheek		
Tongue—anterior two-thirds	Submandibular lymph node	Jugulo-omohyoid, Deep cervical
Floor of the mouth		
Buccal mucosa		
Hard palate		
Gingiva and alveolus		
Upper lip and lateral part of lower lip		
Maxillary and mandibular teeth		
Oral palate		
Cheeks, nose, and anterior nasal cavity		
Tongue—tip		
Center of the lower lip	Submental lymph node	Submandibular
Chin		
Lower incisors		
Tongue—posterior one-third tongue		
Posterior nasal cavity		
Paranasal sinuses	Retropharyngeal	Superficial and deep cervical nodes
Hard and soft palate		
Nasopharynx		
Oropharynx		
Auditory tube		
Tonsil	Upper jugular	Jugulodigastric
Scalp	Mastoid	
Larynx, pharynx, trachea, esophagus	Pretracheal, paratracheal, prelaryngeal, infrahyoid	Deep cervical

Table 17-3: Difference between blood and lymph.

Blood	Lymph
Has all cells RBC, WBC, platelets, plasma contains more fibrinogen and clotting factors	Has WBC predominantly lymphocytes, less fibrinogen and clotting factors Lacks RBCs and platelets
More oxygen and nutrients, more glucose concentration present	Less oxygen and nutrients, glucose concentration present
Red in color	Colorless or light yellow
Coagulates quickly	Coagulates very slowly
Faster flow rate	Slower flow rate
The movement of blood is in circular motion	The movement of lymph is in a single direction

Persistent generalized lymphadenopathy is a condition where lymphadenopathy is persistent for a long time without any apparent cause.

Autoimmune diseases like systemic lupus erythematosus, scleroderma and rheumatoid arthritis are frequently related to lymphadenopathy.

Malformations due to failure of lymphatics to communicate with venous system result in lymphangiomas and majority of which manifest in childhood below 2 years.

Edema accumulates in tissues during inflammation or when lymph drainage is impaired, or lymphatic vessel is blocked.

Points to Remember

- Lymphoid organs are classified as primary, secondary and tertiary lymphoid organs.
- T-lymphocytes and B-lymphocytes form a major component of lymphatic system.
- The clear fluid that circulates in the lymphatic system is called as Lymph.
- Waldeyer's ring consists of the adenoids, pharyngeal tonsil at the roof of the pharynx, the two palatine tonsils between the anterior and posterior palatine pillars, and lingual tonsil at the base of the tongue.
- Lymph nodes are small bean-shaped glands that are responsible for filtering fluid from the lymphatic system.
- Lymph nodes are not seen in central nervous system.
- Inflammation of lymph nodes is known as *Lymphadenitis*.
- Enlargement of lymph nodes is referred as *lymphadenopathy*.
- Lymphoid tissue in the oral cavity is referred to as *mucosa-associated lymphoid tissue* (MALT)

PRACTICE QUESTIONS

1. Classify and discuss various lymphoid organs.
2. Describe the structure of a lymph node.
3. Describe about the lymphatic drainage in the head and neck.
4. Discuss the differences between blood and lymph.
5. Describe the various functions of the lymphatic system.
6. Write a note on clinical considerations of lymph nodes.

MULTIPLE CHOICE QUESTIONS

1. **The lymphocytes, which become immunocompetent in thymus are:**
   a. B lymphocytes
   b. T lymphocytes
   c. NK cells
   d. None of the above
2. **Lymphocytes are of two types namely:**
   a. T cells and erythrocytes,
   b. Erythrocytes and platelets
   c. T cells and B cells
   d. Platelets and B cells
3. **Medulla consists predominantly of:**
   a. Stromal cells
   b. B cells
   c. Dendritic cells
   d. T cells
4. **Which of the following is not a part of lymphatic system:**
   a. Liver
   b. Thymus and spleen
   c. Tonsils
   d. Adenoids
5. **What are large aggregates of lymphatic tissue in the small intestine called as?**
   a. Lymph nodes
   b. Tonsils
   c. Adenoids
   d. Peyer's patches
6. **Where are Peyer's patches located?**
   a. Esophagus
   b. Stomach
   c. Small intestine
   d. Oral cavity
7. **What is the acronym for lymphatic tissue found in the mucosa?**
   a. SALT
   b. MALT
   c. BALT
   d. None of the above
8. **Which lymphoid organ is the primary site of cancer metastasis?**
   a. Adenoids
   b. Lymph nodes
   c. Spleen
   d. Thymus
9. **The outer cortex of the lymph node consists of:**
   a. B lymphocytes
   b. T Lymphocytes
   c. Platelets
   d. All of the above
10. **Waldeyer's ring is comprised of:**
    a. Adenoids
    b. Palatine tonsils
    c. Lingual tonsils
    d. All of the above
11. **Which of the following statements is false–Lymph differs from blood as it:**
    a. Lacks red blood cells
    b. Lacks platelets
    c. Is red in color
    d. Flows back into veins
12. **The indented region of the lymph node is called as:**
    a. Cortex
    b. Paracortex
    c. Afferent lymphatic
    d. Hilus
13. **What propels lymph through lymphatic vessels?**
    a. Skeletal muscle contraction
    b. Breathing movements
    c. Contraction of smooth muscles in vessel wall
    d. All of the above

14. **Which of the following is not a secondary lymphoid organ?**
    a. Thymus
    b. Spleen
    c. Lymph node
    d. Peyer's patch
15. **T-lymphocytes**
    a. Can ingest pathogens and kill them
    b. Can recirculate through blood and lymphoid organs
    c. Are short-lived
    d. Are educated in the bone marrow
16. **What is the function of lymphatic system?**
    a. Immunity
    b. Transport of lipid from GIT to the blood
    c. Drains excess interstitial fluid
    d. All of the above
17. **Lymph nodes are distributed throughout the body but not seen in:**
    a. Groin
    b. Neck
    c. Armpit
    d. Central nervous system
18. **Which of the following cells produce antibodies?**
    a. T cells
    b. NK cells
    c. Plasma cells
    d. Macrophages
19. **Which of the following lymph nodes monitor lymph originating from the head and neck?**
    a. Thoracic lymph nodes
    b. Abdominal lymph nodes
    c. Axillary lymph nodes
    d. Cervical lymph nodes
20. **Compared to blood capillaries, lymph capillaries:**
    a. Have walls of smooth endothelial lining
    b. Are frequently irregular in shape
    c. Are smaller in diameter
    d. Have a basal lamina
21. **The lymphatic system consists of all of the following, *except*:**
    a. Blood
    b. Lymph nodes
    c. Lymphatic vessels
    d. Lymph

ANSWERS

1. b	2. c	3. d	4. a	5. d	6. c	7. b	8. b	9. a	10. d	11. c	12. d	13. d	14. c	15. b
16. d	17. d	18. c	19. d	20. b	21. a									

BIBLIOGRAPHY

1. Agin AMR, Lee MJ. Grant's Atlas of Anatomy, 10th edition. Baltimore: Williams & Wilkins; 1999.
2. Angel CE, Chen CJ, Horlacher OC, et al. Distinctive localization of antigen-presenting cells in human lymph nodes. Blood. 2009;113:1257-67.
3. Avery JK, Chiego DJ. Essentials of Oral Histology and Embryology- A Clinical Approach, 3rd edition. St. Louis: Mosby; 2006.
4. Avery JK. Oral Development and Histology, 3rd edition. St. Louis: Mosby; 2006.
5. Bajenoff M, Germain RN. B-cell follicle development remodels the conduit system and allows soluble antigen delivery to follicular dendritic cells. Blood. 2009;114:4989.
6. Berkovitz BKB, Holland GR, Moxham BJ. Oral Anatomy, Histology and Embryology, 4th edition. US: Elsevier; 2009.
7. Blum KS, Reinhard P. Keystones in lymph node development. J Anat. 2006;209:585.
8. Castellarin P, Pozzato G, Tirelli G, et al. Oral lesions and lymphoproliferative disorders. J Oncol. 2010;2010:202305.
9. Cawson RA, Odel EW. Essentials of Oral Pathology and Oral Medicine, 8th edition. Edinburgh: Churchill Livingstone; 2008.
10. Chandra S, Chandra S, Chandra M, et al. Textbook of Dental and Oral Histology with Embryology & MCQ's, 2nd edition. India: Jaypee Brothers Medical Publishers (P) Ltd; 2010.
11. Chaplin DD. Overview of the immune response. J Allergy Clin Immunol. 2010;125(2):53.
12. Chatterjee K. Essentials of Dental Anatomy and Oral Histology, 2nd edition. India: Jaypee Brothers Medical Publishers (P) Ltd; 2014.
13. Ellis H. Clinical anatomy, 11th edition. London: Blackwell Publishing; 2006.
14. Elmore SA. Enhanced histopathology of the lymph nodes. Toxicol Pathol. 2006;34(5):634.
15. Elmore SA. Histopathology of the Lymph Nodes. Toxicol Pathol. 2006;34:425.
16. Ferrer R. Lymphadenopathy: differential diagnosis and evaluation. Am Fam Physician. 1998;58(6):1313-20.
17. Fu YX, Chaplin DD. Development and maturation of secondary lymphoid tissues. Annu Rev Immunol. 1999;17:399.
18. Guyton AC, Hall JE. Textbook of Medical Physiology, 11th edition. Mississippi: Elsevier; 2006.
19. Harizi H, Gualde N. The impact of eicosanoids on the crosstalk between innate and adaptive immunity: The key roles of dendritic cells. Tissue Antigens. 2005;65(6):507.
20. Iaochim HL, Medeiro JL. Lymph Node Pathology, 4th edition. Philadelphia: Lippincott Williams and Wilkins; 2009.
21. Isselhard DE, Brand RW. Anatomy of Orofacial Structures, 7th edition. St. Louis: Mosby; 2003.
22. Katakai T, Hara T, Lee JH, et al. A novel reticular stromal structure in lymph node cortex: an immuno-platform for interactions among dendritic cells, T cells and B cells. Int Immunol. 2004;16(8):1133.
23. Kumar GS. Orban's Oral Histology and Embryology, 14th edition. India: Elsevier; 2015.
24. Lamont R, Burne R, Lantz M, et al. Oral Microbiology and Immunology, 1st edition. US: ASM Press; 2006.

25. Liu X, Cheng C, Chen K, Wu Y and Wu Z. Recent Progress in Lymphangioma. Front. Pediatr 2021;9:735832.
26. Maini R, Nagalli S. Lymphadenopathy. 2021 Aug 11. In: StatPearls [Internet]. Treasure Island (FL): StatPearls Publishing; 2021 Jan. PMID: 32644344.
27. Meneses A, Verastegui E, Barrera JL, et al. Lymph node histology in head and neck cancer: impact of immunotherapy with IRX. Int Immunopharmacol. 2003;3(8):1083-91.
28. Mills SE. Histology for Pathologists, 3rd edition. Philadelphia: Lippincott Williams and Wilkins; 2007.
29. Mohseni S, Shojaiefard A, Khorgami Z: Peripheral lymphadenopathy: Approach and Diagnostic Tools. Iran J Med Sci. 2014;39:158-70.
30. Paul WE. Fundamental Immunology, 6th edition. Philadelphia: Lippincott Williams and Wilkins; 2008.
31. Pepper S, Islam H, Jayabose S, et al. Neuroblastoma masquerading as cervical lymphadenitis. J Pediatr Hematol Oncol. 2007;29(4):260-1.
32. Randall TD, Carragher DM, Rangel-Moreno J. Development of secondary lymphoid organs. Annu Rev Immunol. 2008;26:627.
33. Richards PS, Peacock TE. The role of ultrasound in the detection of cervical lymph node metastases in clinically N0 squamous cell carcinoma of the head and neck. Cancer Imaging. 2007;7:167.
34. Snell RS. Clinical Anatomy, 7th edition. Washington DC: Lippincott Williams and Wilkins; 2004.
35. Standring S. Gray's Anatomy, 39th edition. Edinburgh: Elsevier Churchill Livingstone; 2005.
36. Waugh A, Grant A. Ross and Wilson Anatomy and Physiology in Health and Illness, 9th edition. Edinburgh: Churchill Livingstone; 2005.
37. Willard-Mack CL. Normal structure, function, and histology of lymph node. Toxicol Pathol. 2006;34:409.
38. Woolf N. Cell, Tissue and Disease—The Basis of Pathology, 3rd edition. Philadelphia: WB Saunders; 2000.

CHAPTER

Age Changes in Oral Tissues

Einstein T Bertin A, B Sivapathasundharam

CHAPTER OUTLINE

- Theories of Aging 273
  - Programmed Theories 274
  - Damage or Error Theories (Non-programmed) 274
- The Cell Biology of Aging 274
  - Effects of Aging on the Cellular Processes 275
  - Effects of Aging on the Cellular Changes 276
- Effects of Aging on the Human Body 276
  - Effects of Aging on the Body Systems 276
  - Effects of Aging on the Regulatory Mechanisms 277
- Effects of Aging on the Oral and Circumoral Structures 277
  - Face 277
  - Bone 277
  - Dental Arch Form 278
  - Salivary Glands 278
  - Oral Mucous Membrane 278
  - Temporomandibular Joint 278
  - Oral Musculature 279
  - Mastication 279
  - Deglutition 279
- Effect of Aging on the Dental Tissues 279
  - Enamel 279
  - Dentin–Pulp Complex 280
  - Periodontium 281
- Forensic Implications of Age-related Changes of the Dental Tissues 283
  - Gustafson's Method 283
  - Age Estimation from Dentin Translucency 283
  - Age Estimation from Incremental Lines of Cementum 283
  - Age Estimation from Pulp-to-tooth Area Ratio 284

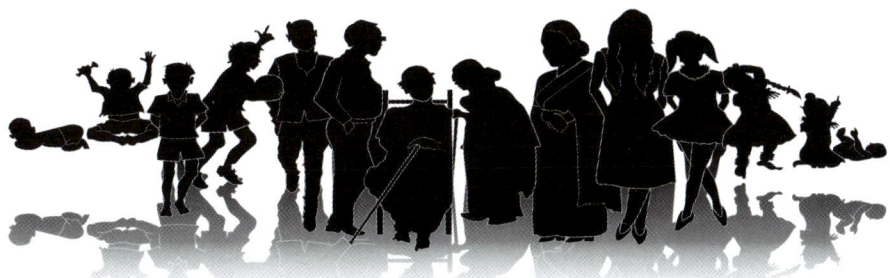

"Life can only be understood backwards; but it must be lived forwards".

—Søren Kierkegaard

Aging, in simple terms, is a time-related deterioration of the physiological functions and tissue structures essential for the continued existence and reproduction. Differentiation of normal aging changes from those of the disease processes related to old age is of paramount importance to avoid over- and underdiagnosis.

THEORIES OF AGING

Many theories have been proposed to explain the process of aging, but still a universally accepted theory with a satisfactory explanation is lacking.

The traditional aging theories consider that aging is neither an adaptation nor is genetically programmed. Modern

biological theories of aging in humans fall into two major categories:
- Programmed theories
- Damage or error theories.

Programmed Theories

The programmed theories imply that aging follows a biological timetable, perhaps a continuation of the one that regulates childhood growth and development and are further categorized into:
- *Programmed longevity theory* that considers aging to be the result of a sequential switching on and off of certain genes, with senescence being defined as the time when age-associated deficits are manifested.
- *Endocrine theory* proposes biological clocks that act through hormones to control the pace of aging.
- *Immunological theory* states that the immune system is programmed to decline over time, leading to an increased vulnerability to infectious diseases and thus aging and death.

Damage or Error Theories (Non-programmed)

The damage or error theories that attribute the cause of aging to environmental assaults to living organisms that induce cumulative damage at various levels, include—
- *Wear and tear theory*, where vital parts in our cells and tissues wear out, resulting in aging.
- *Rate of living theory* supports that faster an organism's rate of basal metabolism, the shorter its life span.
- *Free radicals theory* proposes that superoxide and other free radicals cause damage to the macromolecular components of the cell, giving rise to accumulated damage, causing cells and eventually organs to stop functioning **(Figures 18-1A and B)**.
- *Cross-linking theory*, also referred to as the glycosylation theory of aging, states that it is the binding of glucose (simple sugars) to protein (a process that occurs under the presence of oxygen) that causes various problems **(Figure 18-2)**.

Somatic DNA damage theory highlights the DNA damage accumulation in nondividing cells of mammals, causing cells to deteriorate and malfunction.

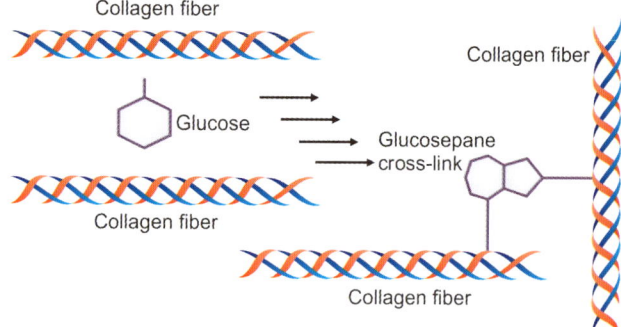

Figure 18-2: Cross-linking of collagen.

THE CELL BIOLOGY OF AGING

Aging is a consequence of the interactions between an individual's lifestyle and molecular processes that occur over the lifetime. A clear understanding of cellular programs responsible for aging and their dysregulation is vital to understand the aging process and to attempt to increase the longevity.

Many checkpoints exist at various stages in the cell function, starting from the nucleus through chromosome organization, transcriptional regulation, and nuclear export/import, ranging outward to protein translation and quality control, autophagic recycling of organelles, maintenance of cytoskeletal structure, and finally maintenance of the extracellular matrix (ECM) and extracellular signaling. An intricate interplay of information between these systems plays a role in regulating the aging process.

The nine hallmarks of aging that are generally accepted include:
- Genomic instability (nuclear, mitochondrial DNA, and nuclear architecture alterations)
- Telomere attrition
- Epigenetic alterations (alterations in DNA methylation patterns, posttranslational modification of histones, and chromatin remodeling and transcriptional alterations)
- Loss of proteostasis (chaperone-mediated protein folding and stability, proteolytic systems)
- Dysregulated nutrient sensing [the insulin- and insulin-like growth factor-1 (IGF-1) signaling pathways, mammalian

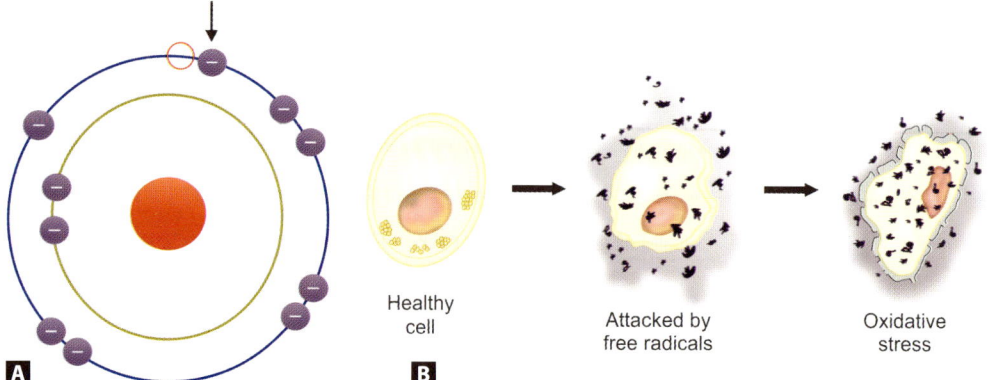

Figures 18-1A and B: Free radical: (A) Unpaired electron causing; (B) Oxidative stress to a healthy cell.

target of rapamycin (mTOR), adenosine monophosphate-activated protein kinase (AMPK), and sirtuins]
- Mitochondrial dysfunction [reactive oxygen species (ROS), mitochondrial integrity and biogenesis, mitohormesis]
- Cellular senescence (telomere loss, INK4a/ARF locus, and p53)
- Stem cell exhaustion
- Altered intercellular communication (inflammation and other types of intercellular communication).

> Reactive oxygen species (ROS) are byproducts of cellular oxidative metabolism. ROS play major roles in the **cell survival modulation, cell death, differentiation, cell signaling, and inflammation-related factor production**.

The cellular processes that are affected during aging and the changes occurring in various cellular components are delineated below.

Effects of Aging on the Cellular Processes

> In the cell nucleus, the deoxyribonucleic acid (DNA) molecule is packaged into thread-like structures called chromosomes. Each chromosome is made up of DNA, tightly coiled around proteins called histones that support its structure. Telomeres are specific DNA–protein structures found at both ends of each chromosome.
> The length of a telomere is proportional to the life span of an individual and the telomere length in early life is predictive of longevity.

Chromosome and telomere regulation: Telomeres protect the genome from nucleolytic degradation, unnecessary recombination, repair, and interchromosomal fusion. However, during cell replication, a small portion of telomeric DNA is lost with each cell division and when a particular limit is breached, the continuous loss of telomeric DNA results in apoptosis or cellular senescence or oncogenic transformation of somatic cells. Thus, telomeric length can be used to determine the life span of a cell or an organism **(Figure 18-3)**.

The average length of telomere shortening in humans was found to be between 24.8 base pairs per year and 27.7 base pairs per year. Further, smoking, obesity, exposure to environmental factors, profession, stress, and diet play a role in aging by accelerating the telomere shortening. This explains the causative role of lifestyle factors in oncogenic transformation.

Transcriptional regulation: Transcription is the process by which the information in a strand of DNA is copied into a new molecule of messenger RNA (mRNA). Insulin/IGF-1 signaling (IIS) and mammalian target of Rapamycin (mTOR) pathways are deemed to play a major role in transcriptional regulation. Pharmacological modulation of IIS/TOR signaling in mammals increases life span and ameliorates several age-related pathologies. mTOR is thus a key modulator in aging and age-related diseases.

Nuclear trafficking and organization: In eukaryotic cells, transport of molecules between the nucleus and the cytoplasm

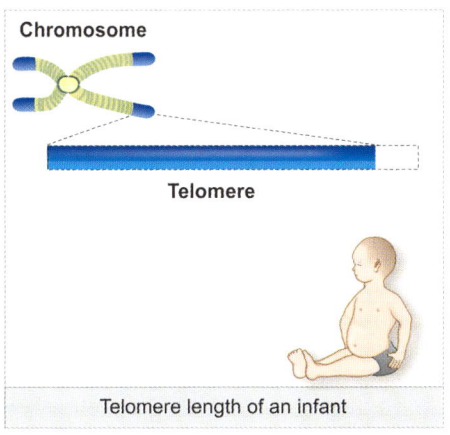
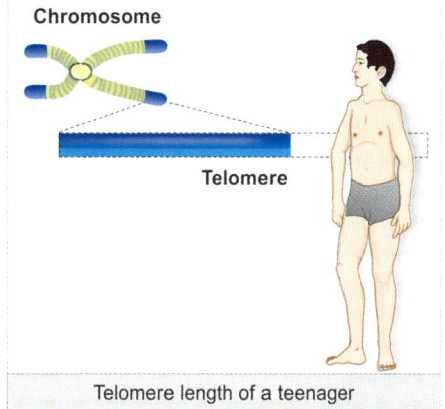
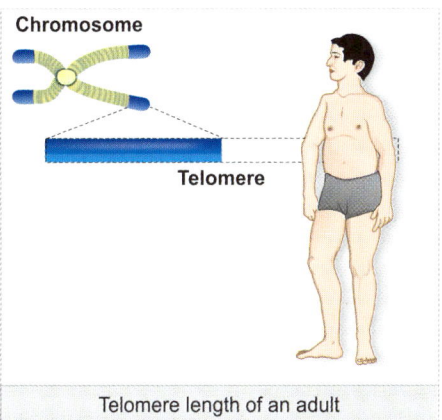
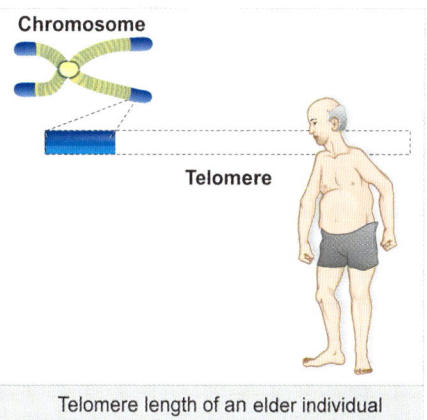

Figure 18-3: Telomere length and aging.

through the nuclear pore complexes (nucleoporins), is very vital for the cellular replication processes and maintenance of viable cellular functions. Nuclear trafficking decreases with cellular senescence resulting in decreased response of the cell to noxious stimuli. Progressive degradation of nucleoporins also results in leakage of proteins and loss of signaling resulting in aging.

> Proteins called laminins perform spatial organization of the nuclear components and any disruption in their organization results in aging and aging-related disorders like progeria and Hutchinson–Gilford progeria syndrome. Disruption in laminin structure and organization results in genomic instability and susceptibility to ROS.

Protein translation and protein homeostasis: Translation is the process by which ribosomes in association with endoplasmic reticulum synthesize proteins from transcribed mRNAs. In continuation with the nuclear organizational deficiencies due to deficient laminin molecule, faulty production of laminin and increased production of faulty laminin A (progerin), have been reported to play a major role in the pathogenesis of premature aging diseases like progeria.

Studies reveal that RNA polymerase III activity is regulated by mTOR pathway and is an important determinant of longevity in experimental animals. Misfolded and damaged proteins activate degradation pathways and signal organismal aging.

Effects of Aging on the Cellular Changes

Mitochondrial changes: Progressive loss of mitochondrial function has been attributed to the production of ROS, which are the by-products of oxidative phosphorylation. Furthermore, mitochondrion can induce apoptosis or necrosis or even cause alterations in mitochondrial DNA by production of ROS, resulting in a decrease in oxidative phosphorylation, which in turn produces more ROS, and thus a vicious cycle is repeated until the cell undergoes senescence or apoptosis.

Cytoskeletal changes: Various factors in environment like stress, ischemia, UV ray exposure or environmental toxins can result in stress to the cytoskeleton and may result in necrosis or apoptosis. Repetitive oxidative stress invariably results in cytoskeletal and cellular damage, which may result in apoptosis, senescence or oncogenic transformation.

Cell membrane and extracellular matrix changes: Similar to the function of nuclear membrane, the plasma membrane of the cell also plays a major role in transport of nutrients and signaling molecules across the cell. Products of the higher level of lipid peroxidation in the aged cells results in a stiffer plasma membrane.

Aging humans experience glycosylation and other proteomic damage to the extracellular matrix proteins, a process that is accelerated in type 2 diabetes patients due to build-up of oxidative damage products and ROS.

■ EFFECTS OF AGING ON THE HUMAN BODY

Aging of the human body includes both the biological and physiological aspects that underlie aging and the general health status. With the probability of death increasing rapidly with advancing age, changes should be happening in an individual, making him or her more vulnerable to disease.

A gradual decline is seen in the performance of many organs such as heart, kidneys, brain or lungs over the life span, partly due to loss of cells from these organs, with a resultant reduction in the reserve capacities of the individual. Also, the cells of an elderly individual might have less active enzymes, thus needing more time to carry out the chemical reactions. Such underperforming cells might ultimately die.

Effects of Aging on the Body Systems

Cardiovascular system: With increasing age, the heart becomes more vulnerable to disease and undergoes deleterious changes, even in the absence of detectable disease. The heart further shows a gradual reduction in performance with advancing age, with nearly a 50% reduction in the amount of blood pumped by the heart between the age of 20 years and 90 years.

Digestive system: Though the secretion of hydrochloric acid as well as other digestive enzymes by the stomach decreases with age, the overall process of digestion is not significantly impaired in the elderly.

Nervous system: There are no striking changes in the structure of the brain due to normal aging. Though a slight loss of neurons can be expected with advancing age owing to the loss of capacity to form new neurons, there is only a minor effect on behavior.

Vision: Visual acuity slightly declines from about middle 20s to the 50s, and then there is an accelerated decline thereafter. There is also reduction in the size of the pupil with age. Aging also brings in presbyopia, reduced night vision, and a higher incidence of ocular diseases such as glaucoma and cataracts.

Hearing: A gradual reduction in the ability to perceive tones at higher frequencies might occur with advancing age, thus interfering with identifying individuals by their voices and with understanding the conversations in a group, but does not ordinarily represent a serious limitation to the individual in daily life.

Other sensory impairments: In elderly individuals, a reduction in the taste sensitivity of the tongue and marginal decrease in pain sensitivity have been reported. The reduction in taste may be due to the decline in the number of taste buds. This along with the nutrition status of the individual, alters the perception of taste. A general slowing of the responses and slightly sluggish reflexes, with a slowing down of the speed of conduction of impulses has been reported, with advancing age.

Skin: In old age individuals, a gradual loss of elasticity and an increasing cross-linking of collagen, along with factors like an exposure to weather and familial traits, lead to the

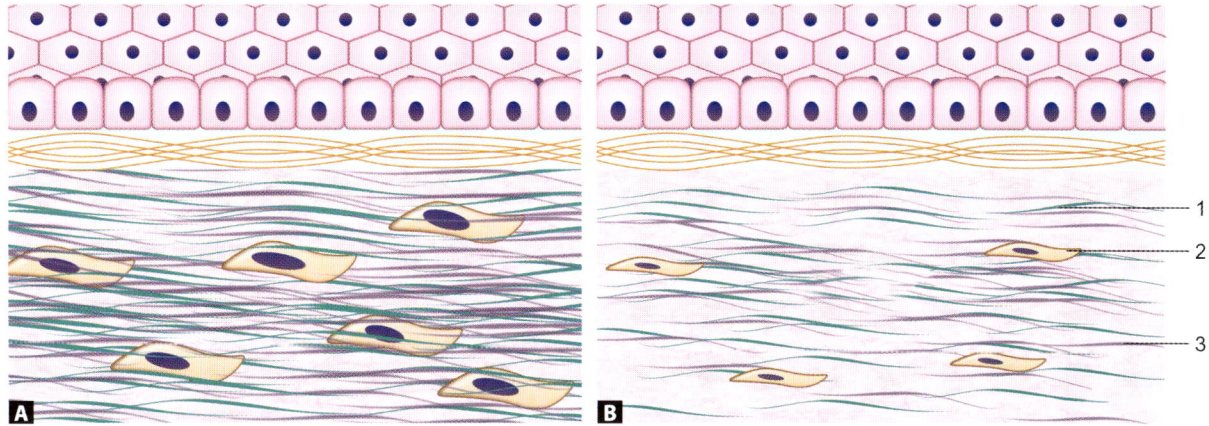

Figures 18-4A and B: Skin of the: (A) Young individual; and (B) Old individual. Note the (1) cross-linked collagen, (2) reduced fibroblasts both in size and number, and (3) reduced elastic fibers.

development of wrinkles and pigmentations associated with senescence **(Figures 18-4A and B)**.

Endocrine system: The significance of the hormones in the regulation of many physiological systems explains the determinant effect of endocrine disorders on the aging process.
- A reduction in the utilization of thyroxine in various tissues of the body results in a decreased basal metabolism rate.
- Reduced function of the adrenal cortex may be attributed to the reduced ability to adjust to stress.
- A reduction in the rate of removal of excess sugar from the blood and a reduced sensitivity of the pancreas so that a higher level of blood sugar is required to stimulate it to action may be observed.
- Secretion of both male and female sex hormones diminishes with age, with a progressive diminishing of sexual activity.

Skeletal system: With increasing age, a gradual loss of calcium resulting in more fragile bones, an increasing incidence of osteoporosis, and slower healing of fractures are common. The mobility of joints diminishes with age and the incidence of arthritis increases.

Respiratory system: Increased stiffness of the bony cage of the chest and decreased strength of the muscles that move the chest during respiration may result in a reduction in vital capacity and an increase in the amount of air that cannot be expelled from the lungs. Formation of cross-links in elastin and collagen with aging reduces the elastic properties of the lung. The lack of appropriate adjustment of the blood flow to the air sacs in the lungs might result in the impairment of oxygen transfer in the lungs of elderly subjects.

Kidney: Elderly individuals lose the concentrating ability of the kidney, so a greater volume of water is required to excrete the same amount of waste material, a change probably partially offset by a decrease in the excretory load because of reduced activity, alterations in food intake, and the reduction in muscle mass of the elderly.

Several changes are observed in circadian rhythm of an individual with aging.

> Systemic aging is controlled by hypothalamus by the mediation of energy homeostasis, hormonal regulation, circadian rhythm, and reproductive functions through the key neuronal regulators such as AgRP/NPY, POMC, AVP, VIP, GHRH, SST, GnRH, SIRTI, BMALI, CLOCK, and KNDy neurons.

Effects of Aging on the Regulatory Mechanisms

Though physiological characteristics, such as the regulatory mechanisms of the acidity of the blood or its sugar level, are adequate to maintain normal levels under resting conditions even in very old people, a longer time is required in the elderly to re-establish normal levels when changes from the normal occur.

EFFECTS OF AGING ON THE ORAL AND CIRCUMORAL STRUCTURES

Less adequate physiological mechanisms for adjusting to changes in environmental temperature result in a preference for more uniform and slightly higher temperatures in the elderly. Also, the incidence of heat prostration in hot weather increases with age.

Lesser exercise in the elderly leads to an increased blood pressure, heart rate, and respiration in the old than in the young. Furthermore, recovery of blood pressure, heart rate, and respiration to resting values takes longer in the old.

Face

Changes occur in the facial appearance due to aging. Face appears flabby due to the loss of muscle tone and thinning of skin. Loss of elastic fibers causes wrinkles. Loss of vertical dimension results in radiating wrinkles at the corners of the mouth **(Figures 18-5A and B)**.

Bone

From a synchronous bone resorption and deposition occurring during the growth and remodeling of bone in the formative years, the bone becomes less active with advancing age.

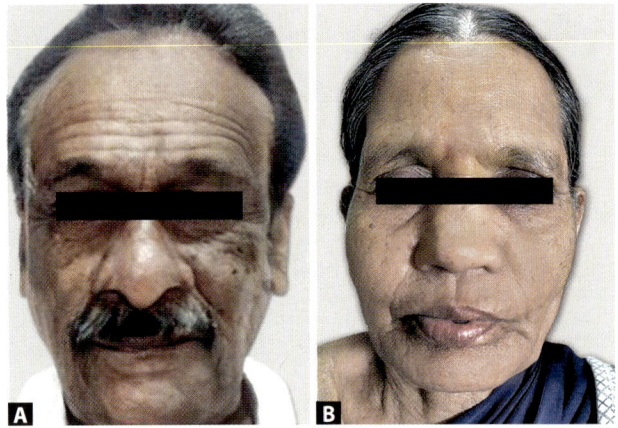

Figures 18-5A and B: (A) Note the wrinkles and pigmentations in aged face; (B) Note the wrinkles at the corner of the mouth due to reduced vertical dimension.

A gradual loss of bone mass at the rate of around 1% per year has been observed after 35–40 years of age. With a decreasing demand for new bone formation associated with the diminishing physical activity in advancing age, resorption exceeds deposition, resulting in a net loss of bone mass.

> In very elderly individuals, slow and continued resorption, along with very little remodeling, results in atrophy of bone along with a reduction in the resilience and an increase in the brittleness and fragility of the bone.

A decrease in the bone-forming precursors or a reduction in the formation of bone matrix proteins may also be contributing to the reduction in bone formation. Further, reduced bone formation may also be due to the dysfunction of the ECM that plays an important role in bone metabolism, a change that might have resulted from the damage of fibronectin by the oxygen-free radicals during the aging process.

In both the maxilla and the mandible, the amount, extent, and uniformity of the bone loss differ with varying etiologies and health status. Maxillary sinus increases in size, corresponding with the loss of maxillary bone.

Dental Arch Form

The phases of eruption of permanent teeth are usually associated with an increase in the dental arch area. However, the arch width, depth, and length decrease as the age advances. This happens till sixth decade. After that, this progressive reduction becomes minimal. With aging, there is a tendency toward more rounding of the arch forms.

Salivary Glands

Significant changes occur in the gland acini and the supporting stroma, with advancing age. Reduction in the volume of acini with a concomitant increase in the ductal volume is a significant change that occurs in aging. Degenerative changes occur in the secretory units and intercalated ducts.

The acinar cells of the major salivary glands are gradually lost up to 60%, being replaced by adipose tissue. The aging salivary acinar cells increase in size and appear eosinophilic, and are referred to as *oncocytes*.

Ductal alterations include an increase in the nonstriated intralobular ducts, dilatation of the extralobular ducts, besides the degenerative and metaplastic changes. An increase in the stromal connective tissue and vascularity is also noticed.

Though there is no direct correlation between the decreased production of saliva in the elderly and the marked changes in the salivary parenchyma, the production of stimulated saliva is reduced. Nevertheless xerostomia (dry mouth) is common in aged individuals. However, it is debatable, whether this is a result of aging or the cumulative effect of the systemic diseases the individual experienced or the medications taken for such diseases. The oral defense mechanisms might be compromised with increasing age, as evidenced by a decrease in the concentration of salivary immunoglobulin A (IgA) in the labial saliva and mucin in mucous saliva.

Oral Mucous Membrane

Compared to the mucosa of a younger individual, the elderly usually have a smoother and drier surface and may appear atrophic or friable. However, this appearance should be more attributed to the effects of systemic diseases or drug therapy or tobacco smoking rather than the aging process. Symptoms such as dryness of the mouth, burning sensation, and abnormal taste are reported frequently in elderly post-menopausal women.

A reduction in the number of filiform papillae imparts a smooth glossy appearance to the tongue, though this change might also be a result of nutritional deficiencies. A gradual decrease in the number of taste buds is noted, a change seen in women ahead of men. The loss of taste buds manifests as an alteration in the taste perception, with the salty and sweet tastes lost initially, followed by the loss of bitter and sour tastes. Development of varicosities is characteristic with advancing age, as seen by the occurrence of nodular varicose veins on the ventral aspect of the tongue (caviar tongue), observed more frequently in patients with varicose veins of the legs.

Microscopical changes observed in the oral mucous membrane include a reduction in the thickness of the epithelium and flattening of the epithelial rete ridges (**Figures 18-6A and B**). Though aging is associated with a decreased metabolic activity, the process of epithelial proliferation and epithelial turnover rate are not affected.

Decreased cellularity along with an increased amount of more cross-linked collagen is observed in the lamina propria, with advancing age. A reduction in Langerhans cells might contribute to a decline in the cell-mediated immunity. An increase in the occurrence of ectopic sebaceous glands (Fordyce's spots) in the labial and buccal mucosa and marked atrophy of the minor salivary glands with fibrous replacement are common features in the elderly.

Temporomandibular Joint

Temporomandibular joint (TMJ) undergoes functional remodeling throughout life, usually in response to changes in articulation of the teeth or alterations in the space between

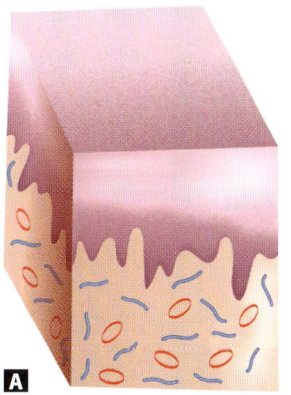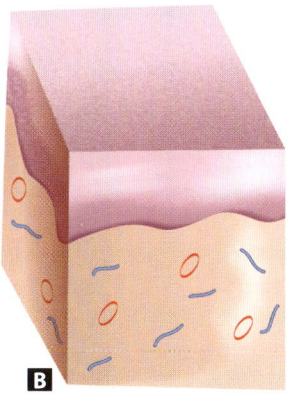

Figures 18-6A and B: (A) Oral mucous membrane in younger individual; (B) Thinned out epithelium with flattening of rete ridges in older individual.

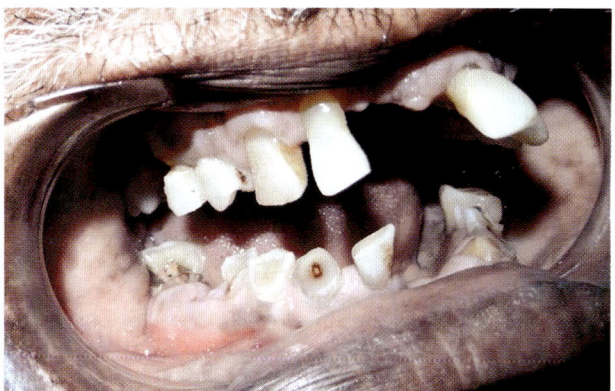

Figure 18-7: Attrition.

maxilla and mandible. Thus, the functional changes in the TMJ are by no means confined to elderly individuals.

Temporomandibular joint changes include—joint clicking, limitation of jaw opening, and deviation of the mandible during function, with the major symptom being pain.

Oral Musculature

Changes in aging oral musculature are consistent with those in aging muscle tissue in the body as a whole, which include reductions in muscle tone, muscle performance, number and activity of muscle cells, and number and size of the muscle fibers. Replacement of the muscle mass by fat or fibrous connective tissue results in generalized atrophy of the musculature attached to the bones in the oral cavity.

Mastication

Atrophy of the muscles of mastication, with age, decreases the biting force and slows the chewing performance. The atrophy is probably caused in part by disuse because less muscular effort is required for chewing as a result of failing dentition or a progressively softer diet or both.

Deglutition

Aging does not significantly affect the transit of the prepared food bolus through the mouth and pharynx. However, a lip seal has to be maintained for swallowing which, due to the decreased muscle mass and tone, can make swallowing difficult. This can alter the ability to form and prepare a bolus in the oral stage of swallowing.

■ EFFECT OF AGING ON THE DENTAL TISSUES

Enamel

Ameloblasts, the formative cells of enamel are lost after the formation of enamel during amelogenesis and thus, enamel cannot regenerate.

Loss of Enamel

The most significant change seen in enamel with increasing age is the progressive loss of enamel due to attrition (loss of tooth substance due to tooth to tooth contact as in mastication) by demineralization and remineralization altering the surface of the enamel. Attrition manifests as wear facets of the occlusal surfaces with a gradual elimination of the pits and fissures and the interproximal wear resulting in a polished surface of the enamel. Prolonged tooth wear may result in loss of significant portions of the enamel, exposing the dentin (**Figure 18-7**).

Loss of occlusal enamel results in a reduction of the vertical dimension of the tooth crown, compensated by formation of cementum at the apex of the root or by an axial movement of the tooth.

Flattening of the proximal contour of the teeth is compensated by mesial or approximal drift, brought about by the anterior component of the occlusal force and contraction of the transseptal ligament.

Discoloration

Darkening of the teeth with increasing age is common. This could be attributed to the continuous addition of organic material from the environment into the enamel and also to the fact that the thickening layer of dentin is seen through the thinning layer of translucent enamel, resulting in deepening of the dentin color.

Reduced Permeability

In the younger enamel, the pores between the crystals permit slow passage of water and substances of low molecular size. With increasing age, the crystals increase their size owing to acquiring more ions, thereby reducing the size of the pores, and rendering the enamel less permeable. This reduction in pore size might result in loss of water from the outer layers of dentin causing its separation from the enamel. As a result the enamel loses its support making it more prone to cracks.

Changes in the Surface Layer

The presence of perikymata and microscopic structures such as enamel pits, enamel rod ends, enamel caps, and enamel brochs confer a rough and irregular surface to newly formed teeth, which is lost when the tooth erupts into the oral cavity. These characteristic structures are lost rapidly in the facial and lingual surfaces than proximal surfaces and in anterior teeth than posterior teeth.

The surface of the enamel mirrors the changes happening within the tissue. With advancing age, the ionic exchange between the enamel surface and the oral environment results in a progressive increase in the content of nitrogen and fluoride. The high content of fluoride offers increased resistance to dental caries and makes the enamel surface extremely hard, though equally brittle. The modulus of elasticity of enamel also increases.

Dentin–Pulp Complex

The embryological, histological, and functional relationship of dentin and pulp are reflected in the age-related changes also, wherein the age changes of pulp are reflected in the dentin.

Age-related Changes in the Dentin

Secondary and tertiary dentin: Attrition of the enamel stimulates the odontoblasts resulting in the rapid deposition of the dentin matrix. The collagen fibers are randomly oriented affecting the arrangement of tubules. This is termed as irregular secondary dentin. With advancing age, there is increased deposition of the secondary dentin, besides the tertiary dentin that is deposited as a response to microbial stress or trauma arising from dental caries, abrasion, attrition, operative procedures, and the like.

Sclerotic dentin: The progressive deposition of intratubular (peritubular) dentin within the dentinal tubules results in a gradual obliteration of the dentinal tubules with apatite crystals, usually leading to complete closure of the tubules. The refractive index of such a dentin is now equal to that of the dentinal tubules, which are predominantly filled with the inorganic content and thus appear translucent in ground sections **(Figure 18-8)**. This transparent or sclerotic dentin is more brittle and less permeable because of the high mineral content and might help in prolonging the pulpal vitality. Sclerotic dentin is common near the root apex of the teeth in middle-aged individuals and is often found beneath worn enamel, such as in the incisal area of anterior teeth, beneath slowly progressing dental caries where reparative dentin is being produced on the pulpal wall, and beneath the Tomes' granular layer in the cervical area of older teeth where the cervical cementum has become exposed to the oral cavity as a result of gingival recession.

Dead tracts: During the aging process, the odontoblasts may completely retract their processes from the dentinal tubules or might die, resulting in empty dentinal tubules that are sealed off. In ground sections, these air-filled dentinal tubules appear black in transmitted light (the light being refracted away by the air molecules) and are hence referred to as dead tracts **(Figure 18-9)**. Dead tracts are more common in the coronal dentin, usually bounded by areas of translucent dentin. Dead tracts probably represent the initial step in the formation of sclerotic dentin.

Age-related Changes in the Pulp

Volume of the pulp chamber: The continued deposition of secondary dentin results in a decrease in the volume of the

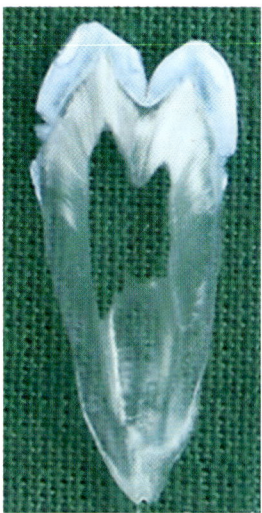

Figure 18-8: Ground section of tooth showing sclerotic dentin.

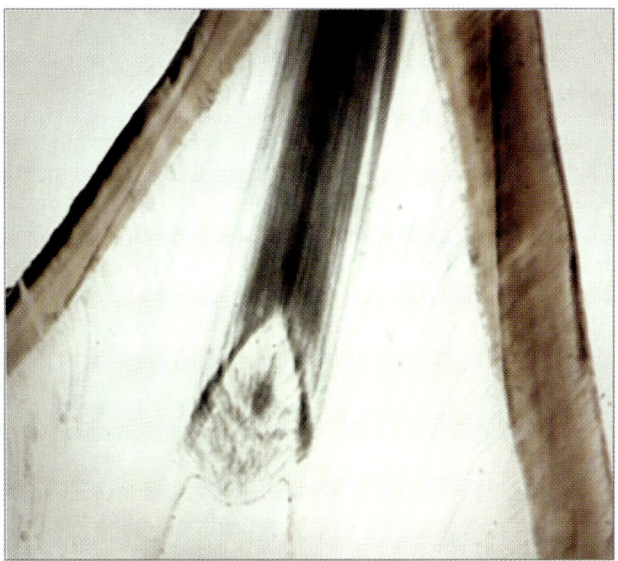

Figure 18-9: Ground section of tooth showing dead tracts.

pulp chamber and the root canal. Root canal dimension is being reduced to thin channels or completely obliterated **(Figures 18-10A and B)**.

Cellular changes: With advancing age, there is a gradual reduction in the density of the odontoblasts and the pulpal fibroblasts, the reduction being more pronounced in the radicular pulp than the coronal pulp. Further, these cells are marked by a reduction in the size and number of the cytoplasmic organelles. The odontoblasts show the presence of intercellular and intracellular vacuoles and develop the 'wheatsheaf' appearance.

Collagen alterations: The aging pulp is characterized by accumulation of both fibrils and bundles of collagen, throughout the pulpal tissue, a change accentuated by the decreasing size of the pulp chamber and the resultant concentration of the fibers. Thus pulp appears fibrosed.

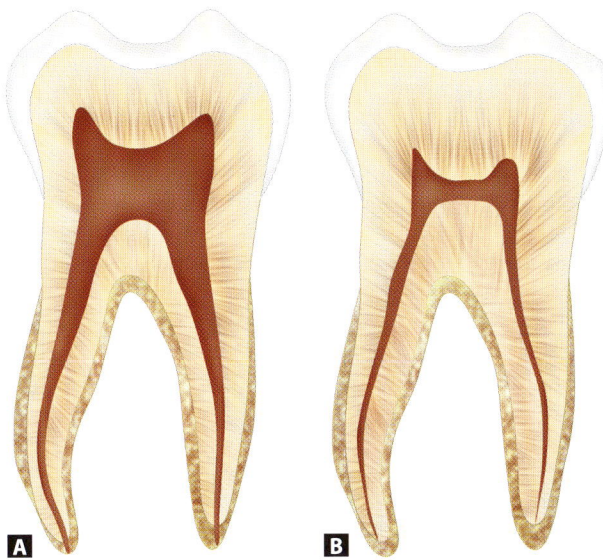

Figures 18-10A and B: Reduction in the volume of the pulp; (A) Young pulp; (B) Older pulp.

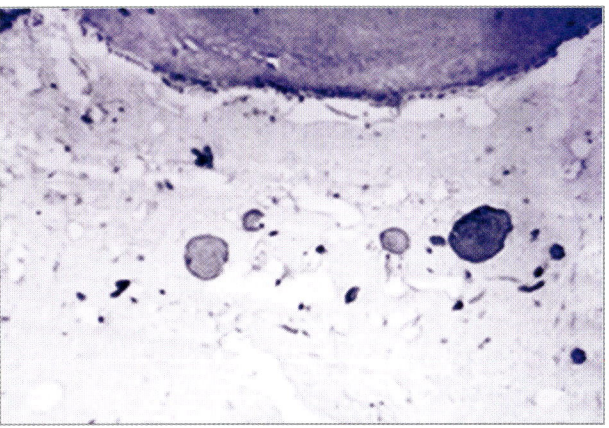

Figure 18-11: Hematoxylin and eosin stained decalcified section of pulp showing pulp stones in the pulp chamber.

Vascular changes: These include a reduction of the pulpal vascularity owing to a decrease in the number of blood vessels and formation of atherosclerotic plaques within the pulpal vessels. An increase in the collagen in the medial and adventitial layers of blood vessels is also a regular finding with age. Age-related changes in the capillary endothelium include discontinuity of the basement membrane that is more thick and homogeneous, presence of an increased number of pinocytic and micropinocytic vesicles with abundant microfilaments in the endothelial cytoplasm, more toward the abluminal side of the cell membrane, and the presence of extensive Golgi complexes with distended cisternae, spherical lipid-like droplets, non-granular glycogen molecules, abundant ribosomes, rough endoplasmic reticulum, multivesicular bodies, and intracytoplasmic bodies called as Weibel–Palade bodies, containing von Willebrand factor and P-selectin.

Neural degeneration: A continued loss and degeneration of the axons (myelinated and unmyelinated) are seen in the aging pulp, rendering the pulp less sensitive.

Calcifications: A characteristic age-related change seen in the pulp is the occurrence of irregular areas of dystrophic calcification, in relation to the blood vessels and seen more in the central pulp or the deposition of diffuse minerals along the collagen bundles. It may be suggested that the areas of the collagen fibers with more cross-linkages are more likely to develop calcifications. Further, the pulp stones are larger and more numerous in the older teeth **(Figure 18-11)**.

Cementum

Compensation for occlusal wear is usually achieved by continued cementum deposition around the apex of the tooth and thus, there is an increase in the thickness of cementum (hypercementosis) with age, with a predilection for the lingual surfaces compared to the other surfaces **(Figure 18-12)**. The aging cementum is less permeable to dyes and ions, which can

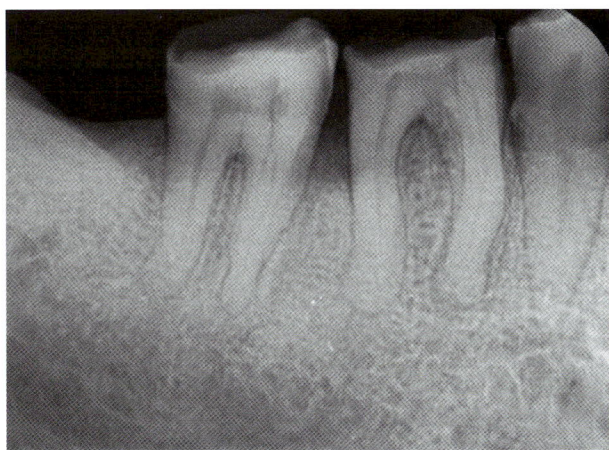

Figure 18-12: Radiograph of hypercementosed molars.
Source: Dr Ragu Ganesh, Meenakshi Ammal Dental College, Chennai, India

explain the loss of viable cementocytes in the deeper layers of cementum (less permeable to nutritive molecules).

Gingival recession exposes cementum and this exposed cementum is quickly worn off with mechanical friction, exposing the deeper dentin, and leading to extrinsic staining and hypersensitivity.

With age, the cementum takes up fluoride and in areas adjacent to periodontal ligament there is higher concentration of fluoride content.

Periodontium

Gingiva

Visible changes in the gingiva with age include a dry and atrophic appearance of the gingiva, a decrease in the gingival width, and the gingiva becomes less resilient and more sensitive to external stimuli. Loss of stippling seen in the elderly can also be attributed to the role of inflammation. There is an apical shift of the junctional epithelium in the elderly individual, with subsequent exposure of more tooth surface and root (gingival recession). The degree of gingival recession is more related to age, tooth movement, inflammatory changes resulting from disease, oral care habits, and heredity.

Microscopically, the gingival epithelium exhibits atrophy, acanthosis (increase in the thickness of spinous cell layer), parakeratosis, and a reduction in the cellular and nuclear diameter and nuclear-cytoplasmic ratio.

Gingival fibroblasts are greatly reduced in number and further, are also morphologically and functionally altered. Production of collagen by the gingival fibroblasts is decreased drastically due to intracytoplasmic phagocytosis, thereby decreasing the fibrous component. Secretion of more heparan sulfate and less chondroitin sulfate by the aging gingival fibroblasts alters the composition of the extracellular matrix.

Periodontal Ligament

Significant changes are observed in the periodontal ligament with advancing age, the most prominent being the marked decrease in the cell density and the fibrous component.

Decreased expression of osteocalcin by the periodontal ligament fibroblasts may impact the progress of cell cycle (G1 to S phase), thereby resulting in a decreased mitotic activity. Reduced expression of C-fos ligand by the aging cells may cause a reduction in the chemotaxis and motility of the ligament cells.

Other age-related changes include an overall decrease in the production of organic matrix, loss of acid mucopolysaccharides, increase in the elastic fibers, and a decrease in the cell rests of Malassez.

With aging, there is a decrease in the masticatory forces, thereby resulting in a reduced periodontal ligament width. Further, the progressive loss of soft tissue attachment with increasing age, leads to exposure of the roots and loosening of the teeth within their bony sockets.

In the elderly, the periodontal ligament fibers are attached to the peaks on the scalloped surface of the cementum and alveolar bone rather than to the entire surface, thereby impacting the periodontium as a whole.

Alveolar Bone

Alveolar bone is one of the first bones to be affected by loss of mass, resulting in a lesser resistance of the periosteal and periodontal surfaces of alveolar bone to harmful local oral trauma, inflammation or disease. This contributes greatly to periodontal disease, loss of teeth, and in the edentulous patient, inability to obtain adequate support and stability for dentures.

Alveolar bone or residual ridge resorption is confounded by such factors as age, sex, race, and health status of the patient when the teeth are extracted, the tooth extraction technique, the diet of the patient, the presence of local factors, and the frequency of denture use.

Besides the gradual reduction in the bone mass, specific changes noted in the alveolar bone with advancing age include an increase in the number of interstitial lamellae, fatty infiltration of the bone marrow, a reduction in the height of the alveolar processes in edentulous jaws, a more open internal trabecular arrangement indicating bone loss, and a marked increase in the distance between the alveolar crest and cementoenamel junction.

Radiographically, the alveolar bone shows loss of lamina dura and a thinner cortical bone at the angle of the mandible.

Due to the increase in the number of vascular spaces, the mandible becomes porous. The smaller blood vessels have thicker walls and this along with lesser canaliculi number, reduces the nutrition to the osteocytes which results in a low osteocytic count.

Summary of the effects of aging on oral and circumoral tissues is given in **Table 18-1**.

TABLE 18-1: Effects of aging on oral and circumoral tissues.

Enamel	• Reduction in thickness of enamel • Color becomes darker • Attrition, abrasion and erosion • Surface becomes shiny and polished • Brittleness and cracks on enamel surface • Resistant to caries
Dentin	• Color becomes darker • Decrease in sensitivity • Increase in bulk • Increased irregular secondary dentin and tertiary dentin deposition • Dead tracts more common in coronal dentin • Sclerotic dentin formation • Increased aspartic acid racemization
Pulp	• Decreased volume of pulp chamber and root canal • Reduced cellular components • Increased fibrous components • Decreased vascularity • Reduced sensitivity • Occurrence of calcifications
Cementum	• Scalloped surface • Increase in cemental thickness • Loss of cementocytes
Alveolar bone	• Residual ridge resorption • Reduced bone mass • Increased osteoporosis • Decreased vascularity • Fatty filtration of marrow
Gingiva	• Decreased gingival width • Gingival recession • Reduced stippling • Thinning of epithelium • Decreased keratinization • Flattened rete ridges • Decreased fibroblasts
Periodontal ligament	• Reduced periodontal ligament width • Decreased cellularity • Increased fibrous component • Decreased mitotic activity • Increase in elastic fibers • Decreased vascularity • Loss of soft tissue attachment leading to mobility • Cementicles

Contd...

Contd...

Salivary glands	• Reduced acinar volume • Acinar atrophy • Ductal dilatation • Increased stromal connective tissue • Fatty infiltration • Presence of oncocytes • Reduced salivary flow and compromised immune mechanism
Oral mucosa	• Atrophy • Dryness, dysgeusia, and burning sensation • Less elastic • Increased fibrosis • Decreased cellularity • Reduced epithelial thickness and flattened rete pegs • Ectopic sebaceous glands
Tongue	• Loss of filiform papillae • Reduction in taste perception • Lingual varicosities
Maxilla and mandible	• Decreased rate of bone formation • Continuous resorption and less bone remodeling • Reduced dental arch width, length and depth • Rounding of arch forms
TMJ	• Clicking sounds • Limited opening movement • Deviation of mandible during function
Face	• Loss of muscle tone • Thinning of skin • Wrinkling • Loss of vertical dimension

FORENSIC IMPLICATIONS OF AGE- RELATED CHANGES OF THE DENTAL TISSUES

Age-related alterations in the dental tissues have been employed historically in the assessment of the age of an individual.

Gustafson's Method

In 1950, *Gustafson G* proposed a method for age estimation based on age-related morphological and histological changes of the teeth. This method assesses the following changes:
❖ Attrition (A)
❖ Secondary dentin deposition (S)
❖ Loss of periodontal attachment (P)
❖ Cementum apposition at the root apex (C)
❖ Root resorption at the apex (R)
❖ Dentin translucency (T)

Gustafson assigned different grades ranging from 0 to 3, for each of these regressive changes or variables. Implying that a tooth can have any of four grades for attrition (A0, A1, A2, or A3) and for the other variables adding the allotted grade for each variable (*e.g.* A3 + S2 + P2 + C1 + R2 + T1 = X), a total score (X) was obtained. It was found that an increase in the total score corresponded with an increase in age. Age was estimated using the formula:

$$\text{Age} = 11.43 + (4.56 \times X).$$

Applying Gustafson's method on Indian population, Pillai and Bhaskar obtained an average error rate of about ± 8 years as against the original Gustafson's method that gave an error of ± 3.6 years. This difference could be attributed to variable dental hygiene and habits such as beetle-leaf and tobacco chewing in Indians.

Further modifications of the Gustafson's method were made later to rectify the statistical errors in the original method. Significant modification was proposed by Johanson G. This has seven grades, viz. 0, 0.5, 1, 1.5, 2, 2.5, and 3, instead of the four grades suggested by Gustafson. Further, the grade for the respective variable was substituted in a multiple regression formula to estimate age:

$$\text{Age} = 11.02 + (5.14 \times A) + (2.3 \times S) + (4.14 \times P) + (3.71 \times C) + (5.57 \times R) + (8.98 \times T).$$

Johanson observed that more the number of teeth used, more accurate was the age estimate.

Age Estimation from Dentin Translucency

Among the regressive changes employed originally by Gustafson, dentin translucency had been identified by many researchers as a better contributor in terms of age estimation.

Bang G and Ramm E reported a predictable increase in root translucency with advancing age. Their methodology included measuring the translucency (as viewed from the proximal side of the tooth) from its apical limit up to the junction of translucent and nontranslucent zone of dentin coronally, approximately midway between the root surface and root canal; if translucency lengths (T) are different on the buccal or labial and lingual or palatal sides, separate measurements are taken and averaged. They further provided a tooth-specific regression formula for age estimation.

Acharya AB and Vimi S adapted the Bang and Ramm formula to the Indian milieu and observed marginally better results. This formula, common to all single-rooted teeth, is as follows:

If the translucency measured is more than 9 mm:
❖ *Formula I*: Age = 35.5619 + (3.4828 × T)

If the translucency measured is less than or equal to 9 mm:
❖ *Formula II*: Age = 29.9074 + (7.4507 × T) + (−0.4369 × T²)

Using these formulae, an average age estimation error of ± 8.3 years was found for Indians, which may be categorized as "moderately good" accuracy.

Age estimation from dentinal translucency is a convenient approach that can be carried out with lesser expertise and can be measured on either intact extracted teeth or ground sections of teeth. However, the junction between translucent and nontranslucent zones can sometimes be highly irregular, making it difficult to measure the length.

Age Estimation from Incremental Lines of Cementum

Counting of the incremental lines of acellular cementum has been employed for age estimation, with an accuracy of ± 2 to ± 3 years of actual age. The accentuated incremental lines of cementum would also serve to indicate events such as pregnancies, skeletal trauma, and renal disorders, which can accurately be dated to an individual's life-history, thus facilitating identification.

Though cementum apposition shows particular promise for aging skeletal remains, shortcomings with the counting of cemental incremental lines include finding a marked difference in the number of incremental lines in different sections of the same tooth as well as in different regions of the same section and the compromise of the precision of aging in periodontal pathologies.

Radiograph is also used as an alternate method for age estimation instead of ground sections as it is nondestructive.

Age Estimation from Pulp-to-tooth Area Ratio

Pulp-to-tooth area ratio refers to measuring the area of the pulp chamber/root canal and the tooth area of canines on radiographs and calculating their ratio. The rationale for this method is based on the continued deposition of secondary dentin with increasing age that reduces the area of the pulp chamber/root canal, which is reflected in the decrease in pulp-to-tooth area ratio.

The ratio is calculated to compensate for and circumvent differences in magnification of radiographs and angulation between X-ray beam and film or sensor. Babshet M *et al.* found that an India–specific formula predicted age better in Indians than the original Italian formulae of Cameriere R *et al.*

The following linear regression formula may be used in Indians: Age = $64.413 - (195.265 \times PTR)$, where PTR is the pulp-to-tooth area ratio. This formula produced an average error of ± 10.76 years, an error rate that borders on what may be considered as "acceptable" in forensic age estimation.

Points to Remember

Aging is a time-related deterioration of the physiological functions and tissue structure essential for the continued existence and reproduction.

- **Theories of aging in humans include** programmed theories and damage or error theories, that include significant theories such as *programmed longevity theory* (aging to be the result of a sequential switching on and off of certain genes), *and free radicals theory* (superoxide and other free radicals cause damage to the macromolecular components of the cell, giving rise to accumulated damage, causing cells and eventually organs to stop functioning).
- **The nine hallmarks of aging** include genomic instability, telomere attrition, epigenetic alterations, loss of proteostasis, dysregulated nutrient sensing, mitochondrial dysfunction, cellular senescence, stem cell exhaustion and altered intercellular communication.
- The effects of aging on the cellular processes include telomere shortening, altered transcriptional regulation, decreased nuclear trafficking and dysregulated protein translation and protein homeostasis. Cellular changes in aging involve mitochondria, cytoskeleton, cell membrane and extracellular matrix.
- **Age-related changes observed in the various body systems** include increased risk for cardiac disease; alterations in food intake; decline in the visual acuity and occurrence of ocular disorders and diseases; gradual reduction in the ability to perceive tones at higher frequencies; reduction in the taste sensitivity; marginal decrease in pain sensitivity; a general slowing of the responses and slightly sluggish reflexes; development of wrinkles and pigmentation; reduced function and utilization of various hormones; more fragile bones, osteoporosis, a slower healing of fractures, and decreased mobility of joints with increased risk for arthritis; a reduction in vital capacity, an increase in the amount of air that cannot be expelled from the lungs, and impairment of oxygen transfer in the lungs; reduction in the kidney function; and several changes in the circadian rhythm.
- **Effects of aging on the oral and circumoral structures** include loss of facial muscle tone, thinning of skin, development of facial wrinkles, and loss of vertical dimension resulting in radiating wrinkles at corners of the mouth; altered bone remodeling, loss of bone mass, atrophy of bone along with a reduction in the resilience and an increase in the brittleness and fragility of the bone, besides an increase in the volume of maxillary sinus, and more rounding of the arch forms; reduction in the volume of salivary gland acini, a concomitant increase in the ductal elements, and reduction in the volume of stimulated saliva; smoother and drier oral mucosa appearing friable with increasing incidence of symptoms such as dryness and burning sensation,
Abnormal taste; atrophy of papillae resulting in glossy tongue, increase in the lingual varicosities; and a decrease in the number of taste buds; increased incidence of TMJ symptoms and signs such as joint clicking, limitation of jaw opening, and deviation of the mandible during function, with the major symptom being pain; changes in oral musculature such as reduction in muscle tone, muscle performance, number and activity of muscle cells, and number and size of the muscle fibers, besides a generalized atrophy of the musculature attached to the bones in the oral cavity; decrease in the biting force and slower chewing performance owing to atrophy of the muscles of mastication; and difficulty in swallowing due to decreased muscle mass and difficulty in achieving a proper lip seal tone.

PRACTICE QUESTIONS

1. Discuss the age-related changes of the oral mucosa and salivary glands.
2. Enumerate and discuss the age-related changes of dental hard tissues.
3. Discuss the significance of age-related changes of dental pulp.
4. Discuss in detail the changes in periodontium with advancing age.
5. Discuss the potential uses of age-related changes in forensic odontology.

MULTIPLE CHOICE QUESTIONS

1. **Which of the following increases with aging?**
   a. Tone of facial muscles
   b. Bone mass of maxilla and mandible
   c. Width of the dental arches
   d. Size of the maxillary sinus
2. **Which of the following statements regarding age-related changes in salivary glands is FALSE?**
   a. Reduction in the volume of acini
   b. Reduction in the ductal volume
   c. Decrease in the concentration of salivary IgA
   d. Decreased production of stimulated saliva
3. **Smooth glossy appearance of the tongue seen with advancing age is due to the reduction in the number of:**
   a. Fungiform papillae
   b. Circumvallate papillae
   c. Filiform papillae
   d. Foliate papillae
4. **Which of the following statements regarding age-related changes in the oral mucous membrane is FALSE?**
   a. Burning sensation of the mucosa
   b. Alteration of the taste perception
   c. Development of lingual varices
   d. Increased thickness of the epithelium
5. **Which of the following statements regarding age-related changes in the enamel is FALSE?**
   a. Loss of enamel due to attrition
   b. Discoloration of enamel
   c. Increased permeability
   d. Increased resistance to dental caries
6. **Progressive deposition of peritubular (intratubular) dentin within the dentinal tubules results in the formation of:**
   a. Dead tracts
   b. Predentin
   c. Secondary dentin
   d. Sclerotic dentin
7. **Which of the following is probably the precursor to the formation of transparent dentin?**
   a. Predentin
   b. Granular layer of Tomes
   c. Dead tracts
   d. Secondary dentin
8. **Which of the following statements regarding age-related changes in the dental pulp is FALSE?**
   a. Decrease in the volume of pulp chamber
   b. Reduced fibrosis of the pulp
   c. Reduction in the density of odontoblasts and fibroblasts
   d. Reduction in pulpal vascularity
9. **Which of the following statements regarding age-related changes in the periodontal ligament is FALSE?**
   a. Decrease in the cell density
   b. Decrease in the elastic fibers
   c. Reduction of the periodontal ligament width
   d. Decrease in the production of organic matrix
10. **Which of the following statements regarding age-related changes in the alveolar bone is FALSE?**
    a. Residual ridge resorption
    b. Reduced vascularity
    c. Reduced osteoporosis
    d. Fatty infiltration of the bone marrow

ANSWERS

1. d   2. b   3. c   4. d   5. c   6. d   7. c   8. b   9. b   10. c

BIBLIOGRAPHY

1. Acharya AB, Vimi S. Effectiveness of Bang and Ramm's formulae in age assessment of Indians from dentin translucency length. Int J Legal Med. 2009;123(6):483-8.
2. Avery JK. Oral Development and Histology, 3rd edition. Stuttgart: Thieme; 2002.
3. Babshet M, Acharya AB, Naikmasur VG. Age estimation in Indians from pulp/tooth area ratio of mandibular canines. Forensic Sci Int. 2010;197(1-3):125.e1-4.
4. Bang G, Ramm E. Determination of age in humans from root dentin transparency. Acta Odontol Scand. 1970;28:3-35.
5. Berdyyeva TK, Woodworth CD, Sokolov I. Human epithelial cells increase their rigidity with ageing in vitro: direct measurements. Phys Med Biol. 2004;50(1):81.
6. Buchwalter A, Hetzer MW. Nucleolar expansion and elevated protein translation in premature aging. Nat Comm. 2017;8(1):328.
7. Cameriere R, Ferrante L, Cingolani M. Variations in pulp/tooth area ratio as an indicator of age: a preliminary study. J Forensic Sci. 2004;49(2):317-9.
8. Cheigo DJ. Essentials of Oral Histology and Embryology: A clinical approach, 4th edition. India: Elsevier; 2013.
9. D'Angelo MA, Raices M, Panowski SH, et al. Age-dependent deterioration of nuclear pore complexes causes a loss of nuclear integrity in postmitotic cells. Cell. 2009;136:284-95.
10. DiLoreto R, Murphy CT. The cell biology of aging. Mol Biol Cell. 2015;26:4524-31.
11. Filer D, Thompson MA, Takhaveev V, et al. RNA polymerase III limits longevity downstream of TORC1. Nature. 2017;552(7684):263.
12. Gabbianelli R, Malavolta M. Epigenetics in ageing and development. Mech Ageing Dev. 2018. pii: S0047- 6374(18)30117-9.
13. Goldsmith TC. Modern evolutionary mechanics theories and resolving the programmed/non-programmed aging controversy. Biochemistry (Mosc). 2014;79(10):1049-55.
14. Gomes NM, Ryder OA, Houck ML, et al. Comparative biology of mammalian telomeres: hypotheses on ancestral states and the roles of telomeres in longevity determination. Aging Cell. 2011;10:761-8.
15. Gourlay CW, Ayscough KR. The actin cytoskeleton: a key regulator of apoptosis and ageing. Nat Rev Mol Cell Biol. 2005;6:U583-5.
16. Gustafson G. Age determination on teeth. J Am Dent Assoc. 1950;41(1):45-54.
17. Heidinger BJ, Blount JD, Boner W, et al. Telomere length in early life predicts lifespan. Proc Natl Acad Sci U S A. 2012;109:1743-8.

18. Hood S, Amir S. The aging clock: circadian rhythms and later life. J Clin Invest. 2017;127:437-46.
19. Jafari Nasabian P, Inglis JE, Reilly W, et al. Aging human body: changes in bone, muscle and body fat with consequent changes in nutrient intake. J Endocrinol. 2017;234(1):R37-R51.
20. Jin K. Modern biological theories of aging. Aging Dis. 2010;1(2):72-4.
21. Johanson G. Age determination from teeth. Odontologisk Revy. 1971;22:1-126.
22. Johnson SC, Rabinovitch PS, Kaeberlein M. mTOR is a key modulator of ageing and age-related disease. Nature. 2013;493(7432):338.
23. Kagerer P, Grupe G. Age-at-death diagnosis and determination of life history parameters by incremental lines in human dental cementum as an identification aid. Forensic Sci Int. 2001;118:75-82.
24. Kim K, Choe HK. Role of hypothalamus in aging and its underlying cellular mechanisms. Mech Ageing Dev 2018 May 2. pii: S0047-6374(18)30050-2. doi: 10.1016/j.mad.2018.04.008. [Epub ahead of print]
25. Kim SK, Allen ED. Structural and functional changes in salivary glands during aging, Microsc Res Tech. 1994;28:243-53.
26. Kim SY, Ryu SJ, Ahn HJ, et al. Senescence-related functional nuclear barrier by down-regulation of nucleo-cytoplasmic trafficking gene expression. Biochem Biophys Res Commun. 2010;391:28-32.
27. Kumar GS. Orban's Oral Histology and Embryology, 14th edition. India: Elsevier; 2015.
28. Melfi RC, Alley KE. Parmar's Oral Embryology and Microscopic Anatomy, 10th edition. Philadelphia: Lippincott Williams & Wilkins; 2000.
29. Miles AEW. 'Sans teeth': changes in the oral tissues with advancing age. Proc Roy Soc Med. 1972;65:801-6.
30. Nanci A. Ten Cate's Oral Histology; Development, Structure and Function, 8th edition. India: Elsevier; 2013.
31. Neville BW, Damm DD, Allen CM, et al. Oral and Maxillofacial Pathology, 4th edition. Missouri: Elsevier; 2016.
32. Pekovic V, Gibbs-Seymour I, Markiewicz E, et al. Conserved cysteine residues in the mammalian lamin A tail are essential for cellular responses to ROS generation. Aging Cell. 2011;10:1067-79.
33. Razak PA, Richard KM, Thankachan RP, et al. Geriatric oral health: A review article. J Int Oral Health. 2014;6(6):110-6.
34. Renz H, Radlanski RJ. Incremental lines in root cementum of human teeth—a reliable age marker? Homo. 2006;57:29-50.
35. Saunders MJ, Yeh C-K. Oral Health in Elderly People. In: Chernoff R (Ed). Geriatric Nutrition: The Health Professionals Handbook, 4th edition. Burlington: Jones & Bartlett Learning; 2013. pp. 163-207.
36. Sivapathasundharam B. Shafer's Oral Pathology, 8th edition. India: Elsevier; 2016.
37. Slack C, Partridge L. Genes, pathways and metabolism in ageing. Drug Discov Today Dis Models. 2013;10(2):e87-93.
38. Trindade LS, Aigaki T, Peixoto AA, et al. A novel classification system for evolutionary aging theories. Front Genet. 2013;4:25.
39. Valdes AM, Andrew T, Gardner JP, et al. Obesity, cigarette smoking, and telomere length in women. Lancet. 2005;366: 662-4.
40. Valenzuela A, Martin-de las Heras S, Mandojana JM, et al. Multiple regression models for age estimation by assessment of morphologic dental changes according to teeth source. Am J Forensic Med Pathol. 2002;23(4):386-9.
41. Zole E, Ranka R. Mitochondria, its DNA and telomeres in ageing and human population. Biogerontology. 2018;28:1-20.

CHAPTER 19

Stem Cells

Shankaranarayanan S, Manimaran K, B Sivapathasundharam, Protyusha Guha Biswas

CHAPTER OUTLINE

- History of Stem Cells 287
  - » Dental Pulp Stem Cells 288
- Classification of Stem Cells 288
  - » Cell Potency 288
  - » Source of Stem Cells 288
  - » Embryonic Stem Cells 288
  - » Induced Pluripotential Stem Cells 288
  - » Adult Stem Cells 288
- Mechanism of Action of Stem Cells 289
- Application of Stem Cells in Regenerative Medicine 290
- Dental Stem Cells 290
- Isolation of Dental Pulp Stem Cells 291
- Applications of DPSCs in Regenerative Dentistry 292

Stem cells, also known as "precursor" or "progenitor" cells are clonogenic cells capable of self-renewal and multi-lineage differentiation. They are unspecialized cells in the human body that are capable of becoming specialized cells, each with new specialized cell functions. The name "*stem cell*" denotes stemness of multiplication. Basically, a stem cell remains uncommitted until it receives a signal to develop into a specialized cell. Stem cells have the remarkable property of developing into a variety of cell types in the human body. They serve as a reservoir of repair system by being able to divide without limit to replenish other cells. When stem cells divide, each new cell has the potential to either remain as a stem cell or become another cell type with new special functions.

Classically the stem cell possesses three properties:
1. *Self-renewal:* The ability to go through numerous cycles of cell division while maintaining the undifferentiated state.
2. *Potency:* The capacity to differentiate into specialized cell types. In the strictest sense, stem cells are to be either totipotent or pluripotent—to be able to give rise to any matured cell type. Multipotent or unipotent progenitor cells are sometimes referred to as stem cells.
3. *Homing:* The capacity of stem cells to find their destination or niche is known as homing. It is a process wherein the stem cells respond to gradients of chemoattractants by locating and migrating to them and lodging within specific tissue areas. Another essential property of stem cells is the flexibility in the use of their functional potentials. Further stem cells are characterized by their ability to respond to actual needs of the system. For this, the cells require communication between each other and with their microenvironment. Some of the adult stem cells possess the property of transdifferentiation or plasticity. Transdifferentiation is the ability of the cell to transform from one cell lineage to another completely different cell lineage. However, transdifferentiation is not a unique property of all stem cells; it is found that some cells such as pancreatic cells can be converted to hepatocytes and vice versa.

HISTORY OF STEM CELLS

The history of stem cell research began in the mid-1800s with the discovery that some cells could generate other cells. Now stem cell research is embroiled in a controversy over the use of human embryonic stem cells for research. In the early 1900s, the first real stem cells were discovered when it was found that some cells generate blood cells. Around this time, the term "stem cell" was proposed for scientific research.

A revolution in medical science happened in the year 1968, with the first successful bone marrow transplant discovered in human umbilical cord blood. Another major breakthrough was derivation of embryonic stem cells (ESCs) from the inner cell mass (ICM) of mouse blastocysts. In 1997, evidence of cancer stem cells (CSC) was presented with leukemia as an example of a stem cell-derived cancer. Human ESC line derived from the ICM of human blastocyst promised great potential for establishing stem cell-based therapies and much effort has since been put into work with ESCs. However, due to ethical considerations and technical difficulties when working with ESCs, other avenues were continuously explored. Hence, in 2006, Japanese researchers Takahashi and Yamanaka published a report of induced pluripotent stem cells (iPSCs) from adult mouse fibroblasts. The Nobel Prize in Physiology or Medicine 2012 was awarded jointly to Sir John B Gurdon and Shinya Yamanaka "for the discovery that mature cells can be reprogrammed to become pluripotent. The manifold applications of human cells and tissues have led to the establishment of the medical discipline called "regenerative medicine".

Dental Pulp Stem Cells

The presence of stem cells in dental pulp tissue primarily has been demonstrated in 1985 and these cells have osteogenic and chondrogenic potential *in vitro*, and could also differentiate into dentin, *in vivo*. Dental pulp stem cells isolated from adult human dental pulp had the ability to regenerate a dentin-pulp-like complex. Stem cells even in the inflamed pulp have the capacity to form mineralized matrix both *in vitro* and *in vivo*.

CLASSIFICATION OF STEM CELLS

Stem cells can be classified based on cell potency:
1. Totipotent
2. Pluripotent
3. Multipotent
4. Oligopotent
5. Unipotent

Cell Potency

Totipotent: These cells have the potential to differentiate into all possible human cell types including an entire functional organism. The first few cells to appear during the division of the zygote are totipotent cells, e.g. Zygote, spore, morula.

Pluripotent: These cells can give rise to almost all cells. However, it cannot give rise to an entire organism. The cells from the early embryo are pluripotent, e.g. Embryonic stem cell.

Multipotent: these cells can give rise to a limited range of cells within a closely related family of cells, e.g. Hematopoietic stem cell, mesenchymal stem cell.

Oligopotent: these cells can differentiate into few different types of cells, e.g. Adult lymphoid or myeloid stem cell.

Unipotent: these cells can only produce cells of their own type with the property of self-renewal, e.g. Adult muscle stem cell.

Source of Stem Cells

Pluripotent stem cells: Cells with ability to differentiate into all types of cells in the body.
* Embryonic stem cells
* Induced pluripotent stem cells

Non-embryonic or somatic stem cells: Tissue specific stem cells found in the body that differentiate to yield limited number of mature cell types to build the tissue in which they reside.
* Adult stem cells

Embryonic Stem Cells (ESCs)

These cells are pluripotent, self-replicating stem cells that have the potential to differentiate into any cell in the body (except the placenta). Pluripotent stem cells have the ability to differentiate into cells of all the three germ layers namely—ectoderm, endoderm and mesoderm. ESCs can be derived from a very early stage in human development, even before implantation would normally occur in the uterus, i.e. from the inner cell mass of the blastocyst stage of human embryos.

In the embryo, three kinds of mammalian pluripotent stem cell types have been described—ESCs, embryonic germ cells derived from primordial germ cells, and embryonal carcinoma cells. ESCs are derived from 4-day-old to 5-day-old embryo (blastocyst). Each blastocyst consists of 50–150 cells and includes three structures—an outer layer of cells (the trophoblasts), a fluid-filled cavity (the blastocyst), and a group of about 30 pluripotent cells at one end of the cavity, called the inner cell mass (the embryoblasts) **(Figure 19-1)**.

Induced Pluripotent Stem Cells

Induced pluripotent stem cells (iPSCs) are a type of pluripotent stem cells that are artificially derived from adult somatic cells by inducing a "forced" expression of specific genes. They are reprogrammed back into natural pluripotent stem cells with an embryo-like pluripotent state with features of pluripotency and differentiability. These cells are a great boon to stem cell research and regenerative therapeutic purposes.

Adult Stem Cells

Adult stem cells are undifferentiated cells, found throughout the body after embryonic development. They have limited differentiation potential compared to ESCs and are mostly lineage-restricted (multipotent) defined by their tissue of

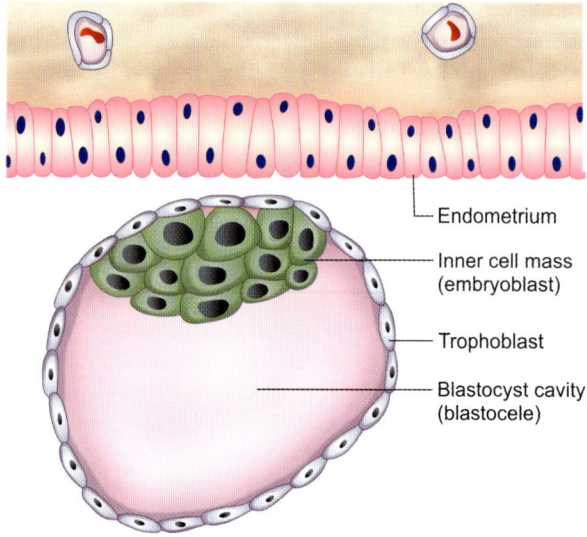

Figure 19-1: Embryonic stem cell.

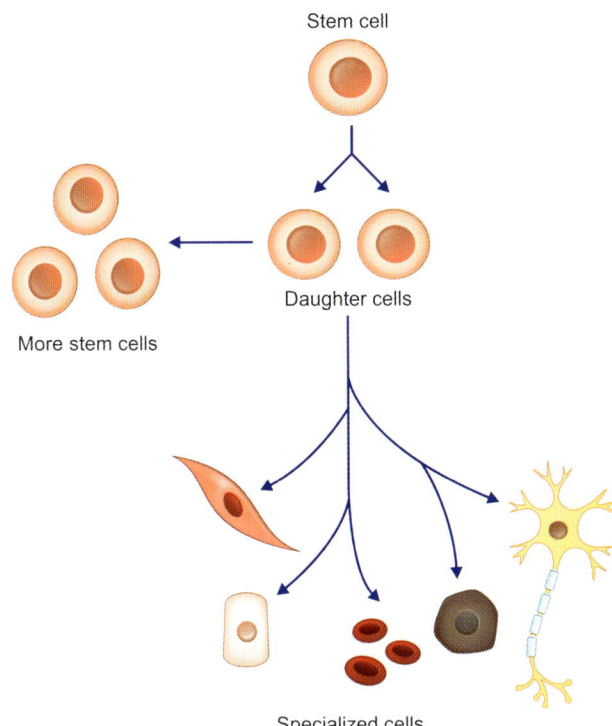

Figure 19-2: Replication of an adult stem cell.

origin (mesenchymal stem cell, adipose-derived stem cell, dental pulp stem cell, etc.). These cells play a major role in replacement of dying cells and regeneration of damaged tissues. They are also known as somatic or tissue-specific stem cells. An adult stem cell undergoes replication by mitosis to produce two daughter cells, one daughter cell differentiates into a cell with characteristic morphology and specialized function and the other cell retains the property of mother cell for long-term cell renewal **(Figure 19-2)**.

Types of Adult Stem Cells

Endodermal origin: Pulmonary Epithelial SCs, pancreatic SCs, hepatic oval cells, gastrointestinal tract SCs, ovarian and testicular SCs, mammary and prostatic gland SCs.

Mesodermal origin: Hematopoietic SCs, mesenchymal SCs, mesenchymal precursor SCs, mesenchymal stroma SCs, multipotent adult progenitor cells, bone marrow SCs, fetal somatic SCs, cardiac SCs, satellite cells of muscle, unrestricted somatic SCs.

Ectodermal Origin: Neural SCs, ocular SCs, skin SCs

The bone marrow contains two types of adult stem cells.

One population is called hematopoietic stem cell (HSC) that differentiates into all the blood cells.

The other population of cells is called nonhematopoietic stem cells from bone marrow that differentiates into bone, cartilage, fat, and connective tissue.

Hematopoietic Stem Cells

The hematopoietic stem cells (HSCs) may be referred to as the paradigmatic tissue specific cells. These cells have the ability to self-renew continuously in the marrow and differentiate into the blood cells and its components. HSCs reside in bone marrow but migrate through blood to various organs on proper signaling. They are also found in liver, spleen, umbilical cord, and blood. There are evidences that these HSCs also have plasticity, i.e. they tend to form tissues other than blood systems. This property may be useful in life-saving regenerative therapies.

Non-hematopoietic Stem Cells

The non-hematopoietic stem/progenitor cells are also termed as mesenchymal stem cells or bone marrow stromal cells.

Mesenchymal stem cells (MSCs) are multipotent adult stem cells that can differentiate into connective tissue, bone, cartilage, marrow-stroma, and adipocytes. MSCs may also give rise to sarcomeric muscle, endothelial cells, and cells of non-mesodermal origin, such as hepatocytes and neural cells.

With this wide range of differentiation potential, MSCs find the possibility in engraftment and immunosuppressive effect. Their expansion through culture led to increasing clinical interest in the use of MSCs, through either intravenous infusion or site-directed administration, in numerous pathologic situations.

> During embryonic development, mesenchyme or the embryonic mesoderm contains stem cells that differentiate into virtually all connective tissue phenotypes such as bone, cartilage, bone marrow stroma, interstitial fibrous tissue, and dense fibrous tissues such as tendons and ligaments, as well as adipose tissue and skeletal muscle.

Mesenchymal stem cells have been isolated from various tissues. The different sources could be umbilical cord blood, chorionic villi of the placenta, amniotic fluid, peripheral blood, fetal liver, lung, and exfoliated deciduous teeth. Increased number of reports is available describing their presence in adipose tissue and dental pulp.

A standard set of criteria have been formulated to identify MSCs.

First, MSC must be plastic-adherent when maintained in standard culture conditions.

Second, MSC must express CD105, CD73 and CD90, and lack expression of CD45, CD34, CD14 or CD11b, CD79 alpha or CD19 and HLA-DR surface molecules.

Third, MSC must differentiate to osteoblasts, adipocytes, and chondroblasts *in vitro*.

■ MECHANISM OF ACTION OF STEM CELLS

The basis of stem cell action is the formation of new tissues to promote repair and regeneration of damaged tissues, thereby restoring normal function. This enables the implication of stem cells in degenerative diseases through remodeling of injured tissues. It was originally hypothesized that stem cells on administration would migrate to sites of damaged area and perform the following functions:

- ❖ Differentiation into replacement cell types.
- ❖ Rescue of damaged or dying cells through cell fusion.

- Secretion of paracrine factors such as growth factors, cytokines, and hormones.
- Transfer of organelles (*e.g.* mitochondria) and/or molecules through tunneling nanotubes (TNTs), Ca^{2+} (calcium), and Mg^{2+} (magnesium).
- Mediate the transfer of proteins or peptides, RNA, hormones, and/or chemicals by extracellular vesicles such as exosomes or microvesicles.

These functions help to increase angiogenesis, plasticity, pluripotentiality, reduce inflammation, activate neighboring resident stem cells, and aid in remodeling. Hence, these functions form the basis for the development of cell-based therapeutics and regenerative medicine.

APPLICATION OF STEM CELLS IN REGENERATIVE MEDICINE

The use of stem cells in medicine can be generalized into three broad categories: cell-based therapies, drug discovery and basic knowledge via research. Given their unique regenerative abilities, stem cells offer new potentials for treating a multitude of diseases. Laboratory studies and research on stem cells continues to advance knowledge and possibilities of their usage in several frontiers of human healthcare.

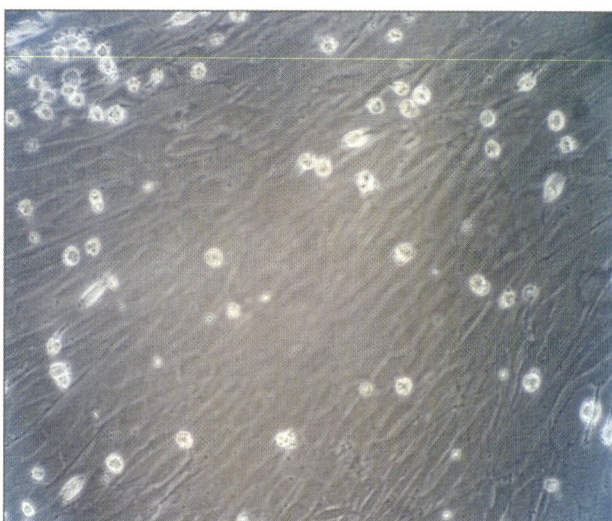

Figure 19-3: Dental pulp stem cell appears spindle-shaped in culture. *Source:* Mother Cell Regenerative Centre, Tiruchirappalli, India.

Potential Uses of Stem Cells
- Cardiovascular disease treatment
- Brain disease treatment including Alzheimer's and Parkinson's disease
- Hematological disease treatment such as leukemia, thalassemia, sickle cell anemia
- Diabetes
- Osteoarthritis and rheumatoid arthritis
- Baldness
- Blindness
- Deafness
- Stroke
- Learning defects
- Spinal cord injury
- Muscular dystrophy
- Liver disease
- Organ transplantation
- Bone marrow transplantation
- Toxicology screening
- Cancer therapy

DENTAL STEM CELLS

The main component of the dental pulp tissue is dental pulp stem cells, which are mesenchymal cells derived from the neural crest. There are strong evidences that cells isolated from this structure of tooth have the ability to form tooth. Recently, dental tissues such as periodontal ligament (PDL), dental papilla or dental follicle have been identified as specific MSC populations **(Figure 19-3)**. Studies show that periodontal ligament stem cell culture exhibits almost 30% higher proliferative rate compared to the cultured bone marrow stromal stem cells. STRO-1, the putative stem cell marker used to isolate and purify bone marrow stromal stem cells is also expressed by periodontal and dental pulp stem cells.

Therefore, dental stem cell biology provides meaningful visions into the development of dental tissues and cellular differentiation processes. The cells isolated from tooth structure can be bioengineered into physiologically whole tooth along with epithelial and mesenchymal population of neural crest germ cells.

The final goal of tissue engineering in dentistry is to develop a functional tooth. Dental stem cells could also be a feasible tool for dental tissue engineering and help in construction of complex structures including periodontal ligament fibers, bone, cementum and dental pulp which could effectively improve modern dentistry. Dental precursor cells are attractive for novel approaches to treat diseases like periodontitis, dental caries or to improve dental pulp healing, and the regeneration of teeth and various craniofacial structures such as mandibular condyles, cranial sutures, calvarial bone and subcutaneous adipose tissue. These cells are easily accessible and, in contrast to bone marrow-derived mesenchymal stem cells, are more closely related to dental tissues.

Sources of dental stem cells are:
- Dental pulp stem cells (DPSCs)
- Dental follicle stem cells (DFSCs)
- Stem cells from human exfoliated deciduous teeth (SHED)
- Periodontal ligament stem cells (PDLSC)
- Stem cells from the apical papilla (SCAP)
- Stem cells derived from gingiva (GSCs).

Dental pulp stem cells (DPSC): Dental pulp stem cells are similar to MSCs in some ways; they are of fibroblastic morphology with selective adherence to solid surfaces, have good proliferative potential, anti-inflammatory property and capacity to differentiate *in vitro*, and the ability to repair tissues *in vivo*. The regeneration of pulp-dentin capacity is greater in DPSCs than the other dental stem cells. Besides dentin and pulp, they can even differentiate into adipocytes and muscle *in vivo*.

Dental follicle stem cells (DFSC): Dental follicle stem cells are derived from dental follicle tissues and possess the ability to differentiate into cementum and bone. They are therefore used in periodontal and bone regeneration therapies. DFSCs have higher proliferative capacity than DPSCs, easily available for cell culture and adhere well to the culture plates. Human third molar teeth serve as a vital niche for DFSCs.

Stem cells from human exfoliated deciduous teeth (SHED): This stem cell population is from the living pulp debris of exfoliated deciduous teeth. SHED are different from DPSCs, in the way that they are "more immature". They are able to differentiate into a variety of cell types, to an extent greater than the DPSCs and are characterized by faster proliferative capacity, higher population doubling efficiency, sphere-like cluster formation, etc. One striking feature that differentiates SHED from DPSCs is their ability to differentiate into bone-forming cells.

Periodontal ligament stem cells (PDLSC): Periodontal ligament stem cells have first been introduced by Seo, Miura et al. in 2004. The stem cells of the periodontal ligament occupy the perivascular region in the periodontal ligament and the adjacent endosteal spaces. PDLSCs have been reported to form adherent clonogenic population of fibroblast-like cells in the culture. They express early MSC markers. A further class of dental ectomesenchymal stem cells is PDL stem cells, which were isolated from the root surface of extracted teeth. These cells could be isolated as plastic-adherent, colony-forming cells, but display a low potential for osteogenic differentiation under *in vitro* conditions. PDL stem cells differentiate into cells or tissues very similar to the periodontium.

Stem cells from the apical papilla (SCAP): Stem cells from dental apical papilla were first identified in human permanent immature teeth. The dental papilla is an embryonic-like tissue that becomes the dental pulp during maturation and formation of the crown. Therefore, SCAP can only be isolated at a certain stage of tooth development. SCAP have a greater capacity for dentin regeneration than DPSCs because the dental papilla contains a higher number of adult stem cells compared to the mature dental pulp. In addition, SCAP are likely to be less differentiated than DPSCs, as they originate from an embryonic-like tissue. Interestingly, only a combination of SCAP and PDL stem cells induced the formation of a dental connective tissue, namely, the attachment of an artificial tooth crown in the alveolar bone.

Stem cells derived from gingiva (GSC): They are derived from the lamina propria of gingival tissue. These stem cells are capable of multilineage differentiation and related gene expression. GSCs have the potential to differentiate into osteoblasts, chondroblasts, adipocytes, endothelial and neural cells. These cells can be isolated from the free and attached gingiva, inflamed gingival tissue and hyperplastic gingiva. GSCs are the best stem cell source for cell-based therapies and regenerative dentistry.

Stem cells of dental origin	Markers
dental pulp stem cells	CD9, CD10, CD13, CD29, CD44, CD49d, CD59, CD73, CD90, CD105, CD106, CD146, CD166, STRO-1, Oct-4, Nanog, SSEA-4, and Vimentin.
Dental follicle stem cells	Nestin, Notch-1, STRO-1, cementum attachment protein and cementumprotein-23, BMP-1, BMP-7, CD9, CD29, CD10, CD13, CD44, CD49d, CD59, CD73, CD90, CD105, CD106, CD166 and HLA-Class I
Stem cells from human exfoliated deciduous teeth	CD13, CD44, CD73, CD90, CD105, CD146, Nanog, STRO-1, Oct-4, fibroblast growth factor 2 (FGF-2), Nestin, SSEA-3, SSEA-4, transforming growth factor-β(TGF-β), TGF-β2, collagen I (Col I), and Col III
Periodontal ligament stem cells	STRO-1, scleraxis, CD9, CD10, CD13, CD29, CD44, CD49d, CD59, CD73, CD90, CD105, CD106, CD146, and CD166
Stem cells from the apical papilla	Mesenchymal surface markers, STRO-1, CD146, and CD24.
Stem cells derived from gingiva	STRO-1, Oct-4, Sox-2, SSEA-4, Nanog, HLA-ABC, Nestin, Tra2-49, and Tra2-54.

ISOLATION OF DENTAL PULP STEM CELLS

There are various methods of isolation of stem cells from dental pulp—(A) enzymatic digestion—where the pulp is digested with collagenase or dispase enzyme and isolated trypsinized cells are plated in culture dishes; (B) explant culture—where small pieces of undigested dental pulp tissue is explanted directly to Petri dishes; (C) combination of enzymatic and explant cultures—dental pulp tissues are initially trypsinized and then small tissue pieces are explanted to Petri dishes for their outgrowth. Once the cells are isolated, they are cultured in Minimum Essential Medium (MEM) supplemented with 20% fetal bovine serum (FBS) at 37°C with 5% CO_2 and 90% humidity in CO_2 incubator; (D) magnetic activated cell sorting (MACS)—it is a simple, inexpensive immune magnetic method used for isolation of stem cell population based on their surface antigens (CD271, STRO-1, CD34, CD45, and c-Kit). This technique can handle large number of cells, however, the degree of purity of stem cells is low using this method. (E) Fluorescence activated cell sorting (FACS)—this is an effective and easy technique for isolation of stem cells based on cell size and fluorescence. Nevertheless, this technique is not suitable for processing large quantities of cells, requires expensive equipment and skilled personnel.

APPLICATIONS OF DPSCs IN REGENERATIVE DENTISTRY

At present, inflammation of the dental pulp is managed by conventional methods such as pulp capping or root canal therapy. However, with advancements in dental research, scientists are focusing on use of tissue engineering approach with cells, biological, and growth factors.

They can use biocompatible material as direct pulp capping agents that can supply growth factors or molecules to stimulate reparative dentin formation.

Dental pulp stem cells are being used for regenerative therapies for bone-related diseases and orthopaedic surgeries, as dental pulp stem cells have the potential to differentiate into osteoblasts and chondroblasts. The clinical studies by d'Aquino, De Rosa et al. (2009) have shown the use of DPSCs cells in oral and maxillofacial (OMF) bone repair. They have used DPSCs along with collagen sponge for providing optimal support in OMF repair. Thus, autologous transplantation of DPSCs can be used in a low-risk and effective therapeutic strategy for the repair of bone defects.

Manimaran, Sharma et al. (2016) have shown bone regeneration in a mandibular ameloblastoma defect with the help of autologous DPSC and buccal pad of fat with more than one year of follow-up proving the safety and bone formation potentials of DPSC. Tricalcium phosphate was used as scaffold and platelet-rich fibrin as growth factors in that case **(Figures 19-4 to 19-6)**.

Side population (SP) of dental pulp cells has the property of vasculogenesis. Vasculogenesis is a potential treatment for ischemic heart disease and it is an exciting area of research in regenerative medicine. These SP cells from dental pulp are positive for *CD31* and *CD146* genes. Thus, it is suggested that SP cells are a new source of stem cells which stimulate angiogenesis or vasculogenesis in tissues and can be used in cell-based treatment of ischemic heart diseases.

Dental stem cells also have the potential to be used in regenerating brain tissues, treating muscular dystrophy and bone regeneration. A recent animal study has also shown reconstruction of large size cranial bone defects in rats using human DPSCs.

Dental pulp stem cells being a source for cell-based therapy to stimulate angiogenesis during tissue regeneration, an unhealed diabetic ulcer was treated with DPSC and platelet-rich plasma by Sankaranarayanan S, Ramachandran et al. **(Figures 19-7A to C)**.

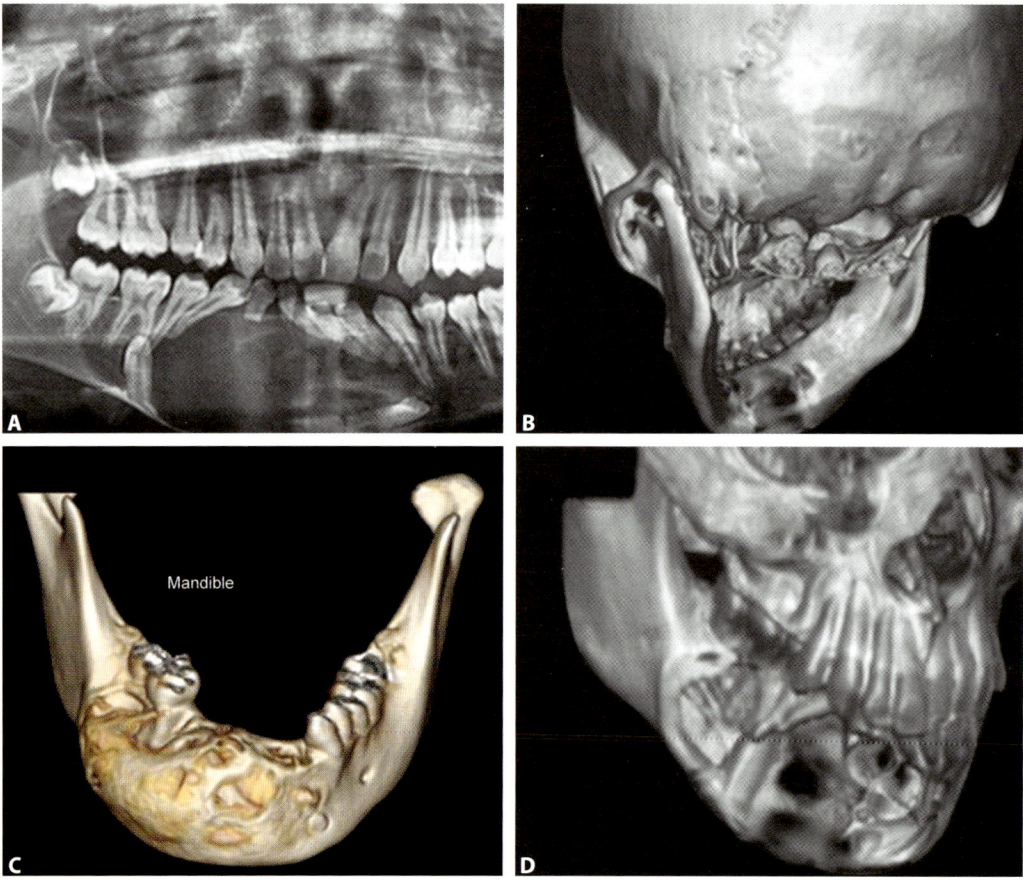

Figures 19-4A to D: (A) Preoperative orthopantomograph; (B) Computed tomography of the mandible showing lingual perforation; (C) Labial expansion; (D) Lateral view of the mandible.
Source: Mother Cell Regenerative Centre, Tiruchirappalli, India.

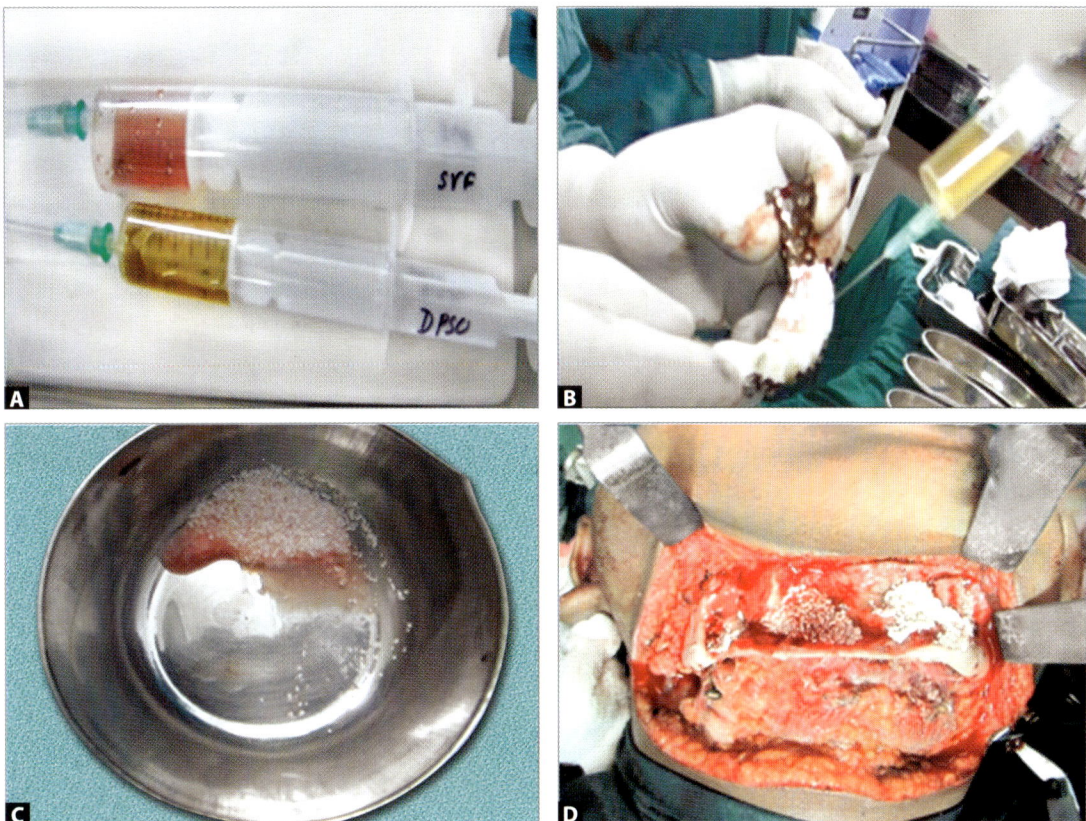

Figures 19-5A to D: Intraoperative procedures: (A) Syringes with stromal vascular fraction and dental pulp stem cells; (B) Placing stromal vascular fraction and dental pulp cells in syboGraft; (C) Stromal vascular fraction mixed with granules; (D) Placing mixed granules over lingual cortex
Source: Mother Cell Regenerative Centre, Tiruchirappalli, India.

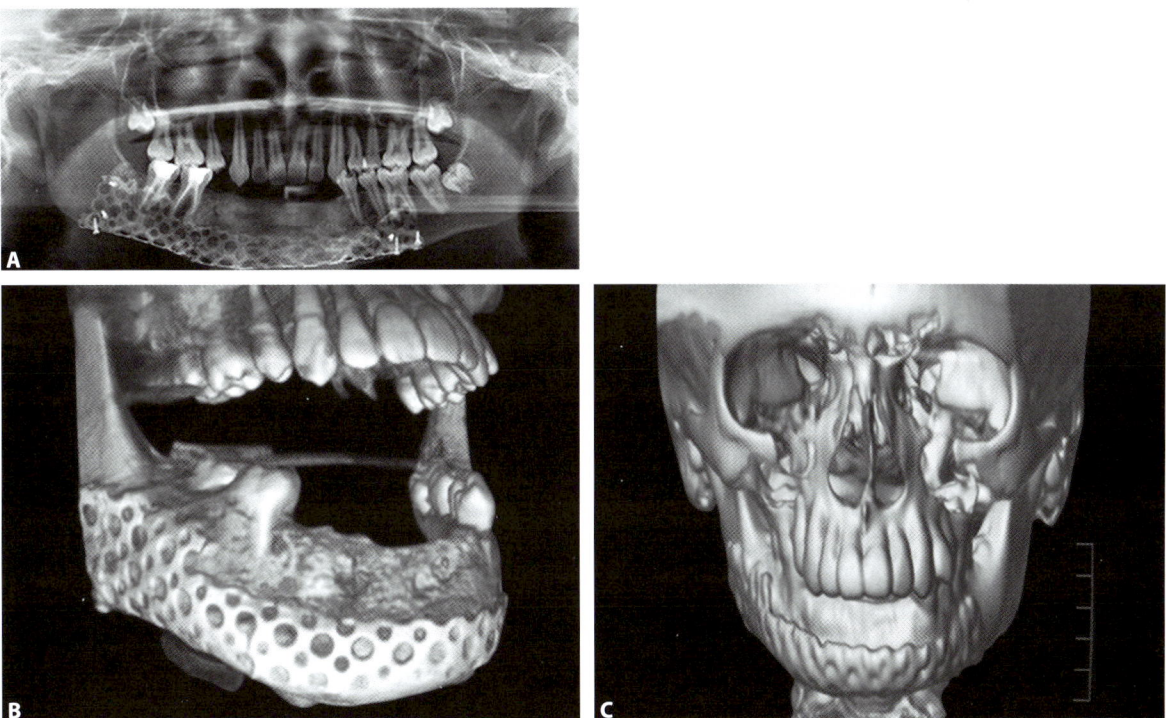

Figures 19-6A to C: (A) Postoperative orthopantomogram at 10th month; (B) Computed tomography of the mandible at 10th month AP view; (C) Mandible lateral view.
Source: Mother Cell Regenerative Centre, Tiruchirappalli, India.

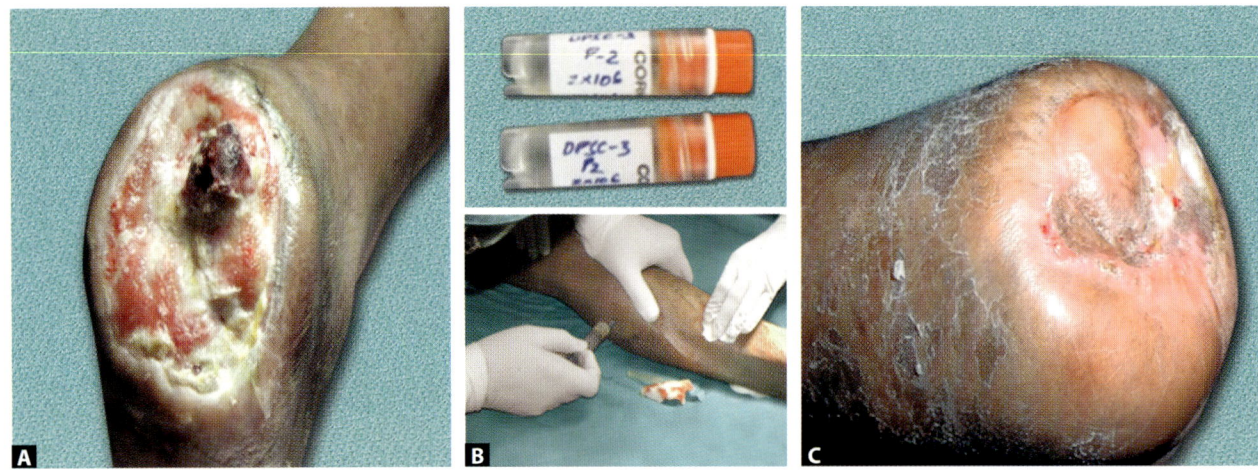

Figures 19-7A to C: (A) Unhealed ulcer; (B) Injection of dental pulp stem cells along the course of artery; (C) Healed stump postoperative 6 months.
Source: Mother Cell Regenerative Centre, Tiruchirappalli, India.

Points to Remember

1. All stem cells regardless of their source have three general properties:
    a. Capable of dividing and renewing themselves
    b. Unspecialized
    c. Can give rise to specialized cell types.
2. There are two main types of stem cells:
    a. Pluripotent stem cells
        – Embryonic stem cells (ESCs)
        – Induced pluripotent stem cells (iPSCs)
    b. Adult or multipotent stem cells
        – Mesenchymal stem cells (MSCs)
        – Neural stem cells (NSCs)
        – Hematopoietic stem cells (HSCs)
        – Cancer stem cells (CSCs)
3. Embryonic stem cells are pluripotent stem cells derived from the inner cell mass of the blastocyst.
4. Cancer stem cells: Cancer stem cells are a type of cancer cells that responds to cancer drug resistance and tumor recurrence. This concept has a significant impact on cancer treatment strategy and anti-cancer medication development.
5. Dental stem cells, which are easy, convenient, and affordable to collect, hold promise for a range of very potential therapeutic applications.
6. Stem Cells have applications in:
    a. Basic medical research
    b. Drug discovery
    c. Cell therapy

PRACTICE QUESTIONS

1. What are stem cells?
2. Elaborate the properties of stem cells.
3. Classify stem cells with examples.
4. Mention few applications of stem cells in regenerative medicine and dentistry.
5. Mention the sources of dental stem cells. Elaborate on dental pulp stem cells.

MULTIPLE CHOICE QUESTIONS

1. Following are the features of stem cells, *except:*
    a. Homing
    b. Brownian movement
    c. Self-renewal
    d. Differentiation
2. Stem cells have the capacity of dividing and renewing themselves for indefinite periods. This property is known as:
    a. Proliferation
    b. Transformation
    c. Culturing
    d. Fermentation
3. Which is the primary role of adult stem cells in tissues where they are found?
    a. Maintaining tissue
    b. Repairing tissue
    c. Mutationing tissue
    d. Both a and b

4. Where are ESCs derived from?
   a. Blastocyst
   b. Morula
   c. Trophoblast
   d. Endometrium
5. Where can scientists obtain stem cells from?
   a. Only embryo
   b. Only from tissues in the body
   c. Only from brain
   d. Both from embryo and tissues in the body
6. What is a stem cell?
   a. Unspecialized cells in the body that are capable of becoming specialized cells, with specialized functions.
   b. A cell that helps fight against infection.
   c. A cell that can produce all the cell types of the body.
   d. A cell that is specialized.
7. What is homing?
   a. The ability to go through various cell divisions
   b. The capacity to differentiate into specialized cells
   c. Flexibility in the use of their functional potentials
   b. The capacity of stem cells to find their destination or niche
8. Which of these is not a property of stem cells?
   a. Self-renewal
   b. Do not serve as a reservoir of repair system
   c. Homing
   d. Potency
9. What is transdifferentiation?
   a. Flexibility in the use of potential functions
   b. Ability of cell to transform from one cell lineage to another
   c. Responding to gradients of chemoattractants
   d. Cells giving rise to one lineage
10. Cell that can give rise to other types of cells but its ability to differentiate is limited:
    a. Totipotent
    b. Multipotent
    c. Monopotent
    d. Pluripotent
11. Embryonic stem cells were derived from:
    a. Inner cell mass
    b. Cancer stem cells
    c. Inner stem cells of mouse blastocysts
    d. Totipotent cells
12. The pulp chamber comprises:
    a. Fibrous pulp
    b. Dental papilla
    c. Vascular network and nerve bundles
    d. Fibrous pulp, dental papilla, vascular network and nerve bundles
13. Which dental tissues have been identified as the source of specific MSC populations?
    a. PDL
    b. Dental papilla
    c. Enamel
    d. Both a and b
14. Which of these is a stem cell marker?
    a. *STRO-1*
    b. CD3
    c. TCR
    d. CCR4
15. How do dental pulp stem cells appear in culture?
    a. Round
    b. Spherical
    c. Spindle shaped
    d. Elongated
16. Which of these are not the similarities between dental pulp stem cells and MSCs?
    a. Fibroblastic morphology
    b. Good proliferative potential
    c. Anti-inflammatory property
    d. Does not repair tissues
17. Dental follicle stem cells differentiate into?
    a. Cementum
    b. Bone
    c. Cementum and bone
    d. Enamel
18. What serves as a vital niche for DFSCs?
    a. 1st premolar
    b. Canine
    c. 3rd molar
    d. Central incisor
19. What is the difference between SHED and DPSCs?
    a. Ability to differentiate into bone-forming cells
    b. Ability to multiply
    c. Ability to double the efficacy
    d. None of the above
20. Dental stem cells can be used in regenerating:
    a. Brain tissues
    b. Treating muscular dystrophy
    c. Bone regeneration
    d. All of the above

ANSWERS

1. b 2. a 3. d 4. a 5. d 6. a 7. d 8. b 9. b 10. b 11. c 12. d 13. d 14. a 15. c
16. d 17. c 18. c 19. a 20. d

BIBLIOGRAPHY

1. Abumaree MH, Al Jumah MA, Kalionis B, et al. Phenotypic and functional characterization of mesenchymal stem cells from chorionic villi of human term placenta. Stem Cell Rev. 2013;9(1):1-16.
2. Akiyama K, Chen C, Gronthos S, et al. Lineage differentiation of mesenchymal stem cells from dental pulp, apical papilla, and periodontal ligament. Methods Mol Biol. 2012;887:111-21.

3. Bensinger WI, Clift RA, Anasetti C, et al. Transplantation of allogeneic peripheral blood stem cells mobilized by recombinant human granulocyte colony stimulating factor. Stem Cells. 1996;14(1):90-105.
4. Bongso A, Lee EH. Stem cells: their definition, classification and sources. Stem cells: from bench to bedside. Singapore: World Scientific Publishing; 2005.
5. Campagnoli C, Roberts IA, Kumar S, et al. Identification of mesenchymal stem/progenitor cells in human first-trimester fetal blood, liver, and bone marrow. Blood. 2001;98(8):2396- 402.
6. Carraro G, Perin L, Sedrakyan S, et al. Human amniotic fluid stem cells can integrate and differentiate into epithelial lung lineages. Stem Cells. 2008;26(11):2902-11.
7. Castrechini NM, Murthi P, Gude NM, et al. Mesenchymal stem cells in human placental chorionic villi reside in a vascular Niche. Placenta. 2010;31(3):203-12.
8. Cawthorn WP, Scheller EL, MacDougald OA. Adipose tissue stem cells: the great WAT hope. Trends Endocrinol Metab. 2012;23(6):270-7.
9. Chou S, Lodish HF. Fetal liver hepatic progenitors are supportive stromal cells for hematopoietic stem cells. Proc Natl Acad Sci USA. 2010;107(17):7799-804.
10. Cordeiro MM, Dong Z, Kaneko T, et al. Dental pulp tissue engineering with stem cells from exfoliated deciduous teeth. J Endod. 2008;34(8):962-9.
11. d'Aquino R, De Rosa A, Lanza V, et al. Human mandible bone defect repair by the grafting of dental pulp stem/progenitor cells and collagen sponge biocomplexes. Eur Cell Mater. 2009;18(7):75-83.
12. Fast EM, Zon LI. Aging hematopoietic stem cells make their history. Dev Cell. 2016;39(4):390-1.
13. Gronthos S, Mankani M, Brahim J, et al. Postnatal human dental pulp stem cells (DPSCs) in vitro and in vivo. Proc Natl Acad Sci. 2000;97(25):13625-30.
14. Iohara K, Zheng L, Wake H, et al. A novel stem cell source for vasculogenesis in ischemia: subfraction of side population cells from dental pulp. Stem Cells. 2008;26(9):2408-18.
15. Kajstura J, Rota M, Hall SR, et al. Evidence for human lung stem cells. New Engl J Med. 2011;364(19):1795-806.
16. Karamzadeh R, Eslaminejad MB. Dental-related stem cells and their potential in regenerative medicine. Regenerative Medicine and Tissue Engineering. InTech. 2013.
17. Karp JM, Leng Teo GS. Mesenchymal stem cell homing: the devil is in the details. Cell Stem Cell. 2009;4(3):206-16.
18. Keating A. Mesenchymal stromal cells: new directions. Cell Stem Cell. 2012;10(6):709-16.
19. Krause DS, Theise ND, Collector MI, et al. Multi-organ, multi-lineage engraftment by a single bone marrow-derived stem cell. Cell. 2001;105(3):369-77.
20. Lagasse E, Connors H, Al-Dhalimy M, et al. Purified hematopoietic stem cells can differentiate into hepatocytes in vivo. Nat Med. 2000;6(11):1229-34.
21. Lanza R, Blau H, Gearhart J, et al. Handbook of Stem Cells, Volume 1-Embryonic Stem Cells; Volume 2-Adult & Fetal Stem Cells. US: Academic Press; 2004.
22. Magnus T, Liu Y, Parker GC, et al. Stem cell myths. Philos Trans R Soc Lond B Biol Sci. 2008;363(1489):9-22.
23. Manimaran K, Sharma R, Sankaranarayanan S, et al. Regeneration of mandibular ameloblastoma defect with the help of autologous dental pulp stem cells and buccal pad of fat stromal vascular fraction. Ann Maxillofac Surg. 2016;6(1): 97-100.
24. Mathiasen AB, Jørgensen E, Qayyum AA, et al. Rationale and design of the first randomized, double-blind, placebo-controlled trial of intramyocardial injection of autologous bone-marrow derived Mesenchymal Stromal Cells in chronic ischemic Heart Failure (MSC-HF Trial). Am Heart J. 2012;164(3):285-91.
25. Miura M, Gronthos S, Zhao M, et al. SHED: stem cells from human exfoliated deciduous teeth. Proc Natl Acad Sci USA. 2003;100(10):5807-12.
26. Nielsen TH. What happened to the stem cells? J Med Ethics. 20087;34(12):852-7.
27. Prentice DA. Adult stem cells. Issues Law Med. 2004;19(3):265-94.
28. Raoof M, Yaghoobi MM, Derakhshani A, et al. A modified efficient method for dental pulp stem cell isolation. Dent Res J. 2014;11(2):244-50.
29. Sankaranarayanan S, Ramachandran P, Ravi VR, et al. Dental pulp stem cells for treating unhealed diabetic foot ulcer: a pioneering attempt. JIDAT. 2012;4(15):27-9.
30. Seo BM, Miura M, Gronthos S, et al. Investigation of multipotent postnatal stem cells from human periodontal ligament. Lancet. 2004;364(9429):149-55.
31. Shetty P, Bharucha K, Tanavde V. Human umbilical cord blood serum can replace fetal bovine serum in the culture of mesenchymal stem cells. Cell Biol Int. 2007;31(3):293-8.
32. Sonoyama W, Liu Y, Fang D, Yamaza T, Seo B-M, Zhang C, et al. Mesenchymal Stem Cell-Mediated Functional Tooth Regeneration in Swine. PLoS ONE 2006; 1(1): e79. https://doi.org/10.1371/journal.pone.0000079.
33. Spath L, Rotilio V, Alessandrini M, et al. Explant-derived human dental pulp stem cells enhance differentiation and proliferation potentials. J Cell Mol Med. 2010;14(6b):1635-44.
34. Spees JL, Lee RH, Gregory CA, et al. Mechanisms of mesenchymal stem/stromal cell function. Stem Cell Research Ther. 2016;7(1):125.
35. Thomson JA, Itskovitz-Eldor J, Shapiro SS, et al. Embryonic stem cell lines derived from human blastocysts. Science. 1998;282(5391):1145-7.
36. Turksen K. "Adult stem cells." Recherche. 2004;67: 02.
37. Wang X, Sha XJ, Li GH, et al. Comparative characterization of stem cells from human exfoliated deciduous teeth and dental pulp stem cells. Arch Oral Biol. 2012;57(9):1231-40.
38. Yu J, Vodyanik MA, Smuga-Otto K, et al. Induced pluripotent stem cell lines derived from human somatic cells. ObstetGynecolSurv. 2008;63(3):154-5.

CHAPTER 20

Evolution of Jaws and Teeth

Mahesh Verma, Priya Kumar

CHAPTER OUTLINE

- Agnathan to Gnathostomes Transition 297
- Hominid Jaw Evolution 298
  - Earliest Hominids 298
  - Archaic Hominids 299
  - Archaic Megadont Hominids 299
  - Pre-modern Homo 299
- Jaw Suspension 300
- Theories of Evolution of Human Dentition 300
  - Hypothesis Explaining Evolution of Teeth 301
  - Dentition Types 301
- Theories of Cuspal Origin 302
- Evolution of Periodontium 303
- Trends in Evolution 304

Evolution is defined as a change in the heritable characteristics of biological populations over successive generations. More simply, evolution is descent with modification. It leads to biodiversity at every level of biological organization which includes species, individual organisms and even molecules. According to the theory of evolution or origin of species, all present life forms have been derived from earlier simpler life forms. Over the last decade, tremendous progress has been made in understanding the developmental aspects of morphological evolution.

One of the major contributors to the science of evolution is Charles Darwin who in the mid-19th century formulated the scientific theory of evolution by natural selection. In its modified form, Darwin's scientific discovery is the unifying theory of the life sciences, explaining the diversity of life.

AGNATHAN TO GNATHOSTOME TRANSITION

Vertebrates (organisms that possess notochord during the embryonic period to be replaced later by bony vertebral column) have been broadly divided into two groups.

Jawless vertebrates/Agnathans: Jawless fish consist of both present (cyclostomes) and extinct (conodonts and ostracoderms) species. Conodonts contained an intricately patterned series of odontodes (tooth-like structures) throughout the oropharyngeal cavity. They appeared at the dawn of vertebrates and may have brought with them the first vertebrate dentition.

Jawed vertebrates/Gnathostomes: They account for 99% of living vertebrates and include the classes Chondrichthyes (sharks), Osteichthyes (bony fish), Amphibia, Reptilia, Aves, and Mammalia. Apart from presence of opposing jaws, the gnathostomes are also characterized by the presence of teeth, paired appendages and a semicircular inner ear canal.

The jawed vertebrates account for majority of the extant (existing) vertebrate species. The evolution of jaws enabled gnathostomes to become effective predators and thus accounted for their subsequent survival and evolution. The classical view holds that jaws evolved via modifications of ancient gill arch cartilages (viscerocranial elements).

In the embryo, the jaw cartilage supports the mouth and is derived from the first pharyngeal (mandibular) arch, which consists of the palatoquadrate cartilage (contributing to the upper jaw) and Meckel's cartilage (forming the presumptive lower jaw). These endoskeletal jaw cartilages form a developmental and evolutionary framework for adult vertebrate jaws. The neural crest, a migratory and multipotent cell population unique to vertebrates are almost entirely responsible for the embryonic origin of jaws, teeth and the visceral skeleton.

The **Devonian period** (Age of fishes) saw the demise of virtually all jawless fishes. This was because the jawless fish had more trouble surviving compared to their jawed counterparts. Lampreys and hagfish are the only surviving jawless vertebrates. Both of these have round mouths and retractable horny teeth (**Figures 20-1A and B**). They are the most primitive of the vertebrates, indicating that they

CHAPTER 20: Evolution of Jaws and Teeth

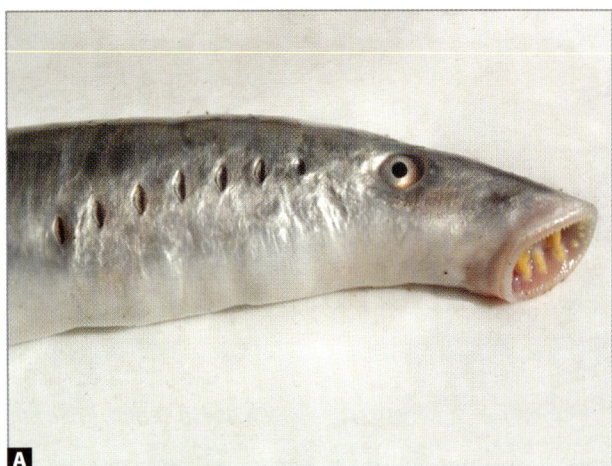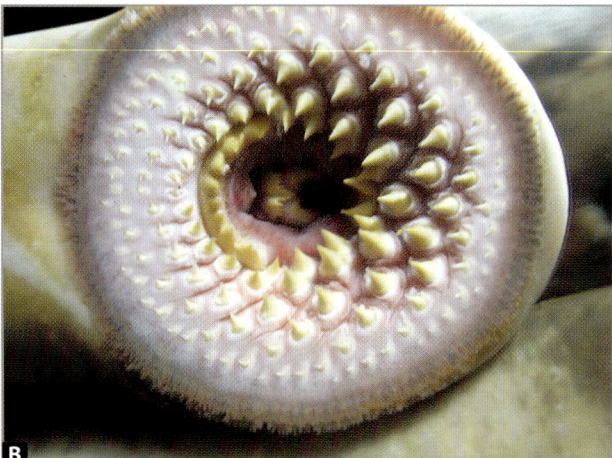

Figures 20-1A and B: (A) Sea Lamprey; (B) Mouth of jawless lamprey with numerous retractable horny teeth

are the least changed from the first vertebrates. Their unique morphological characteristics such as their cartilaginous skeleton, suggest they are the sister taxon of all living jawed vertebrates (gnathostomes), and are thus considered the most basal group of the Vertebrata. Enamel first appeared by around 415 million years ago, close to the boundary between the Silurian and Devonian periods, in a group called the sarcopterygians. This group includes modern-day tetrapods (amphibians, reptiles and mammals) and the lobe-finned fishes, best known for their paired front and back fins, with bones and muscles resembling those in limbs. Enamel was initially limited to the scales, which suggests that like teeth, enamel originated in skin structures and then made the leap to the mouth.

This period also saw the rise of **Labyrinthodonts** (named maze toothed due to the complex pattern of infolding of enamel and dentin), which are considered as the transition between fishes and amphibians **(Figure 20-2)**. The labyrinthodonts are considered the ancestors of all land-living vertebrates.

From amphibians came the first reptiles, and shortly after the appearance of the first reptiles, two branches split off. One branch gave rise to the modern reptiles and birds and the other to modern mammals. One of the earliest mammals like reptiles are the **cynodonts** that evolved more mammal-like characteristics and the jaws of cynodonts resemble modern mammal jaws. From cynodonts came the first mammals that were small shrew-like animals that fed on insects. This egg-laying group of mammals is represented in the modern era by animals like the Platypus. The next evolutionary ladder is held by the primates that are characterized by having large brains relative to other mammals, as well as an increased reliance on stereoscopic vision at the expense of smell (as the skull case enlarges to accommodate the larger brain, the snout reduces in length. As a result, the laterally placed eyes moved toward anteriorly, which enables three-dimensional vision).

The evolution of the mammalian jaw is one of the most important change in vertebrate history, and underpins the exceptional radiation and diversification of mammals over the last 220 million years. In particular, the transformation of the mandible into a single tooth-bearing bone and the emergence

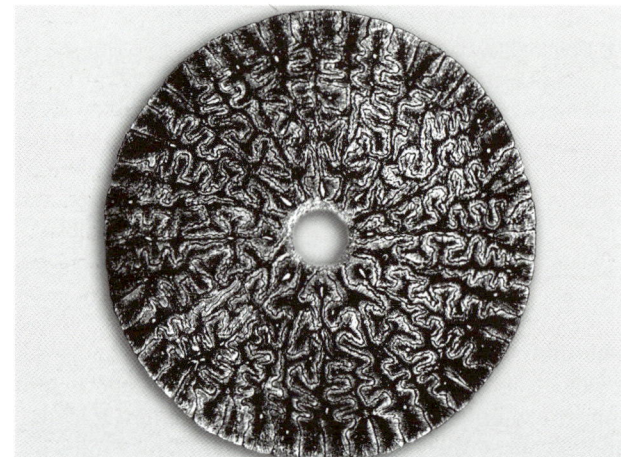

Figure 20-2: Cross section of labyrinthodont tooth with complexly infolded enamel and dentin (Illustration from On The Genesis of Species by St. George Mivart, F.R.S. (1827-1900) London Macmillan and Co. 1871.)

of a novel jaw joint—while incorporating some of the ancestral jaw bones into the mammalian middle ear—is often cited as a classic example of the repurposing of morphological structures.

HOMINID JAW EVOLUTION

Primates are extraordinarily diverse group of mammals having over 50 extant genera and 200 recognized species. Humans and their immediate ancestors have been traditionally placed in the family *Hominidae*. This includes a taxonomic family of primates whose members are known as great apes or hominids and comprise seven extant species. It has been estimated that the human lineage separated from the rest of the hominoids about 5–8 million years ago.

Earliest Hominids

The earliest Hominids lived between 7 and 4.4 million years ago. Their fossilized remains show dental features that included a U-shaped palate and canines similar but

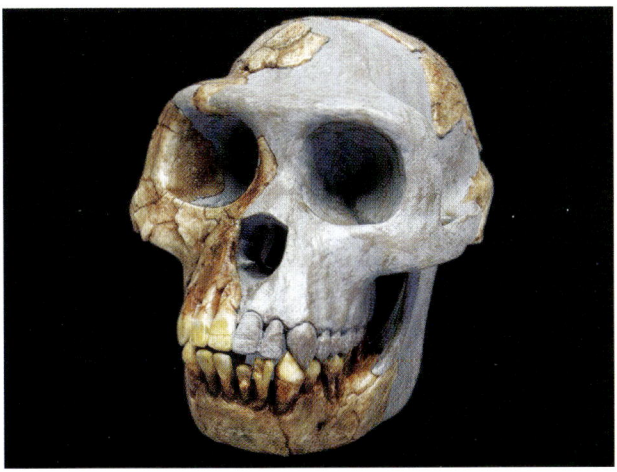

Figure 20-3: *Ardipithecus ramidus*.

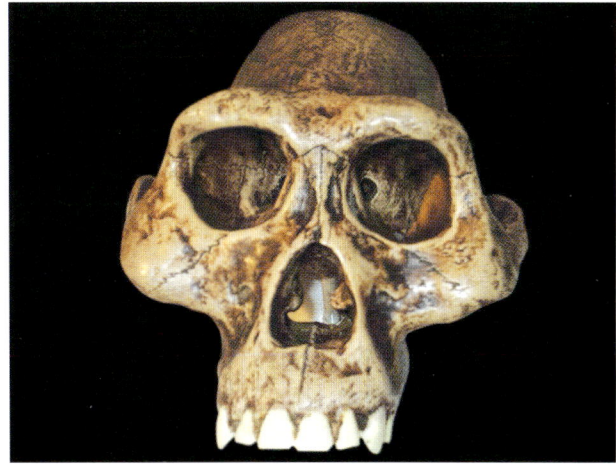

Figure 20-4: *Australopithecus afarensis*.

smaller than those of a chimpanzee's. The overall tooth size was smaller compared to the body size with much thicker enamel. The later species (*Ardipithecus*) had canines that were reduced like the later hominids. They were also less sharp compared to a chimpanzee's, possibly due to them being smaller in general. This indicated that the earliest hominids were probably carnivores with prognathic jaws. In contrast to the social patterns of chimpanzees, the smaller upper canine teeth in *Ardipithecus* suggested that the species was not very aggressive **(Figure 20-3)**.

Archaic Hominids

The *Australopithecus* is the best known archaic hominid and lived about 4 million years ago across eastern and southern Africa. It was a highly successful genus that persisted for around 3 million years. Their brain size was similar to chimpanzees and apes suggesting cognitive abilities at par with modern-day apes. They had prognathic jaws with short blunt and monomorphic canines similar to the earlier hominins; however, the molars were much larger with thicker enamel. This suggested that their diet comprised of hard, coarse plant foods **(Figure 20-4)**.

Archaic Megadont Hominids

The megadont hominids lived about 1.2–2 million years ago and are considered by some as a subgroup of Australopithecus, called the '*Robust Australopithecus*'. They had enormous jaws with powerful masticatory muscles and giant teeth with very thick enamel. Their diet consisted of hard, tough to chew foods. Another species commonly known as the 'Nut cracker Man' had premolars and molars four times the size of those found in present-day humans. This has been interpreted as evidence of hominids predominantly using their posterior teeth for mastication **(Figure 20-5)**.

Pre-modern Homo

The oldest member of the genus *Homo*, *H. habilis* lived about 2 million years ago in East Africa. *H. habilis* is associated with

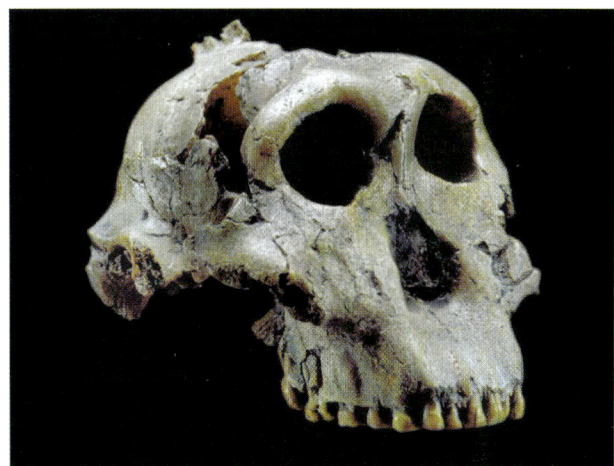

Figure 20-5: *Australopithecus robustus*.

butchered animal bones and simple stone tools. *H. erectus*, a more formidable and widespread descendant persisted from 1.9 million years ago to 100 thousand years ago throughout Africa and Eurasia. It lacked the forelimb adaptations for climbing that was present in *Australopithecus* and showed a major increase in brain size, up to 1,250 cc for later Asian specimens. The incisors showed 'shovel-shape' appearance, which could be attributed to a change towards a hunter-gatherer diet. Molar size was reduced in *H. erectus* relative to *Australopithecus*, reflecting its softer, richer diet, including cooked food.

Neanderthals, although not direct ancestors of Homo Sapiens, are considered close relatives of modern-day humans. Neanderthals lived about 2,50,000 to 30,000 years ago and were named after the valley they were discovered in. They showed more prognathism, resulting in a retromolar space posterior to the third molars, larger molars and canine teeth with no grooves. Compared to modern-day humans, Neanderthals had robust physique, complex behavior and smaller brains **(Figures 20-6A and B)**.

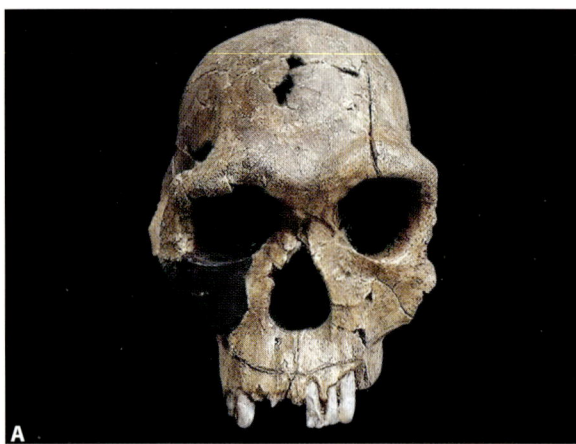 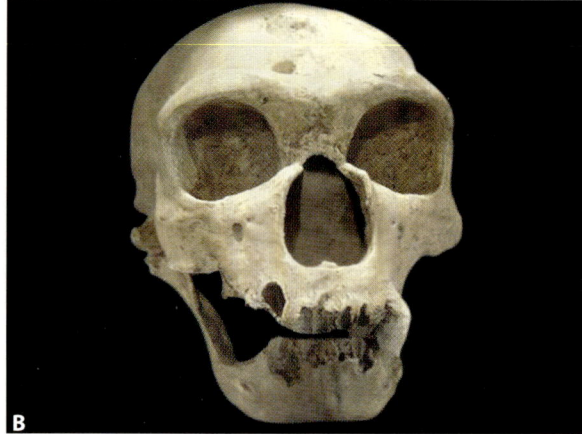

Figures 20-6A and B: (A) *H. habilis;* (B) *H. neanderthalensis*

Homo Sapiens

H. sapiens evolved in Africa around 200 thousand years ago and showed behavioral sophistication as evidenced by a larger brain size. They flourished and spilled into other continents ultimately displacing the other hominins including the Neanderthals. The present-day human dental morphology is characterized by a lack of facial prognathism and parabolic-shaped mandible and maxilla. Humans also display small crowns in relation to body mass and tend to show a reduction in cusp and root number.

The protruding chin, absent in archaic humans and Neanderthals, is one of the evolutionary features which separate *H. sapiens* from our ancestors. They have stated that the appearance of the chin coincides with the appearance of speech 50,000 years ago.

> Chin is believed to have formed from the biomechanical forces associated with mastication. Other researchers believe that repetitive contractions of the tongue and the perioral musculature due to originating speech in the modern humans led to the formation of the chin.

Also the reduction of the dental arches and their retraction under the cranium required axial inclination of the molar roots. It has been proposed that this axial inclination of the teeth in the course of evolution has been paralleled by differential changes in cusp heights in order to keep the masticatory complex functional. Third molars of humans have undergone a forward tilt during evolution due to the displacement of the TMJ in relation to the occlusal plane leading to a more pronounced curve of Spee in humans compared to other Hominids.

Thus, the evolution of our species from an ape-like ancestor to modern-day human was a complex process. The evolutionary process is replete with side branches and evolutionary dead ends, with species like the robust australopiths that persisted for over a million years before fading away **(Figure 20-7)**.

JAW SUSPENSION

Jaw suspension refers to the attachment of the lower jaw with the upper jaw or the skull for efficient biting and chewing. In vertebrates, depending upon the modifications in visceral arches, there are different ways in which these attachments may be attained.

These are:
- **Paleostylic:** None of the arches attach directly to the skull. It is seen in agnathans.
- **Euautostylic:** The mandibular arch is suspended directly to the underside of the skull without involvement of the hyoid bone. This was seen in the earliest gnathostomes.
- **Amphistylic:** The visceral arches are unmodified and made of flexible cartilage. The upper jaw is made of Palatoquadrate and the Meckel's cartilage makes the lower jaw. Hyoid arch is also unchanged. Lower jaw is attached to both palatoquadrate and hyoid arch and hence it is called amphistylic. Amphistylic suspension was seen in the early sharks.
- **Hyostylic:** The mandibular arch is attached to the brain case primarily through the hypomandibula along with the symplectic bone of the hyoid arch. This type of suspension is seen in most modern-day fishes.
- **Metautostylic:** Here the jaw is attached to the brain case directly through the quadrate bone. It is seen in most amphibians, reptiles and birds.
- **Craniostylic:** The entire upper jaw forms a part of the brain case but the lower jaw is called the dentary that is suspended from the dermal squamosal bone of the brain case. It is seen in mammals.

THEORIES OF EVOLUTION OF HUMAN DENTITION

Tooth-like units (odontodes) are described simply as all structures that comprise a mineralized hard tissue unit consisting of attachment bone, dentin, sometimes with a superficial layer of enamel/enameloid, formed from a single papilla. Odontodes can be found in multiple locations around the body of lower vertebrates, whether covering the dermal surface as in extant sharks or as dentition in oral and pharyngeal locations, or lining the oropharyngeal cavity associated with gill arches. They served numerous functions, including protection, sensation and hydrodynamic advantage.

It is believed that teeth and tooth like structures evolved in vertebrates before and independent of oral cavity and

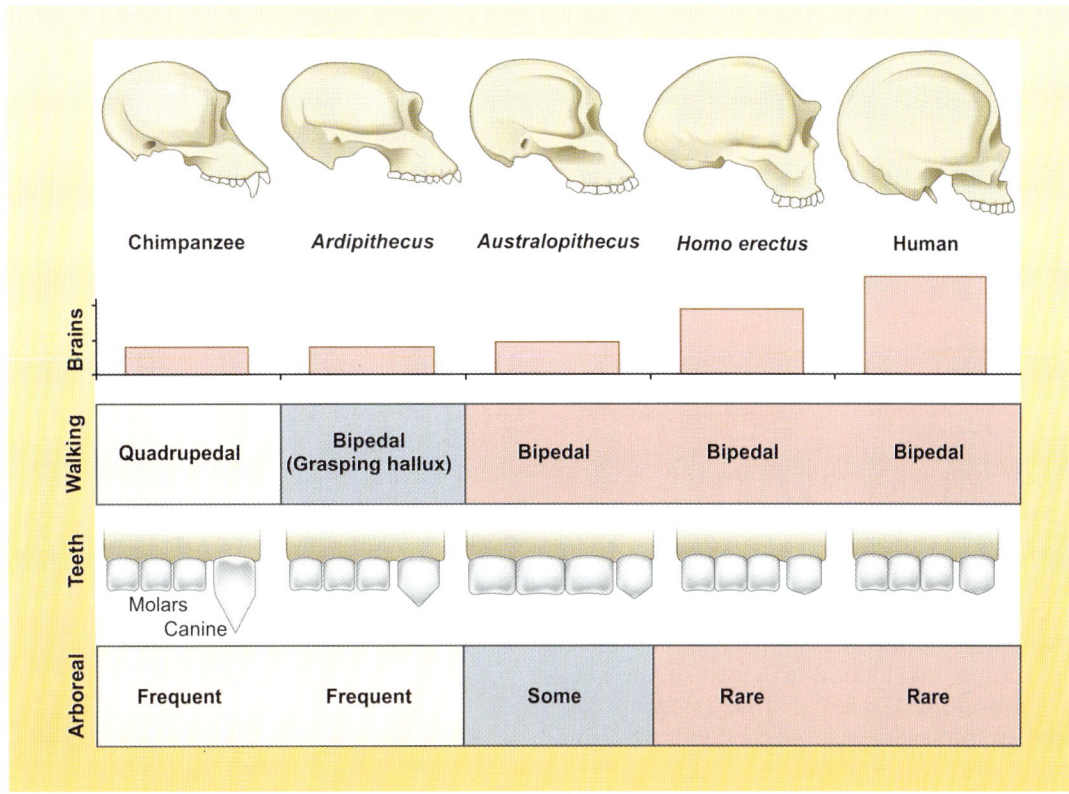

Figure 20-7: Anatomical comparisons of apes, early hominins, *Australopithecus, Homo erectus*, and humans.
Source: Pontzer H. Overview of Hominin Evolution. Nature Education Knowledge 2012; 3(10):8.

jaws. Teeth may be considered as the earliest expression of a fundamental epithelial-mesenchymal interaction as they appeared as skin appendages in the vertebrate fossil records. The dentition is one of the main criteria used by paleontologists to classify fossil vertebrate lineages and mammalian species as it characterizes species.

Hypothesis Explaining Evolution of Teeth

* **'Outside in' model of tooth evolution:** According to this classical hypothesis, teeth came to reside within the oral cavity of jawed vertebrates when odontode-competent tissue layer (containing competent odontome-forming cells) moved from the body surface to the oral cavity. This hypothesis is largely dependent on the similarity of shark skin denticles to teeth.
The 'outside in' model postulates that: (i) odontodes originated on the external surface of an organism in the form of skin denticles; (ii) for oral teeth to evolve, ectodermal cells that form surface denticles must have mixed and been incorporated into the oropharyngeal cavity during development and (iii) only ectodermal cells have the capacity to form odontodes. Thus, according to this theory, teeth are modified skin denticles differing only in the locus of their formation.
* **'Inside out' model of tooth evolution:** This hypothesis suggests that teeth evolved prior to the origin of jaws. It was hypothesized that tooth competence and pattern was co-opted from endodermally derived pharyngeal cavity.

The 'inside out' model postulates that: (1) tooth sets originated inside the posterior pharynx of now extinct agnathans; (2) thereafter, the molecular controls for competence were co-opted anteriorly to the oral jaws; (3) teeth and skin denticles were derived independently from alternative tissue layers, endoderm and ectoderm, respectively; (4) the unique patterning mechanism for a dentition lies specifically within the endoderm of the oropharynx. According to this theory, teeth are not denticles and vice versa.
* **'Modified' 'outside' in model of tooth evolution:** This recently suggested theory states that in accordance with the 'outside in' theory, teeth are derived from odontodes, which were originally ectodermal in origin. These ectodermal odontodes developed inside the oropharyngeal cavity as a result of competent ectoderm migrating inwards—not only via the mouth, but also via each of the gill slits. In accordance with the 'inside out' model, it is suggested that the teeth developed prior to the jaws. This 'modified' hypothesis thus suggests that the initial odontogenic potential of the ectoderm may have been subsequently transferred to endoderm upon contact and cell mixing. Direct contact of both epithelial germ layers is thus a prerequisite for teeth to form **(Figures 20-8A to C)**.

Dentition Types

The dentition of mammals consists of repeated units (teeth) arrayed along curvilinear axes (each jaw quadrant) and is thus

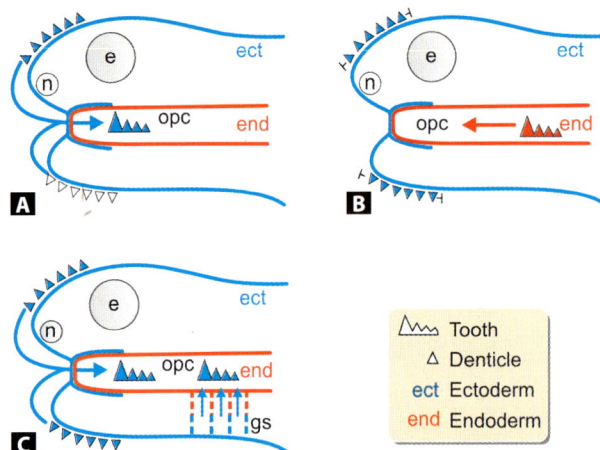

Figures 20-8A to C: (A) 'Outside in 'Model; (B) 'Modified' 'outside in' Model; (C) 'Inside out' Model.
Source: Frazer GJ, Cerny R, Soukup V, et al. The odontode explosion: the origin of tooth-like structures in vertebrates. Bioessays. 2010;32(9):808-17

said to have a segmented organization. The early vertebrate dentition consisted of numerous, similar, simple conical teeth. This condition is still found in many fish and non-mammalian tetrapods and is referred to as *homodonty*. The teeth of homodont species are replaced continuously during life, a condition known as *polyphyodonty*.

In contrast, mammals have a regionally differentiated dental arch, with incisor, canine, premolar, and molar regions, and this is referred as *heterodonty*. This differentiation is typically repeated in each half of both the upper and lower jaws, along a linear axis from mesial to distal. In addition to the heterodonty of mammals, their teeth are typically replaced only once, a condition known as *diphyodonty*. In some mammals, only one set of teeth develops in their lifetime and this condition is called *monophyodonty*, e.g., marsupials retain all their milk teeth except last premolars **(Figures 20-9A and B)**.

The dentition may also be described as *thecodont*, when the base of the tooth is completely enclosed in a deep socket or alveolus of bone. Capillaries and nerves enter the jaw bone and the pulp cavity through the open tips of the hollow roots. This type of dentition is seen in mammals and crocodiles. In contrast, a*crodont* is a type of dentition in which the teeth are fused to the surface of the underlying jawbone. These teeth have no roots and are attached to the edge of the jawbone by a fibrous membrane. Acrodont dentition is seen in fishes, amphibians and reptiles.

The dentition is described as *pleurodont* when the teeth are fused to the inner/lingual surface of the jaw bone through the outer surface of their roots. This type of dentition is found in many reptilian families. In acrodont and pleurodont types of dentition, there are no roots, and nerves and blood do not enter the pulp cavity at the base **(Figures 20-10A to C)**.

Another way of classifying dentition is based on the crown lengths. A dentition is described as *Brachydont* when it has low-crowned teeth. A brachydont tooth has a crown above the gingival line and a neck just below it, and at least one root. The crown is enamel covered whereas the cementum is present below the gingival line. The occlusal surfaces tend to be pointed, well-suited for holding prey and tearing and shredding. Human teeth belong to this category.

A *Hypsodont* dentition on the other hand, is characterized by high-crowned teeth with enamel that extends far past the gingival line, providing extra material for wear and tear. Such teeth are designed for foods that are fibrous and gritty in nature and they continue to grow throughout life. Hypsodont molars lack both crown and neck with a rough, flat occlusal surface adapted for crushing and grinding plant material. The tooth is covered with cementum both above and below the gingival line, below which is a layer of enamel covering the entire length. The cementum and the enamel invaginate into a thick layer of dentin. Hypsodont dentition is seen in cows and horses **(Figures 20-11A and B)**.

> To summarise:
> The dentition may be classified based on:
> - Shape and size: Homodont and Heterodont
> - Succession or replacement of teeth: Monophyodont, Diphyodont and Polyphyodont
> - Mode of attachment of tooth to jaws: Thecodont, Acrodont and Pleurodont
> - Crown lengths: Brachydont and Hypsodont

THEORIES OF CUSPAL ORIGIN

A profound characteristic of mammalian evolution is the progressive complexity in post-canine tooth morphology. However, the driving force for this complexity is uncertain: whether to expand the versatility in diet source, or to enhance structural integrity of teeth. It has been argued that presumably a multi-cusp configuration allows for better food manipulation in situations where good occlusion is maintained during mastication. Thus, evolution of tooth complexity probably represents a balance between structural integrity and food manipulation.

❖ **Theory of concrescence:** According to this theory, the earlier mammalian teeth were Haplodont (simple teeth with conical crown without ridges and tubercles) and the modern multicusped teeth are formed by the fusion of two or more such simple teeth into a compound tooth. This may

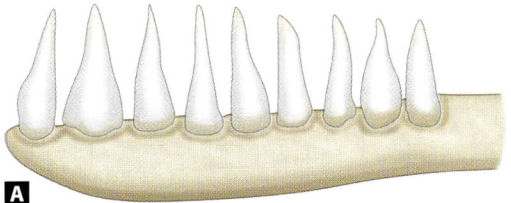
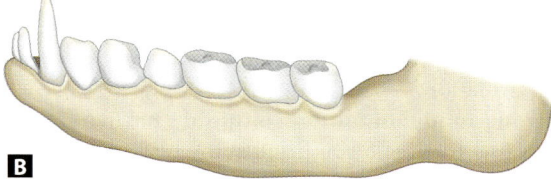

Figures 20-9A and B: (A) Homodont dentition; (B) Heterodont dentition.

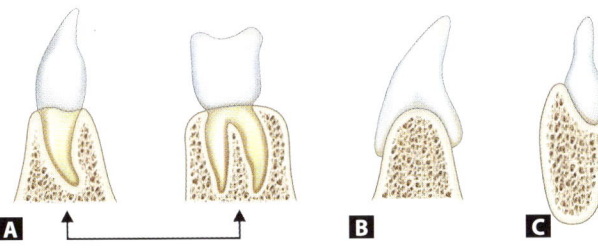

Figures 20-10A to C: (A) Thecodont; (B) Acrodont; (C) Pleurodont

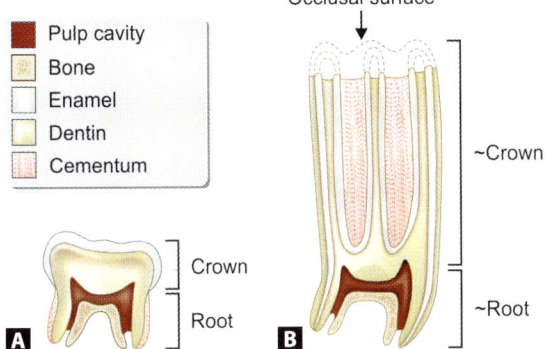

Figures 20-11A and B: (A) Brachydont molar; (B) Hypsodont molar.
Source: Stromberg CAE. Evolution of hypsodonty in equids: testing a hypothesis of adaptation. Paleobiology; 2006; 32(2):236-58.

result from shortening of jaws resulting in a buccolingual fusion of teeth of a similar series.
- **Cingulum theory:** This theory postulates that the cingulum that surrounds the tooth at its neck develops into cusp or cusps explaining the evolution of a complex tooth form.
- **Kinetogenic theory**: This theory states that the tooth originated in its haplodont form and was subject to pressure due to movements of the TMJ and lower jaw. This pressure resulted in flattening of the simple cones and formation of ridges and hollows.
- **Tritubercular theory or Cope-Osborne theory:** This is the most widely accepted theory and states that the multicusped mammalian molar developed from addition of cusps to a simple haplodont tooth. In this, the original haplodont cone is known as the protocone, the cusp that develops in front is called the paracone and the one behind is the metacone. These cusps develop in size until the tooth has three cones/ cusps in a straight line and are called as triconodont teeth.
This triconodont stage underwent further adaptation with the paracone and the metacone becoming external to the original cone (protocone) in the upper jaw and internal in the lower jaw to create a triangular-shaped tooth with a cone at each angle (tritubercular tooth). These tritubercular teeth are a very common occurrence in ancestral mammals. **(Figure 20-12)**
- **Multi-tubercular theory**: This theory does not believe in the origin of multicusped teeth from haplodont teeth. Rather, it states that the modern mammalian molar was derived from multituberculate teeth by reduction in the number of tubercles.

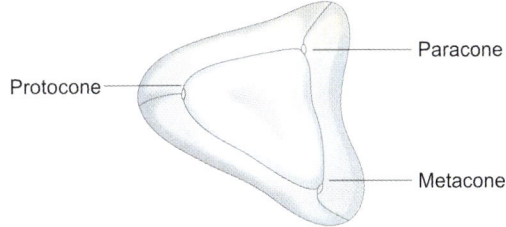

Figure 20-12: Tritubercular tooth with the protocone on the lingual side and the anterior paracone and the posterior metacone on the buccal side.

- **Dimer theory:** This theory proposes that there is one origin for all mammalian teeth whether incisors, canines, premolars or molars.

The stages of tooth development have been divided as:
- **The reptilian stage (Haplodont):** It is represented by the simplest form of a tooth, the single cone. Many teeth are present in each jaw that leads to limited jaw movement in a simple hinge pattern. The teeth lack occlusion and are used primarily for prehension and combat.
- **Early mammalian stage (Triconodont):** This type of tooth is represented by having three cusps arranged in a line. The main (anthropologically original) cusp is located in the center with a smaller cusp located anterior to it and another located posterior to it. This "simplistic" type of dentition has been understood to be either ancestral for mammals or else to have evolved multiple times. Triconodont teeth are well adapted for shearing, and possessing other specifications such as long canines and powerful jaw musculature.
- **Triangular stage (Tritubercular molar):** This stage as explained in the previous section developed from the triconodont teeth by movement of the two smaller cusps resulting in a tritubercular arrangement. The tritubercular molar consists essentially of three cusps, forming what may be called the primitive triangles, so disposed that the upper and lower molars alternate. This type of arrangement is observed in dogs and other carnivorous animals.
- **Quadritubercular molar:** The next stage in the development created projections on the triangular form that finally resulted in occlusion with teeth of the opposite jaw. Thus a fourth cone (hypocone) developed in addition to the protocone, paracone and metacone.

Molars seen in humans, pigs and bears have low rounded cusps that are quadrate in shape and act as efficient effective crushing devices. Such molars are called *bunodont* molars.

EVOLUTION OF PERIODONTIUM

The term periodontium traditionally encompasses the gingiva, periodontal ligament, cementum and alveolar bone. The periodontal attachment has evolved from an attachment wherein the tooth was ankylosed to the bone to a fibrous ligamentous suspension of the tooth within the bone. This allowed for movement of mammalian teeth resulting in continual repositioning as required by the jaw for growth and also to compensate for tooth wear. In the former case, the teeth moved with the jaws whereas in the latter, they were capable of moving as independent units.

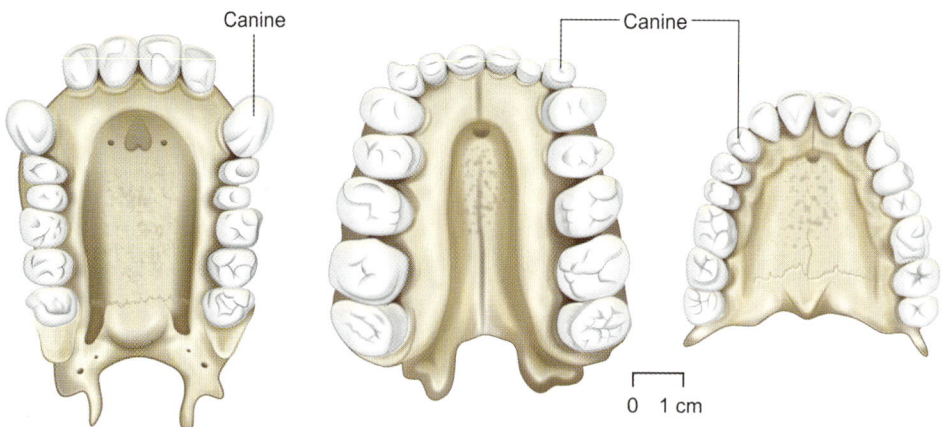

Figure 20-13: Reduction in size of teeth during Hominid evolution.

The means of attachment of teeth in the sockets may be described in four ways:
- **Fibrous attachment:** The teeth are fixed by means of fibrous bands to the submucosa of the fibrous membrane which cover the jaws. It is seen in sharks and rays.
- **Hinged attachment:** A hinged tooth is supported posteriorly by a fibro-elastic ligament, while anterior free edge rests on a buttress of bone.
- **Ankylosed attachment:** The tooth is attached to the jaws by calcified material with no intervention of fibrous or uncalcified tissue. It is seen in eels.
- **Gomphosis attachment:** A membrane exists between the tooth and socket of bone in which it is situated. It is observed in mammals, reptiles and some fish.

The alveolar bone, similar to other bones is known to grow in shape and size in response to frequent and habitual stress and strains and tend to lose mass in the absence of force. This explains the trend in the change in the size of the alveolar process. With decrease in masticatory forces during hominid evolution, the size of the alveoli decreased corresponding to the size of the teeth **(Figure 20-13)**.

TRENDS IN EVOLUTION

The evolution of human masticatory complex is strongly related to diet; the use of tools and fire, and speech. Variations in tooth number may represent an important factor for mammalian diversification. The evolutionary pathway from fish to reptiles to mammals is characterized by a reduction in the number of teeth and of their generations (from polyphyodonty to di- and/or monophyodonty) along with an increase in morphological complexity of the teeth (from homodonty to heterodonty). Some organisms (e.g., killer whales, rats, elephants) develop their dentition only once in their life; others (e.g., turtles, birds, toothless whales, anteaters) have lost their dentition and are characterized by anodontia. Anodontia in many organisms is considered to be secondary, since the embryo possesses tooth germs that undergo apoptosis before birth. Changes in the number and morphology of teeth may reflect a significant factor in the generation of new species in mammals, the most common feature being the loss of various teeth.

Diet and mastication are considered key factors in tooth evolution. There is a strong correlation between teeth form and dietary habits. The modern human diet contains more meat when compared to our early ancestors. Thus, over the course of time, the need for a large, herbivorous dentition was reduced as the requirement of chewing coarse vegetable matter reduced. With the development of stone tools, humans were able to substitute their tools for the sharp teeth, large canines and strong jaws typical of carnivores. With the advent of cooking, food became tender and easier to chew, again reducing the need for a large, robust dentition.

Analysis of ancient calcified dental plaque demonstrates the changes in diet between the Neolithic and Industrial Revolutions. The changes in the oral microbiota and dietary shifts between Neolithic and Industrial era populations have been revealed by sequencing ancient calcified dental plaque. The shift in microbial populations coincided with the new widespread availability of processed food, leading to increased dental caries and gingivitis.

Also, with evolution, the size of the brain increased along with the size of the braincase. This increase occurred at the expense of the jaws, shortening them as a larger brain provided an evolutionary advantage. In short, evolution has produced an increase in brain size at the expense of jaw size. This resulted in decreased space for the third molars to erupt often resulting in their impaction. The third molars in humans are approaching a vestigial condition, since they generally do not appear until relatively late; between the ages of twenty and thirty years, and in many cases do not erupt at all; get impacted due to lack of space.

The evolution of our species from ape-like ancestors has been a complex process. Some human traits, like bipedalism, evolved very early, while others, like large brains, did not evolve until relatively recently. Other traits, like molar size, evolved in one direction only to be pushed back later by changing ecological pressures. Thus, evolution is a complex process resulting from environmental changes, genetic luck, and geological chance.

Points to Remember

- Evolution has occurred from jawless to jawed vertebrates.
- Jaws are developed from first pharyngeal arch with palatoquadrate and Meckel's cartilage which contribute to upper and lower jaw respectively.
- The earliest Hominids displayed dental features that included a U-shaped palate and canines similar but smaller when compared to chimpanzees.
- The *Australopithecus* had brain size similar to chimpanzees and apes with prognathic jaws having short blunt and monomorphic canines and molars were much larger with thicker enamel.
- The megadont hominids had enormous jaws with powerful masticatory muscles and giant teeth with very thick enamel.
- *H. habilis* showed more prognathism, resulting in a retromolar space posterior to the third molars, larger molars and canine teeth with no grooves.
- *H. sapiens'* dental morphology is characterized by a lack of facial prognathism, parabolic-shaped mandible and maxilla, and molars that are the same size as the front teeth.
- Jaw suspensions are of following types: Paleostylic, Euautostylic, Amphistylic, Hyostylic, Metautostylic and Craniostylic.
- 'Outside in' model of tooth evolution, 'Inside out' model of tooth evolution and 'Modified' outside in model of tooth evolution are the three hypothesis explaining evolution of teeth.
- The dentition may be classified based on: Shape and size, succession or replacement of teeth, mode of attachment of tooth to jaws and crown lengths.
- Trituburcular theory or Cope-Osborne theory is the most widely accepted theory among all the theories of cuspal origin.
- The alveolar bone grow in shape and size in response to frequent and habitual stress and strains and tend to lose mass in the absence of force.

PRACTICE QUESTIONS

1. Write a note on dentition types.
2. What is brachydont and hypsodont?
3. Write notes on evolution of teeth.
4. Write notes on theories of the origin of cusps.
5. Write notes on evolution of periodontium.

MULTIPLE CHOICE QUESTIONS

1. Which cartilage is known to form the presumptive lower jaw?
   a. Palatoquadrate cartilage
   b. Meckel's cartilage
   c. Bimaxillary cartilage
   d. Mandibular cartilage
2. Which migratory and multipotent cell population is almost entirely responsible for the embryonic origin of jaws and the visceral skeleton?
   a. Neural crest cells
   b. Pluripotent stem cells
   c. Totipotent stem cells
   d. Embryonic stem cells
3. The present-day human dental morphology is characterized by:
   a. Facial retrognathism
   b. Large molars compared to incisors
   c. Parabolic shaped mandible and maxilla
   d. All of the above
4. Around 50,000 years ago, the appearance of the chin coincided with the appearance of_____?
   a. Moustache and beard
   b. Speech
   c. Small teeth
   d. Large tongue
5. Which of the following jaw suspensions is seen in mammals?
   a. Amphistylic
   b. Hyostylic
   c. Metautostylic
   d. Craniostylic
6. Which type of dentition is seen in mammals?
   a. Acrodont
   b. Thecodont
   c. Homodont
   d. Pleurodont
7. The tooth which is covered with cementum both above and below the gingival line, and underneath a layer of enamel covering the entire length is known as:
   a. Brachydont
   b. Homodont
   c. Hypsodont
   d. Thecodont
8. **Bunodont molars are seen in:**
   a. Humans
   b. Pigs
   c. Bears
   d. All of the above
9. Which of the following theories postulates that the cingulum that surrounds the tooth at its neck develops into cusp or cusps explaining the evolution of a complex tooth form?
   a. Kinetogenic Theory
   b. Cope-Osborne theory
   c. Multitubercular Theory
   d. Cingulum Theory
10. What are the key factors considered in tooth evolution?
    a. Diet and mastication
    b. Genetics and diet
    c. Geological site and mastication
    d. Genetics and geological site

11. **Human teeth are:**
    a. Hypsodont
    b. Homodont
    c. Brachydont
    d. Polyphyodont
12. **Horses and cows have:**
    a. Brachydont
    b. Hypsodont
    c. Homodont
    d. Monodont

ANSWERS

1. b   2. a   3. c   4. b   5. d   6. b   7. c   8. d   9. b   10. a   11. c   12. b

BIBLIOGRAPHY

1. Anthwal N, Joshi L, and Tucker AS. Evolution of the mammalian middle ear and jaw: adaptations and novel structures. J Anat. 2013 Jan; 222(1): 147–160.
2. Brazeau MD, Friedman M. The origin and early phylogenetic history of jawed vertebrates. Nature. 2015 Apr 23;520(7548):490-7.
3. Butler PM. Evolution and mammalian dental morphology. J Biol Buccale. 1983 Dec;11(4):285-302.
4. Cerny R, Lwigale P, Ericsson R, Meulemans D, Epperlein HH, Bronner-Fraser M. Developmental origins and evolution of jaws: new interpretation of "maxillary" and "mandibular". Dev Biol. 2004 Dec 1;276(1):225-36.
5. Cohn MJ. Evolutionary biology: lamprey Hox genes and the origin of jaws. Nature. 2002 Mar 28;416(6879):386-7.
6. Constantino PJ, Bush MB, Barani A, Lawn BR. On the evolutionary advantage of multi-cusped teeth. JR Soc Interface. 2016 Aug;13(121):20160374.
7. Donoghue PCJ, Rücklin M. The ins and outs of the evolutionary origin of teeth. Evolution & Development 2016;18(1):19-30.
8. Emes Y, Aybar B, Yalcin S. On The Evolution of Human Jaws and Teeth: A Review. Bull Int Assoc Paleodont. 2011;5(1):37-47.
9. Fraser GJ, Cerny R, Soukup V, Bronner-Fraser M, Streelman JT. The odontode explosion: the origin of tooth-like structures in vertebrates. Bioessays. 2010 Sep;32(9):808-17.
10. Gaengler P, Metzler E. The periodontal differentiation in the phylogeny of teeth--an overview. J Periodontal Res. 1992 May;27(3):214-25.
11. Gregory WK. A Half Century of Trituberculy the Cope-Osborn Theory of Dental Evolution with a Revised Summary of Molar Evolution from Fish to Man. Proceedings of the American Philosophical Society .1934;3(4):169-317.
12. Huysseune A, Sire JY, Witten PE. Evolutionary and developmental origins of the vertebrate dentition. J Anat. 2009 Apr;214(4):465-76.
13. Koussoulakou DS, Margaritis LH, Koussoulakos SL. A curriculum vitae of teeth: evolution, generation, regeneration. Int J Biol Sci. 2009;5(3):226-43.
14. Kuratani S. Evolution of the vertebrate jaw: comparative embryology and molecular developmental biology reveal the factors behind evolutionary novelty. J Anat. 2004 Nov;205(5):335-47.
15. Lautenschlager S, Gill PG, Luo ZX, Fagan MJ, Rayfield EJ. The role of miniaturization in the evolution of the mammalian jaw and middle ear. Nature. 2018 Sep;561(7724):533-537.
16. LeBlanc AR, Reisz RR. Periodontal ligament, cementum, and alveolar bone in the oldest herbivorous tetrapods, and their evolutionary significance. PLoS One. 2013 Sep 4;8(9):e74697.
17. McCollum M, Sharpe PT. Evolution and development of teeth. J Anat. 2001 Jul-Aug;199:153-9.
18. Novitskaya LI. The problem of the relationship between agnathan and gnathostome vertebrates. Acta Palaeontologica Polonica 26 (1), 1981;26(1):9–18.
19. Peterkova R, Hovorakova M, Peterka M, Lesot H. Three-dimensional analysis of the early development of the dentition. Aust Dent J. 2014 Jun;59 Suppl 1:55-80.
20. Polly DP. Movement adds bite to the evolutionary morphology of mammalian teeth. BMC Biol. 2012; 10: 69.
21. Pontzer H. Overview of Hominin Evolution. Nature Education Knowledge 2012; 3(10):8.
22. Renvoisé E, Michon F. An Evo-Devo perspective on ever-growing teeth in mammals and dental stem cell maintenance. Front Physiol. 2014 Aug 28;5:324.
23. Robinson JT. Prehominid dentition and hominid evolution. Evolution. 1954; 8: 324-334.
24. Rücklin M, Donoghue PC, Johanson Z, Trinajstic K, Marone F, Stampanoni M. Development of teeth and jaws in the earliest jawed vertebrates. Nature. 2012 Nov 29;491(7426):748-51.
25. Shimeld SM, Donoghue PC. Evolutionary crossroads in developmental biology: cyclostomes (lamprey and hagfish). Development. 2012 Jun;139(12):2091-9.
26. Sperber GH. The role of teeth in human evolution. Br Dent J. 2013 Sep;215(6):295-7.
27. Stromberg CAE. Evolution of hypsodonty in equids: testing a hypothesis of adaptation. Paleobiology; 2006; 32(2):236-58.
28. Teaford MF, Smith MM, Ferguson, MWJ. Development, Function and Evolution of Teeth. Cambridge University Press 2000.
29. Wheeler RC, Ash MM. Wheeler's Dental Anatomy, Physiology, and Occlusion (6th ed.). Philadelphia: Saunders, 1984

CHAPTER 21

Tissue Processing for Histological Examination

B Sivapathasundharam, Kavitha B, RJ Vijayashree

CHAPTER OUTLINE

- Types of Preparation 308
- Soft Tissue Processing 308
  » Soft Tissue Processing for Light Microscopy 308
- Tissue Sectioning 311
  » Staining 311
  » Hematoxylin and Eosin Staining 314
  » Processing for Electron Microscopy 315
- Frozen Sections 315
  » Cryosectioning 315
  » Hard Tissue Processing 316
  » Ground Sections 316
  » Decalcified Sections 316
  » Artifacts 318
  » Exfoliative Cytology 318
  » Fine Needle Aspiration Cytology (FNAC) 318
- Digital Pathology 318

Disease is altered or abnormal structure or function occurring in an organism or even plants and manifests with signs and/or symptoms. The alteration in the structure can be studied under microscope. Biopsy is defined as removal of tissue from the living body for microscopic examination to establish the diagnosis. Microscopic examination of the tissue is not only applied to diagnose a disease but also to study the normal cellular architecture of a tissue or an organ. Microscopy plays a significant role in various branches of medicine and science, which include hematology (the study of blood), microbiology (the study of microorganisms), pathology (the study of diseases) and more broadly in the areas of biology, zoology, and botany.

To study the tissue under microscope, it has to be prepared in a specific method to reflect the life-like state. After the removal of tissue from the living body, it undergoes autolysis due to the liberation of lysosomal enzymes and putrefaction (decomposition by the action of microorganisms).

Cells, tissues, and organs cannot be studied properly under microscope unless they are prepared suitably. Though in routine practice the dead cells are examined under the microscope, it is possible and applied on occasions to study the living cells. Accordingly two methods are used for tissue preparation, namely—the methods involved in direct observation of living cells and the methods employed for the study of dead cells.

Live microorganisms and occasionally free cells can be studied directly under microscope. Free cells are colorless and structures within them lack contrast to distinguish the individual structures. Phase contrast microscope may be helpful to overcome this limitation. Human blood cells can be studied in films while surrounded by plasma, in their natural environment.

It is difficult, if not impossible, to preserve the tissue outside the body for a longer period of time due to autolysis and putrefaction. This can be overcome by applying a technique called as tissue culture. Fragments of tissues are removed aseptically, transferred to a physiological medium, and kept at normal temperature. The culture is placed in a thin glass vessel or on a cover glass mounted over a hollow glass slide, which can be observed under microscope. In such culture, growth, multiplication, and in some cases, differentiation of cells into other cell types can be observed directly. Tissue culture is a valuable method for the study of normal development of particular tissue, cancer, and the activity of many viruses.

To enhance the contrast for better visualization, tissue has to be stained. In the study of living tissue, two staining methods, namely—vital staining and supravital staining are applied successfully.

Vital staining involves injection of dyes into the living tissue. The activity of certain cells results in the selective absorption of the coloring materials by these cells, *e.g.* staining of macrophages by trypan blue, on the basis of their ability to phagocytize foreign particles.

Supravital staining involves adding a stain to a medium of cells already removed from the organism, *e.g.* staining of mitochondria in living cells by Janus Green, of lysosome by neutral red, and nerve fibers and cells by methylene blue.

The major drawback of the study of living cells is—it is difficult to handle and available for only limited period of time.

In contrast, dead cells or the tissues taken from an organism, if prepared suitably, can be more or less a permanent preparation.

TYPES OF PREPARATION

In whole-mounts the entire organism or structure is placed directly onto a microscope slide if it is small (*e.g.* a small unicellular or multicellular organism or a membrane that can be stretched thinly on to a slide).

Squash preparations are preparations, where the cells are squashed or crushed onto a slide to reveal their contents (*e.g.* botanical specimens where cells are disrupted to reveal chromosomes).

Smears are used to study the cells suspended in a fluid (*e.g.* blood, semen, cerebrospinal fluid or fluid from a cyst), or where individual cells have been scraped, brushed or aspirated from a surface or from within an organ (exfoliative cytology). Smears are the basis of the well-known "Pap test" (named after George Papanicolaou, who is considered as the father of cytopathology).

Sectioning involves making very thin slices of the tissue. The most effective and convenient way to study the biopsied tissue is to use sections. Sectioning is done by cutting thin slices from a small piece of fixed tissue by using an instrument called microtome. The section is then stained, mounted on a slide, and covered with a glass coverslip.

There are different forms of microscopy but the most common one employed for the study of a sectioned tissue is "bright-field" microscopy. In this, the specimen is illuminated with a beam of light that passes through it. The essential requirements for a specimen to be successfully examined using bright-field microscopy are:
* The cells and other elements in the specimen should be preserved in a "life-like" state, which is obtained by a process called "fixation".
* The specimen should be transparent to allow light to pass through it.
* The specimen should be thin and flat so that only a single layer of cells is present, as in thick sections, the overlapping of the cells obscures the cellular details.
* The components should be differentially stained to achieve the contrast to distinguish clearly.

Specimens submitted for biopsy may be soft, hard or mixed in nature. To appreciate the histological details of these tissues under microscope, they are to be cut into thin sections so that light can pass through them as stated previously. Further, these sections are to be stained to appreciate various components of the cells and tissues.

Thus to visualize the tissue under microscope, tissue has to be subjected to various processes, which is termed "tissue processing". This can be done manually or by an automatic tissue processor **(Figure 21-1)**.

SOFT TISSUE PROCESSING

Routinely, soft tissues are processed for examination under light microscope, which uses visible light. When ultrastructural details are needed, electron microscopy is used. Frozen

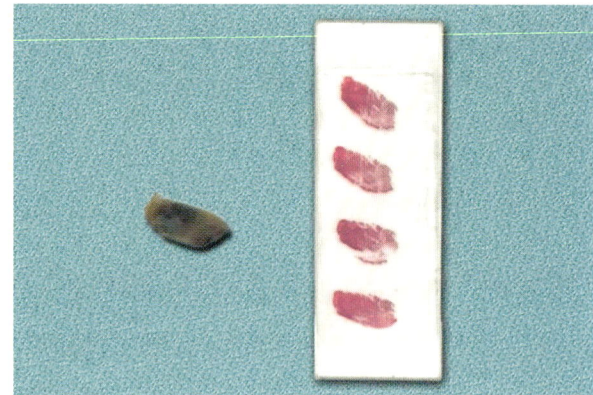

Figure 21-1: Biopsied tissue and its appearance after processing.

sections are prepared for biopsies for quick reporting during the time of surgery. Thus, soft tissue processing can be modified based on the requirement, *i.e.* light microscopy, electron microscopy, and frozen sections.

Soft Tissue Processing for Light Microscopy

Fixation

This is the first step in tissue processing. After biopsy, the tissue is rinsed thoroughly to remove blood, pus or mucus, and immersed immediately in a liquid called fixative. This step is termed as fixation of the tissue.

Fixation facilitates denaturation and coagulation of proteins in the tissues. It enhances the cross-linking (covalent bonds) between proteins and makes the molecules unavailable for further degradation by lysosomal enzymes, thus preventing autolysis and putrefaction, thereby aiding in preservation of the tissue architecture. Thus, the aim of fixation is to preserve the tissue in as life-like a manner as possible without affecting the reactive groups.

Further, fixation helps in hardening the tissue sufficiently to permit them to be handled and manipulated. Formalin is the most commonly used fixative. About 40% formaldehyde is called formalin and 10% formalin is the most preferred fixative. Other fixatives include glutaraldehyde, osmium tetroxide, potassium dichromate, acetone, acetic acid, ethyl alcohol, picric acid, mercuric chloride, chromic acid, etc. Cytological fixatives include Carnoy's fluid, Clarke's fluid, Fleming's fluid, etc. Physical methods like microwave fixation use heat.

Formalin is a saturated solution of formaldehyde gas in water. It contains about 40% (by volume) or 37% (by weight) formaldehyde gas along with a small amount of stabilizer and 10–12% methanol which prevents the formaldehyde polymerization. Thus, formalin contains 37–38% of formaldehyde, 10–15% of methanol, and 48–53% of water.

10% neutral buffered formalin (*i.e.*, 4% neutral buffered formaldehyde) is a best fixative and also the most preferred.

Ideally, the volume of the fixative has to be 20 times the volume of the specimen. Duration of the fixation varies with the size of the specimen. Routinely tissues are fixed for 6–18 hours. Larger specimens have to be cut into smaller pieces to facilitate the entry of the fixative into the inner portion thus preventing autolysis. Formalin penetrates tissue at the rate of 1 mm per hour.

Formalin is the most widely used fixative, since tissues are not damaged or excessively hardened when left in formalin for long periods. The only drawback of formalin is its toxicity. Improper handling of formalin can cause dermatitis and formalin vapor can damage the nasal mucosa and cause sinusitis.

> Formalin toxicity can also cause erosion of gastrointestinal tract and other systemic complications such as metabolic acidosis, acute renal failure and even circulatory shock. It is significant to note that formalin is reclassified as a human carcinogen and is known to cause leukemia and nasopharyngeal carcinoma.

To prepare sections, the tissue specimen has to be held in a medium, which can be cut into thin sections. This medium has to be infiltrated into the specimen thoroughly, even into the micro spaces or the lumen of the vessels or ducts present in the tissue specimen to avoid change in the shape of the specimen during cutting. The basic principle of processing is to embed the tissue into an embedding medium, make the tissue hard, and provide support and protect it from the mechanical forces associated with sectioning. Paraffin wax is one such material. But paraffin cannot replace the formalin directly in the tissue. Thus, the ultimate aim of performing the series of steps in tissue processing is to allow gradual infiltration of paraffin into the tissues. This involves a series of events. In order, formalin is replaced by water, alcohol, xylene, and finally paraffin (xylene is not miscible in water but miscible in alcohol and paraffin). Thus by utilizing the principle of solubility of various agents (water, alcohol, xylene, and paraffin), paraffin infiltration into the tissue is facilitated **(Figure 21-2)**.

Removal of formalin in the tissue and replacement with water: Formalin has to be removed from the tissue after adequate fixation. Inadequate removal of formalin can produce pigment artifacts. The formalin-fixed tissue is kept under running tap water for approximately 10 minutes to remove the formalin. Thus, water replaces the formalin from the tissue.

> If the tissue is kept in formalin for a long time, oxidation of formaldehyde occurs, which results in the formation of a large amount of formic acid. This tends to form artifact in the stained sections, which appear as brown pigments. This can be avoided when buffered formalin is used.

Dehydration

Alcohol is a dehydrating agent. Water is removed from the tissue by immersing it in ascending grades of isopropyl alcohol (70%, 90%, and 100%) for about 30 minutes in each concentration. In increasing grades of concentration, alcohol gradually and completely removes and replaces the water in the tissue. Transferring the tissue directly to the absolute alcohol may cause sudden exit of water molecules, which causes tissue shrinkage.

Clearing

This step involves removal of the alcohol by clearing agent. As stated previously, to cut the tissue into thin slices it has to be held in a medium, whose consistency should not affect the cutting by the microtome. Commonly used embedding medium is paraffin wax. But paraffin is not miscible with the alcohol. So an intermediary chemical, which is miscible with both the alcohol and paraffin, is used in this step. Xylene is the commonly used clearing agent. Other clearing agents are benzene, toluene, eugenol, carbon tetrachloride, cedarwood oil and chloroform. Most of the clearing agents (except chloroform) and the proteins present in the tissue have the same refractive index. As a result, when clearing agent enters the tissue, tissue becomes transparent, and the term "clearing" refers to this property. This change in appearance indicates complete infiltration of the tissue with the clearing agent. The disadvantages of xylene are it is neurotoxic and if the tissue is left in xylene for longer period, it becomes hard and brittle (optimum duration for clearing is 1–2 hours).

Impregnation (Replacement of Xylene with Paraffin Wax)

Since paraffin wax and xylene are miscible, the tissue cleared with xylene is immersed in molten paraffin wax (melting point 54–55°C) and kept in thermostatically regulated wax bath for few hours. Paraffin wax replaces the xylene in the tissue and the tissue is impregnated or infiltrated with paraffin wax.

Embedding

To cut the section, the wax infiltrated tissue has to be embedded in the wax to make into a block. This procedure involves pouring of molten paraffin wax into a rectangular space formed by two "L" mounts **(Figure 21-3)**. This is nothing but the "L" shaped (Leuckhart's) metal blocks arranged to

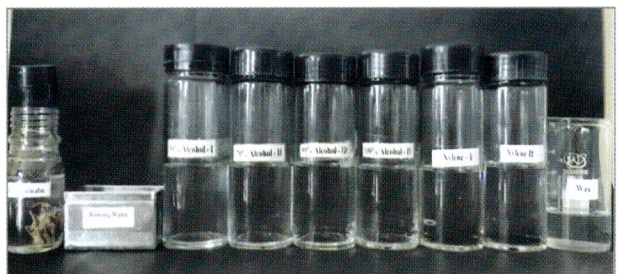

Figure 21-2: Fixation (10% formalin), dehydration (50%, 70%, 90%, and 100% alcohol), clearing (xylene), and impregnation (molten paraffin wax).

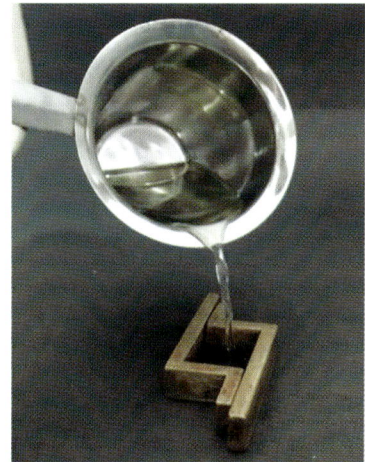

Figure 21-3: Molten wax poured into the space created by arranging the Leuckhart's "L" molds.

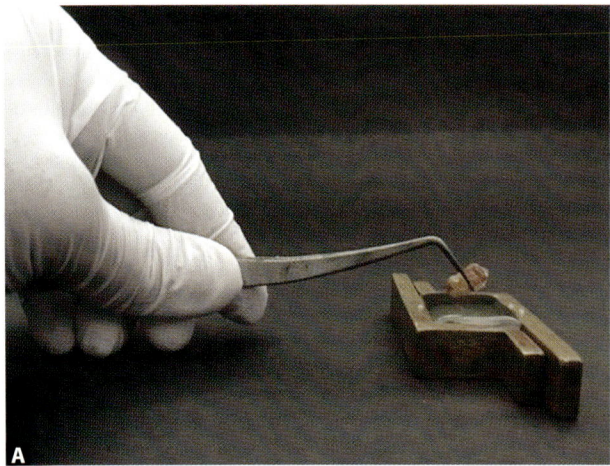
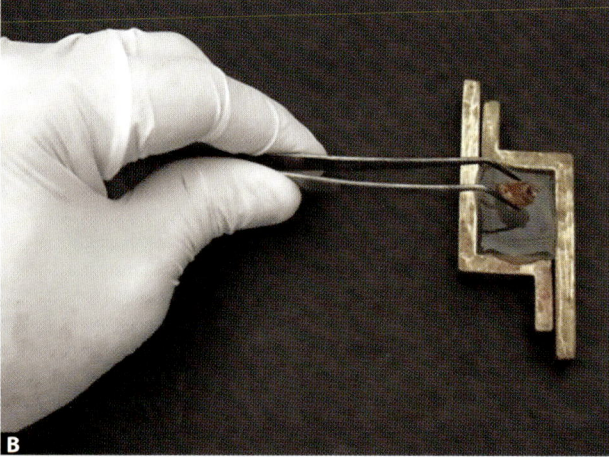
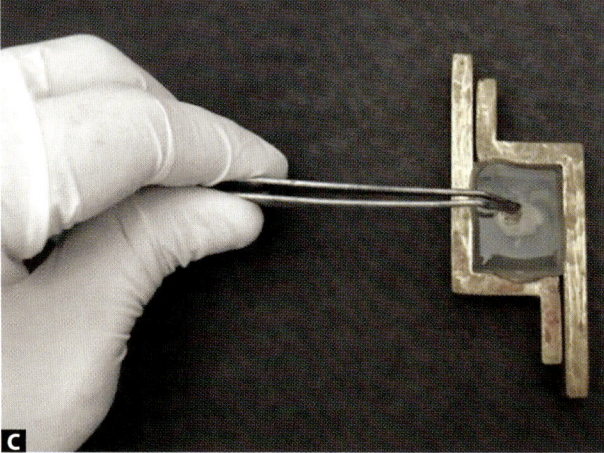

Figures 21-4A to C: Embedding of the tissue specimen into the molten wax.

form a frame of desired size. After arranging two L mounts, the molten paraffin is poured into the space created by the L mounts, the wax infiltrated tissue is oriented in an appropriate manner and the wax is allowed to solidify and harden **(Figures 21-4A to C)**. The metal blocks are then separated thereby forming the tissue blocks **(Figures 21-5 and 21-6)**. Paper blocks and plastic moulds, stainless steel rings, and plastic embedding cassettes are alternate for L mounts **(Figure 21-7)**. Other embedding media are ester wax, gelatin, celloidin, and synthetic resins.

Epoxy resin is used for electron microscopy. Agar agar is used in double embedding and for fine-needle aspiration cytology specimens. Celloidin media is used for cutting hard tissues and gelatin is used when frozen sections are required on friable tissues.

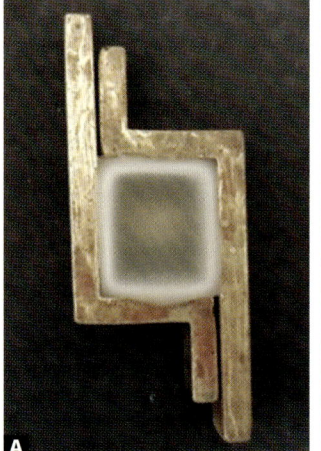
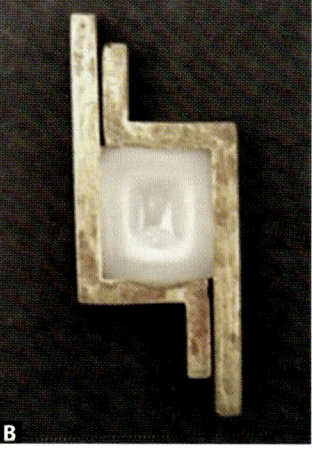

Figures 21-5A and B: Embedded tissue specimen in solidified wax.

MICROWAVE TISSUE PROCESSING

Microwave tissue processing method reduces the turnaround time (duration from the receipt of the specimen to establishing its report), thus making 'same-day diagnosis' a possibility for smaller biopsies. It is done within minutes to hours. Short schedule cycle can be done in 15 minutes, while long schedules involve one hour. The risk of exposure to hazardous chemicals is greatly reduced and also the use of reagents is reduced, thereby being cost-effective. Usage of clearing agent is not required, as the alcohol is evaporated by the microwave energy.

Principle: Microwave tissue processor works on the principle that electromagnetic field causes excitation of molecules which brings about its rotation, resulting in the production of heat energy from within the materials. This heat enhances the rate of diffusion of fluids in and out of the tissue blocks or sections more effectively than the conventional heating.

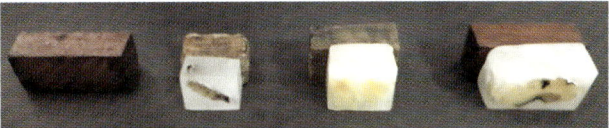

Figure 21-8: Varied sizes of wax blocks attached to respective sizes of wooden blocks upon heating.

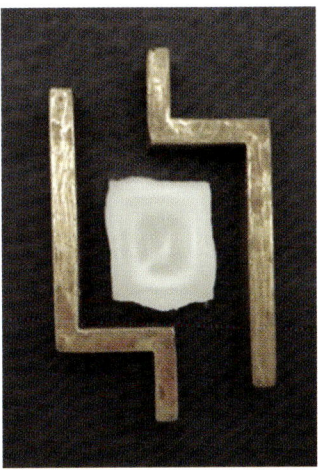

Figure 21-6: Separation of Leuckhart's "L" molds from solidified wax block.

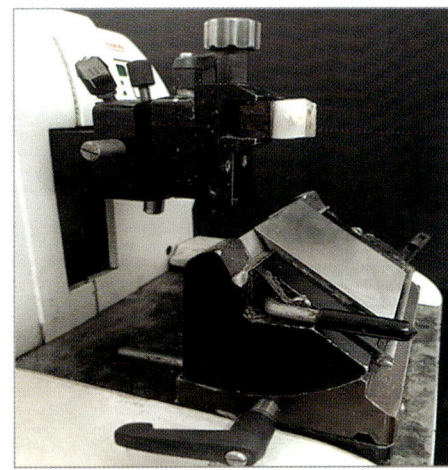

Figure 21-9: Tissue embedded wax block attached to wooden block holder and clamped to the microtome for trimming.

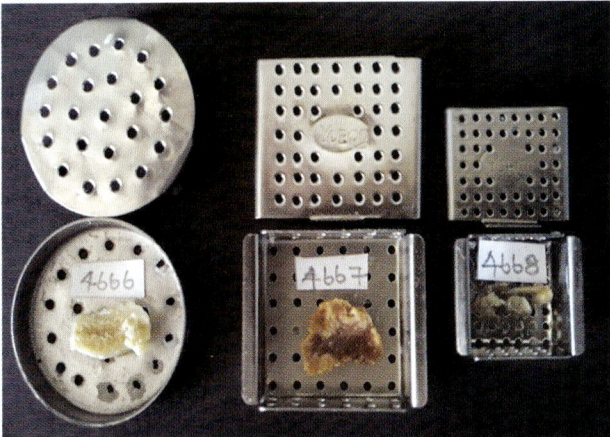

Figure 21-7: Stainless steel cassettes.

TISSUE SECTIONING

Tissue blocks are gently heated, attached to wooden blocks **(Figure 21-8)**, and clamped to the moving arm of the microtome **(Figure 21-9)**. Microtome is a mechanical device for cutting thin uniform slices of tissue (sections). Microtomes are basically of five types, namely—rocking, rotary, sledge, sliding, and freezing microtome. Routinely, paraffin wax embedded tissues are sectioned with rotary microtome **(Figure 21-10)**.

The tissue block is cut to 4 µm thickness with the microtome knife. After few cuts, the section forms a continuous ribbon **(Figure 21-11)**. The ribbon is transferred and spread onto the hot water bath **(Figures 21-12 and 21-13)**. The tissue sections are then transferred onto the glass slide coated with egg albumin **(Figures 21-14 and 21-15)**.

They are placed on a slide warmer for 15 minutes and are dried. When kept on slide warmer, albumin on the glass slide coagulates and fixes the tissue section to the glass slide **(Figure 21-16)**.

Staining

In an unstained section, it is difficult to recognize and differentiate various intracellular and intercellular

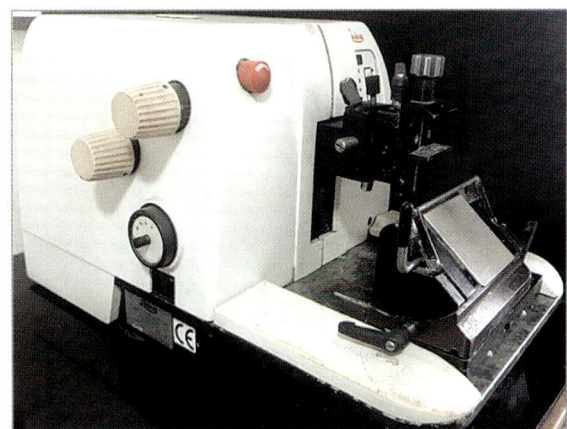

Figure 21-10: Rotary microtome.

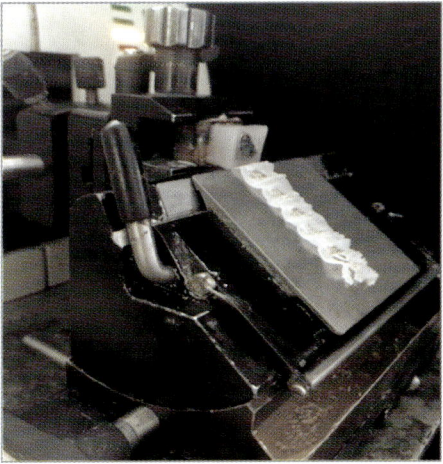

Figure 21-11: Sectioning of the wax block with microtome blade resulting in a wax ribbon.

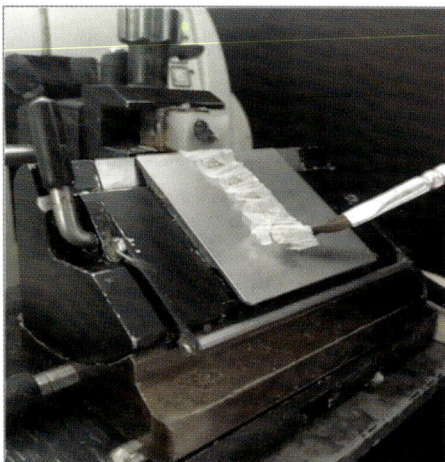

Figure 21-12: Transferring the wax ribbon with the help of a brush.

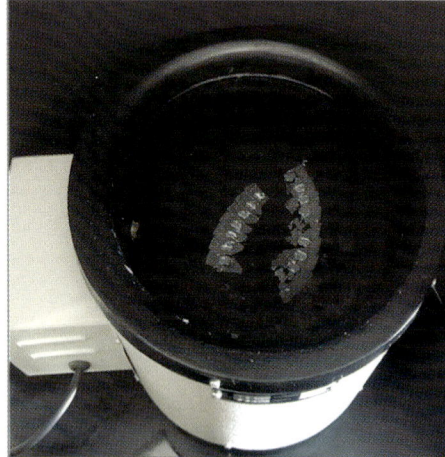

Figure 21-13: Wax ribbon floating in wax flotation bath.

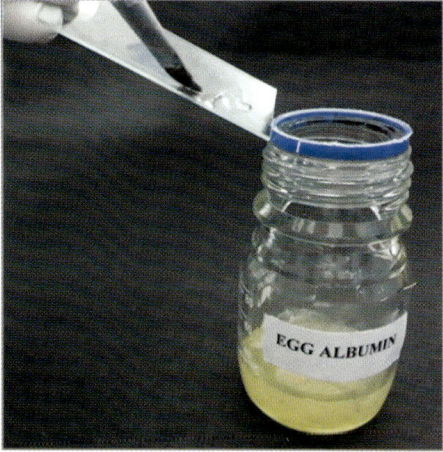

Figure 21-14: Albumin-coated glass slide.

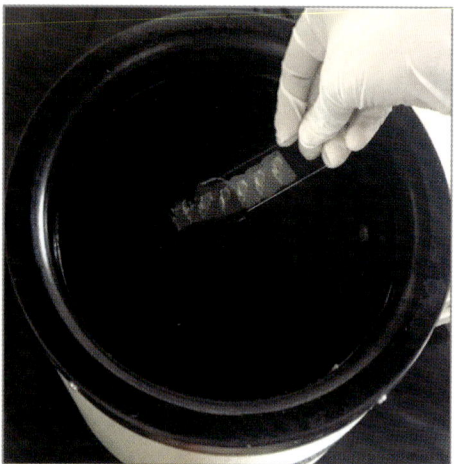

Figure 21-15: Wax ribbon being transferred onto the glass slide.

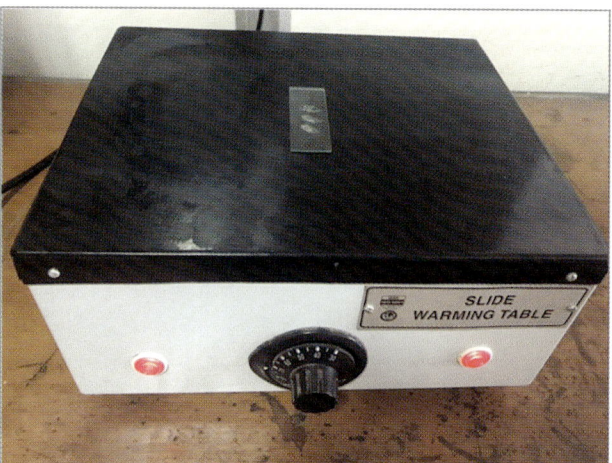

Figure 21-16: Slide with wax ribbon placed on a slide warming table.

components of a tissue. Staining the tissue sections imparts color to the tissue constituents and enhances the contrast for better visualization. Inter- and intracellular composition of the tissue components varies in their physical and chemical nature. This property is utilized in staining.

An ideal stain should not only stain the cell nuclei and cytoplasm but also the intercellular connective tissue.

Routinely used stain is hematoxylin and eosin (H & E).

Routine H & E staining cannot stain the entire tissue components, for example, elastic fibers do not take up H & E stain. To identify certain structures and to enhance visualization, special stains are used. Periodic acid–Schiff (PAS) stain (to demonstrate basement membrane), Verhoeff-van Gieson stain (for elastic fibers), Masson's trichrome stain (to distinguish collagen and muscle), and Ziehl–Neelsen stain (acid-fast bacillus—tuberculous bacillus) are few examples for special stains.

However dark field, phase-contrast, polarized, and interference microscopy do not need staining. They use the physical properties of the visible light photons to demonstrate the subjects to be studied.

> Immunohistochemistry is an auxiliary method for the histopathologists. It works on the principle of detecting the antigens in cells of a tissue by using monoclonal or polyclonal antibodies. The distribution of the antigens can be visualized with the help of this method. Some of the immunohistochemical markers used are Cytokeratin AE1 and AE3 for epithelial cells, smooth muscle actin for detecting myofibroblasts and myoepithelial cells and CD 68 for macrophages.

Tissue processing for light microscopy involves series of steps described in **Table 21-1**.

TABLE 21-1: Steps in tissue processing for light microscopy.

Step 1	Fixation	Fixation of the tissue in formalin
Step 2	Formalin removal	Removal of formalin in the tissue and replacement with water
Step 3	Dehydration	Removal of water in the tissue and replacement with ascending grades of alcohol
Step 4	Clearing	Replacement of alcohol with xylene
Step 5	Impregnation	Replacement of xylene with molten paraffin wax
Step 6	Embedding	Embedding of the specimen in molten paraffin wax
Step 7	Tissue sectioning	Cutting the tissue block with microtome
Step 8	Staining	Staining of sections

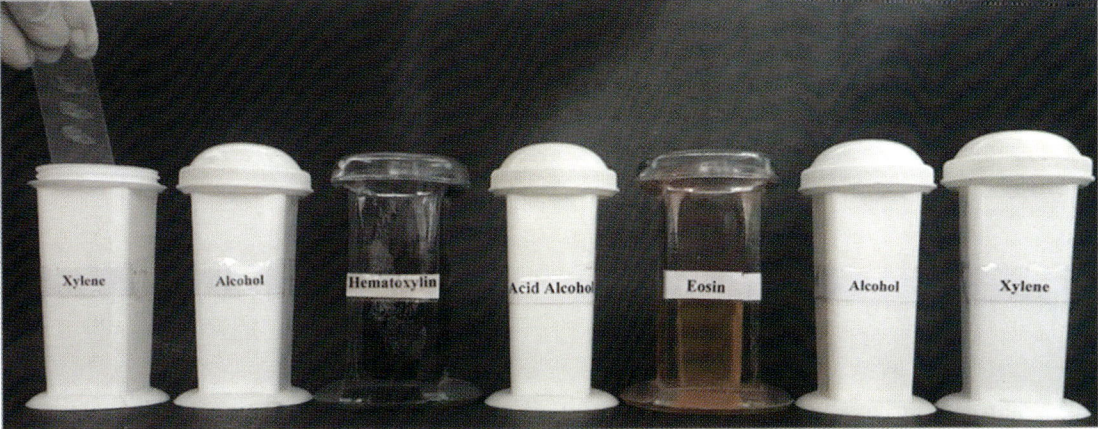

Figure 21-17: Series of reagents for deparaffinization and staining.

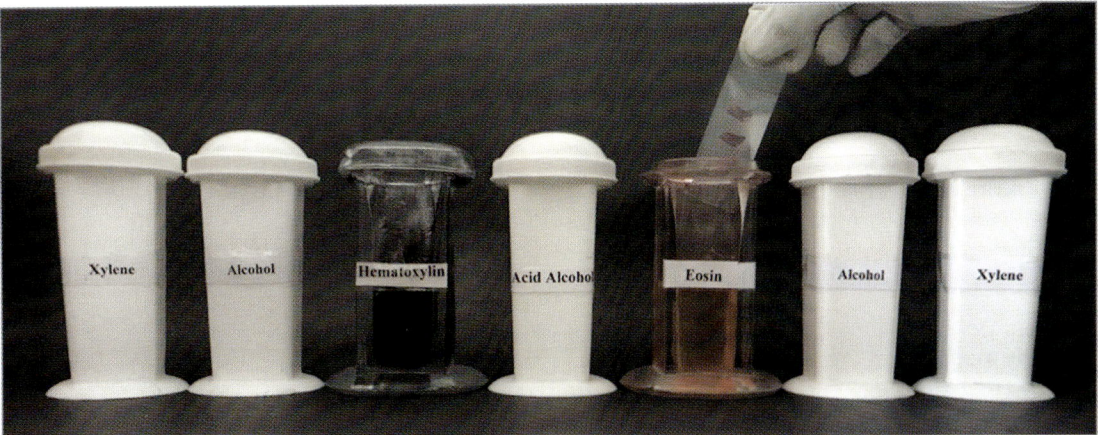

Figure 21-18: Staining in eosin and hematoxylin.

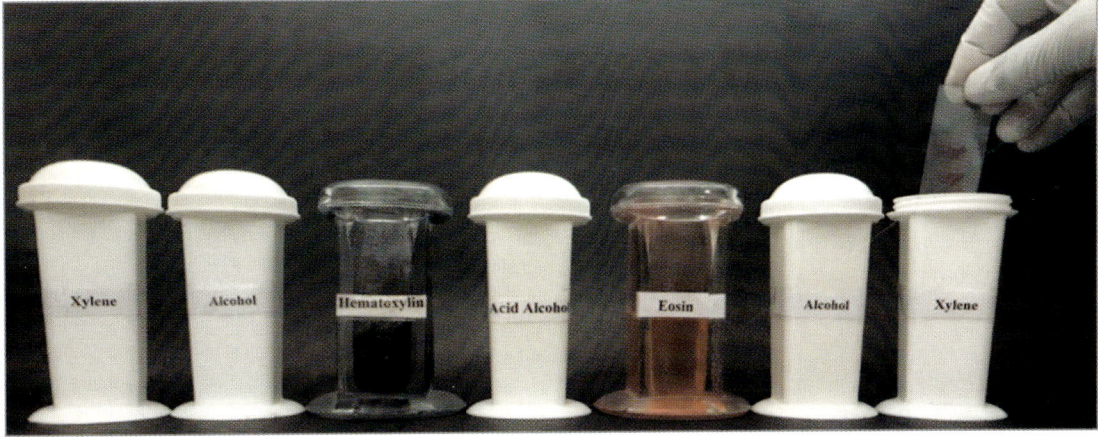

Figure 21-19: The stained section is immersed in alcohol and xylene before fixing the cover slip.

Hematoxylin and Eosin Staining

Hematoxylin and eosin stains are the commonly used stains in histology and histopathology. The principle behind this technique is that basic hematoxylin binds with basophilic substances like DNA or RNA (acidic due to the presence of nucleic acids) and imparts dark blue color to the nucleus. Acidic eosin has affinity for acidophilic substances like most proteins in cytoplasm, intracellular membranes, extracellular fibers, and muscle filaments (basic, due to side chains arginine and lysine) imparting pink color to all these structures.

The steps in H & E-staining technique are as follows (**Figs. 21-17 to 21-19**):
1. Dewaxing
2. Rehydration
3. Nuclear staining: Haematoxylin
4. Blueing
5. Differentiation
6. Blueing
7. Cytoplasmic staining: Eosin
8. Dehydration
9. Clearing
10. Mounting

Dewaxing: Hematoxylin and eosin is a water-based stain. To stain the tissue sections with H & E stain, infiltrated paraffin wax in the tissue sections has to be removed and replaced with water. This process is known as deparaffinization or dewaxing. If not completely dewaxed, the stained sections will have an uneven appearance. Xylene is the most commonly used chemical for dewaxing.

Rehydration: The sections are exposed to descending grades of alcohol, starting from 100%, to 90%, 80%, and 70% alcohol gradually. Finally, the slides are washed in tap water. The section is hydrated so that the aqueous solutions can easily penetrate them.

Nuclear staining: Hematoxylin is the nuclear stain used. It is a natural dye extracted from the wood of *Haematoxylum campechianum*. The haematoxylin has little or no staining capacity. It is oxidized to hematin, which imparts a reddish purple color initially. A mordant such as alum (Aluminium ammonium sulfate) or iron is added to the reagent. This enhances the bonding with the anionic tissue components. Based on the mordant, different types of hematoxylin are available such as Harris hematoxylin, Mayer's hematoxylin, Gill's hematoxylin.

Blueing: Blueing is done to impart a dark blue color to the hematoxylin-stained tissue elements. Ideally, Scott's tap water, a basic solution is used for blueing. However, in places where tap water is alkaline due to its mineral content, the tap water itself can be used for blueing. Blueing can also be repeated after differentiation if required.

Differentiation: Differentiation is the process of selectively removing the excess non-specific background staining from the tissue section by using an acidic solution. Differentiation improves the contrast of the staining. Hydrochloric acid is the standard differentiator. It brings about rapid differentiation. Milder acids like acetic acid are also used for a more controlled and slower differentiation.

Cytoplasmic staining: Aqueous or alcoholic solution of eosin is the widely used cytoplasmic staining. Acetic acid is added to the reagent to improve the sharpness of the pink color.

Dehydration: After staining, the tissue section is dehydrated by immersing in ascending grades of alcohol.

Mounting: The stained slide is immersed in xylene, since it is miscible with both the alcohol and the mounting media. The slide is then covered with glass cover slip by using a mounting media (usually DPX) to protect the stained tissue section. DPX is the commonly used mounting media and is a mixture of distrene, dibutyl phthalate and xylene (**Figures 21-20 and 21-21**). Other mounts used are Canada balsam, fructose syrup, etc. The slides are now ready to be visualized under microscope.

> H & E staining method can be progressive or regressive. In regressive staining, hematoxylin is overstained and a differentiator is used. In regressive staining, hematoxylin is only stained to a point and there is no differentiator employed.

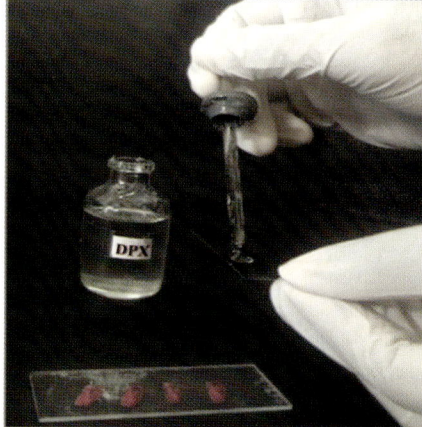

Figure 21-20: DPX is added on a cover slip and placed over the microscopic slide.

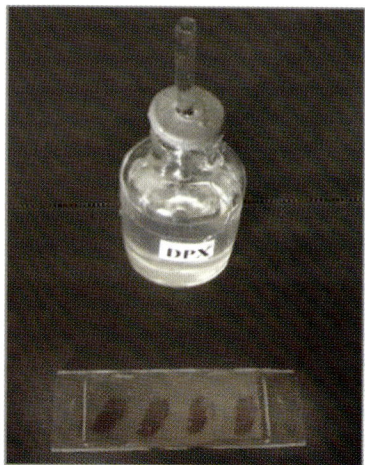

Figure 21-21: Mounted microscopic slide.

Processing for Electron Microscopy

The electron microscope uses accelerated electron beam as the source of illumination, unlike visible light in light microscopy. It produces greater magnification and high resolution to visualize smaller objects with finer details.

In electron microscope, the object can be magnified up to 10,000,000 times, whereas in compound light microscope, the highest total magnification is only 1,000 times, since the resolving power of the optical lens is less. Resolution is defined as the ability to differentiate two adjacent, minute details as separate and individual entities after magnification (minimum distance between two adjacent details that can be distinguished as separate entities). The resolution in light microscope is about 200 nm whereas in electron microscope the resolution is to about 0.2 nm.

Electron microscopes are used to study the ultrastructure of cells, cell organelles, large molecules, microorganisms, crystals, etc. They are of two types—transmission electron microscope (TEM) and scanning electron microscope (SEM). They are expensive—cost and maintenance-wise, extremely thin sections (0.1 µm or 100 nm) of specimens are needed (due to poor penetrating property of electron beam) and technically challenging.

Scanning electron microscope images the surface of the specimen rather than its interior **(Figure 21-22)**. Compared to TEM, the resolution in SEM is lower. Bulky samples that can fit on stage can be imaged thus reducing the need for extremely thin specimen sections for SEM. Also, three-dimensional surface representations of the specimen can be produced unlike two-dimensional images in TEM.

The principles of preparation of tissues are same as that of processing for light microscopy, except the chemical and the instruments used. The processing for electron microscope includes fixation, dehydration, embedding, sectioning, and staining. For electron microscopy, glutaraldehyde is the most commonly used fixative and osmium tetroxide is used as post fixative. Osmium tetroxide fumes are extremely toxic. These fixatives penetrate into the tissues very slowly, necessitating sectioning of the tissues to less than 1 mm thickness. Fixation time is usually 1 hour. Fixation for more than 2–3 hours causes brittleness of the specimen. In electron microscopy, the specimens are very small and slight hardening of tissue is advantageous. Hence, glutaraldehyde is the preferred fixative in electron microscopy, which is not routinely used in tissue processing for light microscopy.

Since thin sections are necessary, tissues are embedded in methacrylates and epoxy resins. Diamond knives are used to section methacrylate blocks and they are unsuitable for epoxy resin blocks, unless the angle of the knife is less than 45°. Comparatively cheaper and easily fabricated glass knives are employed in microsectioning. To increase the contrast, stains using heavy metals are employed, which include lead hydroxide stain, uranyl acetate stain (for fibrous proteins), silver proteinate (protargol), and silver methenamine stain (basement membrane components).

FROZEN SECTIONS

Preparation time for the routine paraffin section is around 3–5 days. On occasions, quick histological examination is required. For example, if a tumor has been resected but it is unclear whether the surgical margin is free of tumor cells, an intraoperative histological examination is needed to assess the marginal clearance or if biopsy is to be reported immediately (on table diagnosis). Sections can be made quickly for histological examination by freezing the tissue, which is known as frozen section or cryosection. Cryosections are also used to detect the presence of substances, which are usually dissolved or lost in the traditional histologic processing technique, for example, lipids. They can also be used to detect some antigens masked by formalin.

The instrument used for cryosection is the cryostat, which is essentially a microtome inside a freezer. Advantages of frozen tissue sections include retention of the natural protein structure of antigens for immunohistochemical studies and the avoidance of usage of formalin, which is a toxic and carcinogenic compound. Drawbacks include a loss of tissue morphology due to freezing artifact and the thickness of cryostat-generated sections. Hence the quality of the slides produced by frozen section is of lower than formalin fixed, wax embedded tissue processing.

Principle: Upon rapidly freezing the tissue sample, the water is converted into ice, which acts as an embedding media allowing the tissue to be sectioned. The tissue becomes firmer if the temperature of the tissue sample is lowered while the tissue softens if the temperature is increased.

Cryosectioning

The biopsied tissue can directly be taken to cryostat or can be fixed with 10% formalin or formol-alcohol. First the tissue is fixed to the metal chuck by using 20% sucrose and a drop of water and it is frozen. Water-soluble glycol medium, solid carbon dioxide gas or liquid nitrogen is used to freeze the tissue. Change in the color of the tissue to glossy white indicates the completion of freezing. Once frozen, the specimen on the chuck is mounted on the cryomicrotome. As stated previously, it is the microtome placed in a freezer.

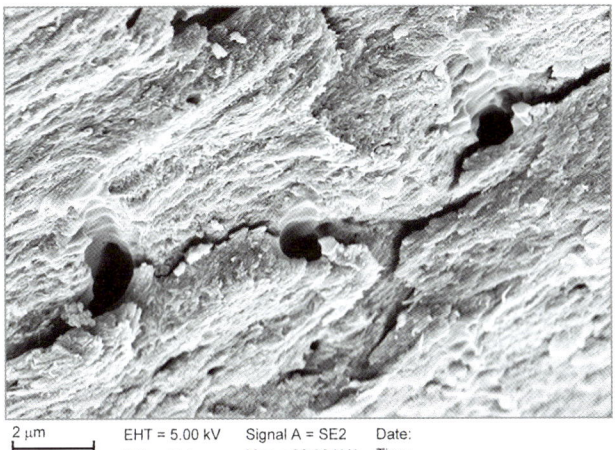

Figure 21-22: Scanning electron microscope picture of dentinal tubules.
Source: Dr Tamarai Selvan.

Once the frozen tissue is mounted onto the microtome, the sectioning is similar to that of paraffin sectioning. Sections up to thickness of 10–15 μm are obtained and can be viewed immediately under light microscope.

> **Tissue microarray**
> The idea was first developed by H.Battifora et al. and later improved by Kononen et al. The word 'array' refers to the orderly arrangement of features. Tissue microarray therefore refers to the method, where a single paraffin block is made with hundreds of separate representative tissue cores arranged in an array fashion allowing multiplex histological analysis. The principle of tissue microarray is numerous cylindrical cores are removed from the different donor tissue blocks and then re-embedding to a single receiver block.
>
> Tissue microarray is used for assessing expression of proteins in around 1000 sections using *in situ* hybridization, immunohistochemistry or fluorescence *in situ* hybridization. As many as 1000 tissue sections can be placed in the same glass slide measuring 45 x 25 mm.

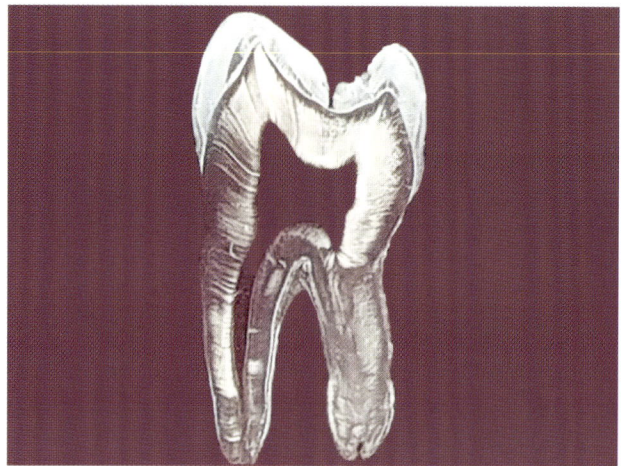

Figure 21-23: Ground section of tooth showing enamel, dentin, and cementum. Pulp chamber appears empty.

Hard Tissue Processing

Hard tissue present in the orofacial region includes teeth and bone. Occasionally, they may need histological evaluation. Hard components of teeth include enamel, dentin, and cementum. Sectioning of the hard tissue is difficult if not impossible with the conventional microtome. To study the hard tissue, it has to be ground to make thin section or it should be made soft by removing the inorganic content (a process called decalcification) to enable sectioning by microtome. Selection of the method is based on the structures to be studied.

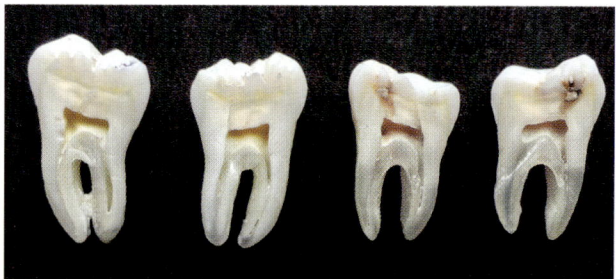

Figure 21-24: Tooth to be ground placed on Arkansas stone.

Ground Sections (Figure 21-23)

Any hard tissue can be studied in ground sections. Enamel is best studied in ground sections. The tooth is cut either longitudinally or transversely with diamond disk and ground by using an abrasive stone with water drops added in intervals to prevent fracture or cracks in the specimen. The commonly used abrasive stone is Arkansas stone. Tooth or bone can be ground as thin as 50 μm **(Figures 21-24 to 21-26)**.

The sections are then placed onto a glass slide and mounted with DPX and coverslip is placed above **(Figure 21-27)**. Ground sections cannot be stained.

Ground section is a simple and quick method to study histology of tissues with maximum mineralization like enamel which is 96% mineralized. Any attempt to study the enamel by decalcification results in total loss of enamel in the acid. Disadvantage of ground section is that staining is not possible and soft tissues like periodontal ligament and pulp cannot be studied.

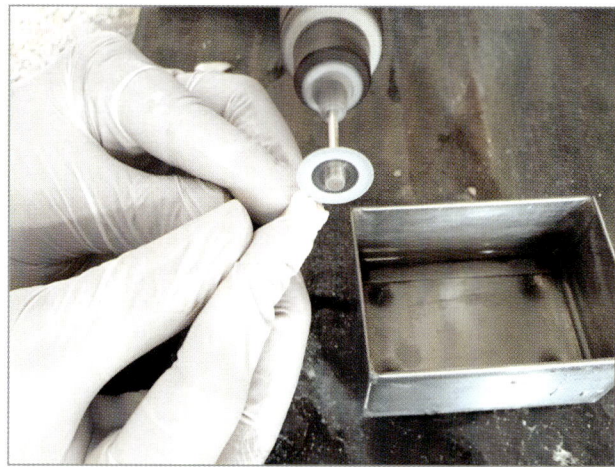

Figure 21-25: Grinding the sliced tooth.

Decalcified Sections (Figure 21-28)

Principle: Calcium and other inorganic components render hardness to the tooth and bone, which prevent sectioning by the conventional microtome. Removal of the inorganic material from the hard tissue converts it into soft, and enables sectioning by microtome. The process of removing the calcium ions from bone and teeth for histological processing is known as decalcification.

Procedure: Thin slices of bone or tooth are obtained by various methods using fine-toothed bone saw, diamond disk attached to air motor, etc. Ideally, thickness of bone slices should not exceed 4–5 mm for effective decalcification.

An ideal decalcifying agent should completely remove calcium in a reasonably short time without damaging the cells or fibers and without interfering with subsequent staining procedures.

Acids: In this method, tooth or bone is immersed in acids, which have decalcifying property. Formic acid, citric acid, hydrochloric acid, and nitric acid are commonly used acid decalcifiers. 5% formic acid is a decalcifying agent with reasonable speed and minimal tissue damage. About 7% citric acid can be used when time is not an important factor. About 0.5% hydrochloric acid has moderate and rapid action. About 5% nitric acid is used by many as routine decalcifying agent as it is rapid. Time of decalcification has to be carefully controlled and its tendency to cause yellow discoloration of tissues can be avoided by addition of 0.1% urea.

Ion exchange resins: These are polymers that act as medium for ion exchange. These are used to deionize or demineralize. Cation resin has a negative functional group and thus attracts positively charged ions. If it is added to the decalcifying fluid, it takes up the calcium ions from the acid decalcifier, thereby enhances the effectiveness of the acid. The advantages of these resins are shortening of the decalcification time, no need to change the acid regularly, and the resin can be reused after washing for a long time.

Ammonium form of sulfonated polystyrene resin is commonly used for the decalcification of teeth and bone. It is layered at the bottom of the container and the specimen is placed on it. This method is limited to the decalcifying fluids, which do not contain mineral acids.

Chelating agents: Certain organic compounds have the property to bind to metals and are termed as chelating agents. Ethylenediaminetetraacetic acid (EDTA) disodium salt has the property to bind to calcium and acts as a chelating agent. EDTA can therefore be used as a decalcifying agent. Artifacts are minimum in tissues decalcified by this method.

Electrophoresis: It is based on the principle of attraction of calcium ions to a negative electrode thereby bringing considerable decrease in the length of time needed for decalcification. This method is not routinely followed compared to other methods.

Excessive decalcification brings loss of tissue details and thereby causing difficulty in diagnosis. Therefore, it is very important that end point of decalcification is to be determined to avoid exposing the tissue to decalcifying agents for longer than necessary period and also to ensure complete removal of calcium. This assessment of completion of decalcification is termed as "end point determination".

The end point determination can be assessed by taking radiographs or by using chemicals. In the chemical method, 1 mL of 5% sodium or ammonium oxalate is added to decalcifying fluid. Turbidity of the fluid indicates the presence of calcium, which means the tissue, is still releasing calcium into decalcifying solution. The decalcifying solution has to be changed and tissue will continue to decalcify. If solution is clear, and absence of turbidity indicates completion of decalcification.

Since 96% of the enamel is mineralized, during decalcification major portion of enamel is lost. Thus enamel cannot be studied upon decalcification. Other hard tissue structures like dentin and cementum of the tooth and bone can be studied after decalcification.

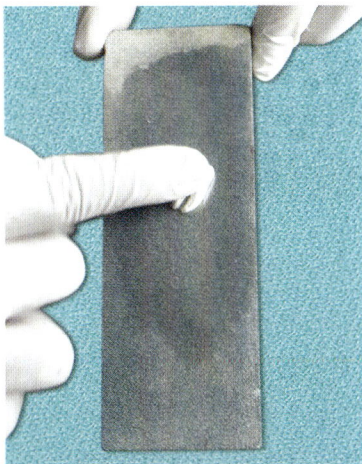

Figure 21-26: Grinding the tooth.

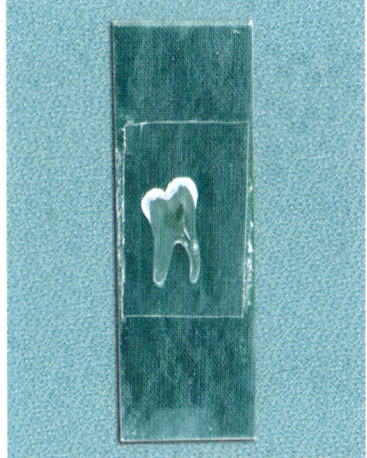

Figure 21-27: Ground section is mounted on a slide.

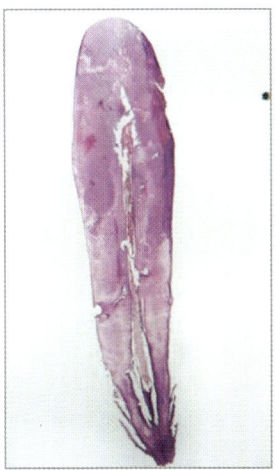

Figure 21-28: Decalcified section of tooth. Total loss of enamel is noticeable. Pulp is visible.

Different methods of decalcification include:
- Acid decalcification
- Ion exchange resins
- Chelating agents
- Electrophoresis.

Various steps in tissue processing for hard and soft tissues are shown in **Flowchart 21-1.**

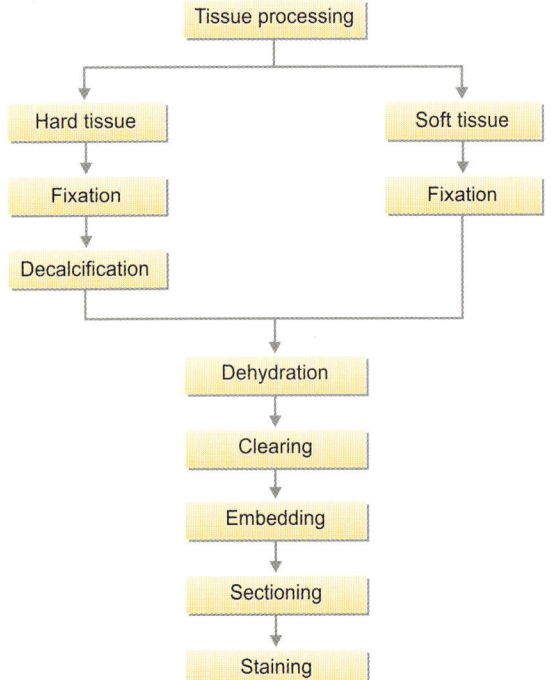

Flowchart 21-1: Steps in tissue processing.

Artifacts

Artifact as defined by Bernstein is 'an artificial structure or tissue alteration on a prepared microscopic slide caused by some extraneous factors'. Such structures are not normally present in a tissue. The accuracy of histopathological diagnosis depends on eliminating or at least minimizing such artifacts. Artifacts can be caused at any of the tissue processing steps or even during biopsy procedures. Based on their time of occurrence, artifacts are classified as:
- Artifacts before fixation
- Artifacts during fixation
- Artifacts during decalcification
- Artifacts during microtomy
- Artifacts during floatation and mounting
- Artifacts during staining
- Artifacts during mounting

Exfoliative Cytology

Exfoliative cytology is the microscopic examination of the shed, desquamated or abraded cells taken from the epithelial surface usually the mucous membrane. It also includes the study of those cells that have been collected from body fluids such as sputum, saliva, urine, etc.

It is a painless, noninvasive, quick, and simple procedure and is suitable for patients who suffer with systemic diseases and are contraindicated for biopsy.

Exfoliative cytology is used in detection of cancer of female genital tract, pulmonary carcinoma, urinary tract lesions, esophageal cancers, oral cancers, and personal identification in the field of forensics.

This procedure is possible only on tissues exfoliating cells into the accessible sites. It should be used as an adjuvant and not as a substitute for biopsy. Interpretation by skilled cytopathologist is necessary.

Physiologically oral epithelial cells undergo maturation starting from basal cells and transforming into mature superficial surface cells and finally shed into the oral cavity. Thus any time, the surface mucosa should exhibit mature cells. But, in malignancy, basal cells due to loss of cohesiveness exfoliate along with superficial cells. These cells exhibit altered morphology in smears.

Exfoliated oral epithelial cells can be obtained by various techniques like cotton tip application, normal saline rinses, wooden spatulas, and cytobrushes.

The obtained material is smeared onto the glass slides and fixed by using alcohol. Various stains like H & E, PAS stain, Gram stain, PAP stain, etc. can be employed to study the exfoliated cells. PAP staining gives good nuclear detail; cytoplasmic transparency and stain color indicate cellular differentiation and degree of cellular maturity of squamous epithelium.

Fine Needle Aspiration Cytology (FNAC)

FNAC is a type of biopsy but minimally invasive. In this procedure a thin gauge needle usually 25–22 G needle is inserted into the lesion to aspirate the content, which may be a solid tissue or fluid for microscopical examination. The aspirated material is smeared onto the glass slide and stained. It is useful in studying the nature of the content of a cyst, abscess or a suspected vascular lesion. The advantage is that it is an inexpensive and quick diagnostic procedure and a valuable tool in cancer diagnosis. The disadvantages are chances of introducing infection and losing of the tissue architecture, so it is not the replacement for biopsy.

DIGITAL PATHOLOGY

The advent of whole slide image (WSI) scanners have revolutionized the field of pathology. An era of digital pathology has begun. Within minutes the WSI can capture multiple images of the entire tissue section present on the slide. These images are then visualized by the pathologists on a computer monitor. The digital pathology has made diagnosis from remote location a possibility and the feasibility for a second opinion from experts anywhere in the world a reality. Scientists are now working on the application of Artificial Intelligence (AI) tools in the field of pathology.

Points to Remember

- Biopsy is defined as removal of tissue from the living body for microscopic examination to establish the diagnosis.
- Vital staining involves injection of dyes into the living tissue.
- Supravital staining involves adding a stain to a medium of cells already removed from the organism.
- In whole-mounts the entire organism or structure is placed directly onto a microscope slide if it is small.
- Squash preparations are preparations, where the cells are squashed or crushed onto a slide to reveal their contents.
- Smears are used to study the cells suspended in a fluid.
- Sectioning involves making very thin slices of the tissue.
- Fixation facilitates cross-linking (covalent bonds) between proteins making the molecules unavailable for further degradation by lysosomal enzymes, thus preventing autolysis and putrefaction, thereby aiding in preservation of the tissue architecture. 10% formalin is the most commonly used fixative.
- Dehydration is the removal of water from the tissue by immersing it in ascending grades of isopropyl alcohol.
- Clearing involves removal of the alcohol by clearing agent, usually xylene.
- Paraffin wax replaces the xylene in the tissue and the tissue is impregnated or infiltrated with paraffin wax.
- To cut the section, the paraffin wax infiltrated tissue has to be embedded in the wax to make into a block.
- Staining the tissue sections imparts color to the tissue constituents and enhances the contrast for better visualization. Routinely used stain is hematoxylin and eosin.
- Basic hematoxylin binds with basophilic substances like DNA or RNA and imparts dark blue color to the nucleus. Acidic eosin has affinity for acidophilic substances like most proteins in cytoplasm, intracellular membranes, extracellular fibers, and muscle filaments, imparting pink color to all these structures.
- Electron microscope uses accelerated electron beam as the source of illumination, unlike visible light in light microscopy. It produces greater magnification and high resolution. In electron microscope, the object can be magnified up to 10,000,000 times, whereas in compound light microscope, the highest total magnification is only 1,000 times. Resolution is defined as the ability to differentiate two adjacent, minute details as separate and individual entities after magnification
- They are of two types—transmission electron microscope (TEM) and scanning electron microscope (SEM). TEM helps to study the inner aspects of the cell, whereas SEM images the surface of the specimen rather than its interior. Also, three- dimensional surface representations of the specimen can be produced unlike two-dimensional images in TEM.
- Hard tissues can be studied microscopically by two methods viz ground sections and decalcified sections.
- Enamel cannot be studied upon decalcification, since 96% of the enamel is mineralized, during decalcification major portion of enamel will be lost. Thus, enamel is best studied using ground sections.
- The process of removing the calcium ions from bone and teeth for histological processing is known as decalcification. Decalcification is usually done by immersion in acids such as formic acid, citric acid, hydrochloric acid, and nitric acid.
- Exfoliative cytology is the microscopic examination of the abraded, shed or desquamated cells from the epithelial surface usually the mucous membrane. Exfoliated oral epithelial cells can be obtained by various techniques like cotton tip application, normal saline rinses, wooden spatulas, and cytobrushes. The obtained material is smeared onto the glass slides and fixed by using alcohol. Stains such as H & E, PAS, Gram stain, and PAP stain are routinely used.

PRACTICE QUESTIONS

1. Write in detail about the steps in tissue processing for microscopical examination.
2. Write notes on fixation.
3. Write notes on clearing.
4. Write notes on frozen sections.
5. Write notes on decalcification.
6. Write notes on ground sections.

MULTIPLE CHOICE QUESTIONS

1. **Fixation is best described as:**
   a. Prevents autolysis and putrefaction
   b. Removes water from the tissue
   c. Compresses the tissue sample
   d. Removes the proteins from the tissue
2. **The step which immediately precedes clearing is:**
   a. Fixation
   b. Dehydration
   c. Impregnation
   d. Embedding
3. **Most commonly used fixative for light microscopy is:**
   a. Xylene
   b. Glutaraldehyde
   c. Isopropyl alcohol
   d. 10% formalin

4. **Fixative of choice for electron microscopy is:**
   a. Formalin
   b. Glutaraldehyde
   c. Osmium tetroxide
   d. Acetone
5. **The most widely used clearing agent is:**
   a. Xylene
   b. Glutaraldehyde
   c. Isopropyl alcohol
   d. Formalin
6. **Melting point of paraffin wax is ___°C:**
   a. 55
   b. 65
   c. 45
   d. 60
7. **Embedding medium of choice for electron microscopy is:**
   a. Agar agar
   b. Liquid nitrogen
   c. Celloidin
   d. Paraffin wax
8. **Embedding medium used for frozen sections is:**
   a. Celloidin
   b. Gelatin
   c. Resin
   d. Agar
9. **Special stain to demonstrate basement membrane is:**
   a. Periodic acid–Schiff stain
   b. Verhoeff–van Gieson stain
   c. Masson's trichome stain
   d. Ziehl–Neelsen stain
10. **Special stain to demonstrate elastic fibers is:**
    a. Periodic acid–Schiff stain
    b. Verhoeff–van Gieson stain
    c. Masson's trichrome stain
    d. Ziehl–Neelsen stain
11. **The hard tissue which is studied best by ground sections is:**
    a. Enamel
    b. Bone
    c. Cementum
    d. Dentin
12. **Pulp and periodontal ligament can be studied microscopically by:**
    a. Ground section
    b. Decalcified section
    c. Frozen section
    d. Cryosection
13. **Studying the shed epithelial cells or scrapping the superficial cells under microscope is known as:**
    a. Biopsy
    b. Exfoliative cytology
    c. Cytomics
    d. Fine needle aspiration cytology

ANSWERS

1. a 2. b 3. d 4. b 5. a 6. a 7. b 8. b 9. a 10. b 11. a 12. b 13. b

BIBLIOGRAPHY

1. Aj A, Mal M. The use of immunohistochemistry in an oral pathology laboratory. 2007;29(2):101-5.
2. Avery JK, Chiego DJ. Essentials of Oral Histology and Embryology—A Clinical Approach, 3rd edition. US: Mosby; 2006.
3. Avery JK. Oral Development and Histology, 3rd edition. New York: Thieme; 2002.
4. Bancroft JD, Gamble M. Theory and Practice of Histological Techniques, 5th edition. New York: Churchill Livingstone; 2002.
5. Berkovitz BKB, Holland GR, Moxham BJ. Oral Anatomy, Histology & Embryology, 4th edition. Elsevier; 2009.
6. Bibbo M. Comprehensive Cytopathology, 2nd edition. USA: Saunders; 1997.
7. Buesa RJ, Peshkov MV. Histology without xylene. Ann Diagn Pathol. 2009;13(4):246-56.
8. Chandra S, Chandra S, Chandra M, et al. Textbook of Dental and Oral Histology with Embryology & MCQ's, 2nd edition. New Delhi: Jaypee Brothers Medical Publishers (P) Ltd; 2010.
9. Chatterjee K. Essentials of Dental Anatomy & Oral Histology, 2nd edition. New Delhi: Jaypee Brothers Medical Publishers (P) Ltd; 2014.
10. Culling CFA. Handbook of Histopathological & Histochemical Techniques, 3rd edition. UK: Butterworths; 1974.
11. Gaunt WA, Osborn JW, Ten Cate AR. Advanced Dental Histology, 2nd edition. Bristol: John Wright & Sons Ltd; 1971.
12. Herzberg AJ, Raso DS, Silverman JF. Color Atlas of Normal Cytology, 1st edition. USA: Churchill Livingstone; 1999.
13. Hewitt SM, Lewis FA, Cao Y, et al. Tissue handling and specimen preparation in surgical pathology: issues concerning the recovery of nucleic acids from formalin-fixed, paraffin-embedded tissue. Arch Pathol Lab Med. 2008;132:1929-35.
14. Jaafar H. Intra-operative frozen section consultation: Concepts, applications and limitations. Malaysian J Med Sci. 2006;13(1):4-12.
15. Kallioniemi O, Wagner U, Kononen J, Sauter G. Tissue microarray technology for high-throughput molecular profiling of cancer. 2001;10(7):657–62.
16. KM, Jayaraj G, Sherlin HJ, KRD Santhanam A. A new rapid tissue processing technique for small oral biopsies - A comparative Study. J Evol Med Dent Sci. 2021;10(1):19-22.
17. Kumar GS. Orban's Oral Histology and Embryology, 14th edition. India: Elsevier; 2015.
18. Kumar K, Shetty DC, Dua M. Biopsy and Tissue Processing Artifacts in Oral Mucosal Tissues. Int J Head Neck Surg. 2012;3(2):92-8.
19. Nanci A. Ten Cate's Oral Histology: Development, Structure, and Functions, 8th edition. India: Elsevier; 2012.
20. Narayan Biswal B, Narayan Das S, Kumar Das B, Rath R. Alteration of cellular metabolism in cancer cells and its therapeutic. J oral Maxillofac Pathol. 2017;21(3):244–51.
21. Odell EW, Morgan PR. Biopsy Pathology of the Oral Tissues, 1st edition. UK: Chapman & Hall; 1998.

22. Parwani A V. Next generation diagnostic pathology: Use of digital pathology and artificial intelligence tools to augment a pathological diagnosis. Diagn Pathol. 2019;14(1):19-21.
23. Provenza DV, Seibel W. Oral Histology: Inheritance and Development, 2nd edition. USA: Lea & Febiger; 1986.
24. Rajkumar K, Ramya R. Textbook of Oral Anatomy, Histology, Physiology & Tooth Morphology, 2nd edition. India: Wolters Kluwer Health; 2017.
25. Rastogi V, Puri N, Arora S, Kaur G, Yadav L, Sharma R. Artefacts: A diagnostic dilemma–A review. J Clin Diagnostic Res. 2013;7(10):2408-13.
26. Renshaw AA. Aspiration Cytology: A Pattern Recognition Approach, 1st edition. China: Elsevier; 2005.
27. Rolls G. An introduction to decalcification. [online] Leica website. Available from https://www.leicabiosystems. com/pathologyleaders/an-introduction-to-decalcification/ [Accessed June 2018].
28. Roskell DE, Buley ID. Fine needle aspiration cytology in cancer diagnosis. BMJ. 2004;329(7460):244-245. doi:10.1136/bmj.329.7460.244
29. Shetty JK, Babu HF, Hosapatna Laxminarayana KP. Histomorphological assessment of formalin versus nonformalin fixatives in diagnostic surgical pathology. J Lab Physicians. 2020;12(04):271-5.
30. Shruthi BS, Vinodhkumar P, Kashyap B, Reddy PS. Use of microwave in diagnostic pathology. J Cancer Res Ther. 2013;9(3):351–5.
31. Sivapathasundharam B, Kalasagar M. Yet another article on exfoliative cytology. JOMFP. 2004;8(2):54-7.
32. Weber DF. A simplified technique for the preparation of ground sections. J Dent Res. 1964;43:462.
33. Wick MR, Mills NC, Brix WK. Diagnostic Histochemistry. UK: Cambridge University Press; 2008.
34. Yang J, Chen X, SU B, et al. A new grossing knife with two parallel blades for preparing uniform thickness gross tissue sections. J Clin Pathol. 2008;61(9):1069-70.

CHAPTER 22

Histochemistry of Oral Tissues

Preethi Murali, B Sivapathasundharam

Chapter Outline

- Oral Tissues and their Chemical Composition 322
- Epithelial Tissue and Derivatives 323
- Connective Tissue 323
- Cells and Fibers 323
    - Fibroblasts 323
- Histochemical Techniques 324
    - Fixation 324
- Specific Histochemical Methods 324
    - Glycogen, Glycoprotein, and Proteoglycan 324
    - Proteins 325
    - Lipids 325
    - Enzymes 325
- Immunohistochemistry 326
- Histochemistry of Oral Hard Tissues 326
    - Carbohydrates 326
    - Proteins 326
    - Lipids 326
    - Enzymes 326
- Histochemistry of Oral Soft Tissues 326
    - Carbohydrates 326
    - Lipids 326
    - Proteins 326
    - Enzymes 327
    - Angiogenic Factor 327
- Advanced Techniques 328
    - Immunofluorescence 328
    - *In Situ* Hybridization 328
    - Polymerase Chain Reaction 328
    - Enzyme-linked Immunosorbent Assay 328
    - Confocal Microscopy 329
    - Flow Cytometry 330
    - Radioautographic Techniques 330
- Clinical Considerations 330

Histochemistry deals with the identification and distribution of biochemical substances in the cells and tissues by means of specialized stains under microscopy. It is simply the chemistry of biological tissues. It combines the techniques of biochemistry and histology. In histochemical procedures, the tissue sections act as the medium in which biochemical reactions are carried out by the addition of substrates, inhibitors, or other chemicals. The aim of histochemical reactions is to localize specific cell structure that expresses given biochemical characteristics, both qualitatively and quantitatively. In histochemical reactions, the site of enzymatic reactions, such as the localization of mitochondrial enzymes or other membrane-bound enzymes, as well as specific cell components can be demonstrated. The subcategory of histochemistry includes enzyme histochemistry, immunohistochemistry, cytochemistry, and *in situ* hybridization.

Oral cavity comprises hard and soft tissues, which possess different biochemical substances in them. Various types of chemicals can stain these biochemical substances. Histochemistry identifies the position and distribution of substances like carbohydrates, lipids, nucleic acids, proteins, enzymes, pigments, and minerals present in a tissue. Histochemical techniques are based on chemical rationales to identify and stain different biochemical materials. There are various innovative techniques, which localize the chemical residues of a large molecule for histochemical application. Thus, physiological as well as the pathological conditions can be diagnosed by these techniques.

Certain advanced techniques are used to understand the biological processes involved in the cells. The biomolecules involved in tissue development, functioning, and pathologies can be detected by these techniques. Recently, these advances help in precise localization of biomolecules. *In situ* hybridization, immunofluorescence, and immunohistochemistry are such techniques which are used both in clinical applications and research.

ORAL TISSUES AND THEIR CHEMICAL COMPOSITION

Epithelium, which lines the oral cavity, supported by the underlying connective tissue, muscles, nerves and associated

salivary glands form the oral soft tissues. The chemical composition of these structures is important in maintaining the integrity of oral health. The chemical composition of the tissues may be altered in disease process. The chemical constituents of these tissues include:
- Proteoglycans
- Glycoproteins
- Proteins
- Lipids
- Enzymes

EPITHELIAL TISSUE AND DERIVATIVES

Superficial epithelial cells contain glycogen along with cytoplasmic components like proteins and carbohydrates.

The lining epithelium and glandular epithelium contains mucin or mucoid content. Mucins are of different types, namely—the strongly sulfated mucins, weakly sulfated mucins, carboxylated mucins, sulfated sialomucins, and neutral mucins. They can be found separately or in combinations. The glycosaminoglycan present in the mucin is usually the component, which determines the staining reaction. Presence of glucuronidase, sulfates and sialic acid determines the acidic nature.

CONNECTIVE TISSUE

Connective tissue is of mesenchymal origin and consists of various cells and fibers. It is found throughout the body and its main function is to support, connect or separate other tissues or organs of the body. They act as a filler substance between the cells and fibers. Connective tissue consists of cells and extracellular matrix. Extracellular matrix is composed of fibers and ground substance. Ground substance is an amorphous gel-like substance into which the cells and fibers are embedded. It consists of water stabilized by glycosaminoglycans, proteoglycans, and glycoproteins, all secreted by the cells of the connective tissue. Apart from functioning as supportive medium, it also helps in intercellular exchange, transport of the products of metabolism, transfer of cell signals and storage of water.

Proteoglycans are macromolecules consisting of a protein core to which 50–100 highly ionic unbranched glycosaminoglycans are covalently attached. They are mainly localized on the cell surface and extracellular matrix. Apart from their function in growth and motility of the cells, proteoglycans influence physical properties of connective tissues such as turgor, resilience, and compressive strength. Through positive and negative modulation of growth factor activity, proteoglycans influence the cellular activity.

Glycosaminoglycan (GAG) chains are attached to the protein core of proteoglycans. The GAG is acidic in nature, which is related with the presence of carboxyl or sulphated groups. Large proteoglycan polymers, named *aggregating proteoglycans* are formed when proteoglycan molecules bind with hyaluronic acid, an unsulfated GAG. *Non-aggregating* proteoglycans are those with less GAG chains.

Some of the non-aggregating proteoglycans are decorin, fibromodulin, perlecan, agrin, and syndecan. Each of these is associated with various connective tissue components.

Morphology of collagen fibrils and their organization are profoundly affected by the nature and amount of proteoglycans present in the connective tissue, since they are closely associated with collagen fibers.

Proteoglycans can either be sulfated or nonsulfated. The sulfated forms are chondroitin sulfates, keratan sulfates, and heparan sulfates whereas the nonsulfated proteoglycan is hyaluronic acid.

Glycoprotein is a type of protein molecule that has a carbohydrate covalently attached to it. It also forms a part of the ground substance in the connective tissue and they contain protein molecules in abundance with less number of carbohydrate moieties than proteoglycans. Glycoproteins are more hydrophilic than ordinary proteins. Fibronectin, laminin, chondronectin, and osteonectin are some of the well-known glycoproteins. Cell surface glycoproteins enhance the cell to cell and cell to extracellular matrix attachment and intercellular communication. Further, they also maintain the cell morphology and function.

Fibronectin is a high-molecular weight glycoprotein present in the extracellular matrix and body fluids. It binds extracellular matrix components such as collagen, fibrin, and heparan sulfate. It also plays a major role in cell adhesion, growth, migration, and differentiation and is important for wound healing and embryonic development.

Laminins are major extracellular matrix protein component of the basal lamina. There are 15 different laminins each consisting of a unique combination of three subchains (α, β, and γ peptide chains). The combination of chains confers some tissue specificity. Laminins are important for the function of the basement membrane and they mediate the essential functions of cells like differentiation, migration, and integrin-dependent cell adhesion and spreading.

Chondronectin is a glycoprotein of cartilage matrix that mediates the adhesion of chondrocytes to type II collagen. The amino acid and carbohydrate compositions of chondronectin are distinct from fibronectin and laminin.

Osteonectin, also known as secreted protein acidic and rich in cysteine (SPARC) or basement membrane protein 40 (BM-40), is a glycoprotein in the bone that binds calcium. It is the most abundant noncollagenous protein in mineralized bone matrix and is implicated in regulating the adhesion of osteoblasts and platelets to their extracellular matrix as well as early stromal mineralization.

CELLS AND FIBERS

Fibroblasts

They are the predominant cell type present in the connective tissue. Fibroblasts help in wound healing and inflammatory process. They play an important role in repair and development. They elaborate collagen, reticular, and elastic fibers, and also the glycoproteins such as fibronectin and proteoglycans. Collagen and reticular fibers stain positively for glycoproteins with silver stains and periodic acid–Schiff (PAS) stain. Elastic fibers are stained by aldehyde fuchsin, resorcin fuchsin, and orcein dye.

The basement membrane, which separates the epithelium from the connective tissue, comprises type IV collagen, laminin, fibronectin, and proteoglycans.

The various cellular enzymatic reactions can be investigated by histochemistry. Most often the enzymes studied are acid and alkaline phosphatases, oxidases, dehydrogenases, esterases, and various other enzymes included in metabolic activities.

HISTOCHEMICAL TECHNIQUES

Fixation

After death, there are alterations in the tissues. Fixation maintains tissue in a life-like condition and helps to study them exactly in the same way as they were in the living state. Fixation of the tissue prevents autolysis and putrefaction. Fixatives decrease the various changes that happen to the cytoplasmic and extracellular macromolecules. These macromolecules include enzymes, structural protein–carbohydrate complexes, lipids and nucleic acids as well.

10% formalin solution buffered to pH 7 is usually used as fixative. This is considered as an ideal fixative. Formaldehyde reacts with major reactive groups of proteins and forms polymeric or macromolecular networks, without affecting their native reactivity to histochemical procedures. Other aldehydes, which are commonly used are acrolein and glutaraldehyde. Glutaraldehyde is routinely used for electron microscopy. Though minimally used in early days, permanganate commonly known as potassium permanganate has been used as a fixative for Electron Microscopy. Tissue density was known to be thick and increased in contrast when fixed with permanganate ions and fine structures were also preserved. Osmium tetroxide was compared and studied among all cytological fixatives used then, for electron microscopy.

Various other fixatives are used for visualizing various other components. *Rossman's fluid* is composed of formaldehyde, picric acid, and acetic acid. Visualization of glycogen, glycoprotein, and proteoglycan is made with Rossman's fluid. *Carnoy's mixture* is composed of ethyl alcohol, acetic acid, and chloroform. Nucleic acids are better visualized with Carnoy's mixture.

If the first or the primary fixation is not effective, it should be supplemented with another fixative to get better staining quality. This is known as secondary or post-fixation. Imidazole buffered osmium tetrachloride is a post-fixative and helps in localizing the lipids rich in unsaturated fatty acids.

Uranyl acetate, a post-fixative is used to preserve the phospholipid membrane and dehydration with acetone minimizes the extraction of phospholipids.

In *frozen sections*, the tissue is frozen and cut into sections for rapid histopathological analysis **(Figure 22-1)**. Cytochrome oxidases are highly labile and not preserved by chemical fixation. Therefore, these are visualized on fresh frozen sections. Freeze drying is done to preserve the *in vivo* status and to prevent diffusion of tissue macromolecules. Freeze dried tissues embedded in glycol methacrylate resin without fixation at lower temperature that ranges from 4–2°C provides better results for enzyme demonstration.

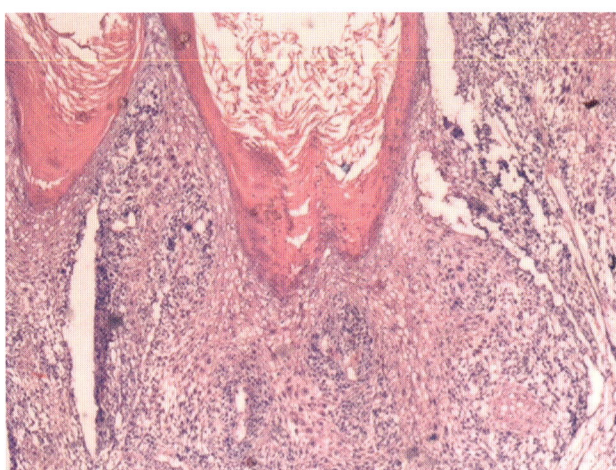

Figure 22-1: Hematoxylin and eosin 20x. A tissue processed as frozen section showing hyperplastic squamous epithelium.

For cerium, lead-based technique of enzyme demonstration Nakan's periodate-lysine-paraformaldehyde and periodate-lysine-glutaraldehyde are found to be superior than classical glutaraldehyde–paraformaldehyde double fixation procedure.

Freeze fracture and freeze-etching technique gives excellent three-dimensional images of the surface of various cell membranes as chemicals are not used in these procedures.

Studying the hard tissue involves careful fixation and decalcification (removal of minerals to make these tissues soft). Formaldehyde or glutaraldehyde and EDTA serve to perform these two steps together.

SPECIFIC HISTOCHEMICAL METHODS

These can be classified into three groups:
1. Glycogen, glycoprotein, and proteoglycan methods
2. Protein and lipid methods
3. Enzyme methods.

Glycogen, Glycoprotein, and Proteoglycan

Periodic acid–Schiff technique is the best known technique for detection of carbohydrate macromolecules (glycogen, glycoproteins, and proteoglycans) **(Figures 22-2A and B)**. Firstly, the periodic acid oxidizes the glycol groups and one of the byproducts is aldehyde. This is demonstrated with Schiff's reagent or leukofuchsin. PAS-positive substance appears as purple–magenta color. A suitable basic stain is used as a counterstain. A substitute for Schiff reagent is anthracene-9-carboxaldehyde carbohydrazide fluorescent reagent.

Periodic acid–Schiff stain may be used in combination with an enzyme called diastase, which breaks down glycogen. Presence of glycogen can be confirmed on a section of tissue by using diastase to digest the glycogen, then comparing a diastase-digested PAS section with a normal PAS section.

Proteoglycans are demonstrated by thiazine dyes like toluidine blue, azure A, and Alcian blue **(Figures 22-3A and B)**

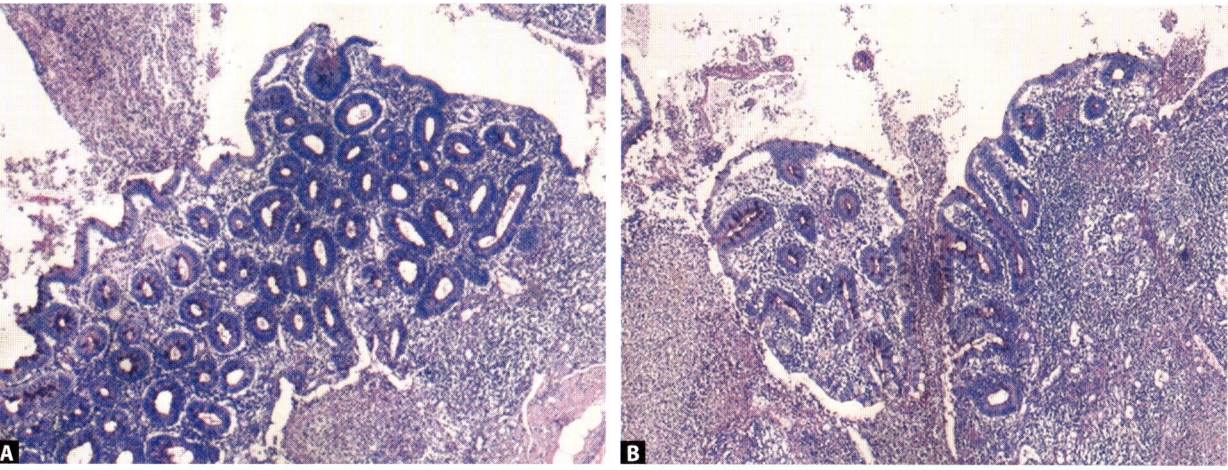

Figures 22-2A and B: Periodic acid–Schiff stain exhibits the presence of mucin in epithelial cells.

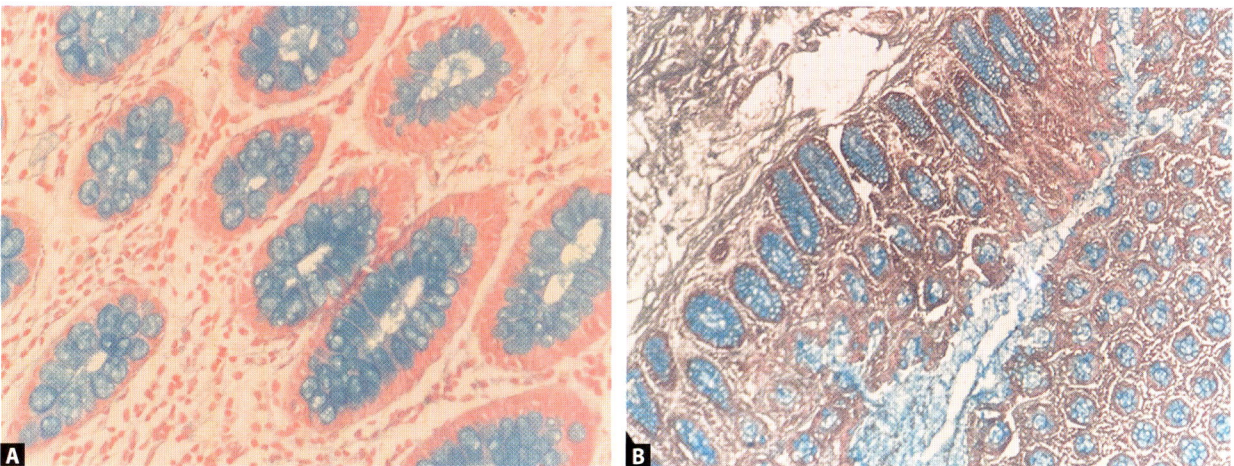

Figures 22-3 A and B: Alcian blue-stained section.

Localization of proteoglycans is done by cationic dyes like:
- Ruthenium red
- Silver tetraphenylporphine sulfonate
- Bismuth nitrate
- Cuprolinic blue.

High-iron diamine thiocarbohydrazide-silver proteinate (HID-TCH-SP) method of Spicer is used for localization of sulfated glycoconjugates. Ruthenium hexamine trichloride is used for the detection of anionic groups of proteoglycans and glycolipids.

Proteins

Various amino acid groups like amino, imine, carboxyl, disulfide, and sulfhydryl groups react to elicit the histochemistry of proteins.

Reagents used for protein histochemistry:
- Dinitrofluorobenzene (DNFB)
- Ninhydrin
- Ferric ferricyanide

Lipids

Lipid dissolves in routine fixation with formalin. So, frozen or freeze-dried sections are needed to study its histochemistry.

Histochemistry of lipids	
Total lipids	Sudan dyes
Phospholipids	Sudan black
Ultrahistochemical reaction of phospholipid	Iodoplatinate
Phosphatidyl serine and sphingomyelin	Malachite green-aldehyde

Enzymes

Enzymes like phosphatases are demonstrated by popular methods like:
- Gomori method
- Coupling azo dye technique
- Wachstein and Meisel's method for glucose-6- phosphatase enzyme.

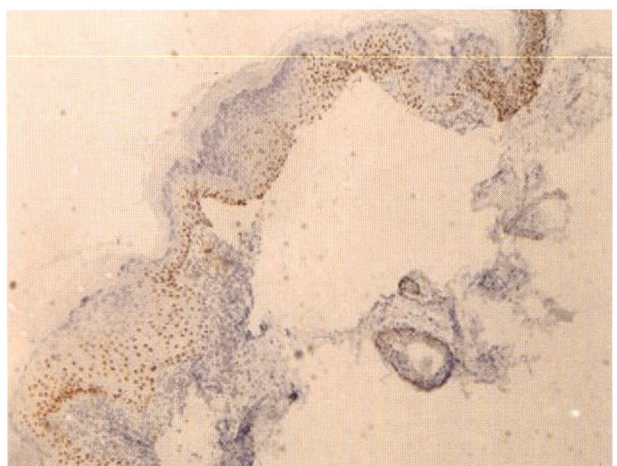

Figure 22-4: Immunohistochemistry—P63 highlights the basal layer of squamous epithelium.

IMMUNOHISTOCHEMISTRY

Paul Ehrlich in 1897 proposed his theory of antigen and antibody interaction. His hypothesis was based on binding of cell surface receptors to toxins in a lock and key type of interaction. This mechanism serves as a trigger for antibodies formation.

Immunohistochemistry combines histological, immunological, and biochemical techniques for the identification of specific tissue components by means of specific antigen or antibody reaction tagged with a visible label. This technique is based on the principle of antibodies binding specifically to antigens in biological tissues.

Immunohistochemistry is widely used in the basic research to visualize the distribution and localization of specific cellular components or biomarkers within a cell or time **(Figure 22-4)**. Apart from that, it has application in diagnosis by typing the cells present in tumors.

HISTOCHEMISTRY OF ORAL HARD TISSUES

Carbohydrates

The ground substance of teeth and bone is best visualized in PAS stain. Developing or resorbing bone and dentin exhibit intense reaction in PAS staining method, whereas ground substance of normal mature bone and dentin do not.

When dentin matrix is less calcified like in interglobular dentin, dentinogenesis imperfecta, and odontome, there is intense reactivity with the PAS stain. When enamel is visualized with PAS, enamel lamellae take the stain but enamel matrix is nonreactive.

Protein

Protein histochemical reactions are visualized intensely in proteins of dentin undergoing decay and in developmental stages of tooth formation. Amino acid groups like amino, carboxyl, or sulfhydryl are identified by specific protein methods.

Dinitrofluorobenzene and ninhydrin–Schiff are of interest in studying teeth and bone.

Dinitrofluorobenzene reagent reacts with α-amino groups of proteins and forms a pale yellow complex. Subsequently, an intense reddish color is formed by reduction and diazotization technique, resulting in formation of azo dye.

Lipids

There is a low lipid content in mature dentin but enamel rod sheath and odontoblastic process have high phospholipid content, hence they are Sudanophilic.

Sudanophilia depends on the solubility of Sudan dyes with lipids. During tooth development, Sudan dye is seen in zone of mineralization and predentin and in the basal zone of the ameloblasts. The role of phospholipids in the process of mineralizing dentin and enamel matrix is looked upon here.

Enzymes

Enzymes associated with teeth and bones include the following:
- Alkaline phosphatase
- Acid phosphatase
- Amino peptidase
- Cytochrome oxidase
- Succinic dehydrogenase

Fresh frozen sections are required for most of the enzyme histochemical techniques.

Alkaline Phosphatase

This enzyme is associated with mineralization and hence its activity is seen in endosteum, periosteum, osteocytes, stratum intermedium, odontoblasts adjoining Korff fibers, and ground substance of developing molars and incisors. Osteoblasts and preosteoblasts show alkaline phosphatase activity, so it is considered as a cytochemical marker in differentiating fibroblasts and preosteoblasts.

Acid Phosphatase

This enzyme is localized in lysosomes of a cell. Acid phosphatase activity is seen in osteoclasts of bone and odontoclasts of resorbing tooth.

HISTOCHEMISTRY OF ORAL SOFT TISSUES

Carbohydrates

The commonly used stain for glycogen, proteoglycans, and glycoproteins is PAS. Salivary mucins are identified by mucicarmine stain **(Figure 22-5)**.

Lipids

Frozen sections are used to study lipid histochemistry. Commonly used stains are:
❖ Sudan black
❖ Oil Red O.

Proteins

In oral epithelium, masticatory mucosa shows keratinization normally. Pathologically, it can occur anywhere in the mouth.

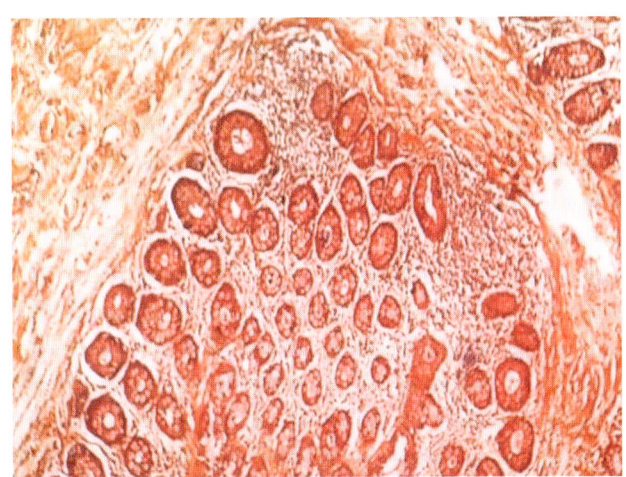

Figure 22-5: Mucicarmine-stained section.

Degree of keratinization can be analyzed by ferric ferricyanide method.

Enzymes

Alkaline Phosphatase

In human gingiva, the capillary endothelium of lamina propria shows alkaline phosphatase activity and so does basement membranes of salivary gland acini.

Acid Phosphatase

This enzymatic activity is high in the zone of keratinization and low in nonkeratinized areas.

Certain other enzymes exhibit low activity in human oral mucosa; however, they can be of significance in specific cases. Enzymes and their localization are listed in **Table 22-1**.

Angiogenic Factor

A 67 kDa protein, an angiogenic factor, was found in macrophages of inflamed gingival tissue and inflamed tissue of rheumatoid origin.

TABLE 22-1: Enzymes and localization.

Enzymes	Reactivity noted
Esterases	♦ Superficial layers of gingiva ♦ Salivary gland ducts ♦ Serous demilunes of sublingual gland
Aminopeptidase	♦ Basal layers of epithelium and connective tissue of gingiva ♦ Salivary gland ducts
β-glucuronidase	♦ Basal layers of oral epithelium
Cytochrome oxidase	♦ Basal layer of free and attached gingiva ♦ Crevicular epithelium and epithelial attachment ♦ Chronic gingivitis ♦ Salivary duct system
Succinate dehydrogenase	♦ Basal cells of gingival epithelium ♦ Salivary ducts ♦ Malignant lesions of oral mucosa

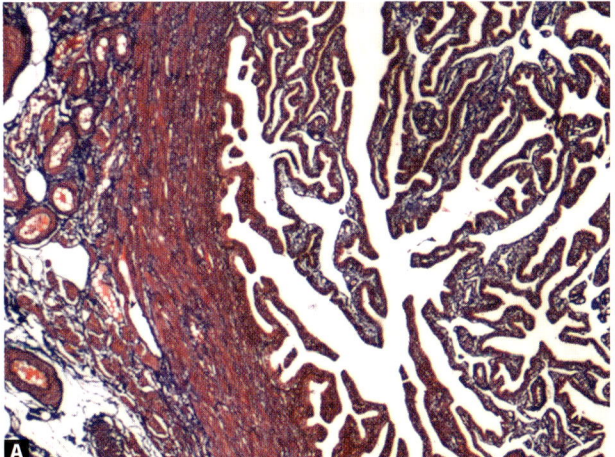

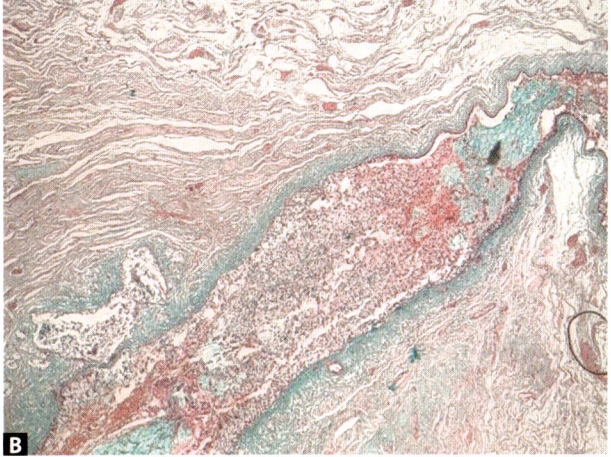

Figures 22-6A and B: Masson's trichrome showing muscle stained in red and collagen in blue.

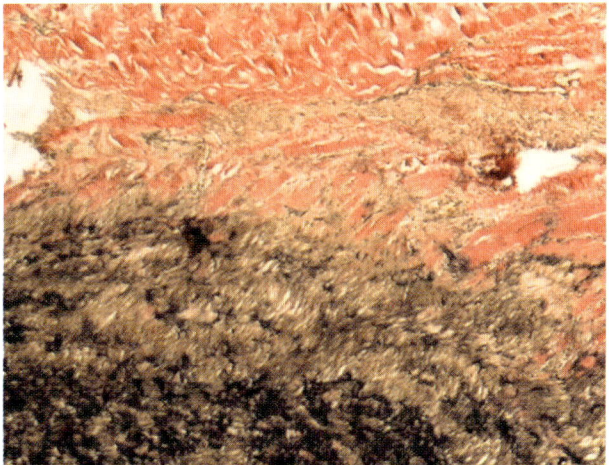

Figure 22-7: Verhoeff–van Gieson stain showing elastin stained in black and collagen in red.

Based on pore size and permeability, differentiation is made between connective tissue components like collagen and muscle. In Masson's trichrome **(Figures 22-6A and B)**, muscle stains red and collagen stains green or blue and in Verhoeff- van Gieson **(Figure 22-7)** elastin stains black, collagen stains red, while muscle stains yellow color.

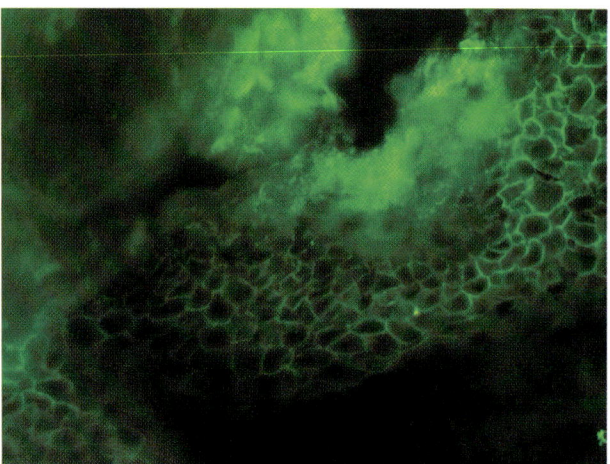

Figure 22-8: Immunofluorescence demonstrating IgG positivity in fishnet pattern of epidermis.

ADVANCED TECHNIQUES

Immunofluorescence

Immunofluorescence is a traditional laboratory technique that uses fluorescent dyes to identify the presence of antibodies bound to specific antigens. It requires a fluorescence microscope, which uses ultraviolet light to visualize.

This helps in detection of biomolecules, antigens, cytoplasmic fibers, and nuclei. It allows visualization of antigen and specific proteins in tissue sections by binding antibody chemically conjugated with a fluorescent dye. These labeled antibodies bind directly or indirectly to cellular antigens.

This technique can be used on tissue sections, cultured cell lines, or individual cells, and may be used to analyze the distribution of proteins, glycans, and other small biological and nonbiological molecules.

The specific antibodies are labeled with a compound that makes them glow an apple green color when observed microscopically under ultraviolet light. It is a standard technique for detection of antibodies **(Figure 22-8)**.

In Situ Hybridization

In situ hybridization (ISH) is a method by which the location of specific nucleic acid targets present in fixed tissue samples is identified. It uses a DNA or RNA probe to detect complementary genetic material in cells or tissues. ISH involves hybridizing a labeled nucleic acid to suitably prepared cells or tissues on microscope slides to allow visualization *in situ*.

Principle of this technique: When a double-stranded DNA is denatured by heating, it becomes single-stranded DNA. It is known as annealing. On cooling, the single-stranded DNA with its complementary sequence becomes double-stranded DNA (reannealing). If a labeled DNA fragment (a DNA probe) is denatured and added to denatured nuclei or chromosomes on a routine, air-dried interphase preparation during reannealing, some of the labeled DNA will hybridize to its complementary sequence in the chromosomal DNA.

Detection of the labeled DNA probe under the microscope identifies the site of hybridization and thus the region of chromosomal DNA complementary to the DNA sequence in the labeled probe.

In situ hybridization provides knowledge about how protein product of target gene is related to the distribution of specific nucleic acid. It helps in mastering wide areas of research such as gene mapping, viral infection, cytogenetics, gene expression, and prenatal diagnosis. The hybridization can be detected by fluorescent dyes in *fluorescent in situ hybridization* (FISH) or with enzymatic probes like in immunoperoxidase or with radioisotope molecules like P_{32}, H_3 or S_{35}.

Polymerase Chain Reaction

Polymerase chain reaction (PCR) is also called molecular photocopying and is used to make numerous copies of a specific segment of DNA quickly and accurately. It is an enzymatic process in which a specific region of DNA is replicated over and over again to yield many copies of a particular sequence. PCR is an inexpensive, fast, and sensitive technique. It enables amplification of tiny amount of DNA into million copies.

This procedure involves first heating the given sample containing the DNA, which denatures the DNA, or separates into two pieces of single-stranded DNA. Next, using the original strands as templates, an enzyme called "Taq polymerase" synthesizes or builds two new strands of DNA. This process results in the duplication of the original DNA, with each of the new molecules containing one old and one new strand of DNA.

Polymerase chain reaction is routinely used in DNA cloning, medical diagnostics, and forensic analysis of DNA. This technique has undergone multiple advancements like pathogens and novel genes identification and nucleotide sequence quantification. It also helps to provide a deep vision into the complicated part of single cells **(Figures 22-9A to C)**.

In real-time PCR, also denoted as quantitative PCR—qPCR (the usage of RT-PCR is inappropriate as this abbreviation is dedicated to reverse transcription PCR), fluorescence is measured after each cycle and the intensity of the fluorescent signal reflects the momentary amount of DNA amplicons (a piece of DNA or RNA) in the sample at that specific time.

Enzyme-linked Immunosorbent Assay

Enzyme-linked immunosorbent assay (ELISA), is a plate-based assay technique designed for detecting and quantifying substances such as peptides, proteins, antibodies and hormones. It is a simple, versatile, sensitive, and quantitative technique. In this technique, an antigen is immobilized on a solid surface and then complexed with an antibody that is linked to an enzyme. This antigen–antibody complex is detected by assessing the conjugated enzyme activity via incubation with a substrate to produce a measureable product. A colored reaction measurable end product results when a substrate is added **(Figures 22-10 A to C)**.

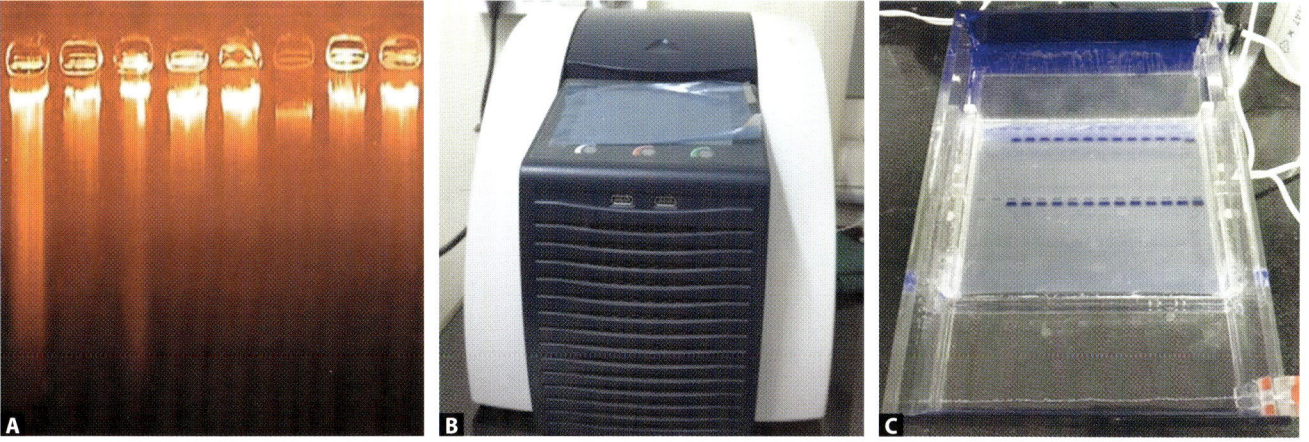

Figures 22-9 A to C: Human genomic DNA isolation in polymerase chain reaction.

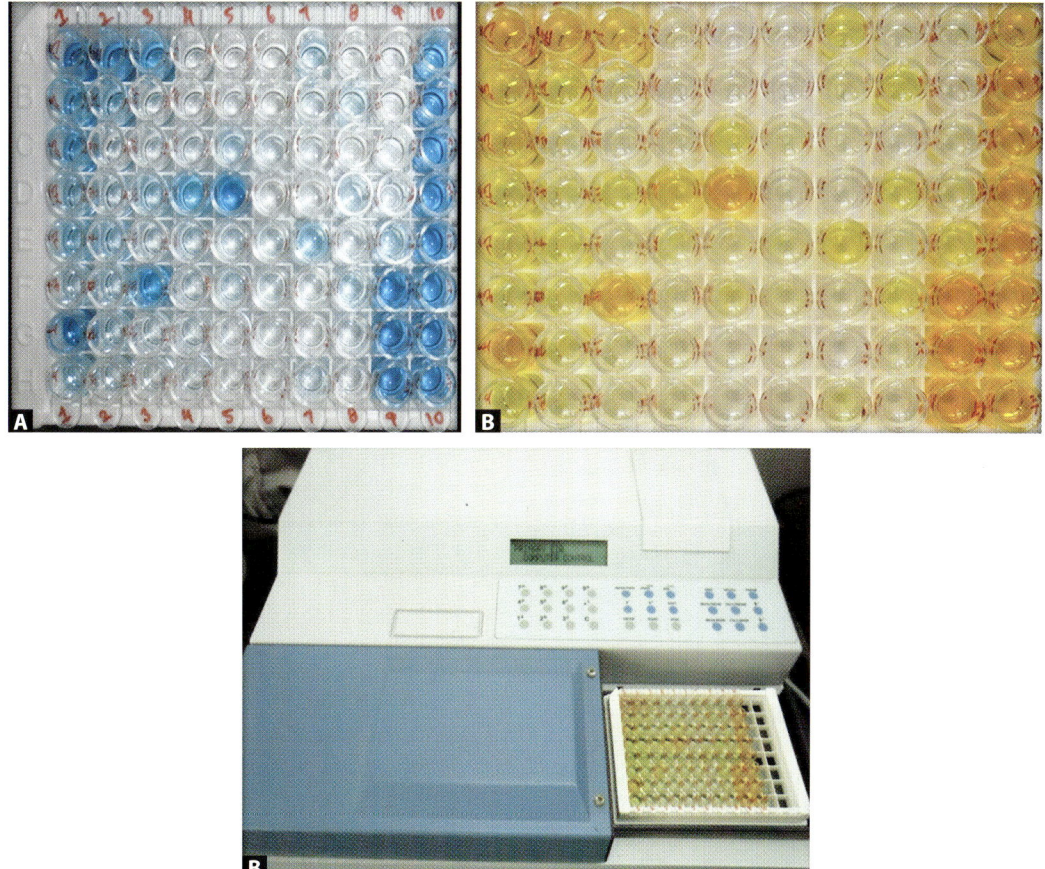

Figures 22-10A to C: (A and B) Enzyme-linked immunosorbent assay plates; (C) Enzyme-linked immunosorbent assay reader.

The application of ELISA ranges from basic research to diagnosis.

Confocal Microscopy

Confocal microscope combines the technologies of laser, computer, and microelectronics. This technique increases the optical resolution and contrast of a micrograph by means of using a spatial pinhole to block out-of-focus light in image formation. Light travels through the sample under a conventional microscope as far into the specimen as it can penetrate, while a confocal microscope only focuses a smaller beam of light at one narrow depth level at a time. It filters the out-of-focus light from above and below the point of focus in the object. It helps in viewing three-dimensional images with better contrast and less haziness. The advantages

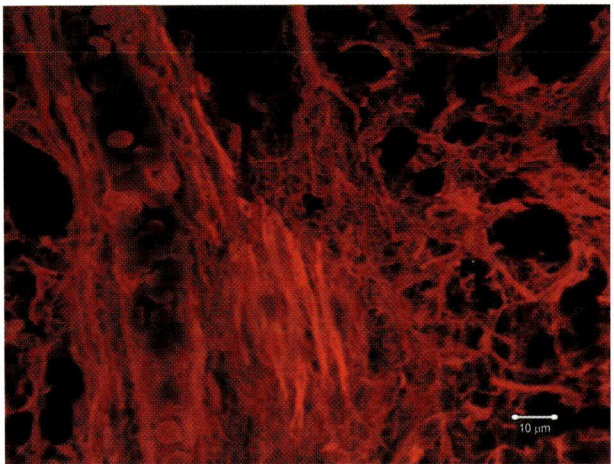

Figure 22-11: Confocal microscopy showing pulp tissue with collagen fibers, blood capillaries and RBCs within the lumen.
Source: Dr N Malathi, Department of Oral Pathology, Sri Ramachandra Dental College, Chennai, India; Dr J Logeswari, Meenakshi Ammal Dental College, Chennai, India.

include shallow depth of field, elimination of out-of-focus glare, and the ability to collect serial optical sections from thick specimens. Both fixed and living cells and tissues that have usually been labeled with one or more fluorescent probes can be imaged in confocal microscopy **(Figure 22-11)**. It also allows examination of fluorescent-labeled thick specimens without physical sectioning.

Flow Cytometry

Flow cytometry is a laser-based technology employed in cell sorting, cell counting, biomarker detection, and protein engineering. It involves suspending the cells in a stream of fluid and passing them through an electronic detection apparatus. This technology allows simultaneous multiparametric analysis of the physical and chemical characteristics of up to thousands of particles per second. Flow cytometry is used in the diagnosis of many diseases. It also has applications in basic research, clinical practice and clinical trials.

Linking the analytical capability of the flow cytometer to a sorting device to physically separate and thereby purify particles of interest based on their optical properties is called cell sorting. The instrument used for this purpose is termed a "cell sorter".

Immunophenotyping through flow cytometry is used to assess CD4T cells, lymphoid, and myeloid neoplasms. It is technique-sensitive and can detect immunophenotype of cells in a specimen with thousand cells. It can also analyze the DNA content of cells.

Radioautographic Techniques

An *autoradiograph* is an image on an X-ray film produced by the radioactive substance present within the tissue. In biology, this technique is used to determine the tissue (or cell) localization of a radioactive substance, either introduced into a metabolic pathway bound to a receptor or enzyme, or hybridized to a nucleic acid.

Standard techniques for radioautography used in biological and medical research can be classified into three categories, *i.e.*, macroscopic radioautography, light microscopic radioautography, and electron microscopic radioautography. These techniques involve: (i) chemical fixation followed by wet-mounting radioautography, which has limited application to only insoluble compounds and (ii) cryofixation followed by dry-mounting radioautography, which is applicable in any kind of compound including soluble compounds.

Wet-mounting radioautography demonstrates insoluble macromolecular synthesis such as nucleic acids, proteins, glucides and lipids. Dry-mounting radioautography demonstrates soluble small molecular compounds such as macromolecular precursors, hormones, neurotransmitters, vitamins, inorganic compounds and drugs or toxins. These procedures are applied for evaluating the various inorganic and organic compounds in living organisms and to elucidate the sites of their incorporation, synthesis, and discharge.

CLINICAL CONSIDERATIONS

There is a definite need for histochemistry to diagnose pathologies arising in oral cavity. Treatment varies for pathologies based on their diagnosis and histochemical stains help in leading to the specific diagnosis. We need histochemical stains for identifying tumors based on their origin and content. For example, lipoma or liposarcoma arise from fat cells and revelation of lipids is needed for its diagnosis. Histochemistry is applied in identifying the nature of the tumor based on its origin, whether from epithelial, or lymphoid tissues or from any other mesenchymal components. Tumor markers aid in accurate identification of tumor based on its tissue of origin.

Recent techniques like PCR and FISH help in identifying chromosomal aberrations and gene products associated with any pathology. ELISA helps in identifying the presence of an antigen in a sample.

With emergence of the pandemic COVID 19, the RT – PCR technique ballooned to an enormous number in detecting viruses, thereby increasing its significance in research as there is capability of the technique to amplify a specific fragment of the nucleic acid.

Detection of important clinical and veterinary viruses using culture methods is time-consuming or impossible, while ELISA tests are not universally available and suffer from comparatively low sensitivity and specificity. Sensitivity and specificity are accurate in qPCR with the inclusion of reverse transcription for the diagnostics of RNA. Moreover, determination of the viral load by (RT)-qPCR is used as an indicator of the response to antiviral therapies. For these reasons (RT)-qPCR has become an indispensable tool in virus diagnostics.

Microbial infections need special stains to identify specific organisms thereby paving way for accurate diagnosis, which helps in appropriate treatment and also avoiding unnecessary antibiotic intake by the patient.

CHAPTER 22: Histochemistry of Oral Tissues

Points to Remember

- Histochemistry deals with the identification and distribution of biochemical substances in the cells and tissues by means of specialized stains under microscope. It combines the techniques of biochemistry and histology.
- Position and distribution of substances like carbohydrates, lipids, nucleic acids, proteins, enzymes, pigments, and minerals present in a tissue is identified.
- There are subcategories in histochemistry like enzyme histochemistry, immunohistochemistry, cytochemistry, and *in situ* hybridization.
- The chemical constituents involved in the oral tissues are:
  - Proteoglycans
  - Lipoproteins
  - Proteins
  - Lipids
  - Enzymes
- Superficial epithelial cells contain glycogen, proteins and carbohydrates whereas lining and glandular epithelium contains mucin or mucoid material.
- Connective tissue is a filler substance between cells and fibers in which ground substance comprises an amorphous gel into which they are embedded.
- *Proteoglycans and glycoproteins are the main components of the ground substance.*
- The sulfated forms of proteoglycans are chondroitin sulfates, keratan sulfates, and heparan sulfates whereas the nonsulfated proteoglycan is hyaluronic acid.
- *Glycoprotein* is a type of protein molecule that has a carbohydrate covalently attached to it.
- Fibronectin, laminin, chondronectin, and osteonectin are some of the well-known glycoproteins
- Fixation maintains tissue in a life-like condition and helps to study them exactly in the same way as they were in the living body preventing autolysis and putrefaction
- A 10% formalin solution buffered to pH 7 is usually used as fixative. Glutaraldehyde is routinely used for electron microscopy.
- Periodic acid–Schiff technique is the best-known technique for detection of carbohydrate macromolecules like glycogen, glycoproteins, and proteoglycans.
- Various amino acid groups like amino, imine, carboxyl, disulfide, and sulfhydryl groups react to elicit the histochemistry of proteins
- Lipid dissolves in routine fixation with formalin. Frozen or freeze-dried sections are needed to study histochemistry of lipids.
- Enzymes like phosphatases are demonstrated by popular methods like Gomori method and coupling azo dye technique.
- Immunohistochemistry is a technique based on the principle of antibodies binding specifically to antigens in biological tissues.
- The ground substance of teeth and bone is best visualized in PAS stain.
- Alkaline phosphatase is present in osteoblasts whereas acid phosphatase is present in osteoclasts and odontoclast cells.
- Most commonly mucins can be identified by mucicarmine, lipids by sudan black and ferric ferricyanide stains for proteins.
- Recent techniques like PCR and FISH help in identifying chromosomal aberrations and gene products associated with any pathology.
- ELISA helps in identifying the presence of an antigen in a sample.

PRACTICE QUESTIONS

1. What is histochemistry, name some advanced techniques used for clinical applications and research.
2. What is fixation? And discuss the various fixatives and their applications.
3. Name the different oral tissues and the chemical constituents present in them.
4. What are the histochemical components of oral hard tissues and mention the stains used for identifying them?
5. What are the histochemical components of oral soft tissues and mention the stains used for identifying them?
6. Mention few clinical applications of histochemistry in diagnosing oral pathologies.

MULTIPLE CHOICE QUESTIONS

1. **Ground substance of the connective tissue is composed of the following features, *except*:**
   a. It is amorphous in nature
   b. It is noncolloidal
   c. It contains proteoglycans and glycoproteins
   d. It helps in adhesion and signaling events
2. **Which of the following is not true about laminin?**
   a. It is a proteoglycan
   b. It is secreted by the epithelial cells
   c. It is present in the basement membrane
   d. It is a glycoprotein
3. **One of the following is a non-sulfated proteoglycan:**
   a. Chondroitin sulfates
   b. Keratan sulfates
   c. Heparan sulfates
   d. Hyaluronic acid
4. **Carnoy's mixture is composed of:**
   a. Ethyl alcohol
   b. Chloroform
   c. Acetic acid
   d. All of the above
5. **Schiff's reagent is:**
   a. Leukofuchsin
   b. Formaldehyde
   c. Glutaraldehyde
   d. Acrolein

6. Rossman's fluid is used to visualize:
   a. Glycoprotein
   b. Glycogen
   c. Proteoglycan
   d. All of the above
7. Freeze-dried specimens are preferred, as formalin fixation dissolves:
   a. Glycogen
   b. Proteins
   c. Lipids
   d. Enzymes
8. Periodic acid-Schiff is used to detect:
   a. Carbohydrates
   b. Lipids
   c. Proteins
   d. None of the above
9. All of the following are used to detect proteins, *except:*
   a. Ninhydrin
   b. Ferric ferricyanide
   c. Dinitrofluorobenzene
   d. Azure A
10. Gomori method is used to detect:
    a. Phosphatases
    b. Lectins
    c. Glycolipids
    d. Proteins
11. PAS recognizes:
    a. Acidic mucins
    b. Basic mucins
    c. Neutral mucins
    d. All of the above
12. Fibronectin, laminin, Chondronectin, and osteonectin are some of the well-known:
    a. Non sulfated proteoglycans
    b. Sulfated proteoglycans
    c. Glycoproteins
    d. Lipids
13. Alkaline phosphatase activity is seen in:
    a. Osteoclasts
    b. Osteoblasts
    c. Odontoclasts
    d. Predentin
14. Sudan Black is commonly used to stain:
    a. Carbohydrates
    b. Lipids
    c. Proteins
    d. Enzymes
15. Basal layers of oral epithelium shows reaction for the following enzyme:
    a. β-glucuronidase
    b. Cytochrome oxidase
    c. Succinate dehydrogenase
    d. Aminopeptidase
16. Masson's trichome stains muscle in:
    a. Red
    b. Blue
    c. Green
    d. Yellow
17. Fluorescent microscope uses:
    a. Visible light
    b. Ultraviolet light
    c. Halogen light
    d. LED
18. The microscopy which uses laser, computer and microelectronics is:
    a. Dark field microscopy
    b. Light microscopy
    c. Confocal microscopy
    d. Stereomicroscopy
19. Numerous copies made from a specific DNA segment is done by:
    a. ELISA
    b. PCR
    c. *In situ* hybridization
    d. Flow cytometry
20. Glucose-6-phosphatase enzyme is demonstrated by:
    a. Wachstein and Meisel's method
    b. Gomori method
    c. Coupling azo dye technique
    d. Nakan's periodate-lysine-paraformaldehyde

ANSWERS

1. b   2. a   3. d   4. d   5. a   6. d   7. c   8. a   9. d   10. a   11. c   12. c   13. b   14. b   15. a
16. a   17. b   18. c   19. b   20. a

BIBLIOGRAPHY

1. Avery JK. Oral Development and Histology, 3rd edition. Thieme: New York; 2002.
2. Bancroft JD, Gamble M. Theory and Practice of Histological Techniques, 5th edition. Edinburgh: Churchill Livingstone Elsevier; 2002.
3. Battifora H. Recent progress in the immunohistochemistry of solid tumors. Semin Diag Pathol. 1984;1:251-71.
4. Beeks JS, Anderson JM. Quantitative methods as an aid to diagnosis in histopathology. Rec Adv Histopathology. 1987;1:255-69.
5. Berkovitz BKB, Holland GR, Moxham BJ. Oral Anatomy, Histology and Embryology, 4th edition. US: Elsevier; 2009.
6. Black C, Allan I, Ford SK, et al. Biofilm specific properties and protein expression in oral Streptococcus sanguis. Arch Oral Biol. 2004;49(4):295.
7. Chandra S, Chandra S, Chandra M, et al. Textbook of Dental and Oral Histology with Embryology & MCQ's, 2nd edition. India: Jaypee Brothers Medical Publishers (P) Ltd; 2010.
8. Cheng H, Caterson B, Yamauchi M. Identification and localization of chondroitin sulphate proteoglycans in tooth cementum. Connect Tissue Res. 1999;40(1):37-47.

9. Culling CFA. Handbook of Histopathological and Histochemical Techniques, 3rd edition. London: Butterworth & Co; 1974.
10. Didonato D, Brasaemle DL. Fixation methods for the study of lipid droplets by immunofluorescence and microscope. Histochem Cytochem. 2003;51(6):773.
11. Edelmann L. Freeze-dried and resin-embedded biological material is well suited for ultrastructure research. J Microsc. 2002;207:5-26.
12. Edelmann L. Freeze-dried and resin-embedded biological material is well suited for ultrastructure research. J Microsc. 2002;207:5-26.
13. Elias JM. Immunohistochemical method. In: Elias JM (Ed). Immunohistology: A Practical Approach to Diagnosis. Chicago: ASCP press; 1990.
14. Enns RK. DNA probes. An overview and comparison with current methods. Lab Med. 1988;19:295-300.
15. Hofler H. What's new in "In situ hybridisation". Pathol Res Pract. 1985;182:421-30.
16. Immunohistochemistry: Basics and Methods by Igor B. Buchwalow, Werner Böcker, 2010
17. Jahanshahi G, Shirani S. Detection of Candida albicans in oral squamous cell carcinoma by fluorescence staining technique. Dent Res J Isfahan. 2015;12(2):115-20.
18. Joshi SR, Mohanty S, Shaw AC. Multicolor digital flow cytometry in human translational immunology. Methods Mol Biol. 2015;1343:53-64.
19. Kralik P, Ricchi M. A Basic Guide to Real Time PCR in Microbial Diagnostics: Definitions, Parameters, and Everything. Front. Microbiol, 2017 8:108. doi: 10.3389/fmicb.2017.00108
20. Kumar GS. Orban's Oral Histology and Embryology, 12th edition. New Delhi: Elsevier India; 2009.
21. Kurec A. Flow cytometry: principles and practices. Med Lab Obs. 2014;46(5):28, 30-1.
22. Lin AV. Indirect ELISA. Methods Mol Biol. 2015;1318:51-9.
23. Luft JH. Permanganate—a new fixative for electron microscopy. The Journal of biophysical and biochemical cytology. 1956 Nov 25;2(6):799.
24. Luzardo-Baptista MJ, García-Tamayo J. Acid phosphatase activity in the small granules of epithelial cells in normal human oral mucosa. Parodontologie. 1971;25(2):49-55.
25. Murray GI, Ewen SW. Enzyme histochemistry on freeze substituted, glycol methacrylate embedded tissue. J Histochem Cytochem. 1990;38(1):95.
26. Nagata T. Techniques and application of microscopic radioautography. Histol Histopathol. 1997;12(4):1091-124.
27. Nagata T. Techniques of radioautography for medical and biological research. Braz J Med Biol Res. 1988;31(2):185-95.
28. Nollau P, Wolters-Eisfeld G, Mortezai N, et al. Protein domain histochemistry (PDH): binding of the carbohydrate recognition domain (CRD) of recombinant human glycoreceptor CLEC10A CD301 to formalin-fixed, paraffin-embedded breast cancer tissues. J Histochem Cytochem. 2013; 61(3):199-205.
29. Nozaka Y. [Anatomical studies of the gingiva. 4. Histochemistry of the connective tissue]. Shikwa Gakuho, 1972;72(2):115-37.
30. Orakzai GS, Waqar-Un-Nisa, Orakzai SH. Oral white lesions— histomorphological assessment and associated risk factors. J Ayub Med Coll Abbottabad. 2015;27(4):865-8.
31. Ragazzi M, Piana S, Longo C, et al. Fluorescence confocal microscopy for pathologists., Mod Pathol. 2014;27(3):460-71.
32. Winckler J. The application of histological and histochemical techniques to freeze-dried cryostat sections. Histochemie. 1970;24(2):168-86.

Appendices

Appendix 1 — Oral Tissues: A Brief Description

Sabarinath B, Preethi S, Manoj Prabhakar, B Sivapathasundharam

Chapter Outline

- Comparison of Hard Tissues 335
- Comparison of Hard Tissue Forming Cells 336
- Comparison of Oral Mucosa 336
- Comparison of Papillae of the Tongue 337
- Comparison of Serous and Mucous Acini 337
- Comparison of Major Salivary Glands 338
- Classification of Cementum 338
- Summary of Molecular Interplay in Tooth Development 338
- Timeline of Tooth Eruption 339
- Differences Between Deciduous and Permanent Dentition 340
- Effects of Aging on Oral and Circumoral Tissues 340
- Abbreviations and Expansions 341
- Glossary 343

COMPARISON OF HARD TISSUES

Features	Enamel	Dentin	Cementum	Bone
Term for formation	Amelogenesis	Dentinogenesis	Cementogenesis	Osteogenesis
Forming cells	Ameloblasts	Odontoblasts	Cementoblasts	Osteoblasts
Derived from	Ectoderm	Ectomesenchyme	Ectomesenchyme	Ectomesenchyme/Mesoderm
Period of formation	During tooth development	Throughout life	Throughout life	Throughout life
Resorbing cells	Odontoclasts	Odontoclasts	Cementoclasts	Osteoclasts
Inorganic content	96%	65%	45–50%	60–70%
Organic content	4%	35%	50–55%	30%
Major protein	Amelogenin	Type I collagen	Type I collagen	Type I collagen
Structural unit	Enamel rods	Dentinal tubules with odontoblastic processes	Acellular extrinsic fiber cementum / Cellular cementum	Osteon or Haversian system
Incremental lines	Lines of Retzius	von Ebner lines	Salter's lines	Resting lines
Reversal lines	Absent	Absent	Present	Present
Resting cells	Absent	Questionable	Cementocytes	Osteocytes
Unmineralized matrix	No specific name	Predentin	Cementoid	Osteoid
Vascularity	Avascular	Avascular	Avascular	Vascular
Innervation	Non-innervated	Innervated	Non-innervated	Innervated
Remodeling	Absent	Minimal	Minimal	Present
Repair	No reparative capacity	Forms reparative dentin	Anatomic and functional repair	Able to repair

Contd...

Contd...

Features	Enamel	Dentin	Cementum	Bone
Types	• Prismatic enamel • Aprismatic enamel	• Primary • Secondary • Tertiary/reparative	• Cellular • Acellular • Intrinsic fiber cementum • Extrinsic fiber cementum	• Compact bone • Cancellous bone • Woven bone
Color	Translucent (yellowish white-grayish/bluish-white)	Light yellow	Light yellow	Yellowish-white, brownish-white
Thickness	2–2.5 mm	Varying in thickness	1.5–2 mm	Varying in thickness
Hardness	Hardest and brittle	Viscoelastic Harder than bone but softer than enamel	Less harder than dentin	Less harder than dentin
Function	Protective covering for the tooth rendering them suitable for mastication	Makes the bulk of tooth	Attaches the tooth to the alveolar bone by means of PDL	Structure and support Storage site for minerals especially calcium
Age changes	• Attrition • Loss of mamelons • Increase in crystal size • Decrease in permeability • Becomes very brittle	• Turns darker in color • Continuous and gradual deposition of secondary dentin • Sclerotic dentin • Reduced permeability	• Increase in thickness • Predominance of acellular cementum	• Gradual decrease in bone formation • Fatty infiltration of marrow spaces • Osteoporosis

COMPARISON OF HARD TISSUE-FORMING CELLS

Features	Ameloblasts	Odontoblasts	Cementoblasts	Osteoblasts
Origin	Ectoderm	Ectomesenchyme	Ectomesenchyme	Ectomesenchyme/mesoderm
Primary function	Formation of enamel	Formation of dentin	Formation of cementum	Formation of bone
Organic matrix	Do not contain collagen	Contain collagen in their organic matrix	Contain collagen in their organic matrix	Contain collagen in their organic matrix
Average size of the cell	40 μm length, 4 μm diameter	40–50 μm in length, 5–10 μm in width	Ranges from 8 μm to 12 μm	Ranges from 20 μm to 30 μm
Shape of the cell	Columnar/tall columnar	Columnar/cuboidal/flat	Cuboidal/ovoid	Cuboidal/ovoid
Cytoplasmic process	Transient cytoplasmic process called Tomes' process	Odontoblastic process with branching that is enclosed within the dentinal tubules	Processes contained within the canaliculi and face toward the periodontal ligament	Processes contained within the canaliculi, face all directions and communicates with neighboring cells
Fate of the cell	After secretion of enamel, they become a part of reduced enamel epithelium and are lost after tooth eruption	Present as the peripheral layer of pulp	Some of them are entrapped in the cementum as cementocytes and remaining in the periodontal surface of the cementum as cementoblasts	Some of the osteoblasts are entrapped in the bone as osteocytes and remaining are present as osteoblasts lining the bony trabeculae

COMPARISON OF ORAL MUCOSA

Types of oral mucosa

Features	Masticatory mucosa	Lining mucosa	Specialized mucosa
Site of oral mucosa	Hard palate and gingiva	Soft palate, buccal mucosa, ventral tongue, floor of the mouth, vestibular fornix, and lips	Dorsal surface of tongue
Type of epithelium	Orthokeratinized and parakeratinized stratified squamous epithelium	Non-keratinized stratified squamous epithelium	Contains papilla that is keratinized in filiform and circumvallate papillae. Non-keratinized in other areas
Functions	Helps to withstand masticatory stress	Resilient. Adapts to the contraction and relaxation of cheeks, lips and tongue and to the movements produced by the muscles	Mastication, deglutition, speech, and taste perception

Contd...

Contd...

Features	Masticatory mucosa	Lining mucosa	Specialized mucosa
Nature of the mucosa	Tightly bound to lamina propria and inflexible	Not tightly bound to lamina propria and flexible	Tightly bound
Layers of epithelium	Stratum basale, stratum spinosum, stratum granulosum, stratum corneum	Stratum basale, stratum intermedium, stratum superficiale	Circumvallate and filiform papillae show features of keratinized epithelium, the rest show features of non-keratinized epithelium
Epithelium connective tissue interface	Long, narrow rete ridges, which sometimes is dove-tailed with one another	Epithelium is thick with short and broad rete ridges	Varies
Taste buds	Absent	Absent (may be present in the soft palate)	Present
Submucosa	Absent in the region of gingiva, mid palatine raphe. Present in lateral aspect of palate	Present	Present
Minor salivary glands	Absent in anterior hard palate and gingiva	Present	Present
Elastic fibers	Less prominent	Present	May be present
Mitotic rate of epithelium	Less	More than keratinized epithelium	Less
Cytokeratin expression	Epithelial stratification exhibits pairs of CK 5 and 14, 1 and 10, 4 and 13	CK 4, 13 and 19	Ventral surface of tongue CK 5, 6 and 14 Dorsal surface of tongue CK 7, 8, and 19

COMPARISON OF PAPILLAE OF THE TONGUE

Features	Circumvallate papilla	Fungiform papilla	Filiform papilla	Foliate papilla
Site	Anterior to sulcus terminalis	Anterior part of the dorsal portion of the tongue especially at the tip	Dorsal surface of tongue	Lateral border of posterior tongue
Shape	Large, cylindrical shaped	Mushroom shaped	Cone or hair shaped	Leaf like
Keratinization	Keratinized in superior surface, nonkeratinized along lateral wall	Nonkeratinized	Keratinized	Nonkeratinized
Taste buds	Present on the lateral wall	Present on superficial surface	Absent	Few
Number	8–12	Around 1,600	Most numerous	Few
Innervation	Lingual nerve and chorda tympani	Lingual nerve and chorda tympani	Lingual nerve and chorda tympani	Lingual nerve and chorda tympani

COMPARISON OF SEROUS AND MUCOUS ACINI

Properties	Serous acini	Mucous acini
Secretory end piece	Spherical	Tubular
Cells per acini	8–12 cells	More than eight cells
Size of lumen	Narrow	Wide
Cell shape	Pyramidal	Cuboidal or columnar
Shape of nucleus	Ovoid	Flattened
Function	Enzymatic	Lubrication
Secretory granules	Zymogen granules	Mucinogen droplets
Staining properties	Dark staining cytoplasm	Pale staining cytoplasm
Type of secretion	Thin watery	Thick mucus
Content of secretion	Protein	Mucoproteins
Cell membrane	Indistinct cell membrane	Distinct cell membrane
Apical microvilli	Present	Absent
Amylase activity	Less	More
Majorly seen in	Parotid gland	Sublingual gland

COMPARISON OF MAJOR SALIVARY GLANDS

Features	Parotid gland	Submandibular gland	Sublingual gland
Size	Largest	Intermediate	Small
Location	Anterior to the ear	Beneath the mandible, near the angle	Anterior floor of the mouth
Capsulation	Entire gland	Entire gland	Minimum
Excretory ducts	**Stensen (Parotid) duct:** Opens on the buccal mucosa opposite to the maxillary second molar	**Wharton (Submandibular) duct:** Opens on the floor of the mouth, near the lingual frenum, at sublingual caruncles	**Bartholin (Sublingual) duct:** Opens in same area as submandibular duct; smaller ducts of Rivinus also open directly along the sublingual folds.
Striated ducts	Shorter	Longer	Rare or absent
Intercalated ducts	Longer	Shorter	Absent
Terminal secretory unit (Acini)	Serous acini	Serous acini; also some mucous acini with serous demilunes	Mucous acini; also some serous demilunes
Secretory product	Purely serous	Predominantly serous (mixed)	Predominantly mucous (mixed)

CLASSIFICATION OF CEMENTUM

Type	Fibers	Composition	Cells responsible for the formation	Location	Function
Primary acellular cementum	Intrinsic	Collagen and ground substance, no cementoid	Follicle, surface cementoblasts	Cervical margin to apical third	Anchorage
	Extrinsic	PDL fiber bundles, no cementoid	PDL fibroblasts	-	
Secondary cellular cementum	Intrinsic	Collagen, ground substance, and cementoid	Bone-like cementoblasts in lacunae	Apical third and interradicular areas	Adaptation
	Mixed	Collagen, ground substance, cementoid, and PDL fiber bundles	Non-follicular	-	
Acellular afibrillar cementum	None	Only ground substance	Follicular cementoblasts	Spurs and patches on the enamel surface	No known function
Intermediate cementum	Intrinsic	PDL fiber bundles	Cementoblasts, trapped HERS cells, and odontoblasts	Near the cementodentinal junction	None

SUMMARY OF MOLECULAR INTERPLAY IN TOOTH DEVELOPMENT

Stages of odontogenesis	Genes and signalling molecules
Tooth initiation	Bmp-4, Msx-1, Fgf-4, Fgf-8 and Fgf-9
Oral aboral axis formation	Fgf-8, Lhx-6, Lhx7 and Gsc
Tooth germ positioning	Bmp-4, Pitx-2, Fgf-8, Pax-9, ActivinβA, Bmp-2
Patterning of dentition	Barx-1, Dlx-1/2, Msx-1, Msx-2 and Alx-3
Regulation of ectodermal boundaries	Shh and Wnt-7b
Dental lamina stage	Bmp-4, Msx-1, Dlx
Bud stage	Wnt, Lef-1, Shh
Bud–cap transition	Bmp-4, Msx-1, Pax-9, ActivinβA, Shh
Enamel knot	Bmp-2, Bmp-4, Bmp-7, Wnt-10b, Fgf-4, Fgf-9, Slit-1 and Shh

TIMELINE OF TOOTH ERUPTION

Deciduous dentition

Maxillary teeth	Eruption period
Central incisor	8–12 months
Lateral incisor	9–13 months
Canine	16–22 months
First molar	13–19 months
Second molar	25–33 months

Mandibular teeth	
Central incisor	6–10 months
Lateral incisor	10–16 months
Canine	17–23 months
First molar	14–18 months
Second molar	23–31 months

Permanent dentition

Maxillary teeth	Eruption period
Central incisor	7–8 years
Lateral incisor	8–9 years
Canine	11–12 years
First premolar	10–11 years
Second premolar	10–12 years
First molar	9–10 years
Second molar	12–13 years
Third molar	17–21 years

Mandibular teeth	
Central incisor	6–7 years
Lateral incisor	7–8 years
Canine	9–10 years
First premolar	10–12 years
Second premolar	11–12 years
First molar	6–7 years
Second molar	11–13 years
Third molar	17–21 years

DIFFERENCES BETWEEN DECIDUOUS AND PERMANENT DENTITION

	Primary dentition	**Permanent dentition**
Development	Develops directly from the dental lamina	Develops as distal or lingual extension of dental lamina
Color	Lighter in color Appear bluish-white	Darker in color Appear yellowish white or greyish white

Number	Twenty in number
	Premolars are absent
	Dental formula: I:C:M
	            2:1:2
		Thirty two in number
		Premolars are present
		Dental formula: I:C:PM:M
		            2:1:2:3

Size	Smaller in size when compared to permanent dentition	Larger in size when compared to deciduous dentition
Shape	Crowns of the deciduous dentition are wider mesiodistally in comparison to their height	Longer as their cervico-incisal height is greater than mesiodistal width
Cervical constriction	More prominent	Not so prominent
Occlusal plane	It is relatively flat	Relatively curved
Contact point	Broad and flat contact area; in molars contact area is situated gingivally	Point contacts. In molars contact point is situated occlusally
First tooth to erupt	Mandibular incisor	Mandibular first molar
Mamelons	Absent	Present on incisal edges of newly erupted incisors.
Thickness of enamel and detnin	Thinner	Thick
Direction of enamel rods	In the cervical area directed occlusally	Directed gingivally
Roots	Roots of multirooted teeth are slender and wide inter-radicular space to accommodate the developing permanent tooth bud	Roots are broad and inter-radicular space is restricted comparatively
Apical foramen	Large	Narrow

EFFECTS OF AGING ON ORAL AND CIRCUMORAL TISSUES

Enamel	• Reduction in thickness of enamel • Color becomes darker • Attrition, abrasion and erosion • Surface becomes shiny and polished • Brittle and cracks on enamel surface • Resistant to caries
Dentin	• Color becomes darker • Decreased sensitivity • Increased bulk • Increased irregular secondary dentin and tertiary dentin deposition • Dead tracts more common in coronal dentin • Sclerotic dentin formation • Increased aspartic acid racemization
Pulp	• Decreased volume of pulp chamber and root canal • Reduced cellular components • Increased fibrous components • Decreased vascularity • Reduced sensitivity • Occurrence of calcifications
Cementum	• Scalloped surface • Increased thickness • Loss of cementocytes
Alveolar bone	• Residual ridge resorption • Reduced bone mass • Increased osteoporosis • Decreased vascularity • Fatty infiltration of marrow

Contd...

Contd...

Gingiva	• Decreased gingival width • Gingival recession • Reduced stippling • Thinning of epithelium • Decreased keratinization • Flattened rete ridges • Decreased fibroblasts
Periodontal ligament	• Reduced periodontal ligament width • Decreased cellularity • Increased fibrous component • Decreased mitotic activity • Increased elastic fibers • Decreased vascularity • Loss of soft tissue attachment leading to mobility • Occurrence of cementicles
Salivary glands	• Reduced acinar volume • Acinar atrophy • Ductal dilatation • Increased stromal connective tissue • Fatty infiltration • Presence of oncocytes • Reduced salivary flow and compromised immune mechanism
Oral mucosa	• Atrophy • Dryness, dysgeusia, and burning sensation • Less elastic • Increased fibrosis • Decreased cellularity • Reduced epithelial thickness and flattened rete pegs • Occurrence of heterotopic sebaceous glands
Tongue	• Loss of filiform papilla • Reduction in taste perception • Lingual varicosities
Maxilla and mandible	• Decreased rate of bone formation • Continuous resorption and less bone remodelling • Reduced dental arch width, length and depth • Rounding of arch forms
TMJ	• Clicking sounds • Limited opening movement • Deviation of mandible during function
Face	• Loss of muscle tone • Thinning of skin • Wrinkling • Loss of vertical dimension • Pigmentations

ABBREVIATIONS AND EXPANSIONS

Abbreviation	Expansion
AgRP/NPY	Agouti-related protein
AIDS	Acquired Immunodeficiency Syndrome
ALCAM	Activated leukocyte cell adhesion molecule
AMBN	Ameloblastin
AMEL	Amelogenin
AMPK	Adenosine Monophosphate-activated Protein kinase
AVP	Arginine Vasopressin
BALT	Bronchus Associated Lymphoid Tissue

Contd...

Abbreviation	Expansion
Barx	BarH1 homolog
BM-40	Basement Membrane protein 40
BMP	Bone Morphogenetic Protein
CAM	Cell Adhesion Molecule
cAMP	cyclic AMP
CAP	Cementum derived Attachment Protein
Cbfa1	Core-binding factor alpha 1
CD	Cluster of Differentiation
CDJ	Cementodentinal Junction
CEJ	Cementoenamel junction

Contd...

Contd...

Abbreviation	Expansion
CFU-GM	Granulocyte Macrophage Colony forming Unit
CICN 7	Chloride Channel 7
CK	Cytokeratin
CSC	Cancer Stem Cells
CSF-1	Colony stimulating Factor 1
DEJ	Dentinoenamel Junction
DGP	Dentin Glycol Protein
Dlx	Distal-less homologue
DMP	Dentin Matrix Protein
DOPA	Dihydroxyphenylalanine
DPP	Dentin phosphoprotein/Phosphophoryn
DPSC	Dental Pulp Stem Cells
DPX	Distrene, Dibutyl Phthalate and Xylene
DSP	Dentin Sialoprotein
DSPP	Dentin Sialophosphoprotein
ECM	Extracellular Matrix
EDTA	Ethylenediaminetetraacetic
EGF	Epidermal Growth Factor
ELISA	Enzyme-linked Immunosorbent Assay
EMT	Epithelial Mesenchymal Transition
ENAM	Enamelin
ESC	Embryonic Stem Cells
FGF	Fibroblast Growth factor
FISH	Fluorescent In Situ Hybridization
GAG	Glycosaminoglycans
GALT	Gut-associated Lymphoid Tissues
GHRH	Growth hormone-releasing hormone
GSC	Stem Cells derived from gingival cells
GTR	Guided Tissue Regeneration
H&E	Hematoxylin and Eosin
Hgf	Hepatic growth factor
HIV	Human Immunodeficiency Virus
HSC	Hematopoietic Stem Cell
ICAM	Intercellular Adhesion Molecule
ICM	Inner Cell Mass
IFA	Immunofluorescent Assay
IFN-C	Interferon-C
IGH	Insulin-like growth factor
IL	Interleukin
Ipsc	Induced pluripotent stem cells
ISH	In Situ Hybridization
KGF	Keratinocyte Growth Factor
KLK	Kallikrein
Lef	Lymphoid enhancer- binding factor (TF)

Contd...

Abbreviation	Expansion
Lhx	Lim homeobox domain gene
MALT	Mucosa-associated Lymphoid Tissue
M-CSF	Macrophage Colony-stimulating Factor
MMP	Matrix Metalloproteinase
mRNA	Messenger RNA
MSC	Mesenchymal Stem Cells
Msx	Msh-like genes in vertebrates (TF)
MtDNA	Mitochondrial DNA
mTOR	Mammalian Target of Rapamycin
NALT	Nose-associated Lymphoid Tissue
NGF	Nerve Growth Factor
OCIF	Osteoclastogenesis Inhibitory Factor
ODAM	Odontogenic Ameloblasts-associated protein
OPG	Osteoprotegerin
PAP	Papanicolaou's stain
PAS stain	Periodic Acid-Schiff stain
Pax	Paired box homeotic gene (TF)
PCR	Polymerase Chain Reaction
PDGF	Platelet-derived Growth Factor
PDL	Periodontal Ligament
PDSC	Periodontal Ligament Stem Cells
PECAM	Platelet Endothelial Cell Adhesion Molecule
PGE 2	Prostaglandin E2
POMC	Pro-opiomelanocortin gene
PRP	Proline-rich Proteins
PTH	Parathyroid Hormone
RANK	Receptor Activator of Nuclear factor kappa B
RANKL	Receptor Activator of Nuclear factor kappa B ligand
ROS	Reactive Oxygen Species
RUNX	Runt-related transcription factor
SCAP	Stem Cells from Apical Papilla
SCPP	Secretory Calcium-binding Phosphoprotein
SEM	Scanning Electron Microscope
SFRP-1	Secreted Frizzled Related Protein 1
SHED	Stem cells from Human Exfoliated Deciduous teeth
Shh	Sonic hedgehog
SMA	Smooth Muscle Actin
SMMHC	Smooth Muscle Myosin Heavy Chain

Contd...

Contd...

Abbreviation	Expansion
SPARC	Secreted Protein Acidic and Rich in Cysteine
SST	Somatostatin
TEM	Transmission Electron Microscope
TF	Transcription factor
TGF β	Transforming Growth Factor β
TIMP	Tissue inhibitors of matalloproteinase
TMJ	Temporomandibular Joint
TNF α	Tumor necrosis factor α
TNTs	Tunneling nanotubes
TOR	Target of rapamycin
TRAP	Tartrate Resistant Acid Phosphatase
VCAM	Vascular Cell Adhesion Molecule
VEGF	Vascular Endothelial Growth Factor
VIP	Vasoactive Intestinal Peptide
Wnt	Wingless homolog

GLOSSARY

Accessory canals: The canals other than the primary pulp canals are called accessory canals. They communicate with the periodontium through accessory foramen.

Acellular cementum: Cementum that does not contain entrapped cementocytes.

Acid phosphatase: It is an enzyme associated with hard tissue destruction and mainly localized to the lysosomes of the osteoclasts. They are more commonly exhibited by an active cell in areas of hard tissue destruction.

Acini: Terminal secretory and functional unit of glands made up of cluster of epithelial cells.

Acrodont: A type of dentition in which the teeth are fused to the surface of the underlying jawbone.

Adherens junction: It is a type of cell junction characterized by the occurrence of protein complexes. It may cover the entire perimeter of the cell or as spots.

Adult stem cells: These are undifferentiated cells, found throughout the body after embryonic development.

Afibrillar cementum: Cementum with a matrix that is devoid of fibrillar type collagen.

Agenesis: Failure of an organ or tissue to develop.

Aging: Progressive biological changes related to the passage of time.

Agnathan: Group of vertebrates without jaw.

Alkaline phosphatase: An enzyme that liberates phosphate under alkaline conditions and associated with hard tissue formation or mineralization. They are capable of hydrolyzing phosphoric acid esters, and therefore, these enzymes readily supply the much required phosphate ion at the site of mineralization.

Allosome: A sex chromosome that differs from an ordinary autosome in form, size, or behavior. The human sex chromosomes are a typical pair of allosomes.

Allograft: Highly processed bone obtained from another human source.

Alveolar crest fibers: This group of periodontal ligament fibers extends from the crest of the alveolar bone obliquely, attaching to the cementum immediately below the dentogingival junction at a position more coronal than their attachment to the bone.

Alveolar process: It is that portion of the jawbone, which houses the roots of the teeth and gives attachment to the principal fibers of periodontal ligament.

Alveologingival fibers: These fibers extend from the crest of the alveolar bone into the lamina propria of the free and attached gingiva.

Ameloblast: An ectodermally derived cell that is responsible for the formation of enamel. They are differentiated from the inner enamel epithelial cells of the dental organ.

Amelogenins: Class of proteins that form much of the organic matrix of the enamel during early development of tooth enamel.

Aminopeptidase: They are enzymes that catalyze the cleavage of amino acids from the amino terminus (N-terminus) of proteins or peptides.

Anatomic repair: It is a type of cemental repair, where the repair reestablishes the former outline of root.

Anchoring fibrils: These are type VII collagen fibrils found near the basement membrane and provide a mechanical attachment for the epithelium with the adjacent connective tissue.

Angiogenic factor: A polypeptide presents in the circulation and plays a role in blood vessel formation.

Anodontia: Absence of the teeth due to failure of development.

Apical fibers: This group of periodontal ligament fibers is arranged radially around the apex of the roots. They originate from cementum of root apex, splaying apically and laterally toward the fundus of the alveolar socket.

Apical foramen: An opening at the root apex, through which the pulp communicates with the connective tissues of the periodontium. Vessels and nerves enter and exit through it.

Apocrine glands: In these glands, the secretory products exit by losing or pinching off the apical portions of the cells, i.e a portion of the cytoplasm is lost (*e.g.*, mammary gland and sweat gland).

Articular disk: A cartilage interposed between two articular surfaces and partially or completely separating the joint cavity into two compartments. In TMJ, the articular disk is a thin, oval plate, which is made up of avascular, fibrous connective tissue, and, placed between the condyle of the mandible and the mandibular fossa. It is also called meniscus.

Atrophy: Decrease in the size of cells, tissues or organs.

Attached gingiva: Portion of gingiva, which extends from the gingival crevice to mucogingival junction. It is firm, resilient and tightly bound to the alveolar bone.

Attrition: Physiological wearing away of the tooth substance as a result of tooth-to-tooth contact as in mastication.

Autocrine glands: Glands that secrete products, which influence the secretion of another product by the same cell (products act on the same cell, which produce them).

Autosome: Any chromosome other than the X and Y sex chromosomes. Humans normally have 22 pairs of autosomes (44 autosomes) in each cell.

Autograft: Transplantation of tissue from one location to another in the same individual.

B cells: These are round and dense basophilic cells depicting a large nucleus with a thin rim of perinuclear cytoplasm. They are responsible for humoral immunity by the production of antibodies.

Bartholin duct: Other name for major sublingual gland duct.

Basal lamina: Ultrastructural term for basement membrane and is a basal complex consisting of lamina and fibers. It has a dark zone called lamina densa and a light zone called lamina lucida.

Basal layer: The layer of the epithelium that is closest to the connective tissue. It provides the epithelial stem cells as well as cells to supplement the epithelial differentiation.

Basement membrane: Thin layer of delicate non-cellular material of a fine filamentous texture that separates the epithelium from the adjacent connective tissue.

Blastocyst: The blastula of the mammalian embryo consisting of an inner cell mass, a cavity, and the trophoblasts. This is formed by the seepage of fluid into the morula.

Bone canaliculi: Branching tubular structure where the osteocytic process is housed. It radiates from each bone lacuna, which contains the osteocytes. Canaliculi of one layer (lamella) communicate with that of another.

Bone morphogenetic proteins (BMP): They are a group of growth factors that belong to the transforming growth factor (TGF) beta superfamily. Initially they are believed to be involved in the formation of bone and cartilage, but are now considered to constitute a group of essential morphogenetic signals and orchestrate the tissue architecture throughout the body.

Bone marrow: Soft tissue present inside the bone. It may be hemopoietic, fibrous or fatty.

Bone remodeling: The phenomena by which the old bone is removed and new bone is formed.

Bone sialoprotein: It is a heterogeneous group of noncollagenous protein, responsible for the proper calcification of hard tissues.

Bone: Vascular and hard connective tissue, which gives the skeletal framework and acts as the reservoir of calcium.

Brachydont: A low crowned tooth with the enamel that extends above the gingival line and a neck just below it with at least one root.

Branchial arch: Six pairs of arched structures that form the lateral and ventral walls of the pharynx of the embryo and gives rise to the structures of the head and neck region. Out of the six pairs the fifth one is rudimentary.

Buccopharyngeal membrane: This is a two-layered membrane formed by the endoderm of the foregut and ectoderm of the primitive oral cavity.

Bud stage: Initial stage of tooth development; gives rise to enamel organ.

Bundle bone: That part of the bone in which collagen fiber bundles are attached.

Cadherin: It is a calcium-dependent transmembrane protein that helps in the attachment of cells to the extracellular matrix.

CAMP or **cyclic AMP:** Second or intracellular messenger of target cells.

Canal of Zuckerkandl and Hirschfeld: Nutrient canal, which houses the interdental and interradicular arteries, veins, lymph vessels, and nerves in the bone.

Cancellous bone (spongy bone): Type of mature bone with large marrow spaces and sheets of trabeculae of bone in the form of bars and plates.

Carnoy's mixture: Mixture of ethyl alcohol, acetic acid and chloroform, used for histochemical staining of nucleic acids.

Cartilage: It is a firm and rubbery avascular connective tissue derived from mesoderm [three types—(1) hyaline,

(2) fibro, and (3) elastic].

Caveolae: Micropinocytotic vesicles located on the plasma membranes of the myoepithelial cells.

Cell-free zone: This zone of pulp is relatively free from cells but contains capillaries and nerves. This zone is also called nuclear free-zone or zone of Weil. This zone is of approximately 40 μm width, seen adjacent to the odontoblastic layer, more prominent in the coronal pulp and inconspicuous in radicular pulp.

Cell lineage: Developmental history of a differentiated cell as traced back to the cell from which it arises.

Cell rests of Malassez: The remnants of the Hertwig's epithelial root sheath are called cell rests of Malassez. They are usually seen in periodontal ligament.

Cell-rich zone: Cell rich zone is present adjacent to the cell-free zone and is seen in coronal and radicular pulp, but less distinct in the apical portion and absent in older teeth. This zone is characterized by numerous fibroblasts, undifferentiated mesenchymal cells, macrophages and dendritic cells.

Cellular cementum: Cementum that contains entrapped cementocytes in their lacunae.

Cemental hyperplasia: Increased thickness of the cementum not correlated with function. This term is usually applied to hypercementosis in a nonfunctional tooth.

Cemental hypertrophy: Increased thickness of the cementum for increased functional needs.

Cementicles: Small, spherical or ovoid calcified masses found in the periodontal ligament.

Cementoblasts: Ectomesenchymally derived cells responsible for the formation of cementum and are differentiated from dental sac cells.

Cementoclasts: Cells that resemble osteoclasts present on the surface of cementum and responsible for resorption of cementum.

Cementocyte: Entrapped cementoblasts within the cementum.

Cementoenamel junction: The junction between the enamel and the cementum at the cervical portion of the tooth.

Cementum: Avascular and mineralized tissue covering the root dentin that gives attachment to the principal fibers of periodontal ligament.

Cementicles: Small, globular calcified masses of cementum seen in the cementum.

Centroblasts: Large round cells with a basophilic rim of cytoplasm and a large vesicular nucleus, produced as the first step toward production of antibodies when mature B lymphocytes encounter an antigenic challenge.

Centrocytes: These cells are smaller than the centroblasts which undergo further division into immunoblasts.

Cervical loop: That part of an enamel organ in which the inner enamel epithelium reflects on to the outer enamel epithelium to form the Hertwig's epithelial root sheath.

Chondroitin sulfate: It is a sulfated glycosaminoglycan composed of a chain of alternating sugars. It is usually found attached to proteins as part of a proteoglycan.

Chromosome: A structure in the nucleus containing a linear thread of DNA, which transmits genetic information from the parent to the offspring.

Cilia: Hairlike processes projecting from epithelial cells, which propel mucus, pus and foreign particles.

Circular fibers: One group of gingival fibers that encircle the neck of the tooth, intermingling with the other fibers in this region and help to hold the free gingiva against the tooth.

Circumferential lamellae: The outer most sheet of bone underlying the periosteum and endosteum.

Circumpulpal dentin: Dentin that lies between the primary dentin and the pulp.

Circumvallate papilla: This is the largest papilla of the tongue and is present anterior to the V-shaped terminal sulcus. A valley-like depression is seen around the entire circumference of this papilla to which minor serous glands discharge their secretion. This papilla contains taste buds.

Clearing: Removal of dehydrating solutions and making the tissue components ready to receive the infiltrating medium (Paraffin wax) in histological processing. Many of the clearing agents except chloroform make the tissue transparent.

Col: Nonkeratinized depressed gingival tissue that lies between the adjacent posterior teeth.

Compact bone (ivory bone): Type of mature bone consisting of tightly packed osteons or Haversian systems forming a solid mass, with less marrow tissue.

Concentric lamellae: They are sheets of bone that surround the central canal (Haversian canal) in an osteon.

Connective tissue: Tissue that supports, connects, binds, and separates other tissues and parts, usually derived from mesoderm.

Contour lines of Owen: Accentuated incremental lines (von Ebner lines) of the dentin are called contour lines of Owen.

Coronal pulp: Part of the dental pulp contained within the pulp chamber or in the crown portion of the tooth.

Cortex: Superficial and outermost layer.

Cribriform plate: Bony plate containing numerous perforations.

Crimping: It literally means to bend or make wavy. In biological context, it denotes a specific type of waviness in collagen fibers of the periodontal ligament observed under polarizing microscope.

Cushion-hammock ligament: Ligament at the base of the socket passing from one bony wall to the other. Its existence is disproved.

Cynodonts: Reptiles that resemble mammal like characteristics and jaws.

Cytochrome oxidase: It is a large transmembrane protein complex found in bacteria, *Archaea*, and in eukaryotes in their mitochondria.

Cytokeratins: Keratin proteins found in the intracytoplasmic cytoskeleton of epithelial cells.

Dead tracts: A dark or black zone in dentin formed by empty or air-filled dentinal tubules caused by retraction of odontoblastic process or death of the odontoblasts.

Decalcification: Process of removal of calcium from the hard tissues such as bone and teeth, to be sectioned and viewed under the microscope. Usually weak acids are used.

Deciduous dentition: Twenty small teeth that appear in the mouth at about six months of age and shed eventually to be replaced by the permanent teeth.

Dehydration: Process of removal of water and fixative from the tissue during histological processing.

Dental lamina: Epithelial ingrowth from the oral ectoderm into the underlying mesenchyme to form the tooth.

Dental papilla: The aggregates of condensed ectomesenchymal cells destined to form dentin and pulp after differentiation into odontoblasts. This occupies the center portion of the dental organ.

Dental pulp: It is a soft connective tissue derived from ectomesenchyme and occupies the central portion of the tooth.

Dental pulp stem cells (DPSCs): They are multipotent stem cells present in the dental pulp that have the potential to differentiate into a variety of cell types.

Dental sac (dental follicle): Condensation of cells and fibers derived from ectomesenchyme destined to form the cementum, periodontal ligament, and alveolar bone.

Denticles: Otherwise known as pulp stones, made up of nodular calcified masses seen in the pulp chamber or root canals of a tooth.

Dentin: First formed hard tissue of the tooth. It is an ectomesenchymal derivative and forms the bulk of the tooth. In the crown it is covered by enamel and in root covered by cementum.

Dentin sialoprotein: A phosphorylated, highly glycosylated protein with high amounts of sialic acid.

Dentinal tubules: Minute wavy channels in dentin, extending from pulp cavity to cementum and enamel and house the odontoblastic process.

Dentinoenamel junction: Scalloped interface between the enamel and the dentin of a tooth crown. Three-dimensionally it is made up of saucer-shaped depressions in the dentin surface.

Dentinogenesis: Formation of dentin by odontoblasts is called dentinogenesis.

Dentogingival fibers: These are the most numerous gingival fibers extending from cervical cementum to lamina propria of the free and attached gingiva.

Dentogingival junction: Anatomical and functional interface between the gingiva and the tooth, wherein the epithelium of the gingiva is attached to the tooth surface.

Dentoperiosteal fibers: Running apically from the cementum over the periosteum of the outer cortical plates of the alveolar process.

Desmosomes: A type of cell junction (Macula adherens) found between adjacent epithelial cells.

Desquamation: Process of shedding of matured epithelial cells from the surface.

Differentiation: The process of changing of one cell type to other during development.

Diffuse calcifications of the pulp: Amorphous, unorganized linear strands of irregular calcific deposits in the pulp tissue paralleling the blood vessels or collagen fiber bundles.

Diphyodont: A condition seen in heterodonty of mammals, where their teeth are typically replaced only once; having two sets of teeth.

DNA: Deoxyribonucleic acid, a self-replicating material that is present in nearly all living organisms as the main constituent of chromosomes and it carries the genetic information.

DPSC: Dental pulp stem cells.

Duct: A narrow tubular vessel or channel lined by epithelial cells that serves to convey secretions from a gland.

Ducts of Rivinus: These are excretory ducts of the sublingual gland, which are eight to twenty in number.

Ectoderm: The outermost of the three primitive germ layers of the embryo.

Ectomesenchyme: Mesenchyme influenced by the migrated neural crest cells.

Elaunin fibers: Immature form of elastic fibers, which are made up of bundles of microfibrils intermingled with small amounts of elastin.

Embedding (tissue): Process of orienting the tissue sample in a support medium and allowing it to solidify during histological processing.

Embryo: Early stage of the development of a multicellular diploid eukaryotic organism is called embryo. From the time of fertilization till 8th week of intrauterine life the fertilized ovum or the zygote is called embryo. After that it is called fetus.

Embryology: A branch of biology that deals with the formation, early growth, and development of living organisms.

Embryonic stem cells: These cells are pluripotent stem cells that have the potential to differentiate into any cell type of the body except the placenta.

Enamel: Ectodermally derived hardest tissue of the human body forming the covering of the anatomic crown of the tooth.

Enamel brochs: These are surface projections of the enamel, made up of radiating groups of hydroxyapatite crystals.

Enamel cord/septum: A vertical extension of the enamel knot in a developing tooth, connecting the enamel knot with the outer dental/enamel epithelium. It may act as reservoir of proliferating cells of the enamel organ. They play a major role in determining the cuspal morphology by acting as signaling center and expressing growth factors.

Enamel cuticle: Two extremely thin layers, covering the entire crown of newly erupted teeth and is subsequently abraded by mastication.

Enamel hypoplasia: A developmental disturbance of teeth characterized by defective enamel matrix formation; may be hereditary or acquired.

Enamel knot: Condensation of cells at the central portion of the inner enamel epithelium at cap stage of tooth development.

Enamel lamellae: It is a hypocalcified defect of enamel characterized by a thin, leaf-like structure that extends from the enamel surface toward the dentinoenamel junction and sometimes crosses the DEJ.

Enamel niche: The epithelial enamel organ is attached to the oral epithelium not by a cord of epithelial cells but by sheet of cells with discontinuities. This discontinuous portion contains ectomesenchyme. Histologically this gives the appearance of a double attachment made up of epithelial cells, which appears like a niche.

Enamel organ: Synonymously used for dental organ. It denotes the epithelial portion of the tooth germ.

Enamel pearl: A developmental anomaly characterized by a small nodule of enamel below the cementoenamel junction, formed by the misplaced ameloblasts.

Enamel rods: Basic structural unit of enamel.

Enamel spindles: It is a hypomineralized structure seen extending from the dentinoenamel junction. It is formed by the extension of odontoblastic process beyond the dentinoenamel junction before the enamel is formed.

Enamel tufts: They are hypomineralized structures originating at the dentinoenamel junction and resemble tuft of grass in ground sections. They extend approximately up to the inner one-third to one-fifth of the enamel. Their formation has been attributed to stress and is considered to be a form of defect.

Enamelins: A class of proteins that form the organic matrix of mature tooth enamel.

Endochondral ossification: A type of ossification, which involves the replacement of a cartilaginous model by bone.

Endocrine glands: They do not have a ductal system; instead their products are directly secreted into the blood and are carried by the blood and tissue fluid to the target area (*e.g.* thyroid gland).

Endoderm: The innermost of the three primary germ layers of the embryo.

Endosteum: It is a thin cellular layer which covers the inner surface of compact and cancellous bone.

Enzyme: Substance, which initiates or accelerates a chemical reaction.

Enzyme histochemistry: Procedure to locate specific enzyme activities in a specimen to aid in confirmatory diagnosis.

Epithelial attachment: The union between junctional epithelium and tooth (dentogingival attachment).

Epithelial pearls: They are concentrically arranged remnants of the epithelium formed in the line of fusion between the palatine processes.

Epithelial rests of Malassez (cell rests of Malassez): During the root formation Hertwig's epithelial root sheath is broken down as soon as the radicular dentin is formed. The remnants of the Hertwig's epithelial root sheath are called cell rests of Malassez. They are usually seen in periodontal ligament.

Epithelium: One of the four basic tissues of the body made up of large cells with little intercellular substance. Covers the body surface, lines the cavities and forms glands.

Eruption: Axial or occlusal movement of the tooth from its developmental position within the jaw to its functional position in the occlusal plane.

Eruptive tooth movement: Occlusally directed movement of the tooth from its developmental position within the bone to its functional position.

Esterase: It is a hydrolase enzyme that splits esters into an acid and an alcohol in a chemical reaction with water called hydrolysis.

Excementosis: A knob-like outgrowth of cementum.

Excretory duct: The largest duct through which the secretion is discharged on to the surface.

Exfoliation: Shedding or falling off of primary set of teeth.

Exocrine gland: Gland that secretes substances onto an epithelial surface directly or by means of a duct (*e.g.* salivary glands).

Extracellular matrix: The substance that is present in between the cells of the connective tissue, usually made up of fibers and ground substance.

Extrinsic fibers of cementum: Cementum having the inserted collagen fibers secreted by the fibroblasts of the periodontal ligament fibers.

False denticles: Localized masses of calcified tissue that do not exhibit dentinal tubules but contain concentric lamellae deposited around a central nidus. May be formed by the calcification of the dead cells.

Fertilization: Fusion of sperm and ova.

Fibroblasts: Connective tissue cells responsible for the synthesis and remodeling of nonmineralized connective tissue.

Fibronectin: Cell adhesion molecule that anchors the cells to collagen or proteoglycan substrates.

Filiform papillae: Fine pointed, cone-shaped papillae on the anterior part of the tongue. The surface of which is keratinized.

Flow cytometry: Is a laser- or impedance-based, biophysical technology employed in cell counting, cell sorting, biomarker detection, and protein engineering, by suspending cells in a stream of fluid and passing them through an electronic detection apparatus.

Foliate papillae: Short vertical folds that are present on the posterolateral border of the tongue. Prominent in animals and vestigial in humans.

Follicular dendritic cells: Inconspicuous cells with many long and slender dendritic cytoplasmic extensions seen in cortical area of lymph node.

Fordyce spots: Enlarged heterotopic sebaceous glands found in the mucosa including the oral cavity.

Free gingiva: The unattached portion of the gingiva that surrounds the tooth and present coronal to the free gingival groove.

Free gingival groove: A faint linear depression parallel to the gingival margin that divides free and attached gingiva.

Freeze-drying: Technique of rapid freezing of fresh tissue and the subsequent removal of water molecules.

Frontonasal process: One of the facial processes in the embryo that forms the forehead and bridge of the nose.

Frozen section: Freezing the tissue with the help of cryostat and cutting into thin slice for microscopical examination.

Functional repair: In this type of cemental repair the cementum is deposited over the damaged area but fails to re-establish the former root outline.

Fungiform papillae: Round, reddish, mushroom-shaped papillae, which are found interspersed between the filiform papillae and containing few taste buds. The surface is nonkeratinized.

Gap junction: A type of cell junction, in which direct cell-cell communication occurs through small pored structures called connexons.

Genotype: A specific combination of alleles at one or more loci on a chromosome.

Germinal center of the lymphatic nodule: Central pale stained area having a heterogeneous population of cells.

Gingiva: That part of the oral mucous membrane, which surrounds the necks of the teeth and covers the alveolar processes.

Gingival fibers: Collagen fibers of the lamina propria of the gingiva, which help in the attachment of the tooth. One end of the fiber starts from the gingiva and the other end is usually attached to the bone or cementum.

Gingival recession: Apical shift of the junctional epithelium with subsequent exposure of more of the tooth surface and root portion.

Gingival sulcus/crevice: Space between the inner aspect of free gingiva and the tooth.

Glenoid fossa: The depression in temporal bone with which the mandible articulates. It is also called mandibular fossa.

Glucuronidase: An enzyme that splits glycosidic linkages in glucuronides.

Glycoproteins: Any of a class of proteins, which have carbohydrate groups attached to the polypeptide chain.

Glycosaminoglycans (GAGs): GAGs are a family of highly sulfated, complex, polydisperse linear polysaccharides that display a variety of important biological roles. They are of four groups, namely heparan sulfate, chondroitin sulfate, keratan sulfate, and hyaluronic acid.

Gnarled enamel: Enamel under the cusp of a tooth characterized by twisted and intertwined enamel rods to withstand the increased masticatory load.

Gnathostomes: Vertebrates, which have a vertically biting device, the jaws.

Goblet cells: A column or goblet-shaped cells found in the respiratory and intestinal tracts, which secrete the main component of mucus.

Gomphosis: The type of joint with limited mobility between two calcified structures with interposed fibrous tissue. A mobile peg and socket joint (*e.g.* TMJ). It is also called as dentoalveolar syndesmosis.

Ground section: A section of bone or tooth prepared for histological study by grinding until it becomes thin enough for microscopic examination.

Ground substance: An amorphous background material that binds tissue and fluids, the latter serving for the diffusion of gases and metabolic substances.

Gubernacular cord: A connective tissue band that connects the tooth germ of an unerupted tooth with the overlying mucosa.

Haplodont: Simplest form of a tooth with the shape of single cone.

Haversian canal: Central canal of the osteon in compact bone, contains blood and lymph vessels, and nerves and surrounded by concentric lamellae.

Haversian system: It is also called as osteon. It is made up of Haversian canal and its concentrically arranged lamellae, constituting the basic structural unit of compact bone.

Hemidesmosomes: Stud-like structures (half desmosome), that attach the keratinocytes to the extracellular matrix/connective tissue.

Heparan sulfate: It is a linear polysaccharide found in all animal tissues. It occurs as a proteoglycan in which two or three heparan sulfate chains are attached in close proximity to the cell surface or extracellular matrix proteins.

Hertwig's epithelial root sheath: An epithelial structure, which plays a major role in the development of root and is made up of outer enamel epithelium and inner enamel epithelium of the dental organ.

Heterodonty: Mammals with regionally differentiated dental arch, with incisor, canine, premolar and molar regions.

Hiatus semilunaris: Semilunar-shaped groove in the external wall of the middle meatus of nasal fossa into which frontal, maxillary, and ethmoid sinuses drain.

Hilum: The depressed area of the surface of a lymph node through which the efferent lymphatics emerge from the medulla and blood vessels enter and leave the node.

Histochemistry: The study of qualitative and quantitative assessment of chemicals within cells and tissues.

Holocrine gland: In this secretion involves death of the cell. The secretory cell is released and as it breaks apart, the contents of the cell become the secretory product. *e.g.* some sweat glands located in the axilla, pubic areas, and around the areola of the breasts and sebaceous glands.

Homing: Tendency of the stem cells to get along with the tissue or organ, when they are given *in vivo*.

Homo sapiens: Systematic name used in taxonomy for the only extant human species.

Homodonty: Early vertebrate dentition with numerous, similar, simple, and conical teeth.

Horizontal fibers: They are located just below the alveolar crest fibers and extend in a more or less horizontal direction from the alveolar bone to the cementum and resist horizontal and tipping forces.

Howship's lacunae: Small bays or depressions in bone, where resorption by osteoclasts takes place.

Hunter–Schreger bands: This is an optical effect of enamel and can be appreciated in longitudinal sections under reflected light. These are alternate dark and light bands of varying widths produced by the change in orientation or direction between adjacent groups of enamel rods.

Hyaline cartilage: One of the three types of cartilage that covers the articulating ends of bones.

Hyaluronan: Also called hyaluronic acid, is an anionic, nonsulfated glycosaminoglycan distributed widely throughout connective, epithelial, and neural tissues.

Hydroxyapatite: Naturally occurring mineral form of calcium apatite with the formula $Ca_5(PO_4)_3(OH)$.

Hypercementosis: An increase in the thickness of cementum.

Hypertrophy: Increase in the size of the tissue or organ due to an increase in the size of the cell.

Hypsodont: A high-crowned tooth with enamel that extends far past the gingival line, providing extra material for wear and tear.

Immunoblasts: An antigenically stimulated lymphocyte with a large nucleus and well-defined basophilic cytoplasm.

Immunofluorescence: It is a technique used for visualization of antigen and specific proteins in tissue sections by binding antibody, chemically conjugated with a fluorescent dye. The specific antibodies are labeled with a compound that makes them glow when observed microscopically under ultraviolet light.

Immunohistochemistry: Identifying cellular and tissue constituents by means of antigen-antibody reactions. The site of antibody binding being identified by direct labeling of the antibody or by use of secondary labeling method.

Impaction: Failure of eruption of the tooth, which has the eruptive force.

***In situ* hybridization:** Histochemical technique that permits identification of a gene or gene product on a tissue section.

Incremental lines of von Ebner: They are fine lines seen in dentin representing the rhythmic deposition of dentin.

Inner enamel epithelium: Tall columnar cells that line the concave surface of the dental organ at cap stage of tooth development. These cells undergo histodifferentiation to become ameloblasts in bell stage and secrete enamel.

Integrins: A group of cell surface proteins that mediate the binding of cells to extracellular matrix proteins to one another.

Intercalated duct: First part of the duct system, arising from the terminal secretory unit (the acini) formed by a short narrow tube lined by a single layer of low cuboidal cells.

Intercellular bridges: They are cell junctions and otherwise called desmosomes.

Interglobular dentin: Hypomineralized dentin found at the junction of mantle dentin and circumpulpal dentin, formed due to the complete fusion calcifying globules.

Interlobular ducts: Ducts located in the connective tissue stroma in between the lobes of the glands.

Intermediate cementum: It is a form of secondary cellular intrinsic fiber cementum restricted to the apex of the tooth near the cementodentinal junction. The thickness of which can be around 10–50 μm and does not resemble either dentin or cementum.

Interradicular fibers: This group of periodontal ligament fibers is seen only in multirooted teeth. They extend radially from the crest of the alveolar bone between the roots of multirooted teeth (interradicular septum) to the cementum in the furcation area of the tooth. They resist forces of tipping and torque and prevent luxation.

Interstitial lamellae: One of the bony plates that fill in between the haversian systems.

Intertubular dentin: It is the dentin located between the dentinal tubules. It forms the bulk of the dentin.

Intramembranous ossification: It is the direct formation of bone within highly vascular sheets of condensed primitive mesenchyme.

Jacobson's organ: A small ellipsoid or cigar-shaped auxiliary olfactory sense organ which undergoes involution during 15th week of intrauterine life.

Junctional complex: Any specialized area of intercellular adhesion.

Junctional epithelium: The epithelium of the gingiva which gets attached to the tooth.

Keratan sulfate: Also called as keratosulfate, is any of several sulfated glycosaminoglycans that have been found especially in the cornea, cartilage, and bone.

Keratinization: Process of keratin formation in the superficial layer of the epithelium by the maturation of the epithelial cells as they differentiate and move from the basal to superficial layer.

Keratinized epithelium: Epithelium having keratin in their superficial layer.

Keratinocyte: Epithelial cell having the potentiality to form keratin.

Keratinosome/Odland bodies: Lamellar granule or a membrane bound granule, which acts as processing and repository area for lipids that contributes to the permeability barrier of the epithelium. It is found in the upper spinous and granular cell layer.

Keratohyaline granules: A substance present in the form of granules (contain keratinosome) in the cytoplasm of cells in stratum granulosum. It is the precursor of keratin.

Labyrinthodonts: Maze toothed due to the complex pattern of infolding of enamel and dentin.

Lacteals: An intestinal lymphatic that takes up chyle and passes it to the lymphatic circulation.

Lamina densa: Dark zone in the basal lamina of the epithelial connective tissue interface, which contains anchoring fibrils.

Lamina dura: A radiographic term used to denote the radiopaque lining of an alveolus that lies adjacent to the periodontal membrane, representing the alveolar bone proper.

Lamina limitans: It is the inner organic lining of the calcified dentinal tubule wall.

Lamina lucida: Clear zone in the basal lamina, which is situated just below the epithelial cells.

Lamina propria: Connective tissue of variable thickness that supports the epithelium.

Lamellar bone: Compact bone containing lamellations/layers (sheets like)

Laminin: Group of extracellular glycoproteins involved in several vital functions including communication, defense, and attachment.

Langerhans cell: Clear cell or dendritic cell in the upper layers of epithelium. They are derived from the bone marrow and play an important role in local defense mechanisms in the epithelium by acting as antigen presenting cells.

Layer of Hopewell-Smith: A thin layer located between the cementum and dentin at the root of the tooth; this layer, elaborated by the inner enamel epithelial layer of the Hertwig's epithelial root sheet, is believed to facilitate the adhesion of cementum to dentin.

Lines of Salter: They are incremental lines of cementum.

Lingual follicles (lymphoid): Irregularly studded, round or oval prominences seen on the posterior most part of the tongue and contain lymphoid tissue. It is also called "lingual tonsil".

Lingual swellings: Appear from the first pharyngeal arches at the floor of the mouth on either side to form the tongue.

Lingual varices: Dilated and tortuous (varicose) veins seen on the ventral aspect of tongue usually occur as a result of aging.

Lingula: A small tongue, like bony projection seen in the medial surface of the mandible, near the orifice of the mandibular foramen.

Lining mucosa: Mucosa having nonkeratinized epithelium found lining the lips, cheeks, vestibule, floor of the mouth, and soft palate.

Lipids: Any one of a group of fats or fat, like substances, characterized by their insolubility in water and solubility in fat solvents.

Lipofuscin: It is a fluorescent, intracellular pigment thought to be a cause for aging.

Lymph: Clear, transparent, colorless alkaline fluid formed by the interstitial fluid and found in the lymphatic vessels.

Lymph node: A rounded body consisting of accumulation of lymphatic tissue found at intervals in the course of lymphatic vessels.

Lymph nodule: A compartmentalized region found within the lymph node composed of a cortical region of combined follicle B lymphocytes, a paracortical region of T lymphocytes, and a basal part.

Lymph spaces: Spaces in connective tissue filled with lymph.

Lymphadenopathy: Enlargement of lymph node.

Lymphatic organ: A structure composed principally of lymphatic tissue, which includes lymph nodes, spleen, tonsil, and thymus.

Lymphatic system: Structures involved in the conveyance of lymph from the tissues to the bloodstream, which includes lymph capillaries, lacteals, lymph nodes, lymph vessels, and main lymph ducts.

Lymphatic vessel: Thin-walled vessels conveying lymph from the tissues.

Lymphoblast: A cell which gives rise to a lymphocyte.

Lymphoid lobule: Structural and functional unit of the lymph node radiating from the hilus to the capsular area in the form of cones.

Lysozyme: Antimicrobial enzyme secreted by the sinus epithelial cells, which may be significant in protection against infection of the nasal mucosa.

Mantle dentin: First formed dentin which is mineralized.

Mantle zone of the lymphatic nodule: Peripheral area of secondary follicle made of closely packed small lymphocytes.

Masticatory mucosa: Mucosa found in the gingiva and hard palate and is immovably attached and covered by keratinized epithelium.

Mast cells: Mononuclear cells which are spherical or elliptical in shape containing histamine and heparin granules.

Maxillary ostium: The opening through which the maxillary sinus communicates with the middle nasal meatus.

Maxillary sinus (antrum of Highmore): Air-filled space of maxilla formed to lighten the weight of the skull and opens into middle meatus of nose.

Meckel's cartilage: Cartilage of the first branchial arch.

Medullary area: Active site of plasma cell proliferation, differentiation and production of antibodies.

Meiosis: Cell division of the reproductive cells that occurs in two phases. The number of chromosomes reduced to half the original number.

Melanocytes: They are melanin-forming cells residing in the basal layer of the epithelium/epidermis. They are derived from the neural crest cells.

Membrana preformativa: The membrane between the inner enamel epithelium and the dental papilla, which will form the future dentinoenamel junction.

Merkel cell: Specialized neural pressure sensitive receptor cell in the basal region.

Merocrine gland: Glandular cells that secrete products from membrane-bound secretory vesicles inside the cell. These vesicles move to the apical surface and coalesce with the apical part of the cell membrane to release the product by exocytosis, *e.g.* salivary glands.

Mesenchymal stem cells: These are multipotent adult stem cells that can differentiate into connective tissue, bone, cartilage, marrow-stroma, and adipocytes.

Mesenchyme: The meshwork of embryonic connective tissue in the mesoderm from which connective tissues of the body are formed.

Mesial drift: Physiological movement of teeth in the mesial direction within the dental arch to maintain tight interproximal contact, brought about by the anterior component of force.

Mesoderm: The middle of the three primary germ layers of the embryo lying between the ectoderm and endoderm.

Metalloproteinases: The group of enzymes those are associated with the breakdown of connective tissue fibers.

Microtome: An instrument used to cut thin sections of the processed tissue for microscopic examination.

Mitosis: Cell division that occur in the somatic cell, results in the production of two daughter cells.

Monophyodonty: Mammals with only one set of teeth that develops in their lifetime.

Morphodifferentiation: A process by which the ameloblasts establish the basic form and relative size of teeth by differential growth. This stage of tooth development, the morphology of the tooth is determined.

Morula: A solid mass of cells resembling a mulberry, formed by cleavage of a zygote.

Mottled enamel: Alterations in enamel structure often due to excessive fluoride ingestion during tooth formation.

Mounting: Process of placing the histological sections under a coverslip with a suitable mounting media (*e.g.* DPX, Canada balsam, etc.) to be examined or to be stored.

Mucin: A glycoprotein found in mucus, which can be present in bile, in salivary glands, skin, connective tissue, tendon, and cartilage.

Mucogingival junction: Line of demarcation between the attached gingiva and alveolar mucosa.

Mucous cells: Specialized epithelial cells, which secrete mucus. They are present in the acini of mucous salivary gland. They have broad base and thin rim of cytoplasm.

Multipotent: Stem cells that can develop into more than one cell type, but are limited than pluripotent cells.

Myoepithelial cells/basket cells: Stellate or spider-like, basket-shaped cells that embrace the secretory and ductal cells in a glandular epithelium, which help in the expulsion of saliva.

Naive B cells: B cells which mature in the absence of foreign antigen and leave the primary lymphoid organ.

Naive T cells: T cells which mature in the absence of foreign antigen and leave the primary lymphoid organ.

Nasal pit: A depression that appears in the olfactory placodes in the early stages of development of the face to form the nose.

Nasmyth's membrane: The reduced enamel epithelium and the basal lamina together constitutes the Nasmyth's membrane. This will be lost as tooth erupts by the degeneration of the epithelial cells and attrition and abrasion.

Natal teeth: Teeth that are present at birth.

Neonatal line: The line of demarcation between prenatal and postnatal enamel and dentin.

Neonatal ring: Neonatal line is otherwise called as neonatal ring.

Neonatal teeth: Teeth that erupt during the first month of life.

Neural crest cells: Specialized cells formed at the lateral portion of the neural tube during the early stages of embryonic development. These cells undergo extensive migration.

Neural crest: Paired longitudinal elevations resulting from the invagination of the neural plate of the ectoderm in the early developing embryo.

Neural groove: Groove formed in the midline of the embryo by the progressive elevation of the neural crest, which leads to the formation of the neural tube.

Neural plate: A thickened band of ectoderm in the midbody region of the developing embryo, which develops into the neural tube.

Nonkeratinocytes: Cells present in the epithelium, but they do not possess cytokeratin filaments and do not have the ability to keratinize, e.g. melanocytes, Langerhans cell, and Merkel cell.

Nucleotide: Nucleotides are the building blocks of nucleic acids; they are composed of three subunit molecules:

(1) a nitrogenous base, (2) a five-carbon sugar (ribose or deoxyribose), and (3) at least one phosphate group.

Nucleotide probes: A labeled fragment of DNA or RNA used to find its complementary sequence or locate a particular clone.

Oblique fibers (of the PDL): They are the largest group of the periodontal ligament fibers, which extend in an oblique direction from the bone coronally and cementum apically.

Occlusal plane: The imaginary surface extending from the tip of the mandibular incisors back along the cusp tips of mandibular molar teeth.

Odontoblast process: Cytoplasmic extensions of odontoblasts enclosed within the dentinal tubules.

Odontoblasts: Cells responsible for the formation of dentin and are differentiated from the dental papilla cells, which in turn are from the ectomesenchyme.

Odontoclasts: Large multinucleated cells associated with resorption of tooth. They are analog to the osteoclasts of the bone.

Odontodes: Tooth-like units that are described simply as structures that comprise a mineralized hard tissue unit.

Osteoprotegerin (OPG): It is a decoy receptor and prevents the binding of RANK and RANKL thereby prevents osteoclast differentiation. It belongs to tumor necrosis factor superfamily.

Orthokeratin: Absence of nuclei or its remnants in the keratin layer.

Osteoblasts: Cells responsible for the formation of bone, usually located on the edges of the bony trabeculae.

Osteoclasts: Multinucleated giant cells responsible for the bone resorption.

Osteocytes: Entrapped osteoblasts within the bone matrix.

Osteodentin: The rapidly formed tertiary dentin that contains entrapped odontoblasts and few dentinal tubules.

Osteoid: Unmineralized bone matrix formed by the osteoblasts, usually found around the bony trabeculae.

Ova: The female reproductive cell, developed in the ovary.

Oxytalan fibers: They are immature elastic fibers composed of microfilaments and have unique staining characteristics.

Paracortex: Densely cellular area extending beneath the cortex and in between the lymphoid follicles forming cellular strands from the capsule to the corticomedullary junction.

Paracrine glands: Glands that secrete products, which influence the secretion of another product by a local gland or cell (products act on neighboring cells).

Paraffin infiltration: Process of permeating the tissue with a support medium, usually paraffin wax during histological processing of tissue.

Parotid gland: One of the three major salivary glands situated in front and below the ear on either side of the face, which is of pure serous type, and transfers its secretion through Stensen's duct.

PDLSCs: Periodontal ligament stem cells.

Perikymata: Horizontal, shallow and parallel grooves seen on the enamel surface of newly erupted tooth, which wear away in course of time.

Periodontal ligament: Connective tissue, which attaches the tooth to the alveolar bone. It was also called pericementum.

Periodontal space: The area occupied by the periodontal ligament. In radiographs it appears as radiolucent band between the tooth root and the alveolar bone proper.

Periodontium: The tissues, which surround and support the tooth. These include the gingiva, periodontal ligament, cementum, and alveolar bone proper.

Periosteum: A specialized connective tissue that covers all bones of the body and made up of inner cellular layer (cambial layer) and outer fibrous layer.

Peritubular dentin: The hypermineralized rim of the dentinal tubule. It is also known as intratubular dentin.

Peyer's patches: Aggregation of lymph nodules found chiefly in the ileum near its junction with the colon.

pH: Measure of hydrogen ion concentration of a solution.

Phenotype: The physical appearance of an organism as distinguished from its genetic makeup.

Pink tooth: Also known as internal resorption of a tooth, which may appear as a pinkish area on the crown, initiated by inflammatory hyperplasia of the pulp.

Plasma cells: A fully differentiated B lymphocyte with a distinct clock-face nucleus, which produces antibody.

Pleurodont: Dentition with the teeth fused to the inner/lingual surface of the jaw bone through the outer surface of their roots.

Plexus of Raschkow: A plexus of myelinated nerve fibers located between the cell-rich zone and the pulp core.

Pluripotent: Type of stem cells which give rise to cells of all the three germ layers of the embryo, *i.e.* endoderm, mesoderm, and the ectoderm.

Pneumatization: Process of formation of air-filled cells or cavities.

Polymerase chain reaction (PCR): The technique used in molecular biology to amplify a single copy or a few copies of a segment of DNA across several orders of magnitude, generating thousands to millions of copies of a particular DNA sequence.

Posteruptive tooth movement: Maintains the position of the erupted tooth in occlusion while the jaws continue to grow and compensate for the occlusal and proximal wear.

Predentin: Unmineralized dentin matrix.

Pre-eruptive tooth movement: Movement of the tooth germs within tissues of the jaw before they begin to erupt.

Premaxilla: Develops from the frontonasal process, carries four incisor teeth and forms a component in palate development.

Preodontoblast: The precursor of an odontoblast.

Primary dentin: Dentin formed before the root completion.

Primary epithelial band: A horseshoe-shaped thickening of the oral ectoderm at about 6th week of intrauterine life in the region of the future dental arch.

Primary lymphoid organ: Area where pre-T and pre-B lymphocytes mature into naïve T and naïve B cells.

Primary palate: It forms the anterior portion of the palate containing the incisor teeth and develops from the median nasal process.

Primates: Extraordinarily diverse group of mammals having over 50 extant (existing) genera and 200 recognized species.

Primitive node: A local thickening of the epiblast at the cephalic end of the primitive streak of the embryo.

Primitive streak: A dense area on the central posterior region of the embryonic disk. It is formed by the morphogenetic movement of a rapidly proliferating mass of cells that spreads between the ectoderm and endoderm, giving rise to the mesoderm layer.

Principal fibers: The major periodontal fiber groups run in different directions and attach the tooth to the alveolar bone proper.

Prochordal plate: A small area immediately rostral to the cephalic tip of the notochord where ectoderm and endoderm are in contact.

Progenitor cell: It is similar to a stem cell, which has a tendency to differentiate into a specific type.

Proteins: Major constituent of cells and tissues which are basically made up of amino acids linked by peptide bonds.

Proteoglycans: A compound consisting of a carbohydrate and protein.

Pseudostratified epithelium: Epithelium made up of single layer of cells that give the appearance of multiple layers, due to the arrangement of nuclei at different levels.

Pulp chamber: The space occupied by the pulp of the crown.

Pulp stones: The calcified masses present in the pulp.

Radicular pulp: Part of the dental pulp contained within the root canal or in the root portion of the tooth.

RANK: Receptor activator of nuclear factor kappa. It is the receptor for RANK-ligand (RANK-L) and part of the RANK/RANK-L/OPG signaling pathway. This signaling regulates osteoclast differentiation and activation. It is associated with bone remodeling and repair.

RANK-L: Receptor activator of nuclear factor kappa-B ligand. It is a member of the tumor necrosis factor (TNF) superfamily. Along with RANK it functions as a key factor for osteoclast differentiation and activation.

Reciprocal induction: The phenomenon by which the cell signals of the epithelium and primitive ectomesenchyme mutually initiates and regulates the formation and differentiation of specialized structures such as enamel, dentin, and cementum.

Reduced enamel epithelium: After the collapse of the stellate reticulum, the ameloblasts, stratum intermedium, remnants of the stellate reticulum and outer enamel epithelium form the reduced enamel epithelium. This protects the enamel until the tooth erupts and plays a role in the formation of dentogingival junction.

Reichert's cartilage: It is the second branchial arch cartilage, which forms the stapes, styloid process, and lesser horns of hyoid bone.

Reparative dentin (tertiary dentin): Dentin that forms around the pulp chamber in response to any abnormal stimulus or irritation.

Resting lines: These are incremental lines representing the interval between the bone formation and rest period.

Rests of Serre: Remnants of dental lamina entrapped within gingiva and jaw bone.

Retained deciduous teeth: Deciduous tooth that is present despite the eruption of permanent tooth.

Reticular network: A delicate meshwork of spindle and stellate-shaped follicular reticular cells and reticular fibers which supports the follicular and parafollicular areas of lymph node.

Reticulin fibers: They are immature collagen fibers associated with the basement membrane of the blood vessels. They can be demonstrated with silver stains.

Reversal line: A distinct basophilic line in stained sections of bone that indicates the location where bone resorption gave way to bone apposition.

RNA: Ribonucleic acid, which acts as a messenger carrying instructions from DNA for controlling the synthesis of proteins.

Saliva: Tasteless, odorless, alkaline watery fluid secreted into the mouth by salivary glands, which helps in providing lubrication for chewing and swallowing.

Salivary gland: Exocrine gland, which produces saliva and is present in the vicinity of oral cavity.

Salivary IgA: Predominant immunoglobulin found in saliva produced by the plasma cells in the connective tissue of the gland.

Salivary pellicle: Thin layer of salivary protein and glycoprotein that quickly forms after teeth are cleaned.

SCAP: Stem cells from the apical papilla.

Schneiderian membrane: Membranous lining of the maxillary sinus.

Sclerotic dentin: Dentin characterized by calcification of the dentinal tubules as a result of injury or aging. This dentin appears transparent. So it is also known as transparent dentin.

Secondary dentin: Dentin formed after the root completion and laid down throughout the life of the tooth.

Secondary lymphoid organ: Area where naïve T and naïve B cells encounter antigenic stimulus and generate adaptive response.

Serous cells: Pyramid-shaped cells with a broad base and a narrow apex facing the lumen present in the serous salivary gland.

Serous demilunes: Crescent-shaped group of serous cells that form a cap-like structure surrounding the mucous acini in mixed salivary glands.

Sharpey's fibers: The embedded portion of the periodontal ligament fibers in the cementum and the alveolar bone.

SHED: Stem cells from human exfoliated deciduous teeth.

Shh: Sonic hedgehog is a protein that in humans is encoded by the *SHH* ("sonic hedgehog") gene. It plays a key role in regulating vertebrate organogenesis, such as in the growth of digits on limbs, development of teeth and organization of the brain. *SHH* gene is located on the long (q) arm of chromosome 7 at position 36.

Somites: One of the paired, block-like masses of mesoderm, arranged segmentally alongside the neural tube of the embryo, forming the vertebral column and segmental musculature.

Specialized mucosa: Mucous membrane covering the dorsal surface of the tongue containing taste buds.

Sperm: It is the male "gamete" or sex cell. It combines with the female "gamete," called ovum, to form the zygote.

Stellate reticulum: The star-shaped cells that lie between the outer enamel epithelium, stratum intermedium and/or inner enamel epithelium. They appear star-shaped because they secrete glycosaminoglycans, which are hydrophilic, and imbibe water. The cells maintain desmosomal contact with the neighboring cells despite the accumulation of water molecules in between the cells and become star-shaped.

Stem cells: Unspecialized cells that are capable of becoming specialized cells, each with new specialized cell functions.

Stem cells from human exfoliated deciduous teeth (SHED): They are mesenchymal cells, originating from the neural crest, which reside within the exfoliated deciduous tooth pulp tissue.

Stensen's duct: It is the other name for the parotid gland duct.

Stippling (gingival): An orange peel appearance of the attached gingiva due to the enlargement of underlying connective tissue papilla.

Stomodeum: Refers to the primitive mouth that appears as a small depression in the early embryo. Also called as stomodeum.

Stratification: Act or process of arranging in layers.

Stratum basale: Innermost layer of the epidermis and other stratified squamous epithelium that lies over the basement membrane.

Stratum corneum: Outermost or superficial horny layer of the epidermis/epithelium having keratin.

Stratum germinativum: Basal and parabasal layer in which proliferation of cells occurs.

Stratum granulosum: Layer of cells containing deeply staining keratohyaline granules.

Stratum spinosum: Prickle cell layer, so called because of the prominent intercellular bridges.

Striae of Retzius: Incremental growth lines in enamel seen microscopically as dark and light bands.

Striated duct: Largest portion of the duct system lined by a layer of tall columnar cells that connects the intercalated to an interlobular duct and is characterized by the folding of the basal plasma membrane.

Sublingual gland: They are smallest of the major salivary glands which is of mixed type, situated in the floor of the mouth between the tongue and mandible on each side.

Submandibular gland: They are paired, mixed, major salivary gland located beneath the floor of the mouth bilaterally.

Submerged teeth: Deciduous teeth present below the occlusal plane that have undergone variable degree of root resorption and then have become ankylosed to the bone.

Submucosa: Connective tissue layer, which lies deeper to the lamina propria.

Succinate dehydrogenase: It is an enzyme complex, found in many bacterial cells and in the inner mitochondrial membrane of eukaryotes. It is the only enzyme that participates in both the citric acid cycle and the electron transport chain.

Sulcus terminalis: It is the separation formed between the anterior two-thirds and posterior one third of the tongue, and marked by a V-shaped depression, just anterior to foramen cecum.

Supraeruption: Condition in which the tooth erupts beyond the occlusal plane due to the loss of the opposing tooth.

Syndecan: A proteoglycan which acts as an adhesion molecule between fibroblast and collagen.

Synovial fluid: A clear thixotropic fluid, which serves as a lubricant in a joint, tendon sheath, or bursa; consists mainly of mucin with some albumin, fat, epithelium, and leukocytes; also helps to nourish the avascular articular cartilage.

Synovial joint: A freely movable joint with a cavity lined by synovial membrane and lubricated by synovial fluid.

Synovial membrane: A connective tissue layer that lines the cavities of joints, tendon sheaths and bursae. The synovial membrane secretes synovial fluid that has lubricating function.

T cells: It is T lymphocyte, a subtype of white blood cell that plays an important role in cell mediated immunity. They are also called as thymocyte.

Taste buds: They are chemoreceptive intraepithelial sensory end organs that mediate the sensation of taste, found around the walls of the circumvallate papillae, on the surface of the fungiform papillae, lateral walls of the foliate papillae, soft palate and epiglottis in small numbers. They are ovoid or barrel shaped and approximately 30–80 µm in length and 50–80 µm in diameter.

Teething: Symptoms of inflammation such as pain, fever and malaise associated with the erupting tooth.

Telomeres: They are specific DNA protein structures found at both ends of each chromosome, and the length is inversely proportional to the lifespan of an individual.

Tertiary dentin: Reparative, response or reactive dentin formed in response to trauma such as caries. It is a defensive reaction of the pulp-dentin complex. Otherwise known as reparative dentin/reactive dentin/irregular secondary dentin.

Thecodont: Dentition with the base of the tooth completely enclosed in a deep socket or alveolus of bone.

Tissue fixation: Process of stabilizing and hardening the tissue with minimal distortion of cells. Fixation prevents autolysis and putrefaction.

Tissue processing: Process of preparing the biopsied/ excised tissue to be examined under the microscope.

Temporomandibular joint (TMJ) ankylosis: The fusion or union of the condyle with the mandibular fossa of the temporomandibular joint by bony or fibrous tissue, resulting in complete/partial immobility.

Tomes' granular layer: This is the granular layer seen in the dentin, adjacent to the cementodentinal junction.

Tomes' process: During the synthesis of enamel, the ameloblast moves away from the enamel, forming a cone-shaped projection, through which the enamel matrix is discharged.

Tonofilaments: They are intermediate filaments that form the cytoskeleton of the epithelial cells and an active component of desmosomes and hemidesmosomes.

Tonsillar crypts: A deep indentation into the pharyngeal surface of a tonsil.

Tonsils: Mass of lymphatic tissue located in depression of the mucous membrane of fauces and pharynx.

Tooth germ: It is the developing tooth made up enamel organ, dental papilla, and dental sac.

Totipotent cells: An undifferentiated cell capable of developing into any type of body cell.

Trabeculae (bone): It is a piece of bone. They anastomose in cancellous bone, which form a meshwork of intercommunicating spaces that are filled with bone marrow.

Transdifferentiation: Conversion of one mature somatic cell into another mature somatic cell without undergoing a pluripotent cell state. It can occur naturally in respone to injury or can be induced experimentally.

Transseptal fibers: A group of principal fibers of the periodontal ligament that extend across the crest of the alveolar bone from the cementum of one tooth to the cementum of the adjacent tooth.

Tartrate-resistant acid phosphatase (TRAP): This is expressed by osteoclasts and is associated with reduced bone resorption.

Triconodont: A type of tooth that is represented by having three cusps arranged in a line.

Trophoblast: The outermost layer of cells of the mammalian blastocyst that attaches the fertilized ovum to the uterine wall and serves as a nutritive pathway for the embryo.

True denticles: Localized masses of calcified tissue seen in the pulp chamber or canals that resemble dentin due to their tubular structure.

Tuberculum impar: A smooth embryonic swelling in the midline of the floor of the primordial mouth between the first and second pharyngeal arches and contributes to the formation of anterior part of the tongue.

Tuftelin: It is an acidic enamel protein, thought to play an important role in enamel mineralization during amelogenesis and implicated in dental caries susceptibility.

Turnover time (epithelial): The time taken for a cell to divide at the basal layer and pass through the entire epithelium to mature and desquamate.

Vermilion border: The red boundary of the lips, which represents the highly vascular, hyalinized epithelial covering between the outer skin and oral mucosa.

Vertebrates: Organisms that possess notochord during the embryonic period to be replaced later by bony vertebral column.

Vestibular lamina: A labial and buccal extension of the oral ectoderm, the cells of which degenerate to form the vestibule.

Volkmann's canal: Small perpendicular canal that connects the adjacent haversian canals of the bone.

von Ebner's glands: They are minor salivary glands and the duct of which open into the valley-like depression surrounding the circumvallate papillae.

von Korff's fibers: The larger diameter collagen fibers with extreme affinity for silver stain composed mainly of type III collagen and found near the future dentinoenamel junction parallel to odontoblastic layer. However, their existence is questionable.

Wharton's duct: Other name for submandibular gland duct.

Woven bone: It is an immature bone in which the collagen fibers of the matrix are arranged irregularly in the form of interlacing networks. It is seen during rapid bone formation as in embryonic development and in repair.

Xerostomia: Dry mouth resulting from reduced or absence in the salivary flow.

Xenograft: Transplant tissue taken from one species to be grafted to another.

Zygote: The cell formed by the union of sperm and ova.

Zymogen granules: Secretory granules that are found in the acinar cells of salivary glands and pancreas.

Appendix 2 Histologic Diagrams

B Sivapathasundharam, RJ Vijayashree

BUD STAGE OF TOOTH DEVELOPMENT

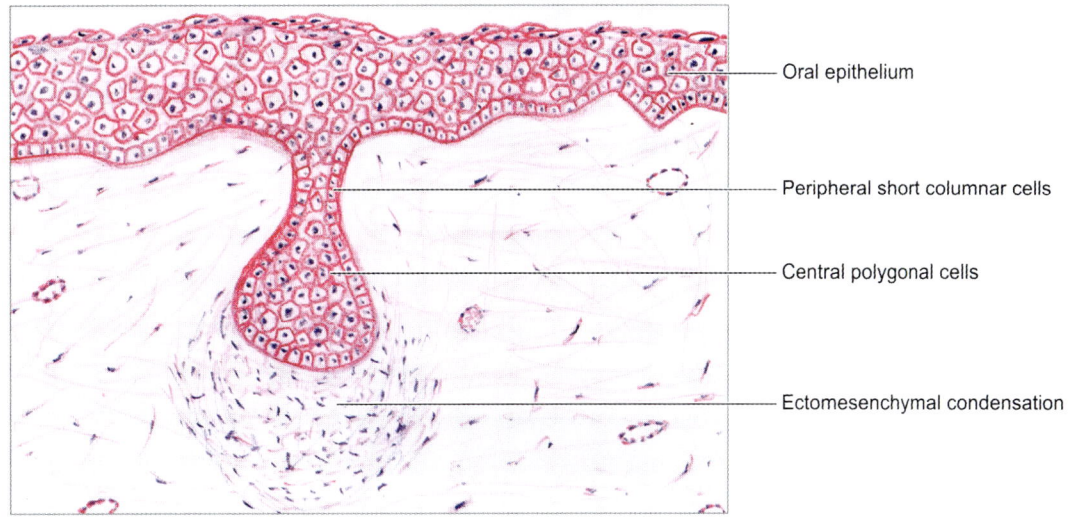

CAP STAGE OF TOOTH DEVELOPMENT

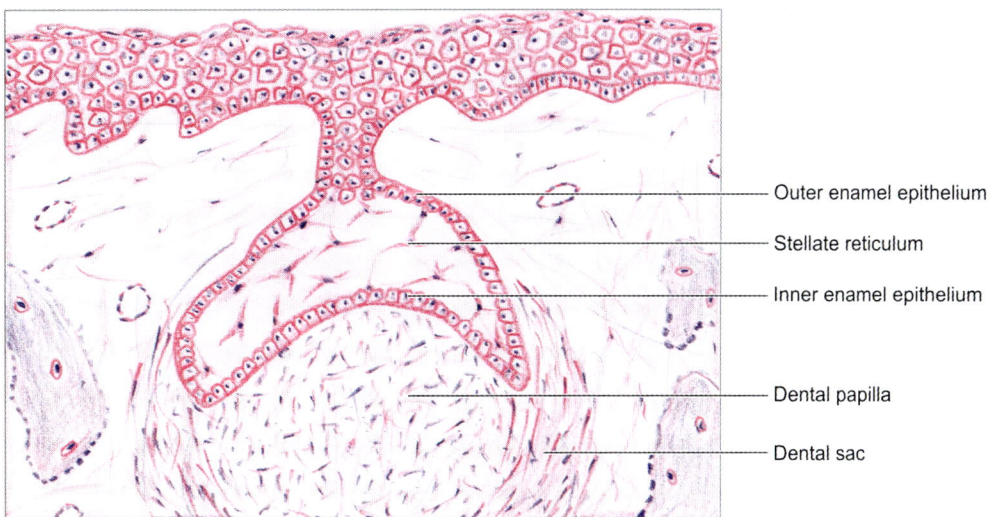

EARLY BELL STAGE OF TOOTH DEVELOPMENT

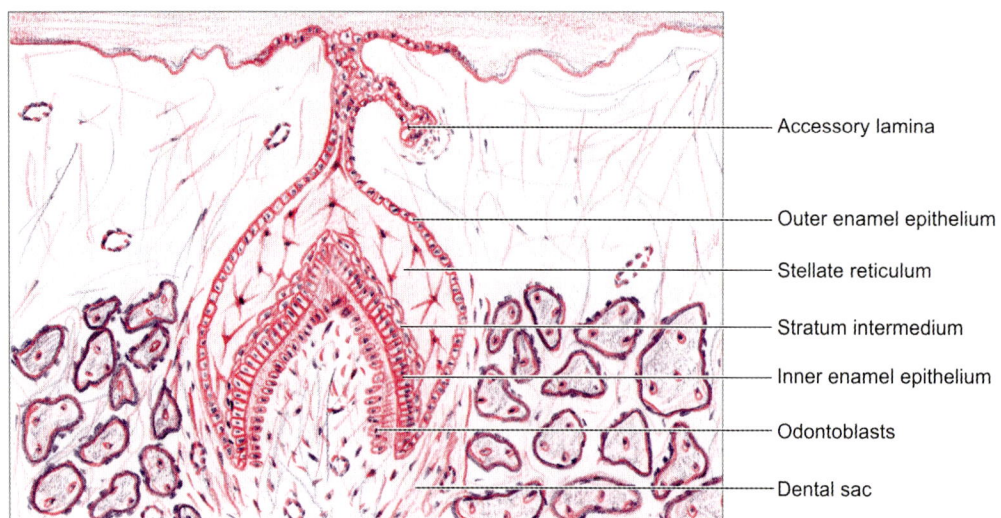

- Accessory lamina
- Outer enamel epithelium
- Stellate reticulum
- Stratum intermedium
- Inner enamel epithelium
- Odontoblasts
- Dental sac

ADVANCE BELL STAGE OF TOOTH DEVELOPMENT

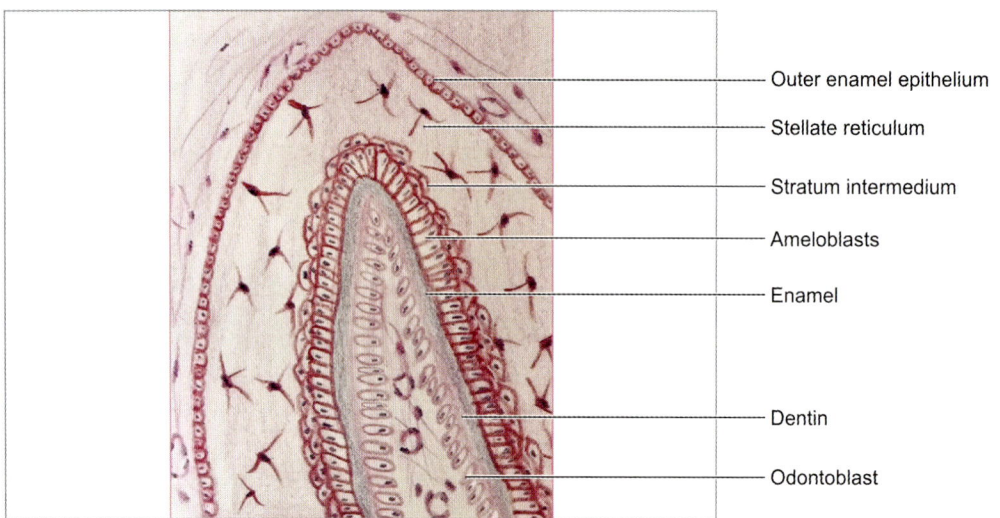

- Outer enamel epithelium
- Stellate reticulum
- Stratum intermedium
- Ameloblasts
- Enamel
- Dentin
- Odontoblast

HERTWIG'S EPITHELIAL ROOT SHEATH

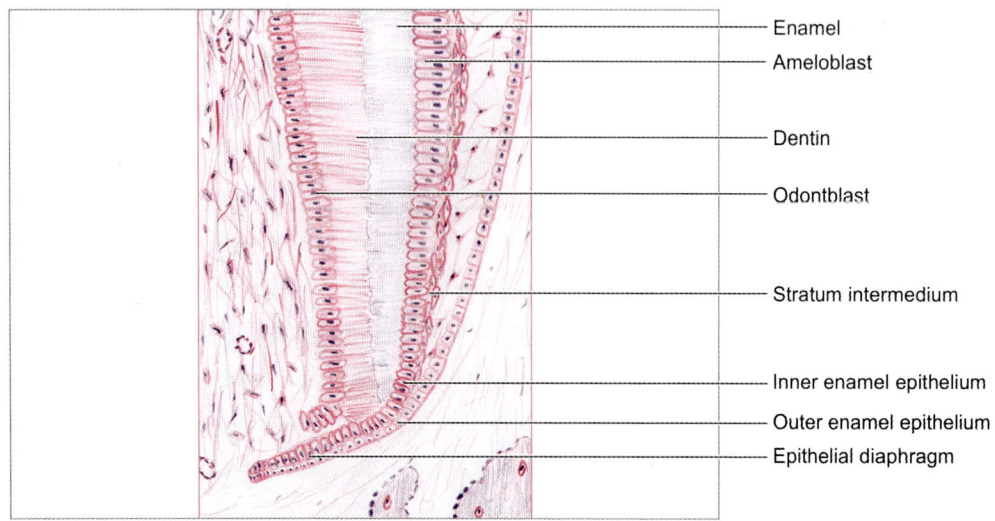

- Enamel
- Ameloblast
- Dentin
- Odontblast
- Stratum intermedium
- Inner enamel epithelium
- Outer enamel epithelium
- Epithelial diaphragm

CROSS SECTION OF ENAMEL RODS

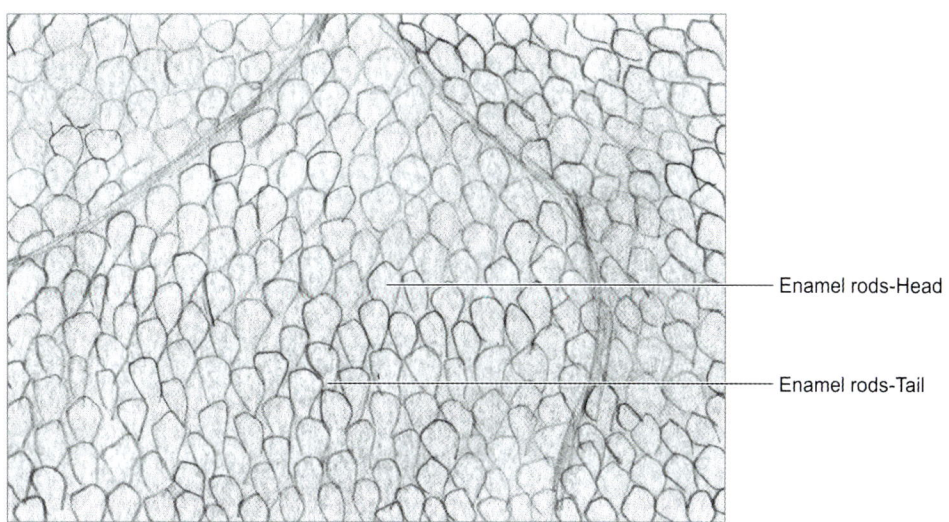

- Enamel rods-Head
- Enamel rods-Tail

CROSS SECTION OF ENAMEL RODS-FISH SCALE PATTERN

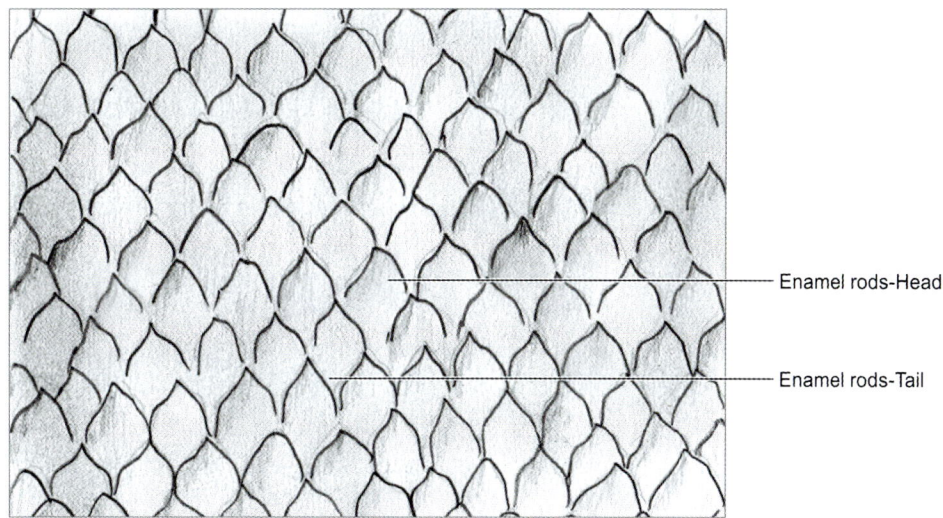

- Enamel rods-Head
- Enamel rods-Tail

ENAMEL RODS EXHIBITING TORTUOUS PATTERN

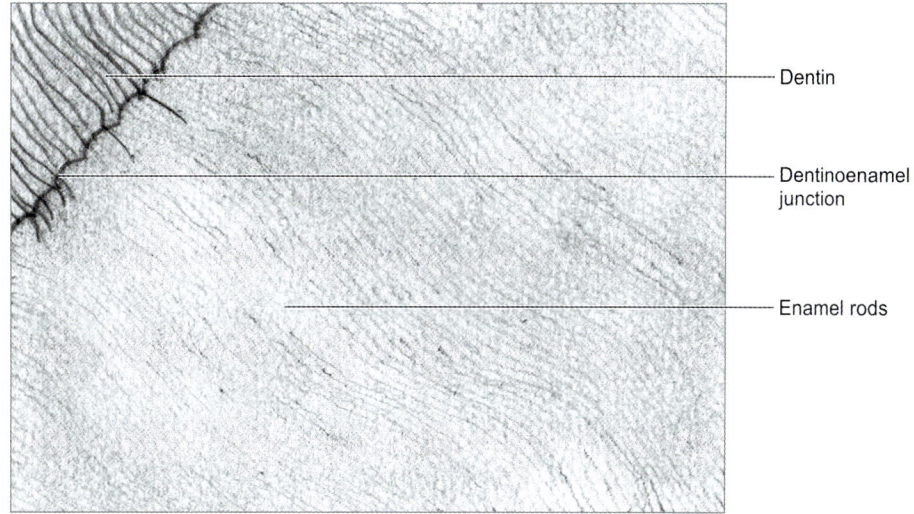

- Dentin
- Dentinoenamel junction
- Enamel rods

INCREMENTAL LINES OF RETZIUS

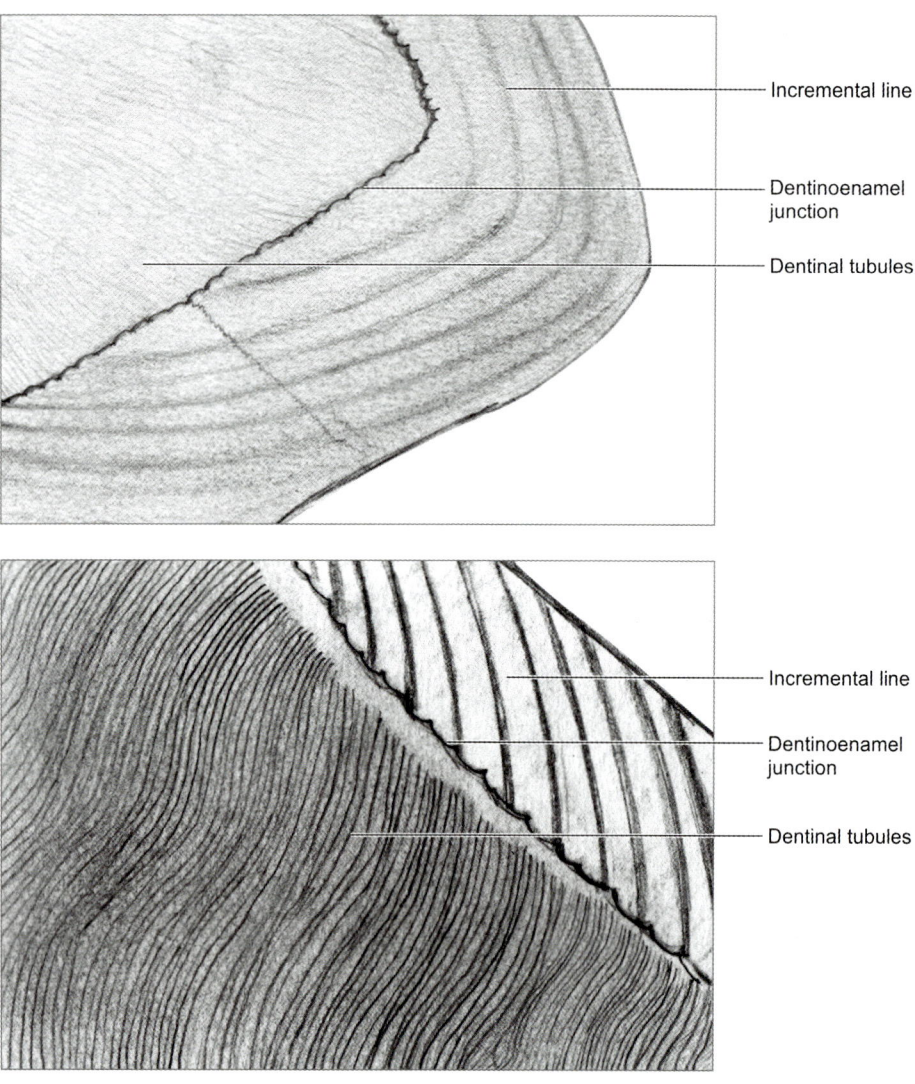

ENAMEL LAMELLAE

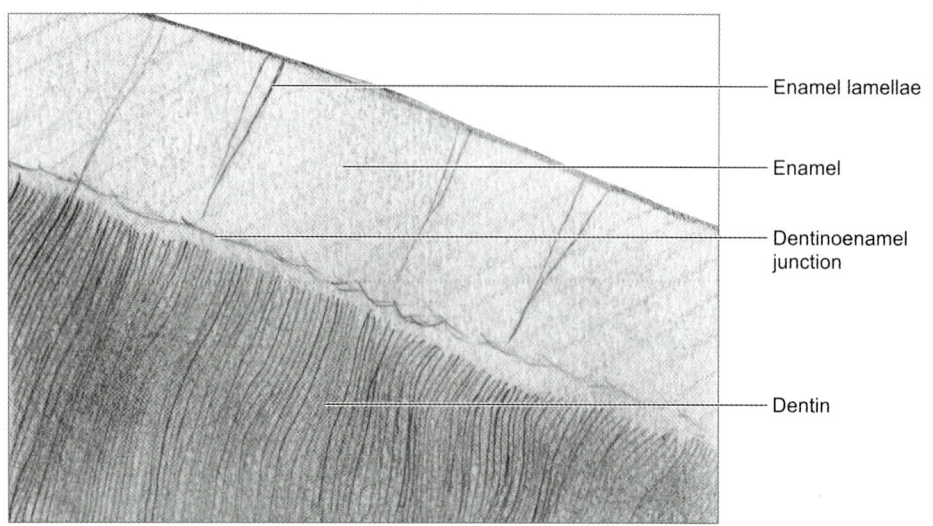

ENAMEL SPINDLES

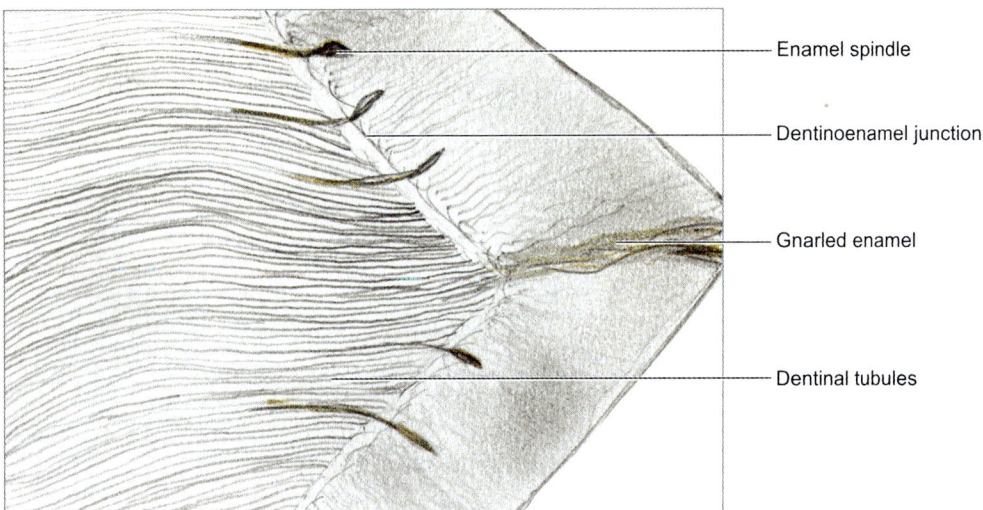

ENAMEL TUFTS

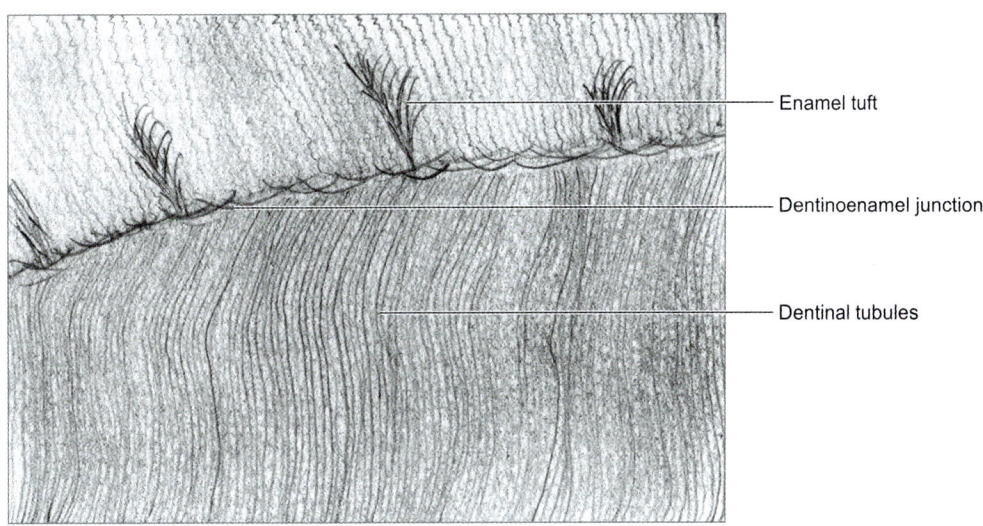

HUNTER SCHREGOR BANDS

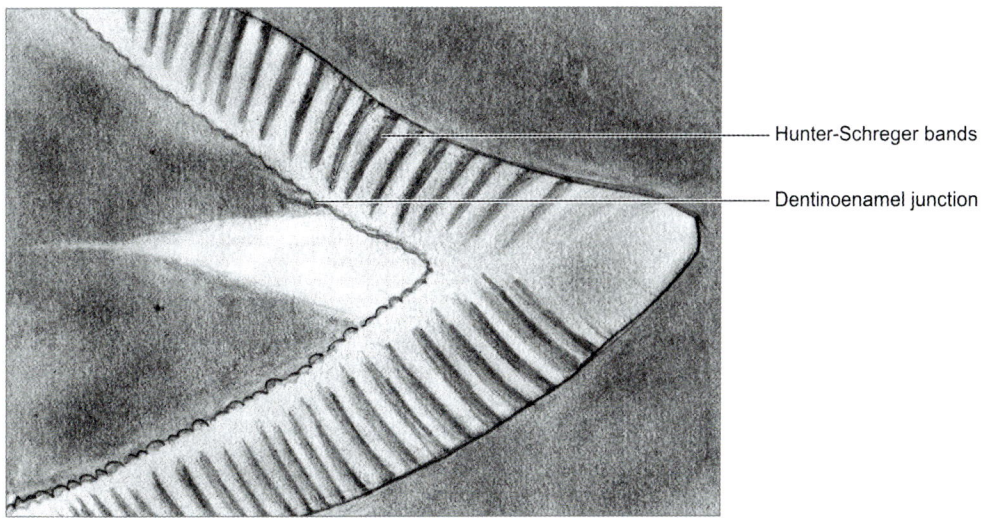

CROSS SECTION OF DENTINAL TUBULES

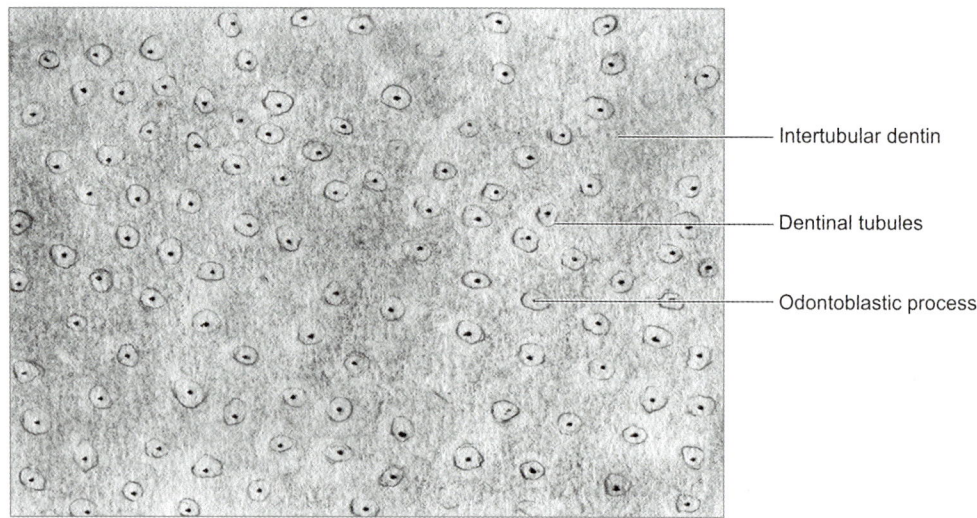

- Intertubular dentin
- Dentinal tubules
- Odontoblastic process

INTERGLOBULAR DENTIN

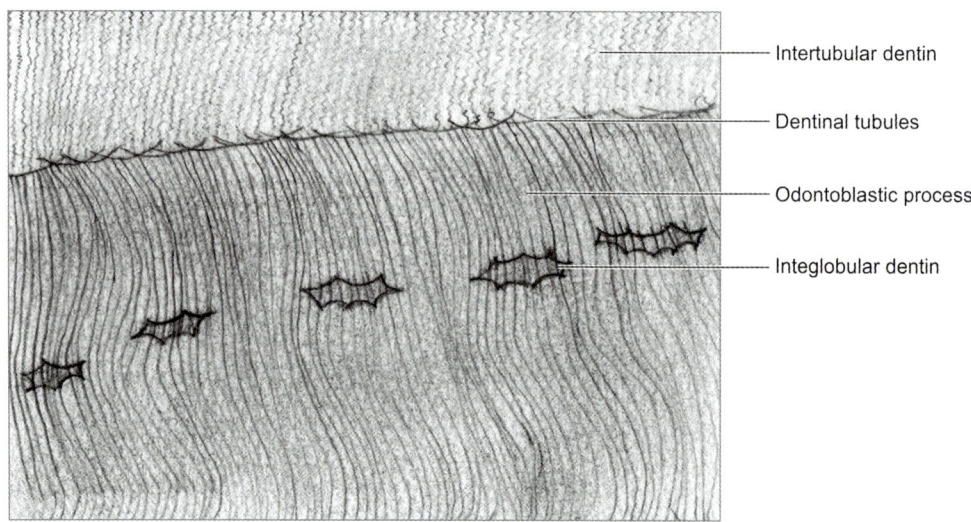

- Intertubular dentin
- Dentinal tubules
- Odontoblastic process
- Integlobular dentin

TERMINAL BRANCHING OF ODONTOBLASTIC PROCESSES

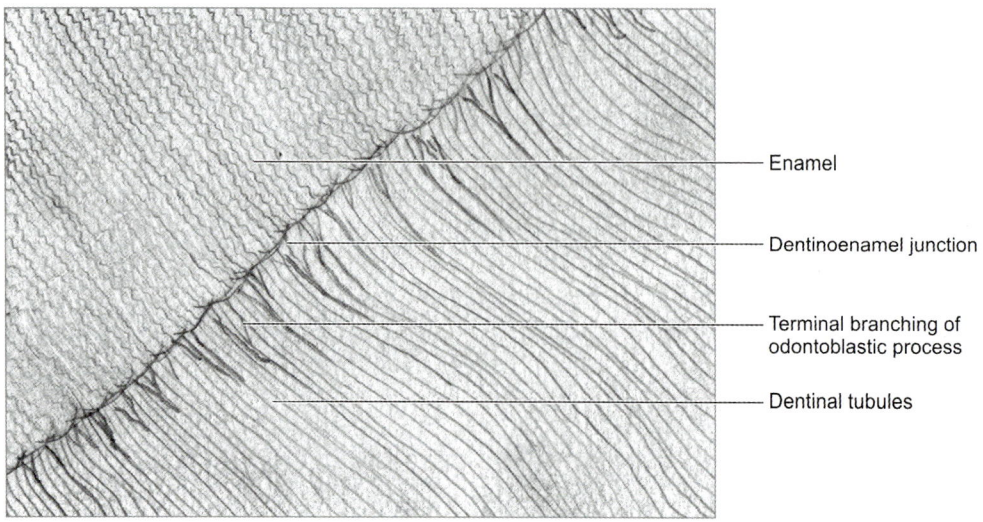

- Enamel
- Dentinoenamel junction
- Terminal branching of odontoblastic process
- Dentinal tubules

DEAD TRACTS

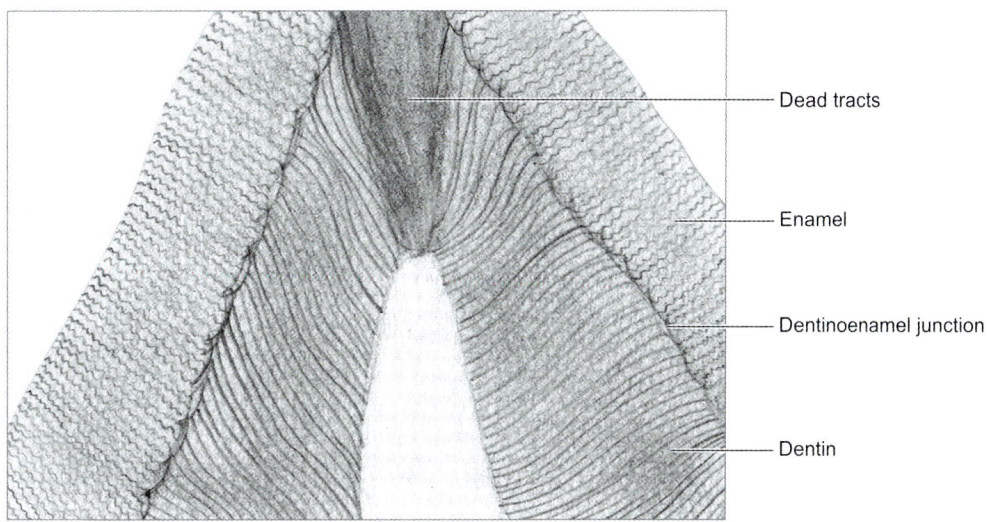

TOMES' GRANULAR LAYER

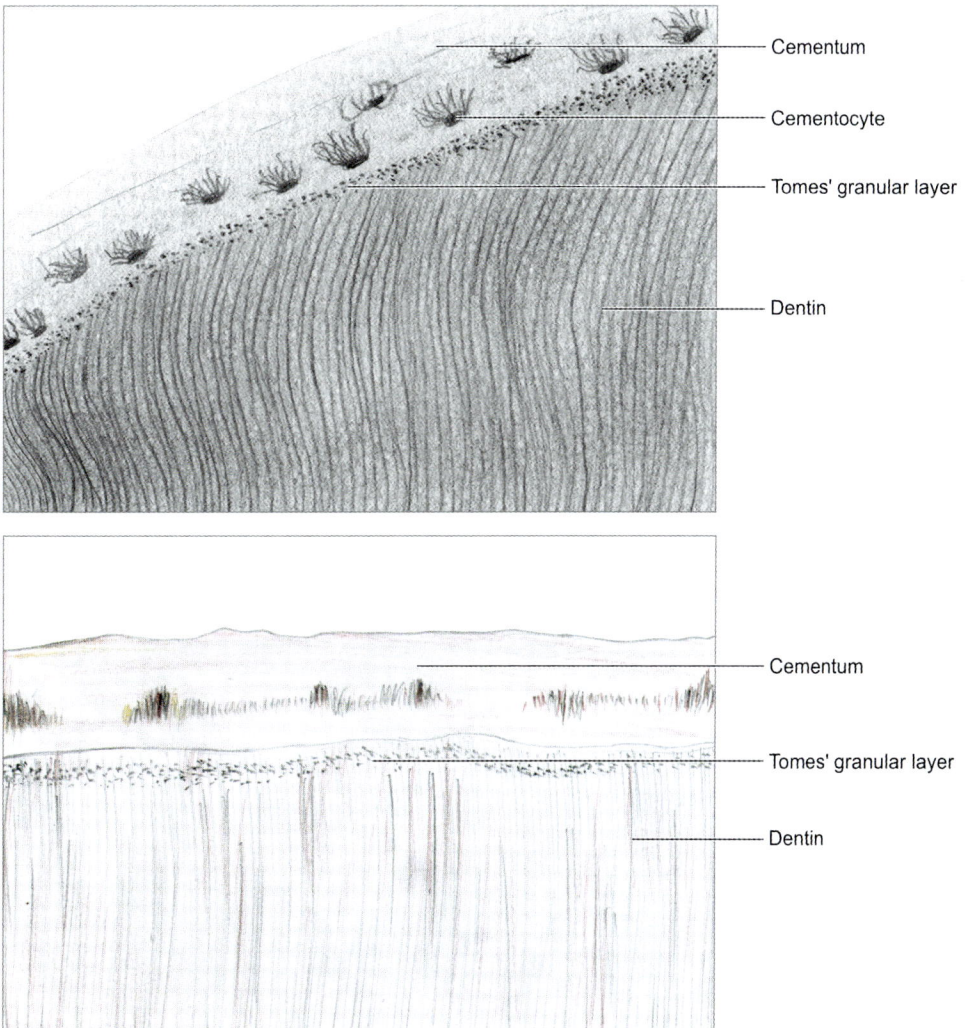

CELLULAR CEMENTUM

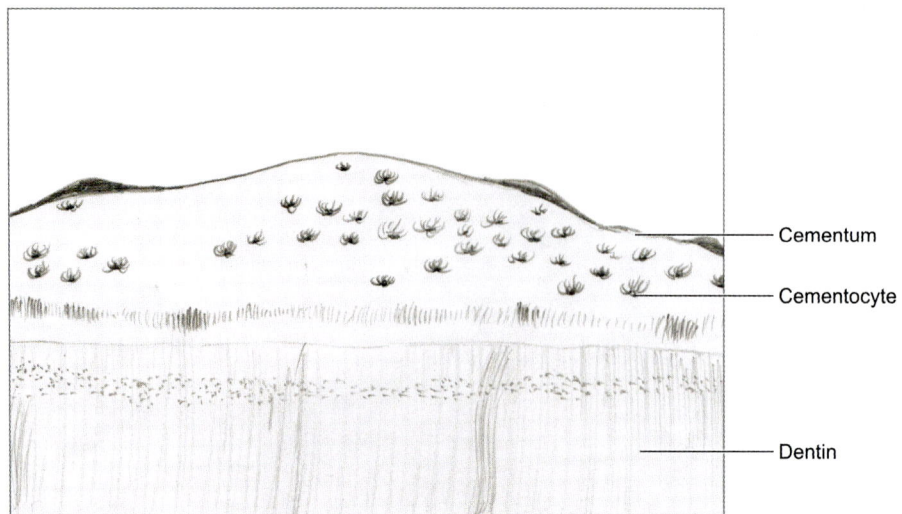

AELLULAR CEMENTUM

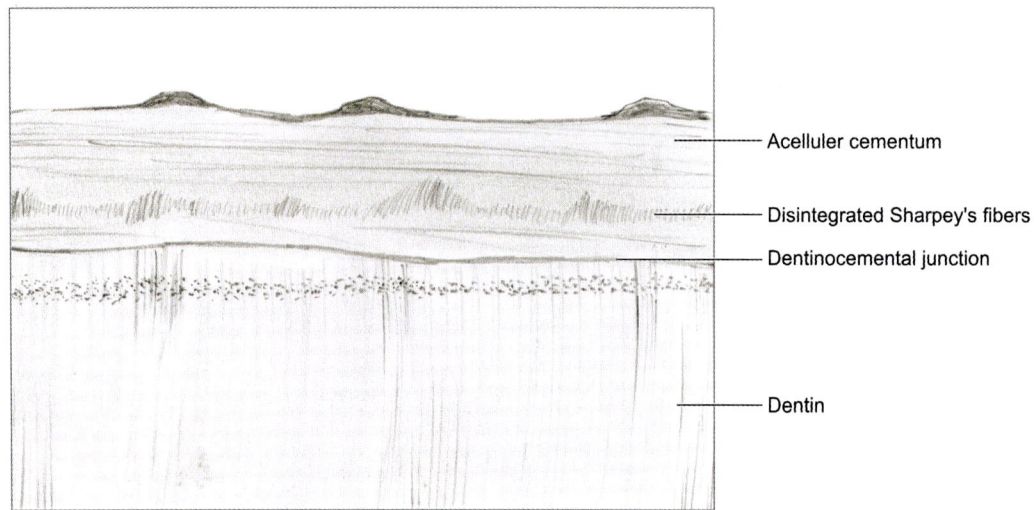

CELLULAR CEMENTUM IN DECALCIFIED AND H&E STAINED SECTION

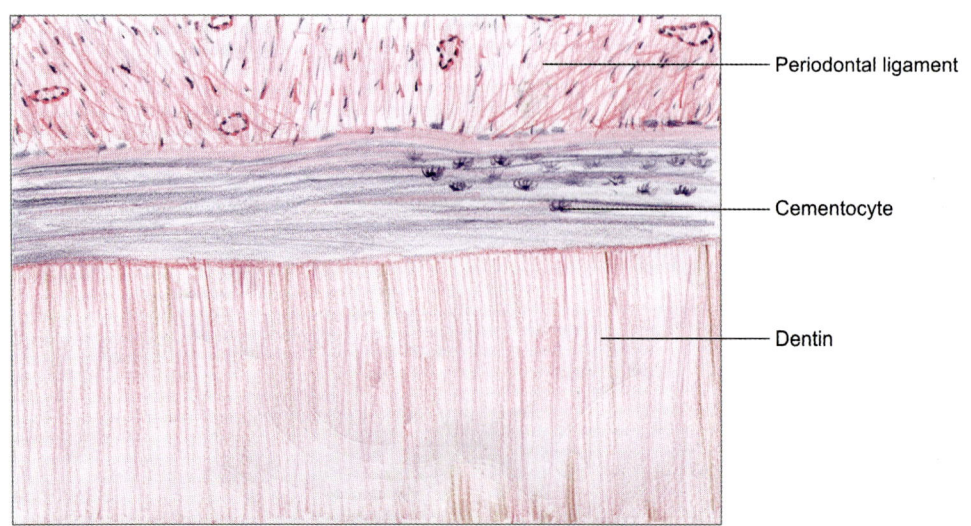

CEMENTOENAMEL JUNCTION-BUTT TYPE

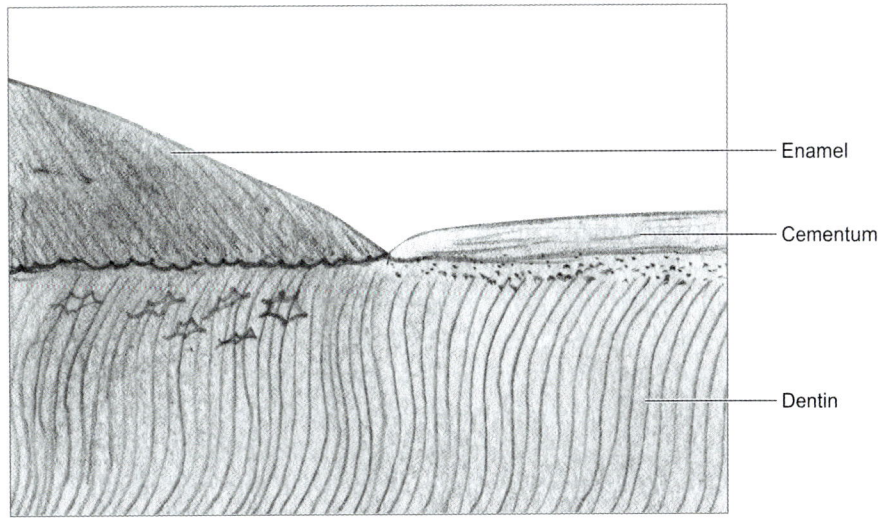

CEMENTOENAMEL JUNCTION-GAP TYPE

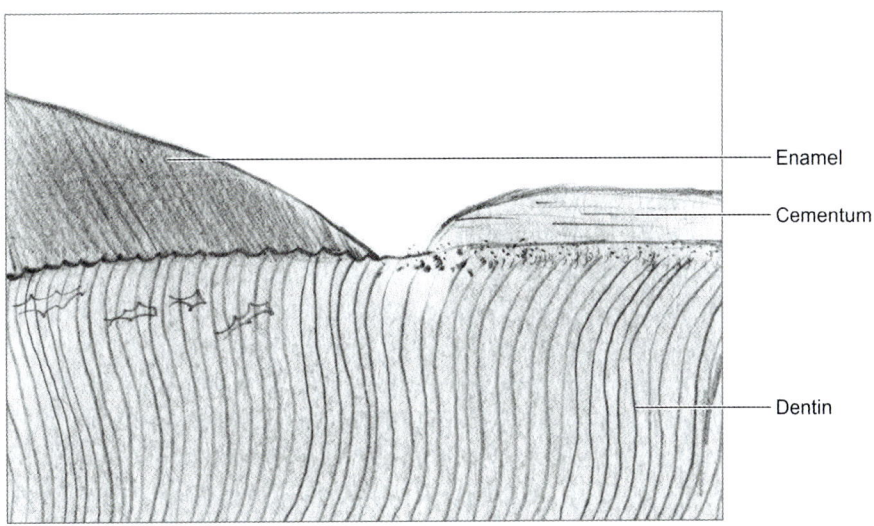

CEMENTOENAMEL JUNCTION-OVERLAPPING TYPE

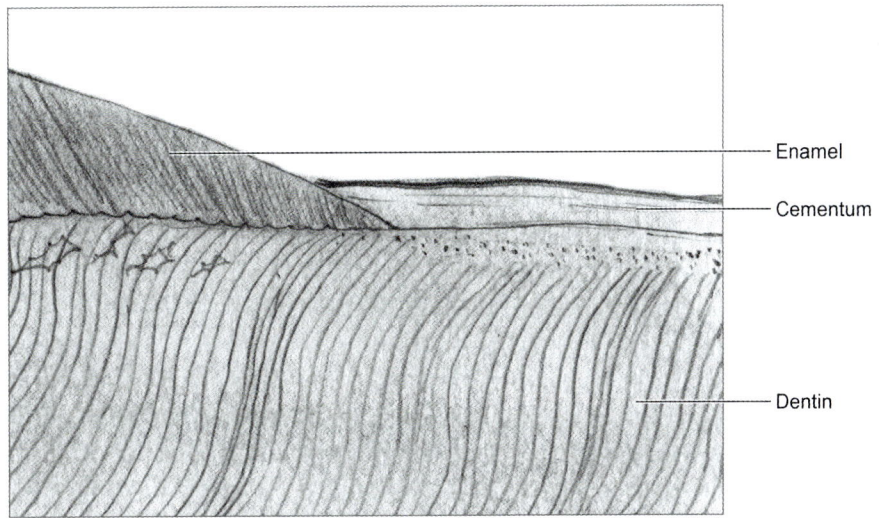

DENTAL PULP

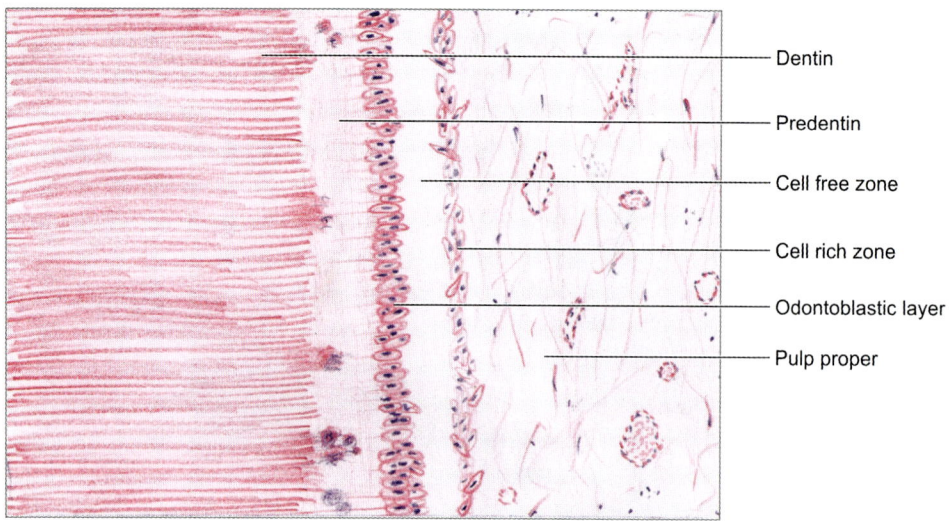

- Dentin
- Predentin
- Cell free zone
- Cell rich zone
- Odontoblastic layer
- Pulp proper

FREE FALSE PULP STONES

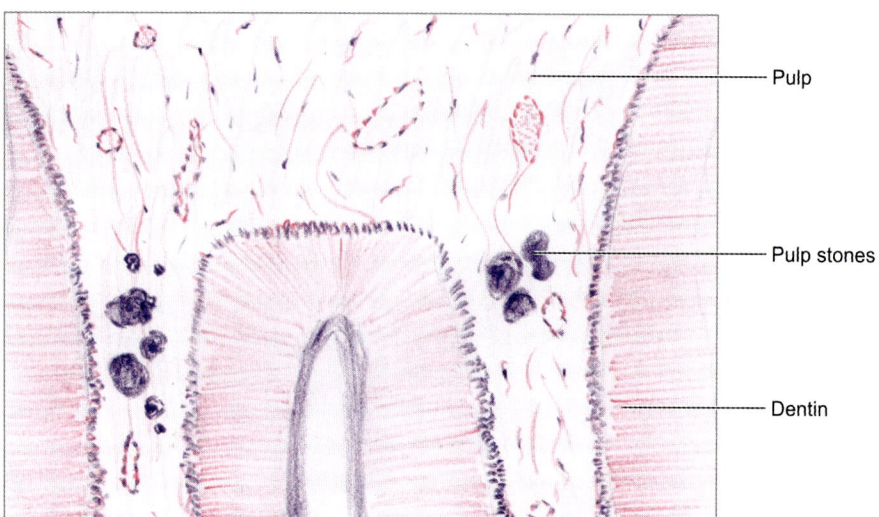

- Pulp
- Pulp stones
- Dentin

LAMELLAR BONE

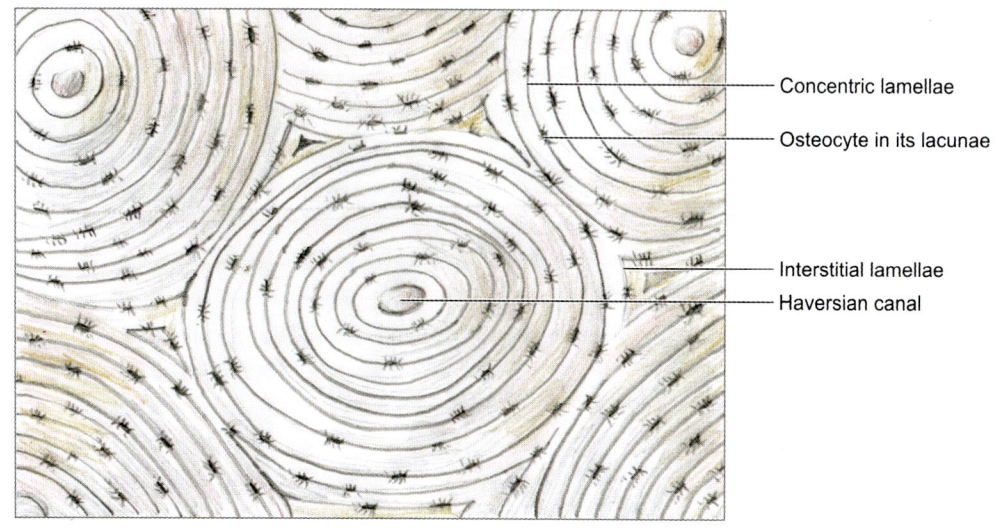

- Concentric lamellae
- Osteocyte in its lacunae
- Interstitial lamellae
- Haversian canal

WOVEN BONE

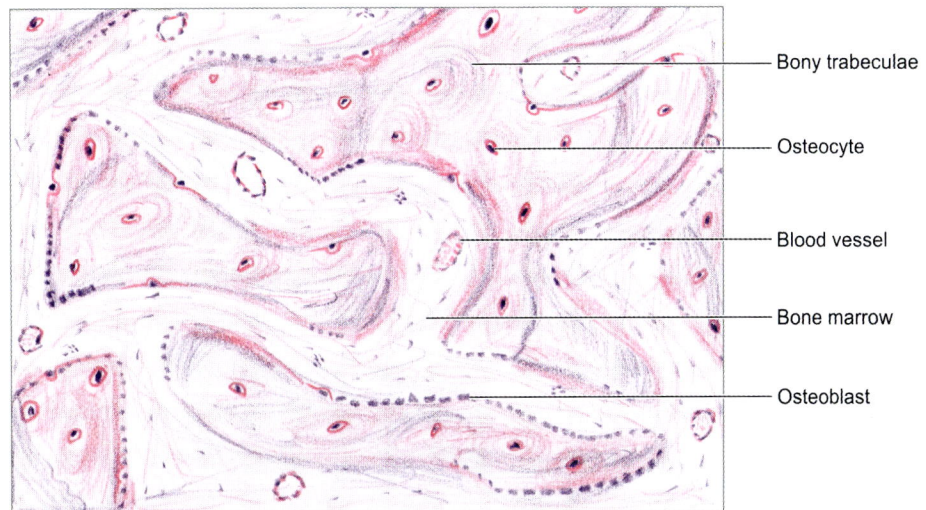

PSEUDOSTRATIFIED CILIATED COLUMNAR EPITHELIAL LINING OF THE MAXILLARY SINUS

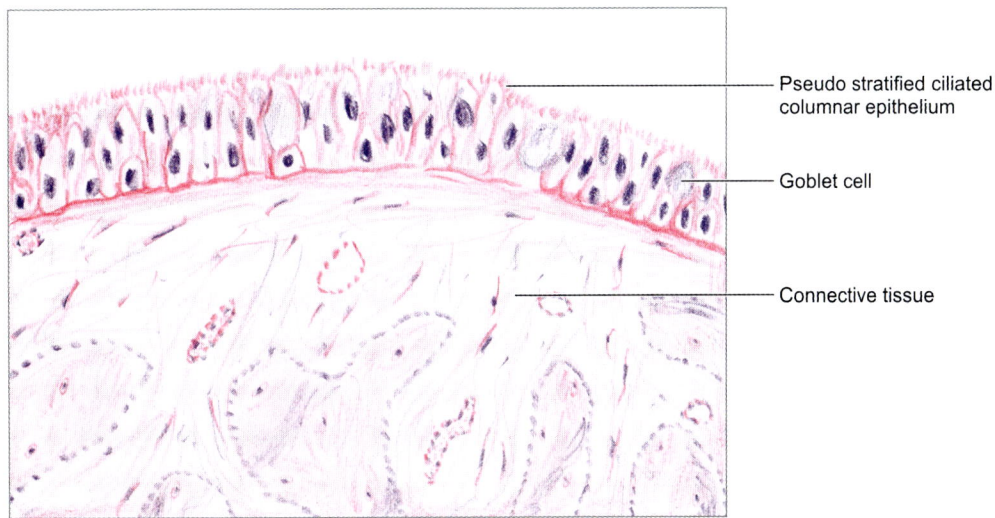

KERATINISED MUCOSA

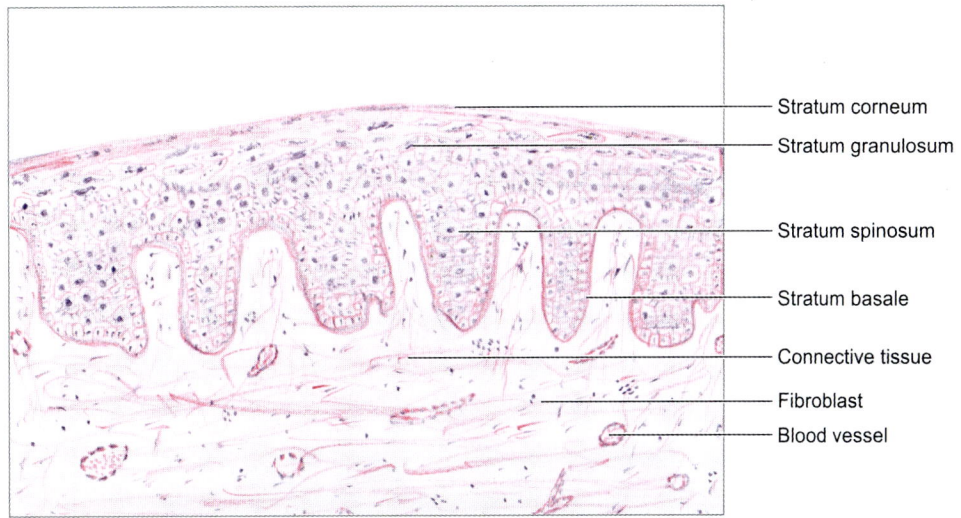

NON-KERATINISED MUCOSA

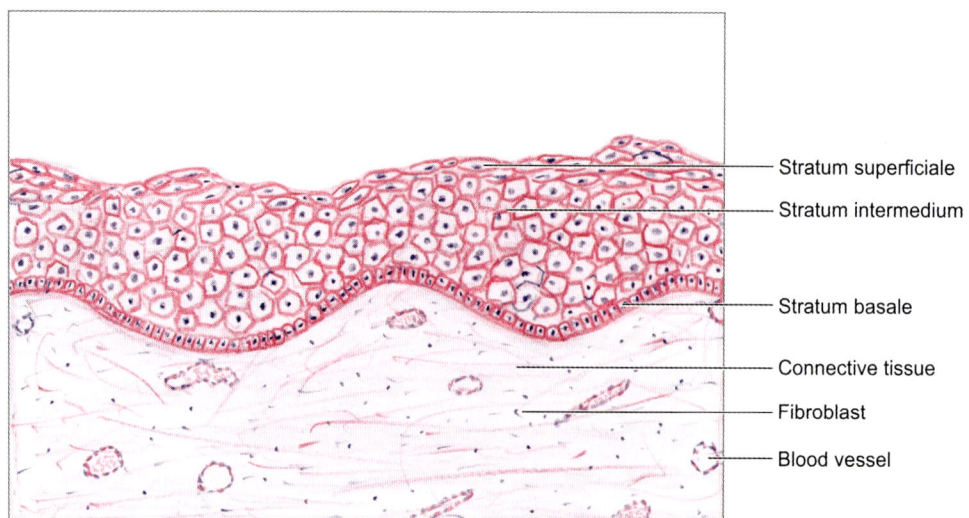

FILIFORM PAPILLAE OF THE TONGUE

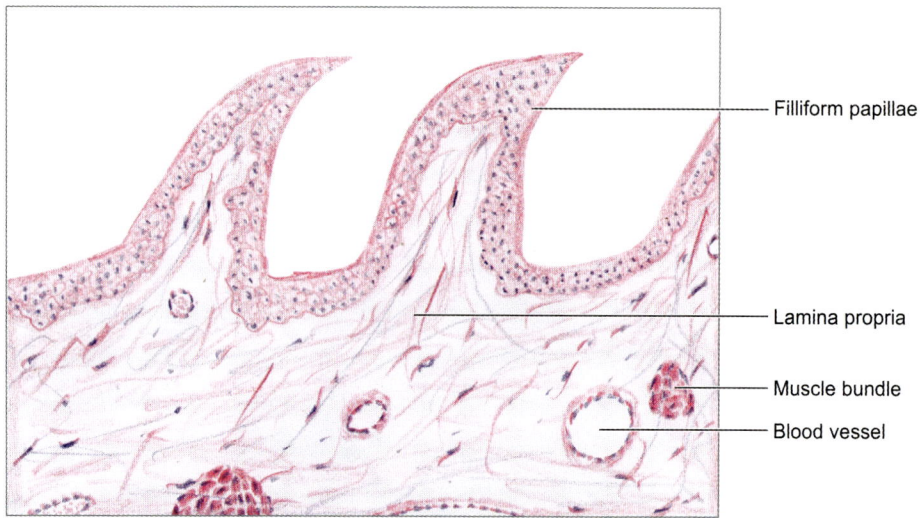

FUNGIFORM PAPILLAE OF THE TONGUE

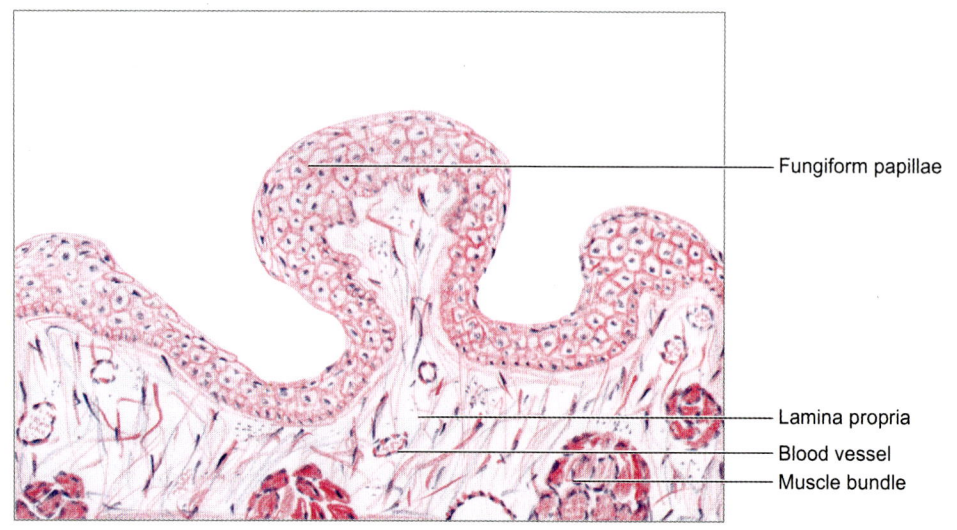

CIRCUMVALATE PAPILLAE OF THE TONGUE

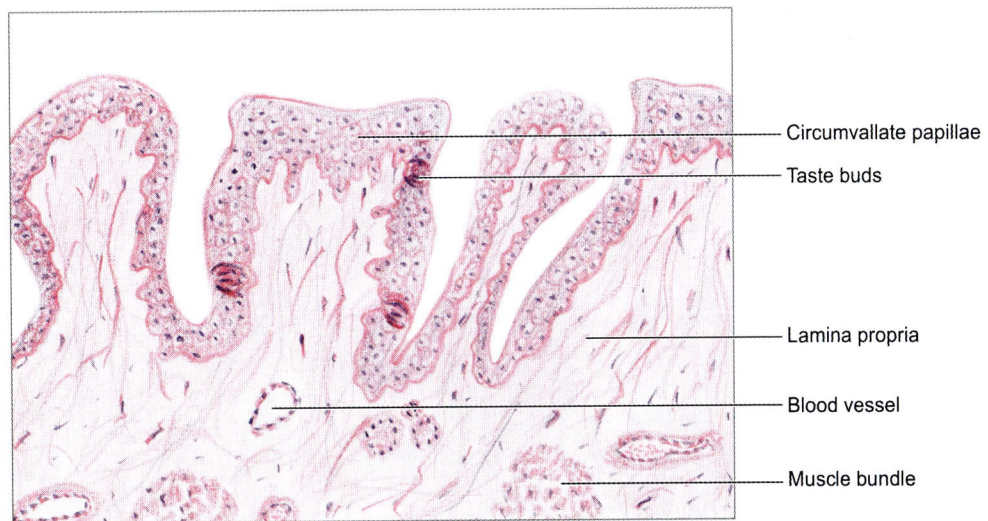

DENTOGINGIVAL JUNCTION

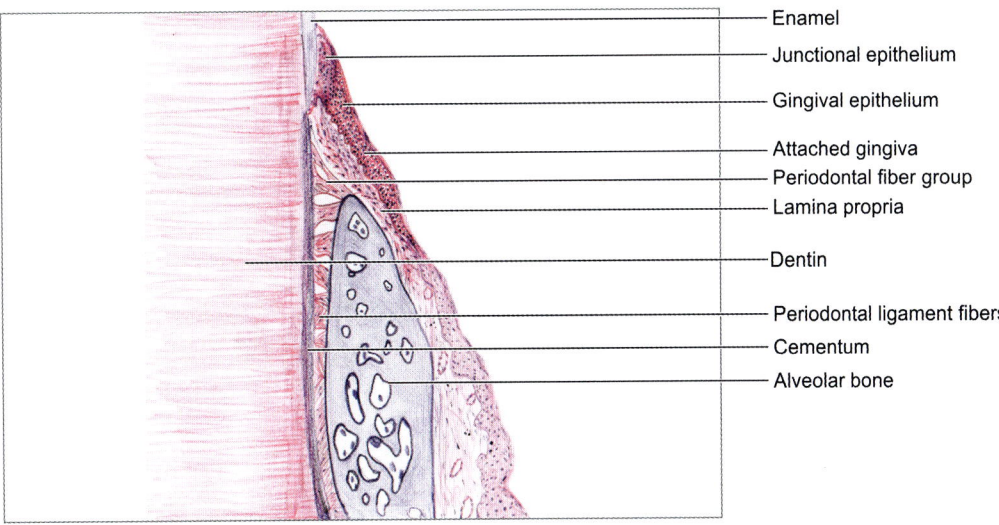

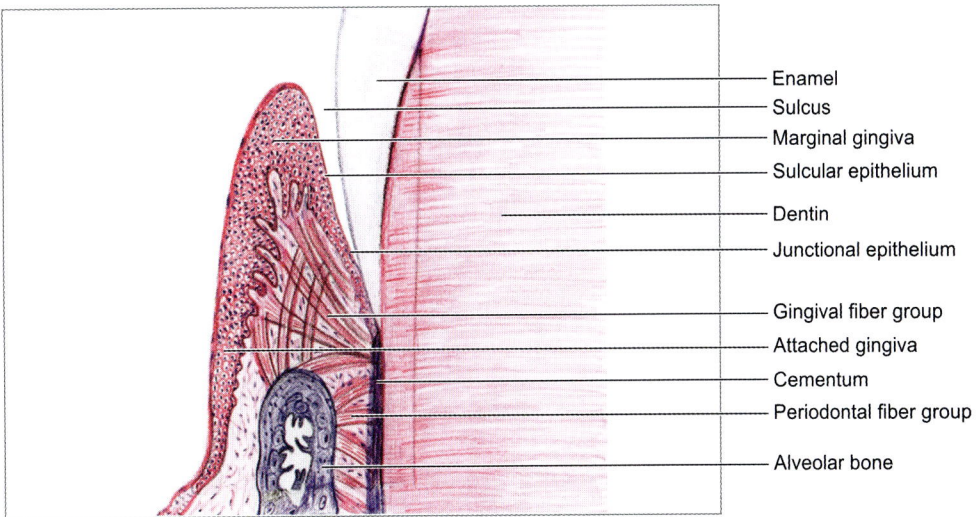

PERIODONTAL FIBER GROUPS

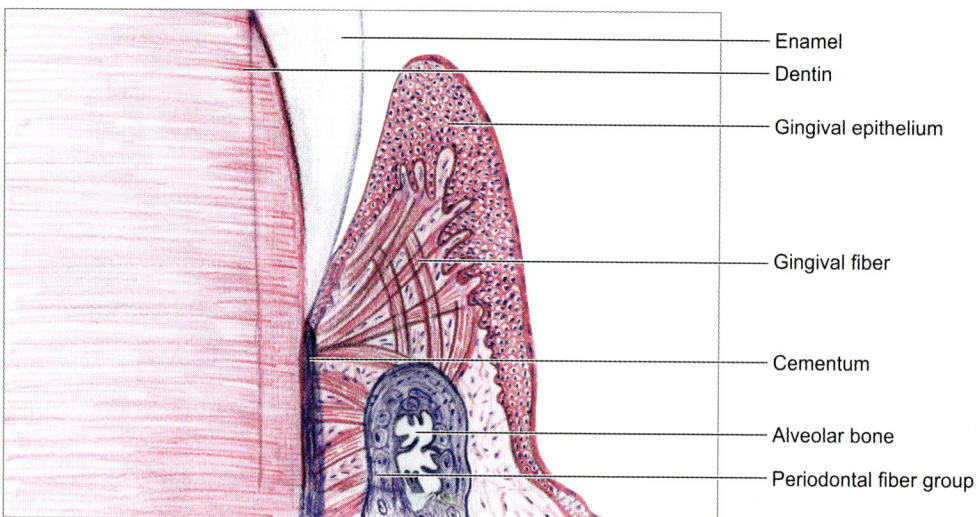

- Enamel
- Dentin
- Gingival epithelium
- Gingival fiber
- Cementum
- Alveolar bone
- Periodontal fiber group

SEROUS SALIVARY GLAND

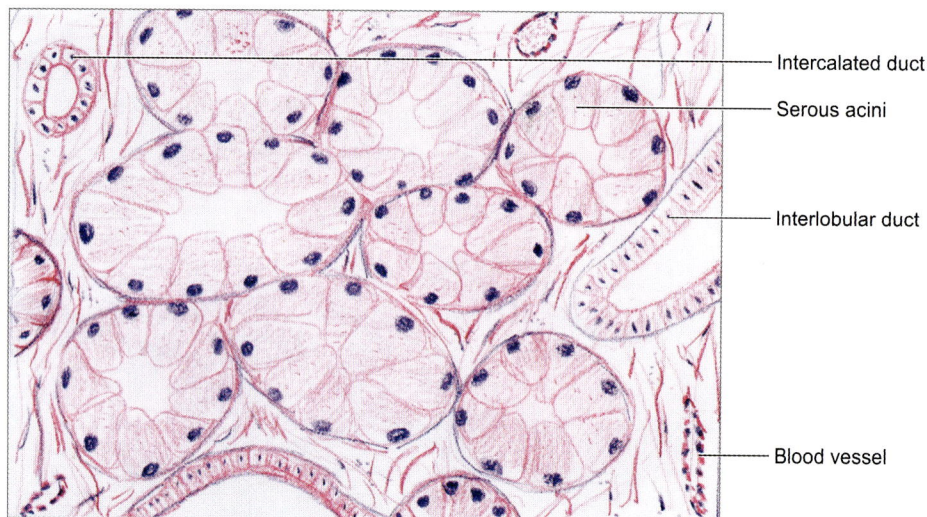

- Intercalated duct
- Serous acini
- Interlobular duct
- Blood vessel

MUCOUS SALIVARY GLAND

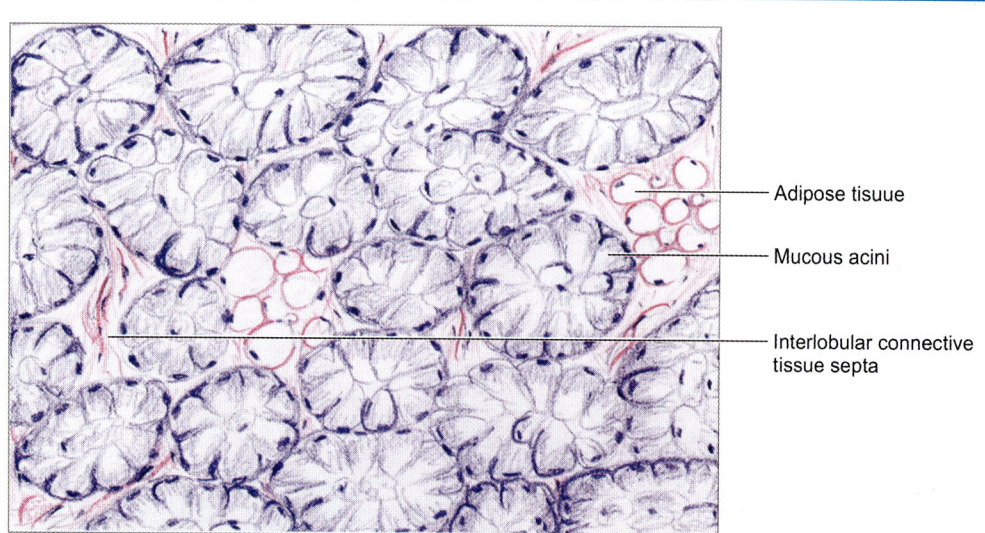

- Adipose tisuue
- Mucous acini
- Interlobular connective tissue septa

MIXED SALIVARY GLAND

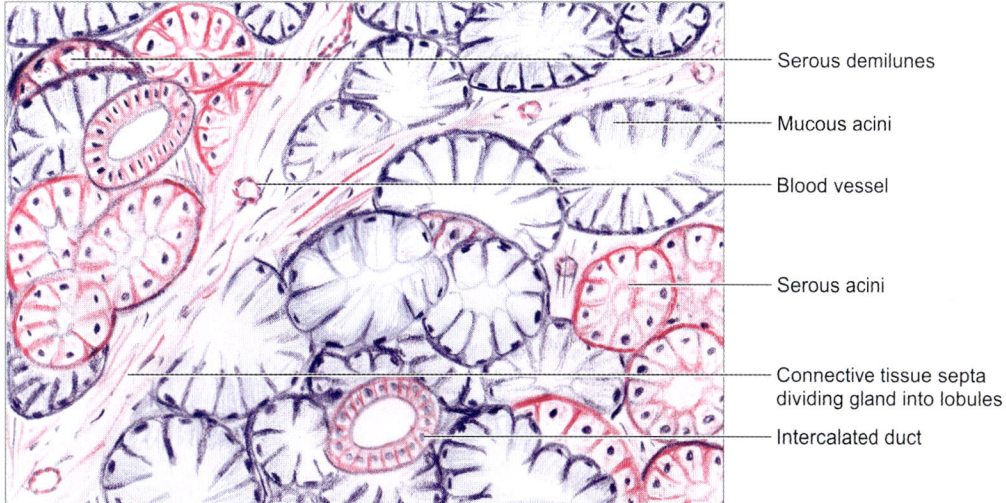

Index

Page numbers followed by *f* refer to figure, *fc* refer to flowchart, and *t* refer to table

A

Abrasion 60
Abscess, periodontal 123, 124*f*
Absorption 175
Abundant elastic fibers 203
Accessory canals 84, 343
Acellular cementum 102, 103, 103*f*, 104, 104*t*, 106, 106*f*, 283, 343
Acetic acid 308
Acetone 308
Acid 317
    decalcification 317
    etching 61
    fast bacillus 312
    phosphatase 326, 327, 343
Acinar
    cells 226, 232, 236
    units 218*f*
Acini 4, 224, 343
Acoustic meatus, external 245
Acquired immunodeficiency syndrome 268
Acrodont 303*f*, 343
Adenoids 263
Adherens junction 343
Adipocytes 13, 231
Adipose
    cells 118
    tissue 202
Adjacent cell membranes 182
Adult stem cell 288, 343
    replication of 289*f*
    types of 289
Afferent lymph vessels 264
Afibrillar cementum 102, 343
Agenesis 259*f*, 343
Agglutinins 232
Agnathan 297, 343
Albright syndrome 161
Albumin-coated glass slide 312*f*
Alcian blue-stained section 325*f*
Alkaline
    phosphatase 99, 326, 327, 343
    salts 129
Allograft 343
Allosome 8, 343

Aluminium ammonium sulfate 314
Alveolar bone 4, 114, 128, 141, 145-147, 169, 199, 282, 340
    destruction of 149
    existence of 147
    part of 4
    remodeling of 146
    resorption of 147, 148*f*
    structure of 145
    turnover 146
Alveolar crest 159
    fibers 115, 119, 343
    group 120*f*
Alveolar mucosa 195, 202
    clinical appearance of 203*f*
Alveolar process 257*f*, 343
    development of 145
    parts of 142*f*
Alveolar socket 128*f*, 142*f*
Alveologingival fibers 120, 199, 343
Amelin 46
Ameloblastin 46
Ameloblastoma 292
Ameloblasts 44, 52, 54*f*, 55, 55*f*, 56*f*, 57, 57*f*, 59, 79*f*, 199, 279, 336, 343
    life cycle of 53, 58, 58*f*
    secreting enamel matrix 35*f*
    transitional 57
Amelodentinal junction 47
Amelogenesis 52, 53, 58
    imperfecta 37, 39*f*, 59
    process of 52
Amelogenins 46, 61, 343
Amelotin 46
Aminopeptidase 326, 327, 343
Anchoring fibrils 189*f*, 343
Angiogenic factor 327, 343
Angiotensin converting enzyme 186
Ankyloglossia 22
Ankylosed tooth 160
Ankylosis 249*f*
Anodontia 304, 343
    partial 37, 38*f*
    total 37
Antigen presenting cells 89, 91, 186
Antroliths 259
Apatite crystals 70

Apocrine glands 218, 219*f*, 343
Apoptosis 32, 85
Aprismatic enamel 51, 58
Arch
    first 21
        branchial 141
        pharyngeal 297
Archaic hominids 299
Ardipithecus ramidus 299, 299*f*
Arthrocentesis 249
    procedure of 249*f*
Articular disk 243, 245, 245*f*, 343
    structure of 246*f*
Articular eminence 245, 245*f*
Atherosclerotic plaques 281
    formation of 92
Atrophy 344
Attached gingiva 194, 195*f*, 196, 344
Attrition 279*f*, 344
Australopithecus 299, 305
    afarensis 299*f*
    robustus 299*f*
Autocrine cells 217
Autocrine glands 217, 344
Autograft 344
Autoimmune diseases 269
Autosome 8, 344

B

Bartholin duct 344
Basal cytoplasm 225
Basal epithelial layer 188, 189*f*
Basal lamina 188, 188*f*, 221, 224, 257, 344
    attachment of 189*f*
    proteins 182
Basal layer 344
Basement membrane 90, 188, 188*f*, 344
Basket cells 226, 351
B-cells 266, 344
    maturation of 263
Bell stage 33, 40
Beta-glucuronidase 327
Bilaminar germ disk 9
    formation of 9, 10*f*
Biopsied tissue 308*f*
Birbeck granules 186

Black hairy tongue 210, 210f
Blastema 242
　temporal 242
Blastocyst 10f, 288, 344
Blood 175, 269t
　capillaries 264
　cells, production of 132
　stream, plasma of 267
　supply 201f, 207, 248, 255
　vessels 84, 90, 121
　　absence of 44
　　development of 92
　　types of 1
Body systems 276, 284
Bone 58, 122, 129, 140, 167, 168, 194f, 277, 335, 344, 355
　apposition 161
　associated cells 116
　canaliculi 344
　cartilaginous 130
　cells 136, 137f
　　populations, dynamics of 147
　changes 147
　classification of 129
　defects 292
　embryonic 133
　formation of 133
　forming cells 133
　growth theory 160
　inorganic portion of 139
　irregular 130, 130f
　long 129, 129f, 135
　loss
　　horizontal 148f
　　vertical 148f
　mandibular 142f
　marrow 263, 263f, 344
　mass 282
　　loss of 278
　matrix, mineralization of 136, 136f
　membranous 130
　mineralization of 136
　morphogenetic protein 117, 129, 137, 140, 344
　osteoclastic 140
　remodeling 140, 140f, 141f, 149f, 344
　resorption 169
　resorptive hormones 170
　short 129, 129f
　sialoprotein 136, 344
　spongy 344
　sutural 130, 131f
　types of 130
Bony fish 297
Brachydont molar 303f
Brain 276
　injury 258

Branched glands 218f
Branchial arch 344
　development of 13
Brush border 101
Brush cells 231
Bruxism 108
Buccal extension, development of 28f
Buccal frena 176, 177f
Buccal mucosa 176, 202, 202f, 203, 209, 209f
　leukoplakia of 210f
　right 211f
Buccopharyngeal membrane 13f, 208f, 344
Bud stage 29, 30f, 40, 344, 357
Bundle bone 4, 344
Bunodont molars 303

C

Cadaveric dissection 256f
Cadherin 344
Caenorhabditis elegans 220
Calciotraumatic line 76
Calcium
　ions 136, 184
　phosphate 57
　　hydroxyapatite crystal 3, 45f, 129, 168
Calcospherites 78
Canaliculi 69, 138
Canalization 223
Canals, primary 84
Cancellous bone 131, 146, 147f, 344
　structure of 133f
Candida albicans 234
Canine
　labial surface of 53f
　upper 159
Capsulitis 249
Carbohydrates 322, 326
Carbon dioxide 315
Carbonate 67, 129
Cardiac bulge 17, 17f
Cardiovascular system 276
Carnoy's fluid 308
Carnoy's mixture 324, 344
Cartilage 118, 344
　forming cells 135
　secondary 144, 144f
Cathelicidins 232
Caveolae 344
Caviar tongue 208, 278
Cavity, vestibular 2f, 27
Cells 88f, 208, 229, 307, 316, 323
　adhesion molecule 90
　apart 32

　biology 274
　body 87
　caveolated 231
　cycle, progress of 282
　eosinophilic 237
　free zone 344
　group of 11, 59, 135
　junctions 175, 180
　lineage 344
　membrane 188f, 276, 281
　migration of 123
　multiplication 9
　number of 94, 217
　polarization 54
　potency 288
　proliferation of 25, 221
　pulpal 3
　rich zone 84, 88, 345
　signaling 6, 6f
　stage 9
　subtypes of 180
　surface receptors 6
　synthetic 116
　types of 1
Cellular cementum 99, 102, 103f, 104, 104t, 345, 364
　formation of 108
Cellular organelles 138
Cementicles 345
Cementoalveolar fibers 115
Cementoblastic processes 99
Cementoblasts 4, 97, 99, 105, 114, 116, 117, 117f, 122, 336, 345
　progenitors 110
Cementocytes 4, 36, 99, 100, 100f, 101, 101f, 101t, 102, 345
Cementodentinal junction 67f, 107
Cementoenamel junction 76, 98, 107, 107f, 108f, 115, 169, 197, 282, 345, 365
Cementogenesis 103
Cementoid 106
Cementum 3, 44f, 58, 67f, 76, 97-99, 100f, 109, 113, 118, 122, 168, 281, 282, 316f, 335, 340, 345
　abnormal thickening of 109
　avascular 98f
　cells of 99
　chemical composition of 99fc
　classification of 103, 338
　derived attachment protein 99
　extrinsic fibers of 347
　fibers of 101
　formation 105f
　functions of 108
　growth of 109
　hypertrophy 109

incremental lines of 106, 106f, 283
intermediate 107, 349
mineralization of 105
types of 98
Central articular disk 242f
Central nervous system 91
Central polygonal cells 32
Centroblasts 345
Centrocytes 345
Cervical
    loop 32, 40, 345
    lymph nodes 268
    sinus 13
C-fibers 91
Chemical composition 67, 68fc, 98, 99fc, 129
Chloride 231
Chloroform 309
Chondrichthyes 297
Chondroblasts 13, 135, 292
Chondrocytes 135
Chondroitin sulfate 345
Chondronectin 323
Chromic acid 308
Chromosome 59, 275, 345
Cilia 345
Ciliated cells 257
Cingulum theory 303
Circular fibers 120, 345
Circulatory system 90
Circumoral tissues 282
Circumpulpal dentin 73, 345
Circumvallate papilla 205, 205f, 206f, 208, 337, 345
Cisterna chyli 264
Clarke's fluid 308
Cleavage 9
Cleft lip 21
Cleidocranial dysplasia 161
Clonogenic cells 287
Coarse woven bone 132, 133
Collagen 191
    alterations 280
    cross-linking of 274f
    fibers 44, 102, 103, 114, 177, 190f, 191, 199, 203, 208, 246, 265
        bundles 192f
        formation 114
    fibrils, morphology of 323
    macromolecule 90
    types of 99
Collagenous fibrous tissue 247
Communication 90
Compact bone 130, 345
    structure of 132f
Computed tomography 256f, 292f, 293f

Concrescence, theory of 302
Condylar
    blastema 242
    cartilage 242
    process 241f
Condyle
    mandibular 244f
    neck of 246
Confocal microscopy 329, 330f
Conjunctiva 264
Connective tissue 116, 188, 194f, 258f, 323, 345
    fibers 122
    papillae 201
    stroma 224
Conodonts 297
Contractile cells 226
Cope-Osborne theory 303, 305
Copper 99
Copula 21
Core binding factor alpha 1 134
Coronal cementum 102
Coronal dentin 66, 77
Coronal pulp 83, 85, 90, 345
    extension of 76
Cortex 345
Cortical plate 141
COVID 19 330
Cranial mesoderm 17
Crest cells 187
Cribriform plate 145, 146f, 345
Cross-linking theory 274
Crown 2f
    formation, completion of 159f
    middle portion of 49f
Crystallites 58
Crystals, long axis of 46f
Cuboidal basal cells 183f
Cushion hammock ligament 159, 345
Cuspal origin, theory of 302
Cyclic adenosine monophosphate 117
Cyclostomes 297
Cynodonts 298, 345
Cystatins 232
Cysts
    mucous extravasation 237f
    odontogenic 37
Cytochrome oxidase 324, 326, 327, 345
Cytokeratin 181, 181fc, 345
    distribution 181t
    profile 195
Cytokines 136
Cytoplasm 86, 89, 118f, 168, 314
    large amount of 116
Cytoskeleton 158

D

Dark colored gingiva 186f
Daughter cells 9, 79f
Dead tracts 75, 76, 280, 280f, 345, 363
Decalcification 316, 346
    methods of 317
Deciduous canine 166
Deciduous dentition 153, 154f, 339, 340, 346
Deciduous mandibular central incisor 166, 166f
    apicolingual resorption of 166f
Deciduous molars 156, 156f, 167f
    crown of 168
    occlusal planes 156f
    shedding of 167
Deciduous teeth 115, 153, 166f, 169, 291
    eruption of 155f
    germ 156
    root 167
Defense cells 118
Deglutition 234, 279
Dehydration 309, 309f, 314, 346
Dendrites 89
Dendritic cells 88, 89
Dens evaginatus 37, 38f
Dental arch 25
    establishment of 27f
    form 278
Dental caries 61, 233
    development of 51
    protection against 233
    risk of 107
Dental cuticle 198
Dental ectoderm 26
Dental fluorosis 60, 60f
Dental follicle 31, 107, 158f, 346
    stem cells 290, 291
    theory 161
Dental hard tissue 36, 129
Dental lamina 26, 26f, 27, 27f, 28f, 29, 40, 71, 158, 346
    development of 28f
Dental origin, stem cells of 291
Dental papilla 28, 32, 33f, 34, 36, 41, 78, 85, 91, 290, 346
    cells 32, 34, 77, 79f
    transforms 91
Dental precursor cells 290
Dental primordium 26
Dental pulp 292, 346, 366
    mature 291
    stem cell 89, 288-290, 290f, 291, 292, 293f, 346
        injection of 294f
        isolation of 291
    tissue 290

Dental sac 31, 33, 34, 346
   cells 36
Dental stalk 32
Dental stem cells 290, 292
   source of 290
Dental tissues 279
   age-related changes of 283
Denticles 346
Dentin 3, 44, 44f, 56f, 58, 66, 67f, 168, 280, 282, 316f, 335, 340, 346
   avascular 91
   chemical
      composition of 68fc
      properties of 66
   color of 66
   complex 71
   dysplasia 79
   formation of 35, 71, 79
   histology of 68
   inner 70
   innervation 72, 72f
   intermingle 48
   irregular secondary 76
   matrix 70, 78
   mineralization of 73, 77, 78
   peritubular 68, 69, 70f, 71, 73, 352
   phosphoprotein 68
   physical properties of 66
   portion of 68
   primary 72, 73, 353
   pulp complex 280
   reparative 76, 353
   secondary 72, 73, 84, 280, 354
   secreting cells 26
   sensitivity 76, 77f
   sialophosphoprotein 55
   sialoprotein 68, 99, 346
   structure of 72fc
   tertiary 76, 280, 355
   thickness 80
   translucency 283
   transparent 75, 75f
   types of 76f
Dentinal
   fluid 68f, 71, 77
   lymph 66, 70
   sclerosis 75
   translucency 283
   tubules 68, 69f, 71f, 72, 73, 80, 87, 91, 280, 315f, 346
      course of 68f
      cross section of 69f, 70f, 362
      primary curvature of 68f
Dentinoenamel junction 47, 49f, 51f, 67f, 77, 346
Dentinogenesis 77, 346
Dentition
   development of 153

   mixed 154f
   permanent 154f, 339, 340
   primary 340
   types of 301, 302
Dentogingival fibers 115, 120, 198, 199, 346
Dentogingival junction 346, 369
   development of 199, 199f
   migration of 170
   shift of 199, 200f
Dentoperiosteal fibers 115, 119, 120, 199, 346
Deoxyribonucleic acid 8
Dermis 177
Desmolytic stage 58
Desmosomes 181, 346
Desquamation 346
Devonian period 297
Diarthrodial joint 241, 242
Diazones 49
Diffuse calcifications 92, 346
Digestion 234
Digestive system 276
Digital pathology 318
Dimer theory 303
Dinitrofluorobenzene 325, 326
Diphyodont 1, 346
Diploid 8
Direct neural theory 76
Discoloration 279
Diskal ligament 247
Distal secretory site 56f
Disulfide bonds 184f
Drosophila 26
   melanogaster 220
Dry mouth 278
Duct 217, 346
   cells 223
   salivary 237
   types of 218f, 229
Ductal epithelial cells 232
Ductal morphology 217
Ductal system 229
Dysfunction syndrome 249

E

Ear
   internal 264
   middle 243
Ectoderm 9, 13, 18, 288, 346
Ectodermal cells, proliferation of 11f
Ectomesenchymal cells 31, 32, 77, 78, 91, 122
Ectomesenchyme 12, 25, 25f, 29, 29f, 221, 346
Ectopic eruption 162
Edema accumulates 269

Elastic fibers 192, 246, 258, 312, 323
   loss of 277
   mature 121
Elastic microfibrils 120
Elaunin fibers 121, 346
Electron microscopy 315
Electrophoresis 317
Embryo 9, 25, 288, 346
   development of 132
   folding of 13, 25
Embryoblast 9, 10f, 288
Embryology 346
Embryonic stem cell 89, 287, 288, 288f, 346
Enamel 3, 35, 44, 44f, 45, 48, 56f, 61, 67f, 76, 168, 279, 282, 316f, 335, 340, 346
   broach 52, 279, 346
      scanning electron microscopic appearance of 52f
   caps 52, 279
   chemical composition of 45fc
   cord 32, 40, 346
   cuticle 51, 198, 199, 347
   development of 59
   epithelium 35f, 40, 51, 57, 102, 104, 157, 199, 353
   formation 44
      genetic control of 59
   hydroxyapatite crystals of 67
   hypomineralized structures of 49
   hypoplasia 59, 347
   inter-prismatic 56
   knot 32, 33, 40, 347
   lamellae 50, 347, 360
      development of 51
   loading of 51
   loss of 279
   matrix formation 54f
   mineral 58
   niche 32, 40, 347
   organ 28, 32, 347
   organic matrix of 45
   pearl 60, 347
   pits 279
   proteins 46
   rods 46, 47f, 48f, 347
      cross section of 359
      direction of 47
      end 51, 279
      exhibiting tortuous pattern 359
      fish scale pattern, cross section of 359
      long axis of 46f
   septum 40
   spindles 49, 71, 347, 361
   structure of 46, 53fc

surface structures of 51
thickness of 45, 56
tuft 51, 347, 361
Enamelin 46, 347
gene 59
Endochondral ossification 135, 135f, 242, 347
Endocrine system 277
Endocrine theory 274
Endoderm 9, 288, 347
Endodermal origin 289
Endoplasmic reticulum 54, 89, 99, 231
Endosteal layer 133f
Endosteum 131, 347
Endothelial cells 90, 116, 189, 191, 264, 289
Endothelial cytoplasm 281
Endothelium, capillary 281
Enzymatic digestion 291
Enzyme 322, 323, 325-327, 327t, 347
histochemistry 347
linked immunosorbent assay 328, 329f
lysosomal 308
Eosinophils 89, 118
Epiblasts 9
Epidermis 177
fishnet pattern of 328f
Epiphyses 129
Epithelial band, primary 28f, 40, 353
Epithelial cells 18, 32, 37, 51, 58, 116, 118, 179, 180, 180f, 188f, 201, 210, 221, 233, 325f
Epithelial connective tissue 178, 198
Epithelial cord
branching of 224
dichotomous branching of 222
formation of 222
growth of 222
terminal parts of 222
Epithelial diaphragm 92
Epithelial enamel organ 29, 31
Epithelial germ layers 301
Epithelial maturation 180f
Epithelial mesenchymal
interaction 221, 301
transition 104
Epithelial pearls 347
Epithelial proliferation 180
Epithelial ridges 178, 179
Epithelial root sheath 114
Epithelial tissue 323
Epithelium 5f, 25, 29f, 175, 178f, 179, 188f, 189f, 196, 246, 347
keratinized 179, 182, 183f, 350
nonkeratinized 185, 185f
orthokeratinized 179f

outer enamel 32, 34, 40
salivary 181t
squamous 326f
thickness of 175
types of 4
Erosion 60
Eruption 5, 155, 155f, 166f, 347
mechanical failure of 162
passive 162
premature 161
Eruptive tooth movement 157, 158, 347
Erythrocytes 264
Esterase 327, 347
Esthetics 175
Ethmoid sinus 253
Ethmoturbinals 255
Ethyl alcohol 308
Ethylenediaminetetraacetic acid 317
Excementosis 347
Excretion 175, 234
Excretory duct 224, 230, 230f, 236, 347
large 234
Exfoliative cytology 308, 318
Exocytosis 231
cytoplasmic 99
Extracellular fibers 314
Extracellular matrix 88f, 89, 189, 191, 221, 274, 347
changes 276
role of 224
Extrinsic fibers 101, 347

F

Face 277, 283, 341
development of 17, 17f, 19f, 21
Facial
cleft 22
deformity 249f
prominences 17f, 21
structures 17
Fat 118
Fatty tissue 237
Fenestration 149f
Ferric ferricyanide 325
Fertilization 8, 9, 9f, 14, 347
Fibers 84, 90, 101, 106, 191, 316, 323
apical 115, 119, 343
horizontal 115, 119, 349
interdental 199
intrinsic 101, 102
longitudinal 199
periodontal 118, 370
system, secondary 120
types of 1
vasoconstrictor 232
vasodilator 232
vertical 199

Fibroblasts 4, 13, 88, 90, 114, 116, 116f, 122, 140, 189, 190, 190f, 231, 323, 347
growth factor 26
like cells 34, 140, 246
oral mucosal 190
phagocytosis 116
Fibrocartilaginous layer 244
Fibro-elastic ligament 304
Fibronectin 99, 323, 347
Fibronexus 116
Fibrosis, oral submucous 210, 210f
Fibrous capsule 242
Fibrous connective tissue 245
Fibrous joint, types of 128
Fibrous matrix 133f
Field theory 30, 31f
Filiform papilla 204, 204f, 208, 337, 347, 368
Fine fiber bundle bone 132, 134t
Fine needle aspiration cytology 318
Fissures 45
Fixation 308, 324
Flat bones 130, 130f
Fleming's fluid 308
Flow cytometry 330, 347
Fluid
components 175
interstitial 175
Fluoride 99
chronic 60
Foliate papilla 205, 205f, 208, 337, 348
Follicles
compartment 265
lingual 350
Follicular cells 114f
Follicular dendritic cells 266, 348
Food manipulation 302
Foramen
apical 36, 84, 343
cecum 21
Fordyce's spots 176, 176f, 209, 209f, 348
Formalin 308
toxicity 309
Free false pulp stones 366
Free gingiva 195, 195f, 348
Free radicals theory 274, 274f
Frontal sinus 253
Frozen sections 315, 324, 348
Fungiform papilla 204f, 205, 205f, 206f, 337, 348, 368
Fusion 37

G

Gametes 9
Ganglion, sphenopalatine 255
Gap junction 32f, 348

Gastrulation 9
Gemination 37
Genes, mutation of 210
Genotype 348
Germ cells 9
    embryonic 288
Germinal center 266, 348
Ghost tooth 79
Gill's hematoxylin 314
Gingiva 180, 179, 193f, 194, 195, 201f, 202, 209, 281, 282, 341, 348
    innervation of 201
    lamina propria of 196
    lingual 176
    mucosa of 175
    vasculature of 201
Gingival connective tissue 121
Gingival crevice 197
Gingival crevicular fluid 200, 201
Gingival epithelium 197, 198, 282
Gingival fibers 119, 198, 198f, 348
Gingival fibroblasts 282
Gingival recession 98, 281, 348
Gingival stippling 196f
Gingival sulcus 195, 195f, 348
Gingivitis 147
Glands 216, 267f
    classification of 216
    compound 218f
    connective tissue component of 231
    endocrine 217, 219f, 347
    eubepithelial 258
    exocrine 217, 219f, 347
    holocrine 219, 219f, 349
    mixed 220, 238
    periphery of 265f
    secretory portion of 234
    simple 217f
    sublingual 236, 236f, 338, 355
    submandibular 235, 235f, 237, 338, 355
Glandular epithelial cells 216
Glandular metabolism, control of 228
Glenoid
    fossa 241f, 242, 243, 244, 244f, 245, 348
    medial 246
Glossitis, benign migratory 209, 209f
Glossopalatine 238
Glucuronidase 348
Glutaraldehyde 308, 324
Glycogen 324
Glycoprotein 258, 323, 324, 348
Glycosaminoglycan 18, 32, 89, 323, 348
Glycosylation 276
Gnarled enamel 49, 348
Gnathostomes 297, 298, 348

Goblet cells 194, 217f, 257, 258f, 348
Golgi apparatus 54, 116, 182, 197, 231, 246
Golgi bodies 139
Golgi complexes 281
Gomphosis 128, 348
    attachment 304
Granular cell layer 184f
Granules
    eosinophilic 118f
    membrane coating 174, 184
    secretory 56f
Grinding tooth 317f
Growth
    factors 233
    maxillary 255
Gubernacular canal 158
Gubernacular cord 158f, 348
Gum pads 153
Gustafson's method 283

H

Haematoxylum campechianum 314
Hairy tongue 210
Haplodont 303, 348
Hard palate 142, 176f, 179, 193, 193f, 194f, 196, 209
    section of 194f
Hard tissue 1, 36, 167, 316, 335
    formation 36
    forming cells 336
    processing 316
    resorption of 165
Hare lip 21
Haversian canal 131, 131f, 348
Haversian system 97, 98f, 101f, 131f, 132f, 348
Head and neck
    lymph nodes 267t
    lymphatics of 267
Hearing 276
Heart 276
    diseases, ischemic 292
Hematopoiesis 132
Hematopoietic stem cell 129, 288, 289
Hemidesmosome 32, 57, 181, 182f, 189f, 348
Heparan sulfate 348
Hertwig's epithelial root 36, 84
    sheath 35, 36, 92, 104, 105, 105f, 114f, 158, 348, 358
    formation of 104f
Heterodont dentition 302f
Hiatus semilunaris 349
High-iron diamine thiocarbohydrazide-silver proteinate 325
Highmore antrum 254, 351

Hilum 349
Hirschfeld canal 145, 146f, 344
His copula 21
Histatin 232
Histiocytes 88, 89, 190, 191f
Histochemical
    stains 330
    techniques 324
Histochemistry 325, 326, 349
Holocrine secretion 219
Homeobox gene 25, 190
Homeodomain 25
Homo sapiens 300, 349
Homodont dentition 302f
Hopewell-Smith, layer of 107, 350
Hormones, metabolic 232
Horseshoe-shaped primary epithelial band 26f
Howship's lacunae 139, 139f, 140, 168, 349
Human blood cells 307
Human chromosome 8f
Human dentition, evolution of 300
Human exfoliated deciduous teeth 291, 354
Human masticatory complex, evolution of 304
Human skeleton 131
Hunter-Schregor bands 45, 49, 50f, 349, 361
Hurler's syndrome 161
Hyaline cartilage 349
Hyaluronan 246, 349
Hydrodynamic theory 77
Hydroxyapatite 349
    crystals 45, 46f, 47f, 55, 67, 129
Hydroxyl ion 45
Hypercementosis 109, 109f, 281, 349
Hyperplasia, cemental 345
Hyperplastic squamous epithelium 324f
Hypertrophy 349
    cemental 345
Hypoblasts 9
Hypobranchial eminence 21
Hypoplasia 259f
Hypsodont 349
    dentition 302
    molar 303f

I

Immature teeth 291
Immunofluorescence 328, 349
Immunoglobulin
    A, salivary 278, 354
    secretory 232
Immunohistochemistry 326, 326f, 349
Immunological theory 274

Index **379**

In situ hybridization 328, 349
Incisive papilla 176f, 193f, 194, 195f
Incisors, lower central 176
Infections, microbial 330
Inferior alveolar nerve 144
Inflammatory cells 89, 91, 187, 189, 191
Inner cell mass 287, 288
Inner enamel 54
    epithelial cells 33, 34, 36, 54, 77
    epithelium 32, 33, 40, 349
Insulin-like growth factor 1 117
Integrins 349
Intercalated ducts 224, 229, 229f, 236, 349
    cells 226
Intercellular bridges 349
Intercellular substance 89, 221
Interglobular dentin 73, 349, 362
    formation of 74f
    ground section of 74f
Interlobular ducts 236, 349
Internal resorption 94
Interradicular fibers 119, 349
Intertubular dentin 68, 70, 349
Intra-articular disk 246
Intrabony tooth movements 157
Intracellular membranes 314
Intramembranous ossification 134, 134f, 350
Intratubular dentin 69, 78
Intratubular nerves 77
Ion exchange resins 317
Iron 99
Ivory bone 345

J

Jacobson's organ 350
Jaw 300
    bone 128
    evolution of 297
    growth 167
    lower 243
    quadrant 301
Joint
    capsule 130, 243, 246f, 248
    cavity 242f
        inferior 245
        superior 245
    compartments 246
    disorders 249
    part of 245
    space 249
Junctional epithelium 197, 197f, 198, 199, 350
    attachment of 199
    cells of 197

K

Keratan sulfate 350
Keratin 184
Keratinization 350
    types of 179
Keratinized stratified squamous epithelium 194f
Keratinocytes 181, 185, 186f, 350
Keratinosome 184, 350
Keratohyalin granules 183, 185, 350
Kidney 276, 277
Kinetogenic theory 303
Korff fibers 73
Krause's bulbs 207

L

Labial expansion 292f
Labial frenum 176, 177f
Labial mucosa 202, 202f
Labyrinthodont 298, 350
    tooth, cross section of 298f
Lacteals 350
Lactoferrin 232
Lacunae 99, 131, 138, 138f
Lamella, interstitial 147f, 349
Lamellar bone 146, 350, 366
Lamina
    cribrosa 145
    densa 188, 188f, 350
    dura 146f, 350
    limitans 350
    lucida 188, 188f, 350
    propria 177, 178f, 187f, 188, 189, 189f, 191f, 196, 198, 200, 350
        cells of 189
        components of 190f
        fibroblasts of 188f
    reticularis 188f
Laminins 323, 350
Langerhans cell 185f, 186, 187, 187f, 197, 350
    origin of 187f
    population 187
    tennis racquet-shaped Birbeck granules of 187f
Lead 99
Lens placodes 18
Leuckhart's L molds, separation of 311f
Leukemia 268
Leukocytes 232, 233
Leukofuchsin 324
Leukoplakia 210, 210f
Ligaments 242
    part of 115
    runs 247
    traction theory 160

Light microscopy 308
Linea alba 176, 176f
Lingual frenum 204f
Lingula 350
Lining mucosa 4, 177, 178f, 179, 201, 336, 350
Lipids 322, 323, 325, 326, 350
    histochemistry of 325
Lipofuscin 350
Lipoma 330
Liposarcoma 330
Lips 201
    lower 209
    portion of 202
    upper 18
    vermilion zone of 202f
Live microorganisms 307
Living cells 307
Living theory, rate of 274
Lobule formation 222
Long-chain sugar polymer 246
Lubricin 246
Lungs 276
Lymph 262, 264, 267f, 269t, 350
    capillaries 90, 264, 265
        structure of 264
    circulation 266
    course of 167, 266
    formation of 264f
    node 263, 265, 266f, 267, 268, 268f, 269t, 350
        capsule of 265, 266f
        cut section of 265f
        distribution of 265
        enlarged 268
        jugulodigastric 268
        regional 186
        structure of 265
        submandibular 255
    nodule 350
    sac 263
    spaces 350
    transport of 264
    vessels 90, 264, 267
        structure of 264, 265f
Lymphadenopathy 350
Lymphatic
    capillaries 265f
    failure of 269
    nodule 263
        germinal center of 348
        mantle zone of 351
    organs 262, 350
        primary 262
        secondary 263
    system 262, 267, 350
        categorization of 267fc

   components of 262fc, 264f
   development of 263
   structure of 264
  types of 1
  vessel 351
Lymphoblast 351
Lymphocyte 88, 89, 191f
  mature 263
  production 262
Lymphoid 350
  cells 266, 266f
  follicles, secondary 266
  lobule 351
  organs 353, 354
   primary 353
   secondary 354
  portion 204
  stem cells 263
  tissue 267
   arrangement of 268f
   bronchus associated 263
   gut-associated 263
   mucosa associated 263
   skin-associated 263
   tertiary 263
Lymphomas 268
Lysosomes 71, 190, 351
Lysozyme 232

M

Macrodontia 37
Macrophages 88, 118, 189, 190, 231
Magnesium 67, 99
Malassez cells rests 105f, 116, 118, 344, 347
Mammalian jaw 298
Mammary gland 219
Mandible 143, 245, 283, 341
  computed tomography of 292f, 293f
  condyle of 243, 244f
  depression of 248
  development of 141, 144f
  growth of 145f
  lateral view of 292f
  neck of 243
  structure of 144f
Mandibular deciduous teeth 166
Mandibular fossa 4, 243-245, 245f
Mandibular incisors 39f
Mandibular permanent central incisors, emergence of 155f
Mandibular teeth 339
Mantle dentin 36, 72, 73, 351
  matrix of 77
Masson's trichrome 312, 327, 327f

Mast cell 89, 118, 118f, 188f, 189, 190, 191f, 231, 351
Mastication 234, 279
Masticatory mucosa 177, 178f, 193, 201, 202, 336, 351
Matrix, cemental 99
Maturation stage 57, 58
Maxilla 141, 283, 341
  development of 141, 143f
  palatine process of 193f
  parts of 142, 142f
Maxillary antral wall 254
Maxillary antrum 259f
  anatomy of 254f
  epithelial lining of 258f
  innervation of 257f
  malignancies of 259
Maxillary arch 142
Maxillary artery, branch of 248
Maxillary bone, loss of 278
Maxillary first molar 38f
Maxillary nerves 18
Maxillary ostium 351
Maxillary sinus 4, 143, 253-255, 256f, 257, 258, 278, 351
  absence of 258
  anatomy of 253, 254
  development of 255, 256f
  enlargement of 255
  invasion of 257f
Maxillary teeth 339
Mayer's hematoxylin 314
Meckel's cartilage 13, 143, 144, 297, 305, 351
  remnants of 247
Medulla 265
Meiosis 9, 351
Meiotic division 9
Meissner's corpuscles 207
Melanin 186f
  pigmentation 175, 186f
Melanocytes 185f, 186f, 197, 351
Melanophages 187f
Melanosomes 186
Melanotic macule 209f
Membrana preformativa 29, 351
Membrane
  bound vesicles 116
  embryonic 13
Meniscus 245
Mercuric chloride 308
Merkel cells 185, 185f, 187, 187f, 197, 198, 207, 351
  nucleus of 187
Merocrine glands 217, 219f, 351
Mesenchymal cells 18, 88, 133

Mesenchyme 12, 351
Mesiodens 38f
Mesoderm 18, 288, 351
Mesodermal origin 289
Metabolism, bacterial 234
Metal replica 161
Metalloproteinases 351
Microglossia 22
Microtome 5, 308, 351
Mid-palatine raphe 193f, 194f
Mikulicz disease 237
Mineralization 58, 73, 77, 78, 105, 136, 136f
Minerals 56, 322
Minor salivary glands 4, 202, 220, 226, 229, 236
  types of 220t
Mitochondria 71, 86, 138, 230, 237
  number of 116
Mitosis 180f, 351
Mitotic index 179
Mitotic spindle 79f
Modern dentistry 290
Modulation 57
Molar
  incisor hypomineralization 60
  permanent 115, 157
  pulp organ 83
  section of 44f
  tritubercular 303
Molten paraffin wax 309f, 310f
Monocytes 88
  derived cells 140
Monophyodonty 302, 351
Morphogenesis 221
Morula 9, 10f, 288, 351
Mouth, floor of 1, 2f, 203, 203f, 204f
Mucin 351
Mucogingival junction 351
Mucopolysaccharides 258
Mucosa
  keratinized 367
  thick 155
Mucous acini 225, 227t, 337
Mucous cells 228f, 236, 258, 351
Mucous glands 194, 220, 227f, 238, 258
Mucous membrane 4
Mucous saliva 278
Mucous salivary gland 370
Multirooted tooth 36
Multi-tubercular
  teeth 303
  theory 303
Mumps 237
Muscles 118, 242, 248
Myelinated nerve fibers 206

Myeloperoxidase 232
Myoepithelial cells 224, 226, 227, 228f, 236, 351
   contraction of 227
   identification of 228
   shape of 227

N

Naive B-cells 351
Naive T-cells 351
Nakan's periodate-lysine-paraformaldehyde 324
Nasal cavity 253
   floor of 194f
Nasal pit 18, 351
Nasal placodes 18
Nasmyth's membrane 51, 57, 199, 352
Nasolacrimal furrow 18
Nasopalatine duct 194
Natal teeth 161, 162f, 352
N-cadherin 12
Nerves 84, 90
   fibers 32, 307
      ingrowth of 92
      pulpal 93
      types of 121
   supply 207, 248, 255
   types of 1
Nervous system 11, 276
Neural crest 25, 352
   cascade 11
   cells 11, 113, 352
      formation of 11
      influence of 25f
Neural degeneration 281
Neural groove 11, 352
Neural plate 352
Neural tube
   formation of 12f
   part of 11
Neuroectoderm 11
Neuromuscular theory 161
Neurons 13
Neuropeptides 232
Neutrophils 201
Night vision 276
Ninhydrin 325
Non-embryonic or somatic stem cells 288
Non-enamel protein genes 59
Non-hematopoietic stem cells 289
Nonkeratinocytes 185, 185f, 186, 352
Nuclear staining 314
Nucleic acids 322
   presence of 314

Nucleoporins 276
Nucleotide 352
   probes 352
Nutritional deficiency 59
Nutritive function 122

O

Oblique fibers 119, 352
Occlusal enamel, loss of 279
Occlusal forces 149
Occlusal wear, compensation for 281
Odland bodies 184, 184f, 350
Odontalgia 93
Odontoblastic layer 85, 85f
   pseudostratified appearance of 86f
Odontoblastic process 68f, 70, 71f, 77, 105
   terminal branching of 362
Odontoblasts 13, 34, 36, 66, 72, 77, 78, 79f, 85-87, 87f, 88, 91, 92, 336, 352
   differentiation of 79f
   life cycle of 85
   number of 92
   process 352
Odontoclasts 94, 168, 169f, 352
   formation of 168f
   resorbing dentin 168f
Odontocyte 86
Odontodes 300, 352
Odontodysplasia, regional 79
Odontogenesis 25, 26t
   stages of 338
Odontogenic apparatus 27
Odontome 155
   forming cells 301
Olfactory organs 194
Oligopotent 288
Oncocytes 237, 278
Oral cavity 1, 1f, 159f, 174, 209, 300, 322
   boundaries of 175
   normal 175f
   parts of 177
   primitive 25
Oral ectoderm 26, 27, 27f
Oral epithelial cells 318
Oral epithelium 29, 58, 159f, 179, 181, 181t, 197
   nonkeratinocytes of 185f, 186
Oral frenum 176
Oral hard tissues, histochemistry of 326
Oral melanotic macule 209
Oral mucosa 177, 178f, 194, 207, 210, 234, 283, 336, 341
   classification of 177
   color of 175

   components of 177
   development of 208
   epithelial ridges 178f
   nerves ending of 207f
   thickness of 175
   types of 336
Oral mucous membrane 4, 174, 278, 279f
   connective tissue of 5f
   functions of 174
Oral soft tissues, histochemistry of 326
Oral tissues 233, 282, 322
   histochemistry of 322
   microscopic structures of 5
   overview of 1
   structure of 5
Orbit 264
Organelles, cytoplasmic 100
Oroantral fistula 259, 259f
Orofacial region, lymphatics of 262
Orthodontic
   tooth movement 123
   treatment 149f
Orthokeratin 352
Osmium tetroxide 308
Ossification, divergent spread of 144f
Osteichthyes 297
Osteoblasts 4, 13, 98, 114, 116, 117, 117f, 118, 122, 133, 136, 137f, 139, 158, 169, 297, 336, 352
   functions of 137
Osteocalcin 99, 129, 136, 282
Osteoclasts 4, 101, 116, 117, 138, 139, 139f, 352
   formation of 139f
   structure of 139f
Osteocytes 36, 86, 100, 101, 101t, 134, 135f, 137, 138, 138f, 352
   structure of 138f
Osteodentin 76f, 352
Osteogenesis 133
Osteoid 72, 134, 137, 137f, 352
   formation 137f
Osteon 131
   primary 140
   secondary 140
Ostconectin 129, 136, 323
Osteopontin 99, 136
Osteoprogenitor cell 136
   derivatives of 136f
Osteoprotegerin 147, 352
   acts 147
Ostia 253
Ostium 255
Ostracoderms 297
Otomandibular ligaments 248
Ova 352

Ovum, fusion of 9
Owen contour lines 75, 75f, 345
Oxytalan fibers 120, 352
Oxytocin 232

P

Pain
　intolerable 93
　myofascial 249
　pulpal 93
Palate 178f
　development of 17, 18, 194
　primary 353
　primitive 18
Palatine
　bone 193f
　glands 194f, 238
　papilla 194
Palatoquadrate cartilage 297
Paleoproteomics 61
Papilla
　apical 290, 291
　cells 92
Papilla
　appearance of 57
　interdental 195f, 196, 196f
Paracone 303
Paracortex 352
Paracrine glands 217, 352
Paraffin infiltration 352
Paraffin wax 309
Paranasal sinuses 253, 257, 258
　　development 255
　　location of 253f
Parathormone 170
Parathyroid hormone 165
Parazones 49
Parenchyma, salivary 237
Parotid
　duct 5f
　gland 220, 233, 234, 235f, 338, 352
Pellicle, salivary 354
Pemphigus 210
Periapical fibers 119
Periapical inflammation, chronic 109
Pericytes 90
Perifollicular cells 114, 114f
Perikymata 49, 52, 61, 279, 352
　scanning electron microscopic appearance of 53f
Periodate lysine-glutaraldehyde 324
Periodic acid-Schiff stain 323, 325f
Periodontal ligament 4, 36, 100, 100f, 105f, 108, 113, 114, 117, 118, 118f, 122, 145, 157, 160f, 167, 170, 282, 290, 291, 341, 352
　cells of 114, 114f

fibers 119f, 282
　attachment of 107, 109
　embedded portion of 129f
　remodeling of 115f
fibroblasts 282
functions of 122
principal fibers of 115f, 120f
role of 160
stem cells 290, 291
thickness of 123
Periodontal pockets 210, 211f
Periodontitis 4, 97, 123, 147, 148f, 281, 352
　aggressive 123
　chronic 123, 123f
Periodontium
　development of 36, 114
　evolution of 303
　marginal 194
　structure of 116
　tissue of 113f
Periosteum 131, 244, 352
　layers of 133f
Peripheral cells 36
Permanent mandibular incisors 166
　eruption of 166f
Permanent mandibular molars 157f
Permanent maxillary molars 157f
Permanent teeth 153, 165
　bud, positioning of 167f
　eruption of 155f
Peroxide, salivary 232
Petrosquamosal suture 245
Peyer's patches 263, 353
pH 233, 353
Phagosome 191f
Pharyngeal arches 13, 14f, 17, 18, 19f, 204
　development of 18
Pharyngeal clefts, fate of 13
Pharyngeal mucosa 234
Pharyngeal pouch 13
Phenotype 353
Philtrum 18
Phosphate 45
　inorganic 136
Phosphoprotein, secretory calcium-binding 59
Pickerill imbrication lines 52
Picric acid 308
Pigments 322
　cells 13
Pink tooth 353
Pits 45
Plasma
　calcium homeostasis 140
　cells 89, 191f, 231, 353
　composition 232
　membrane 198

Platelet derived growth factor 117
Pleurodont 302, 303f, 353
Plexus
　intermediate 121
　subepithelial 207
Plica
　fimbriata 204, 204f
　sublingualis 176, 203, 204f
Plump endothelial cells 266
Pluripotent 288, 353
　mesenchymal cells 134
　stem cells 288
Pneumatization 255, 353
Polygonal cells 179
Polymerase chain reaction 328, 329f, 353
Polymorphonuclear leukocytes 188f, 191f
Polyphyodont 1
Post-canine tooth morphology 302
Posteruptive tooth movement 157, 159, 353
Potassium 99, 231
　dichromate 308
Precementum 106
Prechondroblasts 244
Prechordal plate 9
Precursor cells 287
Predentin 72, 78, 91, 353
　dentin junction 85f
Pre-eruptive tooth movement 156, 157, 353
Premaxilla 353
Premolars
　molars 156
　placement of 167f
Preodontoblast 78, 353
Presbyopia 276
Prickle cell layer 182
Primary saliva 231
　modification of 230
Primitive node 353
Principal fibers 115f, 119, 120f, 353
Prismatic enamel 58
Proacinar cells 224
Prochordal plate 9, 353
　formation 11f
　mesoderm 17
Progenitor cell 116, 118, 182, 190, 287, 289, 353
Progerin 276
Programmed cell death 18, 85, 170
Programmed longevity theory 274
Prostaglandins 136
Protargol 315
Proteases 46
Proteins 56, 322, 323, 325, 326, 353
　basic 233
　extracellular 201

fibrillin 120
fibrous 315
homeostasis 276
noncollagenous 99
translation 276
Proteoglycans 99, 192, 323, 324, 353
aggregating 323
localization of 325
Proteolipids 99
Pseudostratified ciliated columnar epithelium 194f, 258f
Pterygoid
fovea 244f
medial 248
muscle, lateral 242
Pulp 3, 66, 72f, 76, 79f, 80, 83, 89, 91, 168, 280, 282, 340
architecture 85f
canal 83, 84, 94
volume of 92f
cells of 88
central 281
chamber 83, 93f, 281f, 284, 316f, 353
volume of 280
component of 71
core, cells of 85
dentin capacity, regeneration of 290
development of 91
diffuse calcifications of 346
extracellular matrix of 88f
fibers of 90
functions of 91
growth theory 159
horns 94
recession of 94
odontoblastic layer of 72
resorption of 169
space 85
stones 92, 93f, 281f, 353
incidence of 92
structure of 84, 84fc
tissue 330f
volume of 281f
Pulpal architecture, development of 91
Pulpitis 93, 93f

Q

Quadritubercular molar 303

R

Radicular dentin formation 79
Radicular pulp 83, 84, 353
Radioautographic techniques 330
Ramus 241f
Raschkow plexus 353
Regenerative medicine 288, 290

Rehydration 314
Reichert's cartilage 13, 353
Renal disorders 283
Resorption bays 139
Resorptive cells 116, 117
Respiratory epithelium 4
Respiratory system 277
Rete ridges 178, 179
Reticular network 354
Reticulin fibers 121, 354
Retrodiscal laminae 245
Retroperitoneal sac 263
Retzius incremental lines 49, 49f, 360
Retzius striae 45, 49, 354
Rivinus ducts 236, 346
Robust australopithecus 299
Rod
segments 47
sheath 46, 47f
Root
apical third of 84
apices of 254
canal 83, 84, 284
anatomy 93
dimension 280
development 36f
formation 36, 114
fracture 109
growth theory 159
Rossman's fluid 324
Rotary microtome 311f
Rough endoplasmic reticulum 87f
RT-PCR technique 330
Ruffini corpuscles 207
Rugae 193f

S

Saliva 4, 233, 234, 318, 354
composition of 232, 232fc
discharge of 5f
ductal modification of 232
flow of 237
formation of 231
functions of 233
inorganic constituents of 232
primary 231
properties of 233
protects 233
secretion of 231
unstimulated 233
Salivary flow rate 233
Salivary glands 4, 202, 216, 217, 217f, 218, 220, 221, 224, 226, 229, 237, 278, 283, 341, 354
acini 327
anatomy of 237
classification of 220

development of 174, 220, 221, 222f, 223f, 224
discharge 4
epithelial cells 231
histology of 224, 225f, 237
inflammation of 237
major 5f, 220, 220t, 223, 234, 338
mixed 371
neoplasms 237
organs 237
serous 206f, 370
stage of 223
structure of 225f
Salivary secretions, total 233
Salter lines 106, 350
Salts, inorganic 131
Sarcomeric muscle 289
Sarcopterygians 298
Scalloped dentinoenamel junction 48f, 67f
Scarless oral healing 190
Schiff's reagent 324
Schneiderian membrane 257, 354
Schwann cells 13
Sclerotic dentin 75, 75f, 280, 280f, 354
Second maxillary molar teeth 254
Secretions 175, 231
types of 219, 220
Secretory cells 236, 258
Semicircular fibers 199
Sensation 174
Sensory
cortex 93
function 113, 122
impairments 276
innervations 255
nerves 91
Septum, interdental 145
Seromucous acini 225
Serous acini 225, 227t, 337
Serous cells 226, 236, 354
Serous demilunes 226, 354
Serous glands 220, 226f, 238, 258
Serre rests 354
Sesamoid bone 130, 131f
Sex chromosomes 8, 61
Shallow depression 255
Sharp teeth 304
Sharpey's fibers 101, 101f, 102, 102f, 106, 119, 121, 121f, 128, 129f, 146f, 354
Sheathlin 46
Shedding, mechanism of 167
Sialadenitis 237
Sialadenosis 237
Sialic acid 323
Sialorrhea 237
Sialosis 237

Silicon 99, 129
Silver
    methenamine stain 315
    proteinate 315
Single tooth-bearing bone 298
Sinus 253
    bony walls of 257
    cavity 254
    development of 255
    enlarges 255
    polyps 259
Sinusitis 259
Sjögren syndrome 237
Skeletal system 277
Skeletal trauma 283
Skeleton, cartilaginous 298
Skin denticles 301
Skull
    base of 245f
    temporal bone of 241
Small cytoplasmic extensions 70
Smear 308
Smooth ended
    ameloblast 57, 58
    cell function 57
Smooth muscle cells 13, 226
Sodium 231
Soft palate 203, 203f, 205
Soft tissue 1, 131, 308
Somatic cells 275
Somatic DNA damage theory 274
Somites 354
Speech 234
Sperm 9, 354
    fusion of 9
Sphenoid sinus 253
Sphenomalleolar ligament 13
Sphenomandibular ligament 13, 243, 247
Spinous cell layer 184f, 282
Spleen 263
Spore 288
Sputum 318
Squamous cell carcinoma 210, 211f
Stellate reticulum 32, 34, 40, 55, 354
    cells 34
Stem cells 118, 287, 290, 291, 354
    application of 290
    basis of 289
    classification of 288
    derived cancer 287, 291
    history of 287
    mechanism of action of 289
    potential uses of 290
    property of 287
    source of 288
Stensen's duct 354
Stomatodeum 17

Stomodeum 17, 18, 25, 354
Stone 259
    tools, development of 304
Stratified squamous epithelium 179, 179f
Stratum
    basale 180f, 182, 354
    corneum 180f, 184, 185f, 354
    germinativum 182, 197, 354
    granulosum 180f, 183, 354
    intermedium 34, 40, 54, 55f, 56f
    spinosum 180f, 182, 197, 354
    superficiale 185
Striated ducts 224, 230, 230f, 236, 354
Stromal vascular fraction 293f
Stylomandibular ligament 243, 244f, 247
Subepithelial collagen fibers 188
Sublingual fold 203
Submucosa 192, 355
    absence of 177
    presence of 177
Subodontoblastic layer, cells of 79f
Succinate dehydrogenase 326, 327, 355
Sudanophilia 326
Sulcular epithelium 195, 197, 201
Sulcus terminalis 21, 204, 355
Superficial cells 318
Superficial temporal artery 248
Supernumerary maxillary sinus 259
Supraeruption 162, 355
Sweat gland 219
Swellings, lingual 350
Syndesmosis 113
Synovial cells, macrophage-like 246
Synovial fluid 247, 355
Synovial joint 242, 355
Synovial membrane 242, 246, 247, 247f, 355
Synovial tissue 246
Synovial villi 247f
Synovitis 249
Syphilis, congenital 259

T

Tartrate resistant acid phosphatase 117, 355
Taste
    bud 205, 205f, 206, 206f, 208, 355
        number of 276
        structure of 206f
    cell 206f
    pore 206, 206f
    sensation, distribution of 207f
T-cells 355
Teeth 3, 167, 301
    absence of 128
    anatomy of 2f
    anterior 196

apex of 281
cervical constriction of 83
compound 302
crypt 145f
development 25, 28, 28t, 36f, 37, 188, 338
    advance bell stage of 358
    bud stage of 30f, 357
    cap stage of 357
    early bell stage of 358
    initiation of 174
    stages of 29f, 303
    timeline of 27t
displacement of 29
ectodermal derivative of 3
eruption 58, 115, 153, 159
    failure of 161
    theory of 159
    timeline of 339
evolution 297
    model of 301
exfoliates 94
formation 33
functions of 1, 44
germ 27, 157, 355
ground section of 67f, 280f, 316f
hypothesis explaining evolution of 301
initiation 29
morphology of 66
movement 5, 149, 155, 157, 281
    histology of 157
    pattern of 155
neonatal 161, 352
part of 200
patterning 30
permanent 153, 165
posterior 196
presence of 128
primary 153, 156
resorbing cells 122
resorption of 168
secondary 153, 156
sensitivity 80
small 37
socket 116
submerged 162, 355
substance, loss of 279
succedaneous 165
supernumerary 155
surface 61
upper posterior 259
Telomere 355
    length 275f
    regulation 275
Temporal bone 4, 13, 241, 243, 245
    glenoid fossa of 244f
    part of 13

Temporomandibular joint 4, 5*f*, 241, 242*f*, 244*f*, 278, 279, 283, 341
   ankylosis 249, 355
   capsule of 246
   clicking of 249
   development of 242, 243*f*
   dislocation 249
   disorders of 249
   functions of 248
   gross anatomy of 243
   ligaments of 247
   microscopic structure of 243
   movements of 248*f*
   nerves innervations of 248*f*
Temporomandibular ligament 243, 244*f*, 247
Tenascin 99
Terminal tubule cells 224
Thecodont 302, 303*f*, 355
Thermal regulation 175
Thoracic duct 264
Thymus 263, 263*f*
Thyroglossal duct 21, 204
Thyroid
   gland 216, 217
   lingual 210
Tissue 262, 307, 315
   blocks 311
   culture 307
   fibrous 175
   fixation 355
   fluid 265*f*
      loss 267
   fragments of 307
   interstitial 121
   keratinized 197
   microarray 316
   odontogenic 181, 181*t*
   processing 307, 318*fc*, 355
   section 191*f*, 311
   shrinkage 309
T-lymphocytes 197, 263, 266
Tomes' fiber 70, 87
Tomes' granular layer 73, 74*f*, 355, 363
Tomes' process 46, 47, 51, 55, 55*f*, 56*f*, 355
Tomes' resorbing organ 169
Tongue 178*f*, 204, 278, 283, 341
   anterior portion of 22*f*
   body of 204
   circumvalate papillae of 369
   development of 17, 21
   developmental deformity of 22
   differs, innervation of 21
   dorsal portion of 21*f*, 204
   dorsum of 177
   filiform papillae of 368
   fungiform papillae of 368
   large-sized 22
   lateral border of 205*f*
   lymphoid part of 205*f*
   papilla of 204, 337
   part of 21
   posterolateral 237
   small sized 22
   ventral surface of 2*f*, 204, 204*f*
Tonofilaments 355
Tonsillar crypts 355
Tonsils 94, 128*f*, 263, 355
   lingual 205*f*, 206, 207*f*
Toothache 93
Totipotent cells 355
Touch cells 187
Toxins 85
Trabeculae 355
Transcytosis 231
Transduction theory 77
Transgingival fibers 199
Transmission electron microscope 315
Transseptal fibers 120, 199, 355
Trauma, severe 109
Tricalcium phosphate 292
Triconodont 303, 355
   teeth 303
Trilaminar germ disk 9
   formation 9
Tritubercular theory 303, 305
Trophoblast 10*f*, 288, 356
Tropocollagen 90
Tubarial glands 237
Tuberculous bacillus 312
Tuberculum impar 21, 356
Tuftelin 46, 356
Tumor
   cells 268
   necrosis factor 247
Tunica
   adventitia 90
   intima 90

U

Unipotent progenitor cells 287
Uranyl acetate 324
Urine 318
Uvula 178*f*, 203, 203*f*

V

Varices, lingual 350
Vascular pressure theory 159
Vasomotor function 122
Verhoeff-van Gieson stain 312, 327*f*
Vermilion 201
   border 202*f*, 356
   zone 201, 202*f*
Vertebrates 241, 356
Vesicular nucleus, large 116
Vestibular lamina 27, 28*f*, 356
Villi 206*f*
Viral infection 237
Visceral arches 13
Viscerocranial elements 297
Viscosity 233
Vision 276
   three-dimensional 298
Vital cementocytes 100
Volkmann's canal 131, 356
von Ebner's glands 205, 208, 356
von Ebner's incremental line 75*f*, 349
von Korff's fibers 356
von Willebrand factor 281

W

Waldeyer's ring 267, 268*f*
Waste material, amount of 277
Wax
   block, sectioning of 311*f*
   ribbon floating 312*f*
Wear and tear theory 274
Weber glands 237
Weibel-Palade bodies 281
Weil cells free zone 88
Wharton's duct 235, 356
Wheatsheaf' appearance 280
White sponge nevus 209
Wisdom tooth 153
Wormian bones 130
Wound healing 234
Woven bone 133*f*, 134*t*, 356, 367

X

X chromosome 8
Xenograft 356
Xerostomia 237, 278, 356
Xylene, replacement of 309

Y

Y chromosome 8
Yolk sac cavity 9

Z

Ziehl-Neelsen stain 312
Zinc 129
Zuckerkandl canal 145, 146*f*, 344
Zygote 288, 356
   formation of 9*f*
Zymogen 225
   granules 225, 356